Acta Neurochirurgica
Supplements

Editor: H.-J. Reulen
Assistant Editor: H.-J. Steiger

Acta Neurochirurgica
Supplements

Editor: H.-J. Reulen
Assistant Editor: H.-J. Steiger

Intracranial Pressure and Brain Biochemical Monitoring

Edited by

M. Czosnyka, J. D. Pickard, P. J. Kirkpatrick, P. Smielewski, and P. Hutchinson

Acta Neurochirurgica
Supplement 81

SpringerWienNewYork

Dr. Marek Czosnyka
Prof. Mr. John D. Pickard
Mr. Peter J. Kirkpatrick
Dr. Peter Smielewski
Mr. Peter Hutchinson
Addenbrooke's Hospital, Cambridge, UK

Softcover reprint of the hardcover 1st edition 2002

Typesetting: Asco Typesetters, Hong Kong

Printed on acid-free and chlorine-free bleached paper
SPIN: 10845614

With 150 Figures

CIP data supplied for

ISSN 0065-1419

ISBN-13: 978-3-7091-7397-8 e-ISBN-13: 978-3-7091-6738-0
DOI: 10.1007/978-3-7091-6738-0

Preface

The International Symposium on Intracranial Pressure has travelled to many fascinating places and learnt much since its first meeting in Hannover in 1972. This volume contains the extended abstracts presented during the 11th International Symposium on Intracranial Pressure and Brain Monitoring together with the Satellite 3rd International Conference on Neurochemical Monitoring held in July 2000 in Cambridge. The ICP community is multidisciplinary, drawing concepts from and contributing to both basic and clinical neurosciences. ICP now embraces all those techniques which help to elucidate and monitor the pathophysiology of intracranial pressure and interactions between the intracranial CSF and blood circulations in health and disease. The scope of the Symposia continues to expand. New brain modalities derived from tissue monitoring (including microdialysis and oxygenation), brain imaging (positron emission tomography and advanced MRI techniques), and mechanical properties of neural tissue (compliance monitoring and mathematical modelling) keep adding new chapters to the story.

We intended that the Cambridge Symposium would continue the informal and collegiate tradition of previous meetings with a happy blend of the generations and opportunities for lively debate. Over 250 abstracts were submitted and refereed anonymously by the International Scientific Board drawn from 42 scientists still active in the field. Each abstract was assessed by at least three independent board members by a web-based system. Such a system allows as late a deadline as possible in order to maintain topicality of the meeting and also facilitates efficiency of the judging process. The 100 papers that secured the highest grading were then selected for platform presentations. The programme was organised to optimise the time for participants to talk and interact. Professor Marmarou delivered an excellent 'state-of-the-art' opening lecture and Dr Rune Aaslid reviewed the role of transcranial Doppler ultrasonography in clinical research and practice.

This volume contains the short papers with the highest grading, divided into six sections:

- Hydrocephalus
- Clinical management of head injury
- Cerebrovascular dynamics
- ICP analysis
- Experimental (physiology, head injury, subarachnoid haemorrhage, ischaemia, hydrocephalus)
- Brain tissue monitoring and imaging

The seventh section contains the papers presented during the Satellite 3rd International Conference in Neurochemical Monitoring which was organised by Mr Peter Hutchinson.

In order to facilitate contact with the many workers in this field, the meeting website (www.neurosurg.cam.ac.uk/icp2000) has been left open for access to the titles and contact details of all the papers and posters.

We would like to take this opportunity to thank all those involved in Cambridge together with, the International Scientific Board and the International Advisory Board for all their help with the organisation of the meeting. The 12th International ICP meeting will be organised in Hong Kong between 24–29 August 2003 (Website: http://www.surgery.cuhk.edu.hk/icp2003)

Marek Czosnyka
John D. Pickard
Peter Kirkpatrick
Peter Hutchinson
Piotr Smielewski

Contents

Assessment of Cerebrovascular Reactivity

ICP Analysis

Listed in Current Contents

Hydrocephalus

Acta Neurochir (2002) [Suppl] 81: 3–5

How to Select Patients with Normal Pressure Hydrocephalus for Shunting

J. Th. J. Tans and A. J. W. Boon for the Dutch NPH Study Group

Department of Neurology, Westeinde Hospital, The Hague, The Netherlands

Summary

The objective was to compare predictive values of clinical and CT findings, co-existing cerebrovascular disease (CVD) and CSF outflow resistance (Rcsf) for outcome of shunting in NPH. A group of 95 NPH patients was shunted and followed for one year. Gait disturbance and dementia were quantified by an NPH scale (NPHS) and handicap by the modified Rankin scale (MRS). Improvement was defined as a change of at least 15% in NPHS and one grade in MRS at last follow-up. Clinical and CT findings at entry were classified as typical or not typical for NPH. CVD was defined as a history of stroke or CT-scans showing infarcts or moderate to severe white matter hypodense lesions. Clinical and CT findings typical for NPH, absence of CVD and Rcsf > 18 mmHg/ml/min were positive tests and the reciprocal outcomes negative tests. Typical clinical and CT findings were found in 69% and 68%, CVD (history of stroke n = 14, infarcts on CT n = 13, leucoaraiosis n = 32) in 47% and Rcsf > 18 in 38% of patients. The ratio of patients classified as improved in both scales was significantly greater for those with positive than negative tests. Mean improvement differed the most between patients with and without CVD. Using logistic regression analysis Rcsf > 18 was the only significant predictor of improvement in NPHS (OR 4.4, 95% CI 1.3–16.7) and typical CT findings in MRS (OR 5.6, 95% CI 1.8–17.9). We conclude that CVD is an important predictor of poor outcome. The best strategy is to shunt NPH patients if Rcsf is >18 mmHg/ml/min or, when Rcsf is lower, if CT findings are typical for NPH and there is no or limited CVD.

Keywords: Normal pressure hydrocephalus; prediction of outcome.

Introduction

There has been a debate for quite some time about the association between idiopathic NPH and cerebrovascular disease (CVD). The results of shunting in patients with NPH were reported to be unfavorable in the presence of CVD [4, 5] and there is the notion that CVD is the cause of the disease in a subgroup of NPH patients. The role of coexisting CVD in our 95 evaluable patients was examined by determining the prevalence of CVD and four risk factors for CVD and their influence on the outcome of shunting.

The primary result of the Dutch Normal Pressure Study was that the best predictive power of Rcsf is obtained if the limit for shunting is raised to 18 mmHg/ml/min [1]. No less than 92% of patients with an Rcsf above that value showed meaningful improvement after one year of follow-up. The main problem, however, was that Rcsf was below 18 mmHg/ml/min in 60% of patients for whom shunting was successful. Many investigators in the past have stressed the importance of the clinical picture and to a lesser extent that of CT findings for the selection of NPH patients for shunting [2, 3, 6, 7]. Therefore we examined the predictive value of clinical signs and CT findings of the study population and compared them with those of Rcsf and CVD.

Patients and Methods

Gait disturbance was quantified using a gait scale, that evaluates the presence of 10 features of gait and measures the number of steps and seconds required for a 10 meter walk. Dementia was assessed by a dementia scale comprising the 10-word test, digit span, trailmaking and finger tapping. Summation of the gait and dementia scale yielded the NPH scale (NPHS, range 6–80). The modified Rankin scale (MRS) was used as a disability score.

Inclusion criteria were: 1) A gradually developed gait disturbance of both legs, unexplained by other conditions and a GS score ≥ 12; 2) a subcortical dementia, emerging together with or after the gait disturbance and a DS score ≥ 12; 3) an MRS score ≥ 2; 4) a CT-scan showing a communicating hydrocephalus without clinically relevant parenchymal lesions and marked cortical atrophy.

All 95 patients underwent lumbar constant flow infusion to measure Rcsf and received a ventriculo-peritoneal Medos Hakim shunt. The NPHS and MRS were determined prior to and 1, 3, 6, 9 and 12 months after surgery. CVD was defined as the presence of a documented history of stroke, lacunar infarcts on the CT-scan at entry or moderate to severe white matter hypodense lesions (WMHLs). The occurrence of the risk factors hypertension, diabetes mellitus, ischemic heart disease and peripheral vascular disease was recorded. The clinical signs and CT findings were classified as typical or not typical for NPH. Clinical and CT findings typical for NPH, absence of CVD and Rcsf $\geq$ 18 mmHg/ml/min were designated as positive tests for shunt response and the reciprocal outcomes as negative tests.

Outcome measures were the differences between preoperative and last NPHS and MRS scores. Improvement was defined as a change of at least 15% in NPHS and one grade in MRS. We also used the means of the outcome measures for comparison between groups. The results of shunting were studied both univariately and multivariately.

Results

Fifty-three patients had at least one vascular risk factor and these occurred more frequently among patients with CVD. Neither the presence nor the number of the risk factors correlated with outcome. In total 45 patients presented with one or more signs of CVD (history of stroke $n = 14$, lacunar infarcts on CT $n = 13$ and WMHL, s $n = 32$). The severity of the NPH syndrome at entry as reflected in NPHS and MRS scores was not different between patients with and without CVD. Patients with CVD tended to have smaller ventricles and Rcsf was significantly lower in the CVD group.

Mean improvement in NPHS varied from 2.2 to 10.2% and in MRS from 0.15 to 0.51 for the different expressions of CVD. In comparison, the improvement in NPHS ranged from 23.7 to 30.8% and in MRS from 1.08 to 1.35 for NPH patients without coexisting CVD. These differences were highly significant. Outcome was also analysed as the proportion of patients showing improvement in NPHS. Of the 45 patients exhibiting CVD 51% responded to shunting compared to 75% of the patients without CVD, $p = 0.02$.

Univariate analysis of the predictive value of clinical signs, CT findings, CVD and Rcsf showed that both the proportion of shunt responders and the degree of improvement were significantly greater for patients with positive test outcomes. Multiple regression analysis performed to quantify the effect of the four tests on the degree of improvement yielded the following equation: expected mean improvement in NPHS = 4.4Rcsf + 6.4CF + 7.3CVD + 7.7CT + 15.6. (for negative test insert 0, for positive test insert 1). Using logistic regression analysis Rcsf was the only significant factor for shunt response in NPHS (odds ratio 4.4, 95% CI 1.3–16.7) and CT in MRS (odds ratio 5.6, 95% CI 1.8–17.9).

Discussion

Risk factors for CVD did not occur more frequently in patients with NPH than in controls of the same age and these risk factors were not related to outcome after shunting. Signs of CVD were found in almost half of the NPH patients and another 15 cases suffered from ischemic stroke during the one year follow-up. Outcome after shunting was significantly worse for NPH patients with coexisting CVD. The influence of CVD was most pronounced for the degree of improvement. Fifty-one percent of patients with CVD satisfied the criteria for shunt response but marked to excellent improvements were seldomly seen.

Our classification of clinical and CT findings as typical or not typical for NPH was based on the overall impression without using the various clinical scales and CT measurements. Although all patients fulfilled the entry criteria, our population reflected every day practice. We did not include only promising surgical candidates. More than 25% of cases had the 2 highest Rankin grades and there was extensive past and present comorbidity. The multivariate analyses revealed that CVD and CT findings were the most important factors for the degree of improvement and Rcsf and CT findings for distinguishing between shunt responders and non-responders.

On the basis of our results we give the following criteria for shunting patients with a clinical diagnosis of NPH: 1) Rcsf > 18 mmHg/ml/min or 2) Rcsf < 18 mmHg/ml/min if the CT findings are typical for NPH and if there is no or limited cerebrovascular disease. If we had used that strategy for this population we would have realised an improvement ratio of 75%. Better results will be achieved only if the gray area of uncertainty with respect to clinical diagnosis can be reduced.

References

1. Boon AJW, Tans JTJ, Delwel EJ *et al* (1997) Dutch Normal Pressure Hydrocephalus Study. Prediction of outcome after shunting with the resistance to outflow of cerebrospinal fluid. J Neurosurg 87: 687–693
2. Borgesen SE, Gjerris F (1982) The predictive value of conductance to outflow of CSF in Normal Pressure Hydrocephalus. Brain 105: 65–86
3. Greenberg JO, Shenkin HA, Adam R (1977) Idiopathic Normal Pressure Hydrocephalus – a report of 73 patients. J Neurol Neurosurg Psychiatry 40: 336–341
4. Krauss JK, Droste DW, Vach W *et al* (1996) Cerebrospinal fluid shunting in Idiopathic Normal Pressure Hydrocephalus of the elderly: effect of periventricular and deep white matter lesions. Neurosurgery 39: 292–300

5. Larsson A, Wikkelso C *et al* (1991) Clinical parameters in 74 consecutive patients shunt operated for Normal Pressure Hydrocephalus. Acta Neurol Scand 84: 475–482
6. Tans JTJ (1979) Differentiation of Normal Pressure Hydrocephalus and cerebral atrophy by computed tomography and spinal infusion test. J Neurol 222: 109–118
7. Wikkelso C, Andersson H *et al* (1989) Computed tomography of the brain in the diagnosis and prognosis in Normal Pressure Hydrocephalus. Neurology 31: 160–165

Correspondence: J. Th. J. Tans, Department of Neurology, Westeinde Hospital, The Hague, The Netherlands.

Acta Neurochir (2002) [Suppl] 81: 7–10

Agreement Between CSF Flow Dynamics in MRI and ICP Monitoring in the Diagnosis of Normal Pressure Hydrocephalus. Sensitivity and Specificity of CSF Dynamics to Predict Outcome

M. A. Poca[1], J. Sahuquillo[1], M. Busto[2], A. Rovira[2], J. Capellades[2], M. Mataró[3], and E. Rubio[1]

[1] Department of Neurosurgery, Vall d'Hebron University Hospitals, Barcelona, Spain
[2] Magnetic Resonance Unit, Vall d'Hebron University Hospitals, Barcelona, Spain
[3] Neuropsychology, Vall d'Hebron University Hospitals, Barcelona, Spain

Summary

Objectives. The aims of the study were 1) to assess the degree of agreement between CSF flow dynamics determined by MR and ICP monitoring in the diagnosis of NPH, and 2) to determine the sensitivity and specificity of CSF flow dynamics studied by MR in predicting improvement after shunting.

Patients and Methods. A prospective study was carried out in 35 consecutive patients with suspected NPH. CSF velocity (Phase Contrast) through the aqueduct was determined in sagittal plane. Patients were classified as "normal" or hyperdynamic in comparison with a control group of 27 healthy volunteers. Continuous extradural ICP monitoring was performed for at least 72 hours and patients were classified as having active, compensated, or ex-vacuo hydrocephalus. Patients with active or compensated hydrocephalus were shunted.

Results. The degree of agreement between MR dynamics and ICP monitoring was 82%. Sensitivity of CSF velocity was 90% and specificity was 50%.

Conclusions. The degree of agreement between ICP monitoring and CSF velocity is high. High CSF velocity through the aqueduct is a good predictor of improvement after surgery. However, patients with normal velocity in MR required additional tests before a diagnosis of NPH is ruled out.

Keywords: CSF dynamics; non-invasive CSF flow dynamics; ICP monitoring; Normal Pressure Hydrocephalus.

Introduction

The prevalence of dementia has increased with longer life expectancy. Normal pressure hydrocephalus (NPH) is a treatable cause of dementia that should be considered in patients with an increase in ventricular size, specially since Albeck *et al.* have demonstrated that the resistance to CSF outflow rises with age [1]. The main difficulties associated with this entity involve making correct diagnosis and finding reliable variables that predict outcome after shunting. Several types of investigations have been proposed to study, select and differentiate patients who would benefit from shunting from those who would not. Currently, continuous ICP monitoring and conventional studies of CSF dynamic are considered the most powerful methods for the diagnosis of NPH. However, these techniques are invasive and not always available. In the last years, CSF flow dynamics have been studied non-invasively by MRI. Nevertheless, the value of this method in selecting candidates for shunting is still controversial, and the sensitivity and specificity of CSF flow dynamics determined by MRI have not yet been defined.

The aims of the study were: 1) to assess the degree of agreement between CSF flow dynamics determined by MRI and ICP monitoring in the diagnosis of NPH, and 2) to determine the sensitivity and specificity of CSF flow dynamics studied by MR in predicting improvement after shunting, considering improvement after shunting as the "gold standard".

Patients and Methods

A prospective study was carried out in 35 consecutive patients with suspected NPH (16 women and 19 men, mean age 68.6 ± 8.6, range 51–85). All patients presented with gait disturbances, memory impairment, urinary incontinence, and an increase in ventricular size (Evans' index > 0.30 measured by CT scan or conventional MR images) [11].

Non-invasive CSF flow dynamics were determined by MR. CSF velocity through the aqueduct in the sagittal plane was quantified using Phase-Contrast Velocity MRI with Retrospective Cardiac Gating (1.5 MR Imager; Magnetom SP 63 Siemens; 2D-FISP.TR 70 msec. TE 13 msec; flip angle 130; section thickness 4 mm; matrix

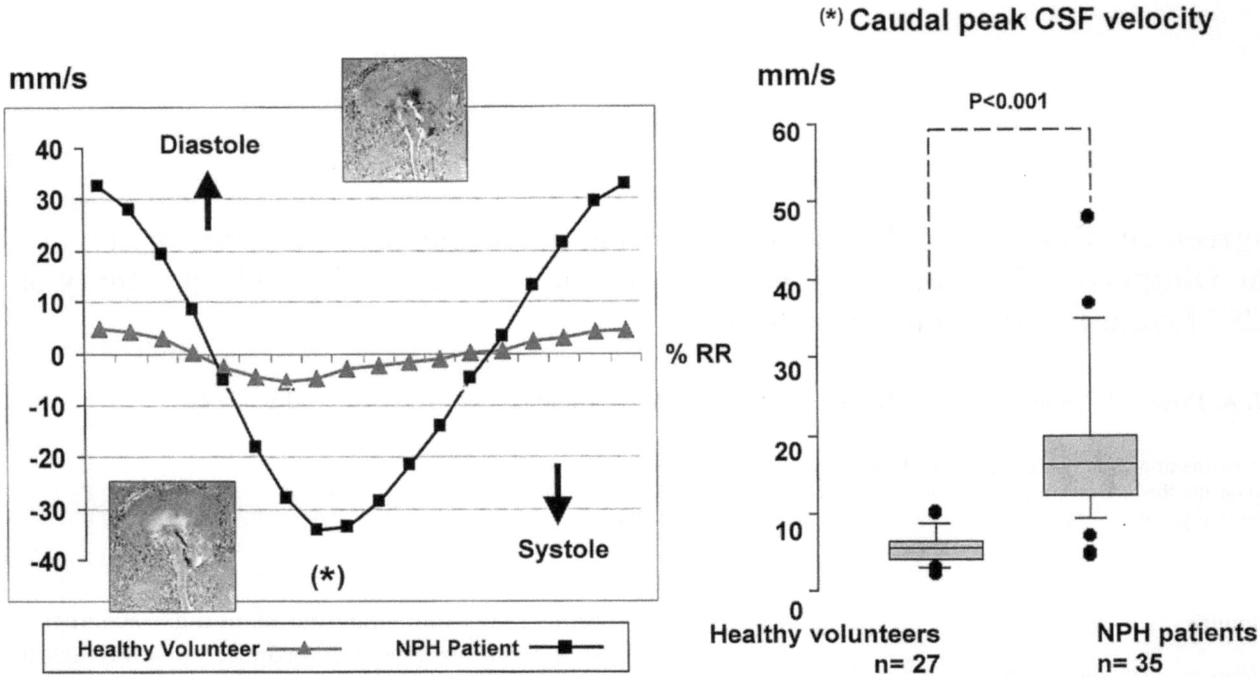

Fig. 1. Figure 1 shows an example of the CSF flow velocity curve of a healthy volunteer and an NPH patient. The sinusoidal morphology of both curves is very similar. The only statistically significant difference was in the caudal and in the rostral peaks of the aqueduct flow velocity, which were significantly increased in patients with NPH compared with those of healthy volunteers ($P < 0.001$). The X-axis denotes percentage of cardiac cycle (%RR), and the Y-axes denote CSF flow velocity in mm/s

192 × 256; POV 250 mm; velocity sensitivity 100 mm/sec; measuring time 7.4 min). Patients were classified as *normal* or *hyperdynamic* in comparison with a control group of 27 healthy volunteers (mean age 31.1 ± 11, range 21–66 years) (Fig. 1). Patients were considered normal when aqueductal CSF peak velocities were between the 2.5 and 97.5 percentiles of the control group. Patients were considered hyperdynamic when aqueductal CSF peak velocities were above the 97.5 percentile of the control group.

Continuous extradural ICP monitoring was performed in all NPH patients for at least 72 hours using a fiberoptic extradural sensor (LADD Research Industries, Inc., Burlington, Vermont). According to their ICP findings, patients were included in one of the following categories: 1) *Active Hydrocephalus*: patients with a mean ICP above 12 mm Hg; 2) *Compensated Hydrocephalus*: patients with a mean ICP below or equal to 12 mm Hg but with abnormal ICP waves; 3) *Brain atrophy* (ex vacuo hydrocephalus), patients with a mean ICP below or equal to 12 mm Hg without any pathological waves during the total recording time [11]. Patients with active or compensated hydrocephalus were shunted.

Clinical changes after shunting were assessed by several functional scales and neuropsychological tests performed in NPH patients before and 6 months after surgery.

Results

Fifteen patients presented with active and 18 presented with compensated hydrocephalus. Brain atrophy was diagnosed in the remaining two patients. Twenty-nine patients were considered hyperdynamic and six normal on the basis of CSF velocity measurements (Fig. 1). The degree of agreement between MR dynamics and ICP monitoring was 82% (Fig. 2). Twenty-eight of the 29 hyperdynamic patients and three of the four patients with normal CSF velocity improved after shunting. The sensitivity of CSF velocity was 90% and the specificity was 50% (Fig. 2).

Discussion

Complete NPH syndrome is characterised by the clinical triad of dementia, gait apraxia, and urinary incontinence, associated with an increase in ventricular size. In these patients, ICP monitoring shows abnormal B-wave activity and CSF dynamics often show increased *Rout*. Both a high percentage of B-waves and high Rout have been reported to be good predictors of outcome. However, both diagnostic methods are invasive and not available in all neurological or neurosurgical departments. MR imaging offers the possibility of non-invasive indirect measurement of CSF dynamics with the use of pulse sequences, specially designed for velocity mapping of slow flow rates [6, 7,

A n= 35

	PIC (+) Active and Compensated Hydrocephalus	PIC (-) Brain Atrophy	
Hyperdynamic Patients	29	0	29
Normal Patients	4	2	6
	33	2	

B n= 33

	Clinical Improvement	No Clinical Improvement	
Hyperdynamic Patients	28	1	29
Normal Patients	3	1	4
	31	2	

Fig. 2. Contingency tables which summarise: A) the agreement between non-invasive CSF dynamics determined by MRI and continuous ICP monitoring, and B) the association between non-invasive CSF dynamics determined by MRI and results after shunting (sensitivity and specificity of CSF dynamics to predict outcome)

10]. This could be a promising method in the diagnosis and management of patients with NPH. Bradley *et al.* correlated a prominent CSF flow void within the aqueduct, revealed by proton-density-weighted images, with positive response to CSF shunting, while normal flow void was linked to a negative response [3, 4, 5]. Gideon *et al.*, however, found that in two of nine patients CSF flow within the aqueduct was within the normal range, despite alterations in ICP recording (*false negatives*) [8]. In our study we found that high CSF velocity through the aqueduct was a good predictor of improvement after shunting. However, in our series there were also patients with normal CSF velocities in which a high percentage of B-waves was found. These patients also improved after shunting. Therefore, in patients with normal CSF dynamics determined by MR imaging and with clinical and radiological findings compatible with NPH, additional tests to rule out this syndrome should be performed.

Craniospinal CSF motion is pulsatile, with a small net craniocaudal component at the level of the aqueduct related to the cardiac cycle. In the aqueduct, caudal flow occurs in systole and a reversal (cranial flow) occurs in diastole. The CSF flow volume through the aqueduct is derived from measurements from phase-contrast CSF velocity in MR images. Specifically, CSF flow volume is the product of the measured velocity of a pixel (in millimetres per second) and the area of the pixel (in square millimetres), integrated over the cross-sectional area of the aqueduct integrated in time over mechanical systole or diastole [5]. In our study we used velocity of CSF flow rather than flow volume because both variables are inter-dependent. Moreover, velocity measurements can be determined quickly, an advantage in older patients who are sometimes disoriented or uncooperative.

In every cardiac cycle, CSF flow draws a curve that is nearly sinusoidal with several curve harmonics. The morphology of this curve was not significantly different in patients with NPH compared with controls (Fig. 1). There was no significant difference between patients and controls in the time to peak flow within the cardiac cycle. The only statistically significant difference was in the caudal and in the rostral peaks of the aqueduct flow velocity (flow amplitude), which was significantly increased in patients with NPH compared with healthy volunteers. Similar results have been reported by other authors [5].

Another methodological point to consider is that in this study patients with NPH were older than controls. Gideon *et al.* [8] found slightly higher mean aqueductal CSF peak velocities in both the rostral and the caudal directions within the cardiac cycle in elderly healthy volunteers compared with young healthy volunteers. These findings, however, were not statistically significant [9]. In our series, aqueductal CSF peak velocities in the two patients older than 60 years were not significantly different from those of the remaining 25 healthy volunteers younger than 60 years. Moreover, additional studies using a similar MRI phase method have demonstrated that ageing or gender have no significant effect on aqueductal CSF dynamics [4, 5, 2].

MRI revealed ICP abnormalities in all hyperdynamic patients, with a percentage of B-waves between 10 and 65%. All hyperdynamic patients except one improved after shunting. The hyperdynamic patient showing no improvement after shunting had a considerable percentage of high amplitude B-waves (30%), but the neuropsychological study suggested that this patient had mixed dementia, with a quick evolution of associated Alzheimer's disease. Four of the six non-hyperdynamic ("normal") patients also presented B-waves (between 5 and 53%), and three of them improved after shunting. The remaining patient who did not improve after shunting also presented with mixed dementia with severe cognitive impairment and urinary incontinence, as well as less evident gait disturbances. An interesting observation is that the ICP recordings of patients evaluated as "normal" by MR dynamics were more difficult to interpret. Basically, the ICP tracings were irregular, presenting greater difficulties in the quantification of B-waves. These patients also presented with considerable cortical atrophy. Another aspect to consider is that one hyperdynamic patient did not improve despite correct functioning of the shunt. Thus, like other methods, this non-invasive method also produces false positives and false negatives.

In conclusion, the degree of agreement between ICP monitoring and CSF velocity is high. High CSF velocity through the aqueduct is a good predictor of improvement after surgery. However, patients with normal velocity revealed by MR require additional tests before a diagnosis of NPH can be ruled out.

Acknowledgments

The authors wish to thank Gail Craigie for correcting the manuscript. This study was supported by *Beca Mutual Mèdica* 1998 and grant FIS 99/968 from *Fondo de Investigación Sanitaria de la Seguridad Social* (FIS).

References

1. Albeck MJ, Skak C, Nielsen PR, Olsen KS, Borgesen SE, Gjerris F (1998) Age dependency of resistance to cerebrospinal fluid outflow. J Neurosurg 89: 275–278
2. Barkhof F, Kouwenhoven M, Scheltens P, Sprenger M, Algra PR, Valk J (1991) Cine RM-phase study of aqueductal CSF pulsatility in normal controls. The absence of effect of aging and the relation to CSF-void on ungated modulus MR (abstr). Book of abstracts: society of magnetic resonance in medicine. Berkeley, CA, pp 299
3. Bradley WG, Jr, Kortman KE, Burgoyne B (1986) Flowing cerebrospinal fluid in normal and hydrocephalic states: appearance on MR images. Radiology 159: 611–616
4. Bradley WG, Jr, Whittemore AR, Kortman KE, Watanabe AS, Homyak M, Teresi LM, Davis SJ (1991) Marked cerebrospinal fluid void: indicator of successful shunt in patients with suspected normal-pressure hydrocephalus. Radiology 178: 459–466
5. Bradley WG, Jr, Scalzo D, Queralt J, Nitz WN, Atkinson DJ, Wong P (1996) Normal-pressure hydrocephalus: evaluation with cerebrospinal fluid flow measurements at MR imaging. Radiology 198: 523–529
6. Enzmann DR, Pelc NJ (1991) Normal flow patterns of intracranial and spinal cerebrospinal fluid defined with phase-contrast cine MR imaging. Radiology 178: 467–474
7. Feinberg DA, Mark AS (1987) Human brain motion and cerebrospinal fluid circulation demonstrated with MR velocity imaging. Radiology 163: 793–799
8. Gideon P, Stahlberg F, Thomsen C, Gjerris F, Sorensen PS, Henriksen O (1994a) Cerebrospinal fluid flow and production in patients with normal pressure hydrocephalus studied by MRI. Neuroradiology 36: 210–215
9. Gideon P, Thomsen C, Stahlberg F, Henriksen O (1994b) Cerebrospinal fluid production and dynamics in normal aging: an MRI phase-mapping study. Acta Neurol Scand 89: 362–366
10. Nitz WR, Bradley WG, Jr, Watanabe AS, Lee RR, Burgoyne B, O'Sullivan RM, Herbst MD (1992) Flow dynamics of cerebrospinal fluid: assessment with phase-contrast velocity MR imaging performed with retrospective cardiac gating. Radiology 183: 395–405
11. Sahuquillo J, Rubio E, Codina A, Molins A, Guitart JM, Poca MA, Chasampi A (1991) Reappraisal of the intracranial pressure and cerebrospinal fluid dynamics in patients with the so-called "normal pressure hydrocephalus syndrome. Acta Neurochir (Wien) 112: 50–61

Correspondence: Dra. M. A. Poca, Ferran Puig 70-72, 1-2, 08023 Barcelona, Spain.

Acta Neurochir (2002) [Suppl] 81: 11–14

Shunting to the Sagittal Sinus

S. E. Børgesen, F. Gjerris, and N. Agerlin

University Clinic of Neurosurgery, Rigshospitalet, Copenhagen, Denmark

Summary

Objectives. To develop a shunt that drains CSF from the ventricles to the sagittal sinus under normal-physiological conditions. This shunting principle will not lead to any over-drainage, and a large proportion of the known shunt-complications will be avoided.

Methods. On the basis of the normal values for ICP, resistance to outflow and the production rate of CSF we have developed a shunt that drains CSF to the sagittal sinus and restores normal condition for the CSF dynamics. The shunt consists of two unidirectional valves, a pre-chamber, a resistance tube made of titanium, and a titanium tube leading CSF into the sagittal sinus. The shunt has been tested in 18 patients. Observation time ranged from 2 to 430 days, mean time 54 days.

Results. The first results from the use of the new shunt are very promising. It has an immediate effect on the clinical symptoms, it restores CSF dynamics (investigated with the shunt inserted) and the size of the ventricles is only gradually diminished. Slit ventricles have not yet been observed. In all patients the symptoms of hydrocephalus were relieved. No occlusion or thrombosis of the sagittal sinus have been observed. This is in agreement with the reports in the literature of shunting to the sagittal sinus, where 99 cases have been presented with an observation period of up to 6 years. The shunt has proven easy and safe to implant.

Conclusions. Shunting to the sagittal sinus has proven easy and safe with regard to short term results. By using a dedicated shunt that drains at normal physiological parameters for the CSF dynamics any over-drainage is avoided, and it may be expected that the complication rate will be substantially smaller than with existing shunting systems.

Keywords: Hydrocephalus; drainage into sagittal sinus.

Introduction

The treatment of hydrocephalus is based on shunt implantation or III ventriculostomy when appropriate. Shunt implantation is connected with an unacceptable high incidence of reoperations due to shunt failure [5, 2]. In the present paper a new shunting principle by a physiologic drainage of CSF into the sagittal sinus is described.

Physiologic Principles

Shunting cerebrospinal fluid (CSF) means leading CSF from the site of accumulation to a resorption site outside the cerebrospinal cavity. The purpose of shunting CSF is to circumvent an obstruction which inhibits the outflow of CSF through its normal pathways during normal pressure/flow conditions.

The goal of CSF shunting is to restore the normal intracranial pressure balance. Shunting CSF to another cavity in the body, e.g. peritoneal cavity or the right atrium of the heart, inherits a disturbance of the normal CSF flow conditions. The draining systems used for diverting CSF from the cranio-spinal cavity to another resorption site are therefore constructed with the aim of re-establishing the normal intracranial pressure level. Shunting devices deploy a uni-directional flow mechanism and some sort of flow restriction working by a variety of principles but always depending on the differential pressure level across the shunting device. As the differential pressure is the resultant of the pressure in the CSF containing cavity and the pressure in the receiving compartment, the flow of CSF through the shunt depends on the pressure in both compartments [6].

Knowledge about the normal physiology of the CSF dynamics has made it possible to describe the pressure and flow conditions of the CSF from the production site to the receiving site. Comparison of the parameters of the normal CSF dynamics with the parameters obtained by shunting CSF to different receiving compartments explain some of the problems connected with shunting of hydrocephalus.

The intracranial pressure (ICP) depends on the CSF production, resorption resistance and pressure in the

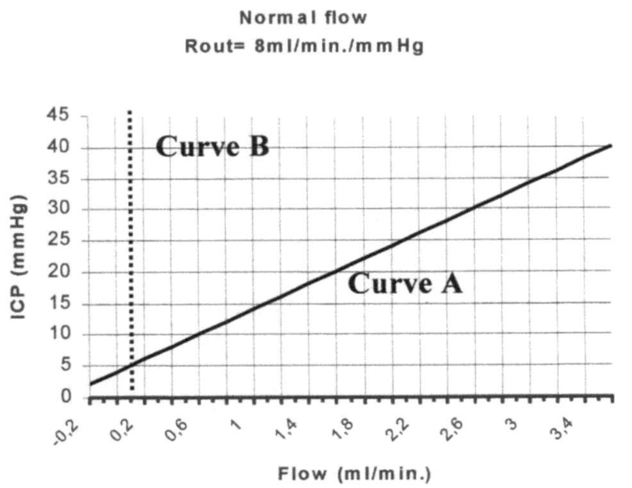

Fig. 1. The relation between ICP and Flow when the receiving compartment pressure is independent of the ICP (*Curve A*) and when the pressure in the receiving compartment (i.e. sagittal sinus) co-varies (*Curve B*)

receiving compartment. The relationship of these parameters are given by the Davson equation:

$$ICP = FR \times R_{out} + Pss,$$

where FR is the formation rate of CSF, R_{out} is the resistance to CSF outflow and Pss is the pressure in the sagittal sinus [6].

From the normal values of FR, R_{out} and ICP the relationship describing a steady state balance of CSF dynamics is shown in Fig. 1. The 2 curves demonstrate the flow of CSF when the ICP is increased i.e. by loading during infusion test where the pressure in the receiving compartment is unincreased (i.e. steady Pss level) (Curve A). The second curve illustrates flow in conditions where the pressure in the receiving compartment co-varies with the ICP (for example): the flow remains stable and the CSF volume in the CSF compartments remains unchanged (Curve B). With the normal formation rate of 0,3 ml/min. and the normal pressure difference between production and receiving compartments, the ICP will constantly be around 10 mmHg. Increasing ICP without increasing receiving compartment pressure will result in increased outflow of CSF.

From knowledge of the normal intracranial pressure [10, 11], the pressure of the sagittal sinus [3, 4], and the normal resistance to outflow of CSF [1, 8] a shunt designated for draining CSF into the sagittal sinus has been developed (SinuShunt [1]*). It has been designed to comply with these data for normalcy and thereby providing a near to normal physiological drainage of the CSF.

Methods

The shunt consists of a ventricular catheter made of silicone rubber, a valve mechanism preventing back-flow from the SS to the shunt or the ventricles, a pre-chamber made of silicone rubber for punctuation and testing the performance of the shunt, a resistance tube made of titanium and dimensioned to create a resistance to outflow equal to normal values (8 ml/min./mmHg), a housing for the valves and the resistance tube made of either polycarbonate or silicone rubber, and a silicone rubber drain leading to the titanium tube for insertion into the SS.

The shunt functions by diverting the CSF from the ventricles to the SS. It is based on the principle that there will always be a pressure difference between the ventricles of the brain and the SS, the pressure being higher in the ventricles than in the SS. If this pressure difference was negative the CSF would not be resorbed. It is possible that the pressure difference is reversed (i.e. the pressure in the SS being higher than the pressure in the ventricles) in short periods of time, but on average the pressure must be higher in the ventricles. Because of these possible reversed pressures, the shunt must be provided with an effective valve mechanism. By inserting two valve mechanisms on each side of the pre-chamber, it is possible to test the shunt by pumping the pre-chamber.

The shunt has been inserted in patients with obvious symptoms of hydrocephalus and expected immediate response to CSF-diversion. The objective of the clinical investigation was to establish the performance of the shunt, the safety of the surgical procedure, and the short time safety of the implantation of a drain in the sagittal sinus. The patients were followed for three months or more. Obligatory endpoints were improved consciousness, validated by Glasgow Coma Scale, disappearance of papillary edema, disappearance of headache and other pressure symptoms, and normalization of intracranial pressure and resistance to outflow of CSF in patients where the clinical improvement was unsatisfactory.

Results

The shunt has been implanted in 18 patients: 5 patients had hydrocephalus following subarachnoid haemorrhage, 4 had tumour in the III ventricle, 4 had cerebellar metastasis, and 5 had normal pressure hydrocephalus. The mean observation time was 132 days, range from 2 to 430 days.

One patient developed infection immediately after implantation, and the patient was withdrawn from the

* SinuShunt®, CSF-Dynamics, Naverland 2, 2600 Glostrup, Denmark

study. One patient developed a large haematoma in the frontal lobe around the ventricular catheter, the drain occluded and the shunt was removed. In 3 patients the drain was not placed correctly in the sagittal sinus (angled prototype of titanium tube was not suitable for insertion in the sinus). In one patient the drain in the sagittal sinus was occluded.

The remaining 12 patients were relieved from their symptoms and signs of hydrocephalus.

Paired T-test on Evan's ratio showed statistically significant decrease in the size of the ventricles ($p < 0{,}001$). It is noteworthy that while the ventricles were diminished by the shunts, they were never observed to become very small. 6 patients were observed to have edema of the optical papillae. The edema resolved in all cases. The pre- and postoperative headache was recorded as unknown, none, moderate and severe. Paired samples T-test on the whole series shows significant reduction of the headache ($p < 0{,}001$).

No adverse effects were observed. No patients had developed occlusion of the sagittal sinus.

Discussion

It is unanimously agreed that the main bulk of CSF is resorbed into the sagittal sinus. It is obvious that leading CSF to the sagittal sinus by a shunt that imitates the normal CSF outflow resistance and thus to reestablish near to normal physiological CSF-dynamics will lead to an optimal by-pass of the CSF-obstruction. It will not inherit all the problems that arise from overdrainage, and it will besides this not be inflicted by the mechanical problems of long drains to the peritoneal cavity, diverse connectors, mechanical stress, etc. connected with normally used shunting systems.

The SinuShunt employed in the present study seems to fulfill the requirements for an optimal shunting system. It has been shown that the shunt provides sufficient CSF-drainage in patients with clinical hydrocephalus. It normalizes the intracranial pressure level, but it does not lead to over-drainage. The symptoms of hydrocephalus are immediately relieved. It is safe and technically simple to implant. The present study is not aiming at proving the long-term effect of shunting to the sagittal sinus. Three patients have been observed for more than one year without showing any signs of occlusion of the sagittal sinus.

Shunting to the sagittal sinus is well known from the literature. A total of 99 cases are reported [9]. When placed correctly, a shunt from the ventricles to the sagittal sinus relieves symptoms of hydrocephalus. As in all literature on treatment of hydrocephalus, patients are included/treated who do not respond to shunting due to either dominating symptoms from the basic disease leading to hydrocephalus (making judgement of the effect of the shunt impossible or in only a very short period of time) or due to misinterpretation of the condition (typically shunting patients with symptoms of normal pressure hydrocephalus who in fact was not in need for a shunt). The shunt-types used for shunting CSF to the SS have been pressure regulated shunts with a range from 2–8 cm water with some sort of valve mechanism. In some cases in the literature there was an unexplained failure of the shunt. The reason may have been a too high opening pressure for the shunt. Two papers give information on long term observation of patients after shunting to the SS. In the series of Hash *et al.* [9] the mean observation period was 7 months in 22 patients who could be followed. No thrombosis of the sagittal sinus was observed. 5 patients underwent autopsy, where no thrombosis was observed. In the series of Wen [12] 17 patients were followed from 2 to 6 years without observation of occlusion of the sagittal sinus.

It can be concluded from the literature that it is possible to treat hydrocephalus by shunting the CSF to the SS. The shunts that have been used have not been especially designed for this specific use, and the CSF-draining principle has not been considered in relation to the normal, physiological CSF-dynamics. The results concerning ventricular size are not reported systematically. The number of complications seem to be smaller than that normally reported. Thrombosis of the SS has not been reported in one single case.

Conclusion

The investigation has shown that shunting to the sagittal sinus using a designated shunting system (SinuShunt®) is technically simple and safe, and it restores the normal CSF dynamics. Occlusion of the sagittal sinus has not been observed in the present series or in the cases reported in the literature. As the shunting principle mimics the normal, physiological CSF-drainage, over-drainage is avoided, and the number of reoperations due to shunt failure may be expected to be markedly reduced.

References

1. Albeck MJ, Børgesen SE, Gjerris F *et al* (1991) Intracranial pressure and cerebrospinal fluid outflow conductance in healthy subjects. J Neurosurg 74: 597–600
2. Borgbjerg BM, Gjerris F, Albeck MJ *et al* (1998) A comparison between ventriculo-peritoneal and ventriculo-atrial cerebrospinal fluid shunts in relation to rate of revision and durability. Acta Neurochir (Wien) 140: 459–464
3. Borgesen SE, Gjerris F (1987) Relationships between intracranial pressure, ventricular size, and resistance to CSF outflow. J Neurosurg 67: 535–539
4. Børgesen SE, Gjerris F, Fedders O *et al* (1997) Measurement of resistance to CSF outflow – Clinical experience in 333 patients. In: Hoff JT (ed) ICP VII. Springer, Berlin Heidelberg New York Tokyo
5. Czosnyka M, Czosnyka Z, Whitehouse H *et al* (1997) Hydrodynamic properties of hydrocephalus shunts: United Kingdom Shunt Evaluation Laboratory. J Neurol Neurosurg Psychiatry 62: 43–50
6. Davson H, Hollingsworth G, Segal MB (1970) The mechanism of drainage of the cerebrospinal fluid. Brain PY 93: 665–665
7. de Jong DA, Delwel EJ, Avezaat CJ (2000) Hydrostatic and hydrodynamic considerations in shunted normal pressure hydrocephalus. Acta Neurochir (Wien) 142: 241–247
8. Ekstedt J (1978) CSF hydrodynamic studies in man. 2. Normal hydrodynamic variables related to CSF pressure and flow. J Neurol Neurosurg Psychiatry 41: 345–345
9. Hash CJ, Shenkin HA, Crowder LE (1979) Ventricle to sagittal sinus shunt for hydrocephalus. Neurosurgery 4: 394–399
10. Magnaes B (1976) Body position and cerebrospinal fluid pressure. Part 1: clinical studies on the effect of rapid postural changes. J Neurosurg 44: 687–697
11. Magnaes B (1976) Body position and cerebrospinal fluid pressure. Part 2: clinical studies on orthostatic pressure and the hydrostatic indifferent point. J Neurosurg 44: 698–705
12. Wen HL (1982) Ventriculo-superior sagittal sinus shunt for hydrocephalus. Surg Neurol 17: 432–434

Correspondence: S. E. Børgesen, University Clinic of Neurosurgery, Rigshospitalet, Copenhagen, Denmark.

Acta Neurochir (2002) [Suppl] 81: 15–17

Why Valve Opening Pressure Plays a Relatively Minor Role in the Postural ICP Response to Ventricular Shunts in Normal Pressure Hydrocephalus: Modeling and Implications

S. W. Cook and **M. Bergsneider**

UCLA Division of Neurosurgery, Los Angeles, CA

Summary

Objectives. In normal pressure hydrocephalus, there is no clear evidence that the opening pressure of differential pressure valves influences outcome. In this study, the objective was to determine whether the relationship between valve opening pressure and post-operative postural ICP changes was predictable.

Methods. Eight adult-onset hydrocephalus patients were evaluated using an intraparenchymal ICP microsensor. Postural ICP measurements were obtained before and after placement of a ventricular shunt (VP or VA) with a Codman Hakim programmable valve.

Results. Valve opening pressure had a poor correlation with ICP at any head-of-bed elevation across subjects (best $r = 0.25$). The degree of negative ICP encountered for any given patient did not appear to be determined by the valve pressure, and varied significantly between patients at the same valve pressure. Each individual's ICP correlated well to opening pressure ($r > 0.76$), but the response is more sigmoidal than linear, and the opening pressure at which ICP changed most was markedly different between patients.

Conclusions. The hydrodynamic pressures generated by shunts with different pressure valves are unpredictable. Our data supports the use of programmable valves in patients with adult onset hydrocephalus and suggests that ICP be measured post-operatively to achieve an optimal clinical outcome.

Keywords: Intracranial pressure; ventriculoperitoneal shunt; Codman-Hakim programmable valve; normal pressure hydrocephalus.

Introduction

The application of the differential pressure valve (DPV) as a method of controlling CSF drainage represents one of the greatest breakthroughs in the treatment of hydrocephalus [8]. These valves were designed primarily with the aim of treating pediatric patients – a situation in which the goal was to simply lower intracranial pressure (ICP).

The use of differential pressure valves in adult patients, however, has not been associated with a similar degree of efficacy and safety. Because both over-drainage [7] and under-drainage [1, 6] states occur more frequently in adults, it can be difficult choosing the optimal valve for any given patient. Although several studies have reported conflicting results when comparing various opening pressures of DPVs [2, 4], it is believed by many that low pressure valves are more likely to result in clinical improvement in patients with normal pressure hydrocephalus (NPH) [4]. This benefit must be balanced against an increased likelihood of complications such as subdural hygromas, hematomas, and slit ventricles.

For many neurosurgeons, the choice of which valve opening pressure to use is largely based on the preoperative ICP measured by lumbar puncture or the ventricular pressure measured at the time of the shunt operation. A valve opening pressure lower than this baseline ICP is chosen, with the intent of decreasing ventricular size by generating a gentle pressure gradient. Recently, programmable valves with various opening pressures have added a new dimension in patient management. For patients with NPH, some have advocated beginning with the highest opening pressure and sequentially lowering this setting until a clinical benefit is seen. The presumption is that an initial high pressure will decrease the risk of over-drainage complications.

In this study, we have sought to determine whether there is a good correlation between the valve opening pressure of a DPV and the post-operative ICP. Our second aim was to determine whether changing the opening pressure resulted in a predictable change in ICP.

Materials and Methods

We studied eight patients with normal pressure hydrocephalus who underwent ventriculoperitoneal or ventriculoatrial shunts at UCLA Medical Center between 11/98 and 6/00. Four of the patients were male, and the mean age was 73 ± 13 years. All patients underwent pre-operative intraparenchymal implantation of a Codman microsensor ICP monitor (Codman and Schurtleff, Inc., Randolph, MA). The ICP was measured relative to atmospheric pressure with the patients supine in bed, with the head of the bed flat and raised to 10, 20, 30, 45, and 60 degrees. Adequate time was allowed at each head of bed angle for equilibration of ICP.

Patients then had a ventriculoperitoneal or ventriculoatrial shunt placed with an in line Codman Hakim programmable valve. The open ended peritoneal catheter provided with the valve was used in all patients. The ICP monitor was retained in the patient post-operatively for 48 hours. On the second post-operative day, ICP was again measured over the same range of postures as pre-operatively. Each time the shunt valve opening pressure had to be changed based on clinical findings, the ICP was again measured over the full range of postures. Three patients agreed to let us measure the postural ICP profile at 30, 50, 80, 110, 140, 170, and 200 mmH_2O. The ability to accurate set of valve was confirmed by an x-ray in each patient.

The correlation between valve opening pressure settings and ICP across patients, with multiple valve settings for each patient, was considered independent and estimated by a Pearson regression. Differences between ICP measurements were assessed by a t-test.

Results

Although the supine ICP at a valve setting of 200 mmH_2O averaged 7.2 ± 4.4 mmHg and was greater than at 50 mmH_2O (2.5 ± 5.3 mmHg), this difference was not statistically significant ($p = 0.19$) due to the broad range of ICPs encountered at each valve setting. When the HOB was raised to 60°, the differences in ICP between the 200 and 50 mmH_2O valve settings was again not significant (-5.4 ± 7.0 mmHg and -10.3 ± 6.3 mmHg, respectively: $p = 0.32$). The mean ICP at each valve setting was, however, significantly lower at HOB 60° compared to the flat position ($p < 0.01$).

The correlation between ICP and the valve opening pressure setting at any given head of bed (HOB) elevation was poor. When supine (HOB 0°), this correlation using pooled data was only $r = 0.23$, and at HOB 60° $r = 0.25$. This gross lack of correlation is illustrated in Fig. 1 where the postural ICP profiles for individual patients are plotted for valve settings of 200 and 50 mm H_2O.

Based on within subject analysis, there was a generally strong correlation between the ICP (HOB 0° and 60°) and valve opening pressures ($r = 0.72$–0.96). When analyzing this relationship graphically, however, this correlation appeared to be sigmoidal across the tested range of valve settings (Fig. 2). The region of

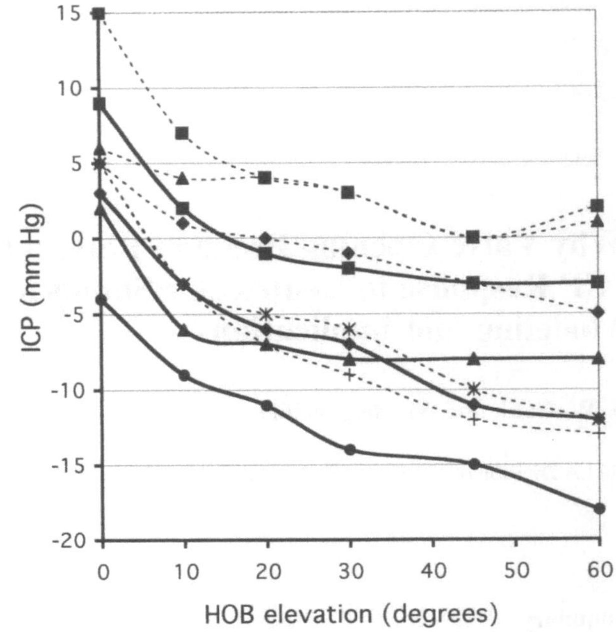

Fig. 1. Postural ICP profiles for individual patients with valve opening pressure set to 50 mmH_2O (solid lines) or 200 mm H_2O (dashed lines). —■— Pt A, 50 mmH_2O —◆— Pt B, 50 mmH_2O; —●— Pt C, 50 mmH_2O; —▲— Pt D, 50 mmH_2O; ---■-- Pt A, 200 mmH_2O; --◆-- Pt B, 200 mmH_2O; ---▲-- Pt C, 200 mmH_2O; ---✳-- Pt E, 200 mmH_2O; ---+-- Pt F, 200 mmH_2O.

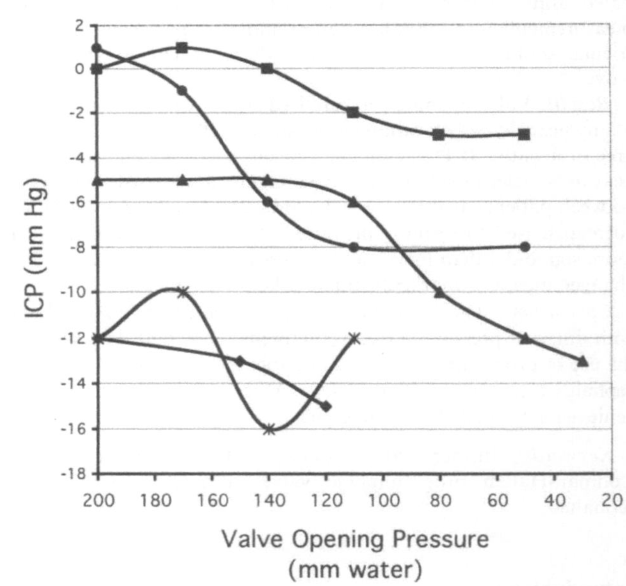

Fig. 2. Relationship of ICP to valve opening pressures for individual patients with the head of bed at 60°

linear response varied markedly between patients and sometimes occurred near the extreme of the possible valve settings.

Discussion

To date, there is still no reliable way to pre-operatively predict a patient's optimal opening pressure in terms of efficacy and safety for the treatment of NPH. The results of studies comparing outcomes using valves with different opening pressures remain controversial and inconclusive [2, 4]. Our data suggests that the major reason why is that there is a poor correlation between ICP and valve opening pressure.

One explanation that shunts with DPVs are unpredictable in adults may be related to the phenomenon of siphoning. It is well known that most patients with DPV shunts experience significantly negative intracranial pressures when upright [3, 5]. When a patient with a ventriculoperitoneal (VP) shunt stands, a hydrostatic fluid column is established equaling the distance between the point of ventricular drainage and CSF egress into the peritoneal cavity. For an adult of average height, the pressure generated by this fluid column is approximately 480 mm H_2O. This pressure head is more than twice the opening pressure of commercially available DPVs (200 mm H_2O). Miyake recently measured intraabdominal pressure in a group of patients and proposed that post-operative ICP follows a linear relationship based on adding the abdominal pressure to the opening pressure of the valve and subtracting the hydrostatic fluid column pressure [5].

Our data suggests that the above linear relationship occurs over only a narrow range of valve opening pressures along a sigmoidal curve (Fig. 2). More importantly, the range of valve opening pressures where the linear portion occurs varies considerably from patient to patient. For some patients, this linear portion of the curve occurs near the extremes of possible valve settings of the Codman Hakim programmable valve.

In summary, it remains unclear how to reliably predict the post-operative ICP profile for any given opening pressure of a DPV shunt. If the management plan is to gradually lower ICP, our data suggest that ICP should be measured both pre- and post-operatively and that a programmable valve is a necessity. In this way, the opening pressure can non-invasively be individualized based on symptomatic improvement and occurrence of overdrainage complications. Future similar studies will be required to relate post-operative ICP to clinical outcome and other valve types.

References

1. Bergsneider M, Peacock WJ, Mazziotta JC *et al* (1999) Beneficial effect of siphoning in treatment of adult hydrocephalus. Arch Neurol 56(10): 1224–1229
2. Boon AJ, Tans JT, Delwel EJ *et al* (1998) Dutch Normal-Pressure Hydrocephalus Study: randomized comparison of low- and medium-pressure shunts. J Neurosurg 88(3): 490–495
3. Chapman PH, Cosman ER, Arnold MA (1990) The relationship between ventricular fluid pressure and body position in normal subjects and subjects with shunts: a telemetric study. Neurosurgery 26(2): 181–189
4. McQuarrie IG, Saint-Louis L, Scherer PB (1984) Treatment of normal pressure hydrocephalus with low versus medium pressure cerebrospinal fluid shunts. Neurosurgery 15(4): 484–488
5. Miyake H, Ohta T, Kajimoto Y *et al* (2000) New concept for the pressure setting of a programmable pressure valve and measurement of in vivo shunt flow performed using a microflowmeter. Technical note. J Neurosurg 92(1): 181–187
6. Pang D, Altschuler E (1994) Low-pressure hydrocephalic state and viscoelastic alterations in the brain. Neurosurgery (Baltimore) 35(4): 643–656
7. Pudenz RH, Foltz EL (1991) Hydrocephalus Overdrainage by Ventricular Shunts A Review and Recommendations. Surg Neurol 35(3): 200–212
8. Pudenz RH, Russell FE, Hurd AH *et al* (1957) Ventriculoauricolostomy. A technique for shunting cerebrospinal fluid into the right auricle. Preliminary report. J Neurosurg 14: 171–179

Correspondence: Marvin Bergsneider, M.D., UCLA Division of Neurosurgery, Box 957039, Los Angeles, CA 90095-7039.

Acta Neurochir (2002) [Suppl] 81: 19–21

Dynamic Shunt Testing Applying Short Lasting Pressure Waves – Inertia of Shunt Systems

M. U. Schuhmann[1], C. G. Schneekloth[1], P. Klinge[1], M. Engel[2], M. Samii[1,2], and T. Brinker[2]

[1] Department of Neurosurgery, Medical School Hannover, Germany
[2] Department of Neurosurgery, Nordstadt Hospital Hannover, Germany

Summary

Laboratory shunt testing often comprises only static pressure flow and flow pressure tests. We applied shorter acting pressure waves using a computerised shunt testing rig to investigate shunt behaviour under conditions that might occur in the clinical situation, e.g. during nocturnal vasogenic pressure waves or shorter rises in ICP at movements or exercise. Additionally the influence of a human-like compliance situation compared to a fixed pressure/volume relationship was investigated. Shunts behaved very differently than seen in static tests and demonstrated a marked inertia the shorter pressure waves acted. Although some valves opened at higher pressure, all valves showed marked hysteresis and none did close – if at all – at the specified pressure level. This behaviour might be a cause of shunt overdrainage not related to siphoning. The simulation of a human-like variable pressure-volume relationship with higher compliance at lower pressures had a positive effect on shunt function by decreasing the amount of drained volume. We therefore suggest to include dynamic pressure wave testing if hydrodynamic properties of shunts are to be evaluated.

Keywords: Shunt evaluation; hydrocephalus; pressure waves; intracranial compliance.

Introduction

The conventionally used pressure-flow and flow-pressure tests are a rather static way to determine the basic hydrodynamic characteristics of shunt systems. Tests last from minutes to hours with relatively small changes of pressure or flow over time. In the human, however, either due to movements, coughing or nocturnal vasogenic pressure waves, fast pressure or flow changes will act on the shunt system in a dynamic fashion. We evaluated the drainage behaviour of shunts exposed to shorter pressure waves using a computerised shunt testing rig. We further compared a standard in-vitro test situation with linear pressure-volume relationship and fixed compliance to a human-like situation with non-linear third order pressure-volume characteristic and variable compliance.

Materials and Methods

3 PS Medical Valves (PSM low, medium, high pressure) and 3 Medos Hakim Precision valves (Medos low, medium, high pressure) connected to the original distal drain were investigated. Details of the used shunt testing rig are described elsewhere [3]. The computer controlled peristaltic pump was connected in series to a pear-shaped fluid container (human compliance simulator = HCS), or alternatively, to a standard ascending pipe (SAP) with constant inner diameter, and to the valve under investigation. The pump generated, by adjusting the flow rate, pressure waves from 1 mm Hg to 11 mm Hg. Pressure wave length was 40s, 90s and 180s. The resulting flow through the shunt system was determined by weighting the out-flowing fluid increments with an electronic high-precision balance. Vaporisation deficits of fluid from the container during the test were corrected. Deaerated destilled water was used. All runs were repeated 4–5 times resulting in 160 pressure-flow plots. Pressure waves were generated in a "standard situation" using an ascending pipe (SAP) and, second, in a "human-like situation" using the HCS. The HCS had a filling volume of 135 ml as described for the human CSF system. Opening and closing pressure (Po, Pc), flow and hysteresis at pressure 6 mm Hg (F6, H6), maximum flow (Fmax), and total drained volume (Vtot) were determined. Statistics: 2-way ANOVA followed by non-parametric tests (Mann-Whitney U). Differences were accepted if $p < 0.05$.

Results

The Medos high pressure valve did not open in any test. Therefore only 130 test runs resulted in flow pressure plots for further analysis. Fig. 2 shows as an example pressure-flow plots of pressure waves lasting 40s, 90s and 180s (SAP and Medos medium pressure valve). Most obviously the valve opened and closed far away from "regular" Po and Pc as determined pre-

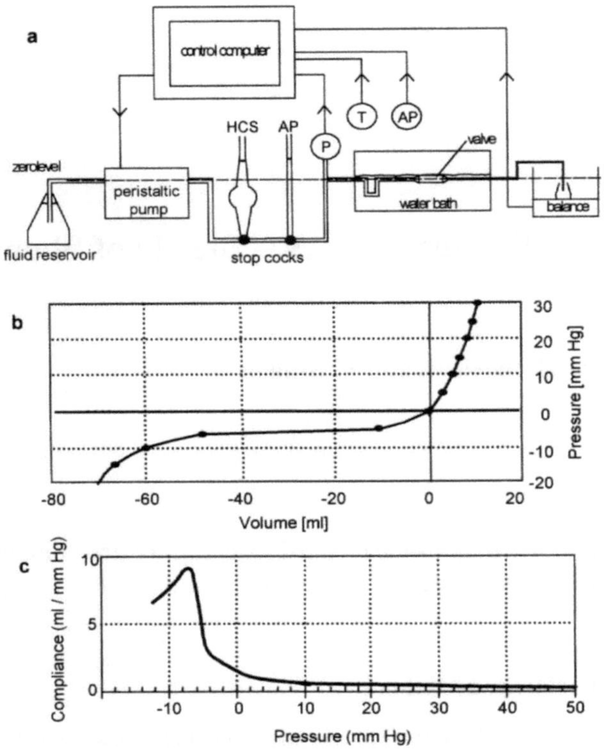

Fig. 1. (a) Shows construction principles of shunt testing rig. (b) Pressure/volume graph underlying construction of Human Compliance Simulator (HCS) (c) displays compliance of HCS as a function of pressure

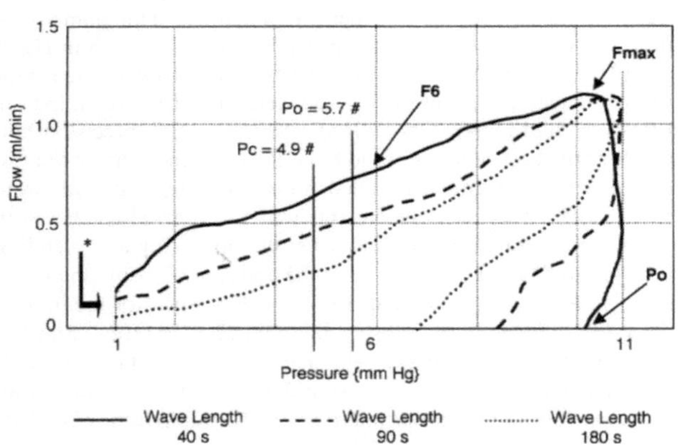

Fig. 2. Pressure flow plot of three pressure waves with duration of 40s, 90s, and 180s in Medos medium pressure valve. *Po* Opening pressure; *Pc* closing pressure; *Fmax* maximum flow; *F6* flow at 6 mm Hg; # Po & Pc as previously determined in flow-pressure and pressure flow tests; * valves had not closed when pressure of 1 mm Hg was reached

viously in flow-pressure (FP) and pressure-flow (PF) tests. A large hysteresis was evident.

Opening pressure (Po): both low pressure valves and the PSM medium opened just above 1 mm Hg. Po of these valves in FP tests was 1.2, 1.4, and 4.9 mm Hg respectively. The other two valves opened above "regular" Po. Valves showed a repeatable pattern: The shorter the pressure waves the higher Po, the later opened the valve.

Closing pressure (Pc): low pressure and medium pressure valves did not close, although Pc of the latter two in PF-tests was 4.0 and 4.8 mm Hg. The shorter the pressure waves, the further was Pc below the value determined in PF-Tests.

Flow and hysteresis at 6 mm Hg (F6, H6) were higher at shorter pressure waves.

Maximum flow (Fmax) was the lower the higher the working pressure of the valve. It was independent of speed of pressure wave, however. In medium and high pressure valves it tended to be lower if the HCS was used.

Total drainage volume (Vtot) was lower in higher pressure valves. It was the higher the slower waves acted and always significantly lower with the HCS system.

Discussion

Applying dynamic pressure waves onto a shunt valve resulted in very different hydrodynamic parameters of shunt function as obtained for the same valves in standard PF and FP tests in other independent laboratories [1] or according to own unpublished data. The speed of the pressure wave influenced results most significantly and thus the inertia of the shunt system plays an important role. In two valves Po was markedly higher, on the other hand hysteresis increased and all valves closed at much lower pressures if at all. The totally drained volume with maximum values of 3–4 ml might seem small, however it exceeded the production rate of 0.3 ml/min.

Compared to coughing the applied pressure waves were still rather slow. For the clinical situation these results imply that shunt inertia might be protective in case of very short lasting pressure waves as generated during coughing. In case vasogenic pressure waves introduce a behaviour of shunts as simulated here, the prolonged opening of valves below the closing pressure, the hysteresis and the demonstrated increase in total drainage volume should consequently lead to overdrainage the longer these pressure waves act. Measurements of in-vivo in-shunt flow confirm this interpretation by demonstrating higher than average shunt flows during the night [2]. As published previously, the use of the HCS enables simulation of patient recorded pressure patterns in the shunt testing work bench [3]. In the present investigation a higher volume was moved per time to produce the same pressure wave using the HCS compared to the SAP. Nevertheless the total drained volume was lower with the HCS demonstrating the influence of a higher compliance at lower pressure range on shunt function.

In summary, shunt testing with dynamic pressure waves revealed a different behaviour of hydrodynamic shunt characteristics compared to results of regular PF and FP tests. The tendency for medium and high pressure valves to open the later the shorter pressure waves act might be protective. On the other hand open valves closed much later at lower pressures and showed marked hysteresis. This behaviour promotes overdrainage which is independent of posture related siphoning.

References

1. Czosnyka M, Czosnyka Z, Whitehouse H, Pickard JD (1997) Hydrodynamic properties of hydrocephalus shunts: United Kingdom Shunt Evaluation Laboratory. J Neurol Neurosurg Psychiatry 62: 43–50
2. Kadowaki C, Hara M, Numoto M, Takeuchi K, Saito I (1995) CSF shunt physics: factors influencing inshunt CSF flow. Childs Nerv Syst 11: 203–206
3. Schuhmann MU, Engel M, Runge L, Samii M, Brinker T Application of clinically recorded ICP patterns – an extension of conventional shunt testing. Accepted for publication at Childs Nerv Syst

Correspondence: Dr. med. Martin U. Schuhmann, Neurochirurgische Klinik, Medizinische Hochschule Hannover, Carl-Neuberg-Str. 1, D-30625 Hannover, Germany.

Acta Neurochir (2002) [Suppl] 81: 23–26

Factors Determining Mean ICP in Hydrocephalic Patients with Hakim-programmable Valve: Implications of the Parallel Arrangement of the CSF Outflow Resistance and Shunt

R. Taylor, Z. Czosnyka, M. Czosnyka, and **J. D. Pickard**

Academic Neurosurgical Unit, Addenbrooke's Hospital, Cambridge UK

Summary

Objective. Measurement of CSF pressure is used clinically to test shunt function in vivo in hydrocephalic patients. Criteria for appropriate shunt function have never been validated.

Method. Hakim-Programmable valve was tested in a model of CSF circulation with variable resistance to CSF outflow (from 12 to 50 mm Hg/ml/min), increased hydrodynamic compliance (> 1.5 ml/mm Hg), and constant perfusion of a rate of 0.4 ml/min, i.e. conditions typical for hydrocephalus. The main question was how the simulated CSF pressure was influenced by the shunt setting and the residual resistance to CSF outflow.

Results. Measured baseline CSF pressure correlated well with shunt operating pressure only when high resistance to CSF outflow (50 mm Hg/(ml/min)) was used. For the medium resistance (20 mm Hg/(ml/min)) operating pressure was strongly affected by system's absorption capacity. For low resistance (12 mm Hg/(ml/min)) operating pressure through the valve was independent on valve's settings and no fluid drainage through the valve was recorded.

Conclusion. Patients with moderately elevated resistance to CSF outflow (12–18 mm Hg/(ml/min)) cannot possibly react to changes of the valve's settings above 100 mm H_2O. Mean CSF pressure results both from shunt setting and patient's own re-absorption capacity.

Keywords: Hydrocephalus; shunt; CSF pressure.

Introduction

Under strictly controlled experimental conditions, CSF reabsorption behaves according to the 'Ohms Law' equivalent formulated by Davson [4]. However, there is a complex and ill understood relationship between CSF reabsorption, alternative and probably slower mechanisms of interstitial fluid absorption, and the active response to various components to the cerebrospinal bed [2].

It is surprising that 'the rigid' behaviour of most shunts helps as many patients as they do. However, there is a subset of patients in whom no shunt appears to render them completely symptom-free. 80% of shunts fail within the first 12 years through obstruction, infection or overdrainage [3]. The ability to externally programme a valve has avoided some revisions in such patients. ICP monitoring or CSF infusion studies have been useful in providing an objective information about individual patient's CSF pressure-flow relationship but the results may not always be easy to interpret.

In shunted patients, baseline CSF pressure in horizontal body position should result from the parallel flow of CSF through the shunt and along CSF reabsorption pathway. We intended to investigate this point more accurately to demonstrate how non-linear behaviour of the programmable shunt may alter this simple relationship.

We used a well-established laboratory shunt testing methodology (UK Shunt Evaluation Laboratory) to construct a model of the hydrocephalic patient and to evaluate the influence of the setting of the Hakim-Programmable Valve and residual reabsorption capacity on operating pressure (i.e. patient's CSF pressure in horizontal body position).

Materials and Methods

The Testing Equipment

The test has been modified from that used in the UK Shunt Evaluation Laboratory [3] as illustrated in Fig. 1. The shunt under in-

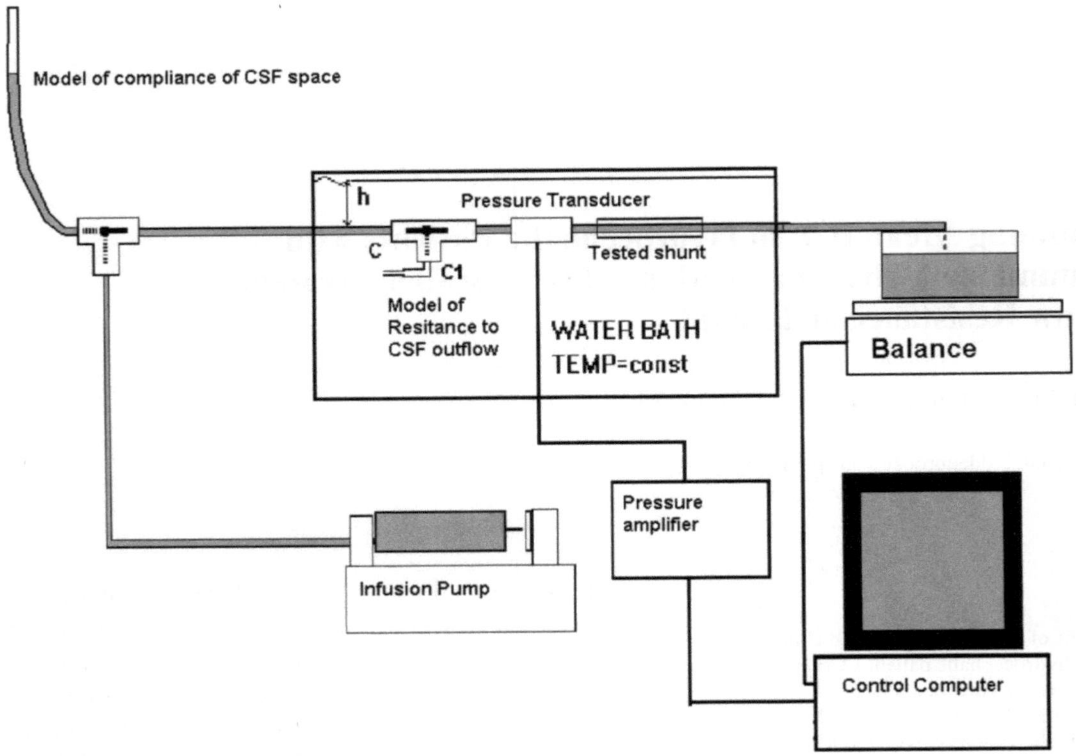

Fig. 1. Schematic diagram of testing rig

vestigation is submerged in a water bath at 37 °C and infused with de-ionised and de-aerated water (with physical properties that represent CSF under normal conditions) by an infusion pump (55-2222; Harvard Apparatus, Southnatick, MA). A model of CSF outflow resistance has been placed in parallel to the shunt to enable the shunt to be investigated in conditions mimicking the environment in vivo. The model of CSF outflow resistance are lumbar puncture needles of three resistances: 12, 20, 50 mm Hg/(ml/min).

Brain compliance was simulated by exponentially-bent open tube filled with water. Compliance of the system decreases linearly with pressure from 2 ml/mm Hg at pressure of 10 mm Hg to 1 ml/mm Hg at a pressure of 25 mm Hg). The input pressure to the shunt is measured with a Luer lock pressure transducer (Gaeltec Ltd., Dunvegan, Scotland) which is submerged in the water bath.

Measurement was controlled by a standard IBM PC with the software designed in house [3]. The pressure waveform is analysed by the computer using a spectral analysis algorithm. This minimises the influence of mechanical disturbances such as vibrations, gravitational waves and vortices in the water bath.

Protocol

The differential mean pressure and flow through the shunt were investigated at different settings of the valve (from 30 to 200 mm H_2O), with a continuous infusion of 0.4 ml/min (simulating CSF formation rate). Resistance to CSF outflow was changed from 12 to 20 and then 50 mm Hg/(ml/min). Every measurement was independently repeated 4 times and results were demonstrated graphically in form of mean values with a standard deviation vertical bar.

Results

Flow rates through the shunt and through the needle for three needles used (simulating variable resistance to CSF outflow 12,20 and 50 mm Hg/(ml/min)) were plotted on Figs. 2a and b respectively with the programmed valve setting along the x axis. For the high resistance needle, flow through the shunt responded linearly to change in the valve's setting. A proportion of the flow through the shunt to patient's own absorption rate changed from 8 (for setting 20 mm H_2O) to 0.5 (for the setting 200 mm H_2O). However, for the lower simulated resistance to CSF outflow (20 mm Hg/(ml/min)), above the valve's setting of 100 mm H_2O, previously observed linear relationship saturated. Above this setting all fluid flew through the resistance to CSF absorption and shunt remained closed. For the lowest resistance (12 mm Hg/(ml/min)), flow through the shunt was almost zero, with an exception of the lowest shunt's settings (below 50 mm H_2O).

As a result, the simulated pressure depended on shunt's settings only when the highest resistance needle was used (see Fig. 3). For the medium resistance

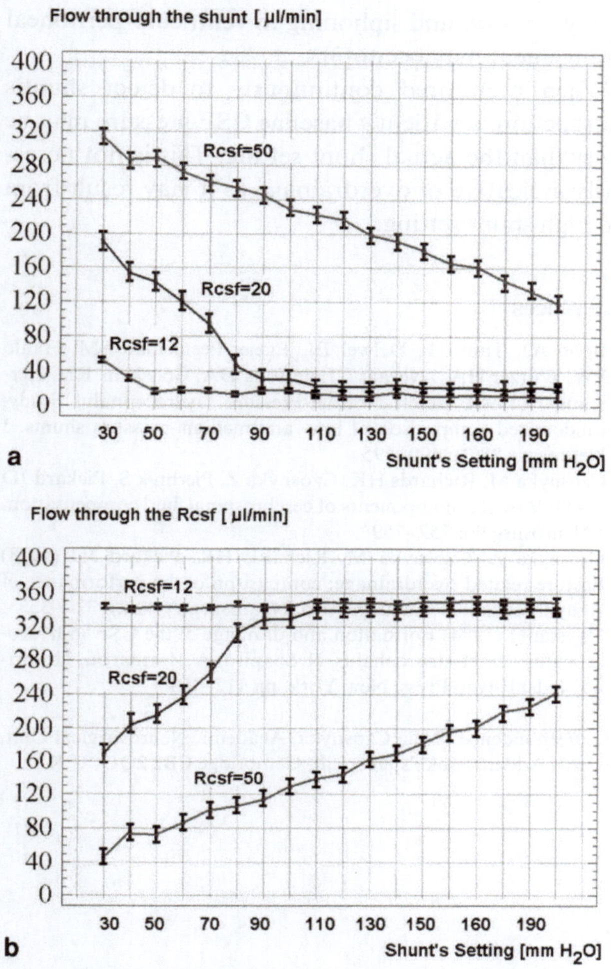

Fig. 2. Relationship between the flow (y axis) through the shunt (a) and through the needle (b) and set shunt operating pressure (x-axis) expressed in mm H_2O. The relationship has been evaluated for three used resistances of needles, simulating patient's own resistance to CSF outflow (Rcsf = 12, 20, 50 mm Hg/(ml/min) as indicated on the graph). Vertical bars show standard deviations of four independent measurements

(20 mm Hg/(ml/min)) operating pressure never increased above 10 mm Hg. For the lowest resistance it was virtually independent on shunt's settings, being continuously equal to 4.7 mm Hg.

Discussion

Conventional knowledge states that the role of programmable valves is to control patient's mean CSF pressure at the level equivalent to set operating pressure. Our laboratory study demonstrated clearly that it was not always the case.

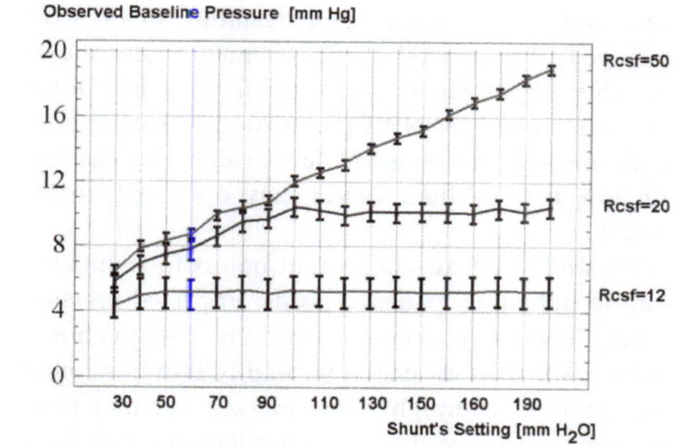

Fig. 3. Relationship between simulated baseline CSF pressure (y axis) and shunt's settings (x-axis) for three different resistance of needles. Vertical bars show standard deviations of four independent measurements

Baseline CSF pressure can be calculated from Davson's formula, that is:

$$\textit{Baseline pressure} = P_{SS} + \{\textit{CSF flow rate} * \textit{combined resistance to CSF outflow}\}$$

where P_{ss} is sagittal sinus pressure.

For low pressures, below the programmed shunt opening pressure the combined resistance to CSF outflow was equal to patient's own CSF outflow and varied from 12 mm Hg/(ml/min) to 50 mm Hg/(ml/min). Remaining variables were: $P_{SS} = 0$ and CSF flow rate 0.4 ml/min. Therefore all drainage was conducted through the resistance needle when the *Baseline pressure < Set shunt opening pressure.*

Only when the baseline pressure exceeded the shunt opening pressure, the combined resistance of the shunt and outflow path can be calculated from the formula, based on two resistors placed in parallel:

$$1/R_{combined} = 1/R_{shunt} + 1/R_{CSF\ outflow},$$

As R_{shunt} for the Hakim-Programmable shunt is 3 mm Hg/(ml/min) [3], combined resistance was low (between 2 and 3 mm Hg/(ml/min) for all CSF outflow resistances used). Low resistance indicates a good ability to stabilise the pressure at a level of shunt operating pressure.

This simple model demonstrates that with moderately increased resistance to CSF outflow (12 to 18 mm Hg/(ml/min)) the programmable shunt set for higher value may never open, resulting in nil CSF drainage and poor level of improvement under shunting. This phenomenon may explain why in 'Dutch trial' on shunting for NPH [1], medium valves were so significantly worse than low level valves. In patients with low ICP medium valves may open only occasionally.

This study indicates important points for matching shunt to individual patient's needs. For fixed pressure shunts, the opening pressure should be always chosen a little lower than measured normal ICP in horizontal body position overnight. Too low an opening pressure may cause overdrainage (particularly with low-resistance valves [3]), too high may render the valve permanently closed. From this point of view, programmable valves are useful for choosing 'optimal' CSF drainage condition. Ideally, they should be set after implantation little above patient's CSF pressure. Then, setting should be stepwise decreased until satisfactory improvement is noticed, which results from optimal proportion of CSF drainage through the shunt system and own CSF reabsorption. This is not always possible to attain, as CSF pressure is grossly related to day activity, and siphoning in ventriculo-peritoneal arrangement may occur [3].

When monitored continuously to detect shunt's malfunction, a patient's baseline CSF pressure may be lower than the actual shunt setting. This is not necessarily indicative of overdrainage as it may result from too high shunt setting.

References

1. Boon AJ, Tans JT, Delwel EJ, Egeler-Peerdeman SM, Hanlo PW, Wurzer HA, Avezaat CJ, de Jong DA, Gooskens RH, Hermans J (1998) Dutch Normal-Pressure Hydrocephalus Study: randomized comparison of low- and medium-pressure shunts. J Neurosurg 88(3): 490–495
2. Czosnyka M, Richards HK, Czosnyka Z, Piechnik S, Pickard JD (1999) Vascular components of cerebrospinal fluid compensation. J Neurosurg 90: 752–759
3. Czosnyka Z, Czosnyka M, Richards HK, Pickard JD (1998) Posture-related overdrainage: comparison of the performance of 10 hydrocephalus shunts in vitro. Neurosurgery 42(2): 327–333
4. Davson H (1984) Formation and drainage of the CSF in hydrocephalus. In: Hydrocephalus, K Shapiro, A Marmarou, H Portnoy (eds) Raven Press, New York, pp 112–160

Correspondence: Zofia Czosnyka, Academic Neurosurgical Unit, Box 167, Addenbrooke's Hospital, Cambridge CB2 2QQ, U.K.

Acta Neurochir (2002) [Suppl] 81: 27–30

Shunt Testing in-Vivo: A Method Based on the Data from the UK Shunt Evaluation Laboratory

Z. H. Czosnyka, M. Czosnyka, and J. D. Pickard

Academic Neurosurgical Unit, Addenbrooke's Hospital, Cambridge, UK

Summary

Objectives. The objective of the UK Shunt Evaluation Laboratory was to perform an independent testing of hydrodynamic performance of hydrocephalus shunts and provide systematic reviewing for neurosurgeons and patients.

Methods. Valves were tested long-term in a computer-controlled rig to evaluate their pressure-flow performance both at baseline and under conditions mimicking phenomena, which may alter CSF drainage in vivo. The operating pressures ($P_{operating}$) and hydrodynamic resistances (R) of all types of valves, currently in use in the UK, have been evaluated (Codman: Hakim-Precision, Hakim-Programmable, Uni-Shunt, Accu-flo, Holter. Medtronic PS Medical: Delta, Flow Control, Lumbo-peritoneal. NMT: Orbis-Sigma, Omni-shunt, Hakim Valve. Heyer-Schulte: In-line, Pudenz-Flushing, LowProfile. Radionics ContourFlex. Sophy Programmable). 67 patients, who had improved in the past following shunting but had recent recurrence of their clinical symptoms, were admitted to undergo a computerized infusion test through the shunt pre-chamber or Ommaya reservoir implanted prior to shunting. The criterion used to detect shunt underdrainage was an increase in ICP during constant infusion above $P_{operating} + R * \text{Infusion rate} + 5$ mm Hg. The validity of this formula has been confirmed in a laboratory study.

Results. 35 patients met the criteria for shunt underdrainage while in 24 normal drainage was demonstrated. Mean ICP achieved during the test was 24 mm Hg in patients with underdrainage versus 14 mm Hg with normally functioning shunts ($p < 0.01$). Out of 35 patients 25 improved and 10 were seen again to have the test repeated. In 7 patients shunt was blocked again. Only 3 patients with primarily confirmed shunt underdrainage did not improve following revisions. In 8 patients overdrainage related to body posture was confirmed using tilt-test.

Conclusions. Shunt testing in-vivo is easy, clinically useful and has good prediction power (90%).

Keywords: Hydrocephalus; shunt; complications.

Introduction

Patients who never improve or improve and then get worse after shunting for hydrocephalus constitute a difficult group to decide about their further management. Is shunt revision always a good strategy and can it be recommended solely on the basis of clinical symptoms and brain imaging?

In clinical practice we use constant rate infusion study [1] to reveal patient's CSF circulatory reserve. We investigated in laboratory hydrodynamic properties of most commonly used shunts [2]. Laboratory study confirmed that most of classic-differential shunts limit CSF pressure rise recorded during constant rate infusion test. We studied whether this shunt-specific pressure rise can be used for the assessment of shunt performance in-vivo.

Method

Laboratory Tests

A typical result obtained with the model of the CSF circulation in hydrocephalic patient, both with and without the shunt, is shown in Fig. 1. This demonstrates that 1.5 ml/min increase in infusion rate gives a stereotyped pressure-time curve. Pressure increases in a $(1 - e^{-x})$ manner to the end equilibrium value. At the end of the infusion, the pressure falls exponentially towards the baseline level.

The upper panel represents the model without the shunt in place. In our model the patient's resistance to CSF outflow was 20 mm Hg/(ml/min), the upper limit of normal being approximately 13 mm Hg/ml/min [1]. In response to the infusion a large increase in ICP is recorded. This increase in pressure is not as great when the shunt is in place. This demonstrates that the role of the shunt is to cut the end equilibrium pressure to a value determined by its hydrodynamic properties.

Systematic laboratory studies revealed that the end equilibrium pressure achieved during constant rate infusion is the most stable parameter characterising shunt function in vivo. The pressure should not increase above the value given by the equation;

$$\textit{Maximum end equilibrium pressure} < \textit{shunt operating pressure} + \{\textit{resistance of shunt} * \textit{infusion rate}\} + 5 \textit{ mm Hg}.$$

The 5 mm Hg is a safety factor that has been used in a considerable number of in vivo studies.

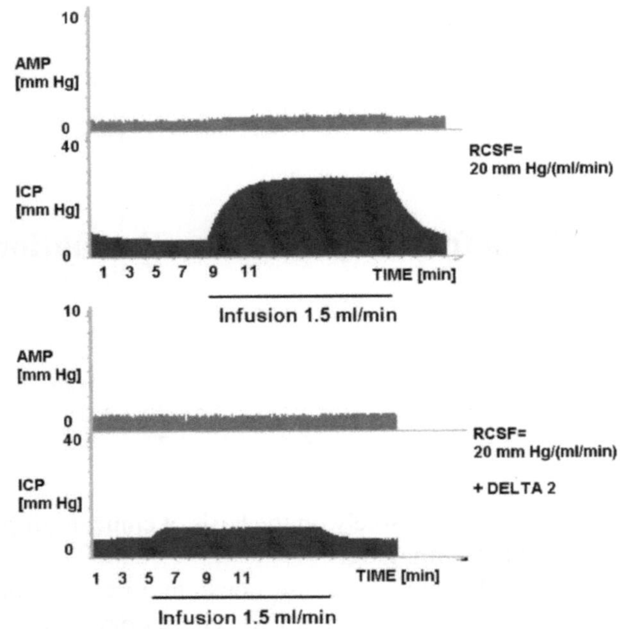

Fig. 1. Infusion study simulated in-vitro without a shunt (upper panel) and with a shunt (lower panel)

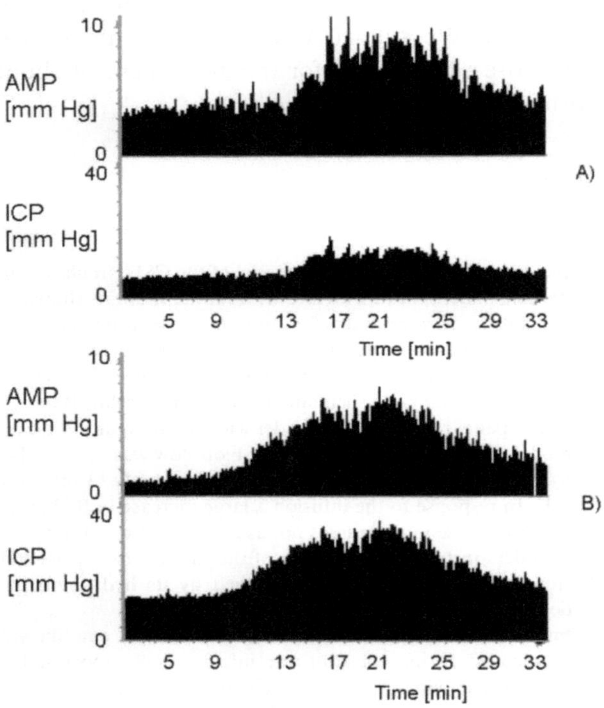

Fig. 2. Infusion test performed to test shunt function in-vivo: (A) Patient with Delta Valve level 2, no evidence of shunt blockage according to formula discussed in the text. (B) Patient with Medos Valve set for 150 mm H_2O. Opening pressure was in norm, but the end-pressure reached during the test was much higher than resulting from the laboratory measurement. Shunt was revised and patient subsequently improved

Table 1. *Critical Thresholds of ICP Rise During Constant Rate Infusion Test (1.5 ml/min) in 12 Types of Fixed-Pressure Valves*

	The Shunt	Performance level	Critical pressure for infusion 1.5 ml/min
1	Delta Valve	level-1	13.8
		level-2	18.65
2	Low Profile Heyer-Shulte	low	15.7
		med	23.1
		high	29.9
3	Pudenz-Flushing Heyer-Shulte with ASD	low	16.1
		med	18.9
		high	24.4
4	In Line H-S	low	20.0
		med	31.6
		high	45
5	Contour-Flex Radionix	low	14.2
		med	18.9
		high	23.8
6	Holter-Valve Codman	low	25.5
		med	31.05
		high	36.7
7	Hakim-Precision Codman	v. low	14.9
		low	17.28
		med-low	19.75
		med-high	21.95
		high	26.0
8	Accu-Flow Codman	low	17.1
		med	18.9
		high	21.5
9	Omni-shunt NMT (Cordis)	low	16.25
		med	19.05
		high	21.25
10	Codman Uni-shunt regular	low	12.2
		med	15.36
		high	26.25
	Codman Uni-shunt elliptical	low	16.15
		med	18.2
		high	32.2
11	CSF-Flow Control standard	low	11.17
		med	17.1
		high	22.5
	CSF-Flow Control contoured	low	12.5
		med	19.6
		high	24.15
	CSF-Flow Control burr-hole	low	11.4
		med	15.95
		high	20.85
	CSF-Flow Control button	low-low	9.01
		low	13.4
		med	11.65
12	Hakim Valve NMT (Cordis)	v. low	14.65
		low	16.8
		medium	18.75
		high	23.15
		v. high	28.75

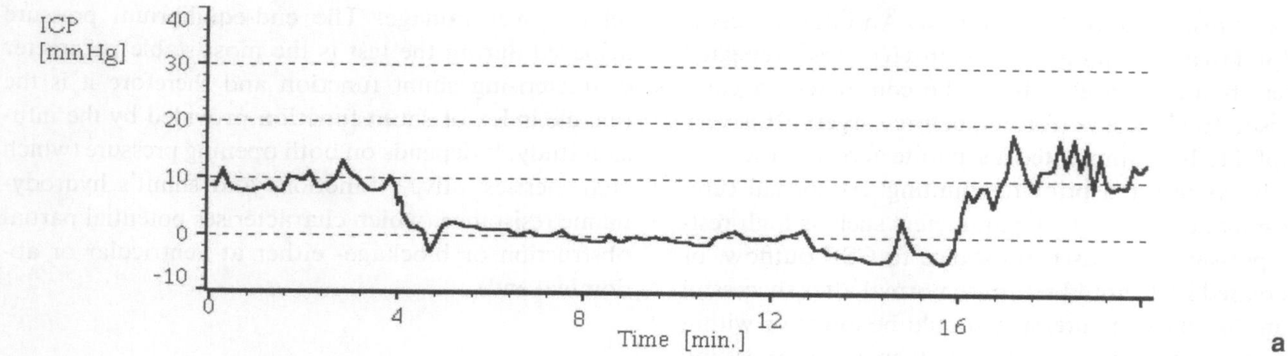

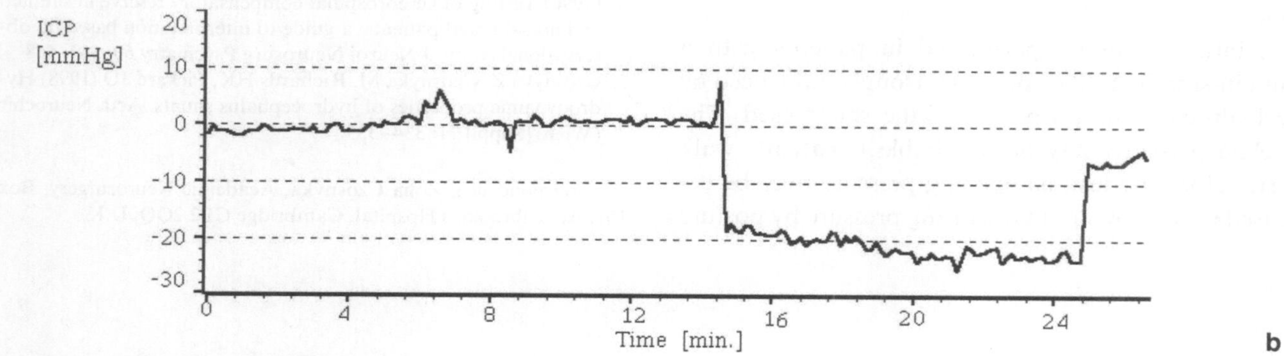

Fig. 3. Tilting tests in patients with overdrainage-like symptoms and different type of shunts: (a) Patient with the Delta valve, tilting from 4 to 16 min, ICP decreased to 0 and returned to the baseline value after the test. Posture-related overdrainage has been excluded. (b) Patient with a shunt with siphon-preventing device (tilting from 14 to 26 min). Pressure decreased to below 20 mm Hg with significantly negative values after the test. Posture – related overdrainage was possible

Critical values of end-equilibrium pressure for all tested fixed-pressure shunts and infusion rates of 1.5 ml/min were given in Table 1. For programmable valves the following formulae were derived:

Hakim Programmable: 12.85 + set level (cm H_2O)/1.356

Sophy Valve: 13 + set operating pressure (in mm Hg)

Results

In total, 67 patients, who had improved in the past following shunting but had recent recurrence of their clinical symptoms (in 1998–1999), were admitted to undergo a computerized infusion test through the shunt pre-chamber or Ommaya reservoir implanted prior to shunting. The criterion used to detect shunt underdrainage was an increase in ICP during constant infusion above critical pressure discussed in the previous section. Figs. 2a and 2b contain examples of reports from infusion studies performed in shunted patients referred to the Neurosurgical Clinic with a degree of recurrence of symptoms.

35 patients met the criteria for shunt underdrainage while in 24 normal drainage was demonstrated. In 8 patients overdrainage related to body posture was confirmed using tilt-test (see Fig. 3). Mean ICP achieved during the test was 24 mm Hg in patients with underdrainage versus 14 mm Hg with normally functioning shunts ($p < 0.01$). Out of 35 patients 25 improved (at discharge) following revision and 10 were seen again to have the test repeated. In 7 patients shunt was blocked again. Only 3 patients with primarily confirmed shunt underdrainage did not improve following revisions. We can assess that positive predictive power of the test was in the range of 90%.

Discussion

The symptoms of underdrainage may vary from lack of a noticeable improvement after shunting to an extremely acute increase in ICP, which, if not managed properly, may cause death within a few hours. A properly functioning shunt stabilizes ICP and usually decreases resistance to CSF outflow. An infusion test is helpful to assess shunt function in-vivo. Tests repeated after shunting should always be considered in comparison to the test performed before surgery. It is very helpful to have implanted a separate access to the CSF pathways inserted prior to shunting. Abnormal cerebrospinal compensatory parameters such as high resting pressure, increased resistance to CSF outflow, or decreased PVI should return to normal after successful shunting. Baseline pressure should be lower or within the measured range of the shunt operating pressure. The end-equilibrium pressure should not exceed critical pressure given by the formula in the previous section.

In infusion studies performed in patients with a shunt in-situ the ICP response is strongly influenced by the hydrodynamic properties of the shunt used. The baseline pressure may be unreliable if patients walk or sit before the test, as opening pressure may be decreased well below shunt operating pressure by posture related overdrainage. The end-equilibrium pressure achieved during the test is the most stable parameter characterising shunt function and therefore it is the reliable index of shunt function provided by the infusion study. It depends on both opening pressure (which characterises valve's function) and shunt's hydrodynamic resistance (which characterises potential partial obstruction or blockage- either at ventricular or abdominal end).

References

1. Czosnyka M, Whitehouse H, Smielewski P, Simac S, Pickard JD (1996) Testing of cerebrospinal compensatory reserve in shunted and non-shunted patients: a guide to interpretation based on observational study. J Neurol Neurosurg Psychiatry 60: 549–558
2. Czosnyka Z, Czosnyka M, Richards HK, Pickard JD (1998) Hydrodynamic properties of hydrocephalus shunts. Acta Neurochir (Wien) [Suppl] 71: 334–339

Correspondence: Zofia Czosnyka, Academic Neurosurgery, Box 167, Addenbrooke's Hospital, Cambridge CB2 2QQ, U.K.

Acta Neurochir (2002) [Suppl] 81: 31–33

Compensatory Mechanisms in Patients with Benign Intracranial Hypertension Syndrome

S. S. Gasparian, N. K. Serova, E. Ya. Sherbakova, and **T. N. Belova**

Burdenko Neurosurgical Institute, Moscow, Russia

Summary

135 patients from 16 to 59 years old with benign intracranial hypertension syndrome (BIH) due to postinflammatory processes (A), venous outflow disorders (V), and endocrinological disorders (G) were investigated by CT, MRI, MRI-Ag, carotid-Ag and constant pressure infusion test. All the obtained data were analyzed and possible relationships between the parameters of CSF dynamics and the clinical data were evaluated. Correlative analysis of the obtained data was performed and the main mechanisms of compensation of BIH syndrome were established. In patients of group A disturbances of CSF absorption system with high level of CSF outflow resistance (R) and secondary elevation of brain elastance (EL) were common. In patients of this group venous disorders were of secondary nature and appeared in a later period of the disease. The patients of group V showed increased intrasinus pressure, which correlated to high R and EL. In patients of group G we found the signs of CSF hyperproduction with high level of EL. Increased R in patients of this group seemed to be a secondary reaction.

The investigation identified the main stages of evolution and compensation of hypertension in the patients with BIH syndrome. The obtained data may be used in optimizing the conservative therapy and indications for lumboperitoneal shunting.

Keywords: Benign intracranial hypertension; CSF dynamics.

Introduction

The benign intracranial hypertension (BIH) syndrome is characterized by severe papilledema and increased CSF pressure without a neurological deficit [3, 4, 5]. The evolution of clinical signs of the BIH syndrome is caused mainly by venous and CSF outflow disorders and low absorbtion of arachnoid membranes. However, the relationships between clinical data, parameters of CSF dynamics, and compensatory mechanisms are still unknown. In order to define these mechanisms, we have analyzed the clinical data, CT, MRI, MRI-Ag and carotid Ag data, parameters of CSF dynamics by constant pressure infusion test (CPIT), changes of CSF flow by radionuclide cysternography and sinusography.

Material and Methods

The material of the investigation were 135 patients with BIH syndrome (117 females and 18 males), from 16 to 59 years old. The patients were divided into three main groups: A – with arachnoditis, postinflammatory processes and trauma [64], G – with endocrinological problems [45], and V – the patients with venous outflow disorders caused by sinus thrombosis [24] and arteriosinus fistulas [2]. All patients were investigated by standard neurological and ophthalmologic methods, carotid angiography (CA), CT and 27 patients by MRI and MRI-angiography. In order to study the parameters of CSF dynamics we used modified CPIT [1, 3] with evaluation of CSF pressure (Po), CSF outflow resistance (R), elastance of cerebrospinal system (El), intrasinus pressure (Pis), and CSF production rate (F).

Results

All the patients had severe papilledema, which was more remarkable in patients of groups G and A, fast decrease in visual acuity during a period of 2 to 10 weeks in the patients of group V. Visual acuity was decreased in 96 patients: group V in 80% cases, in group G – in 65% and in group A – in 70% patients. Periventricular lucency (PVL) on CT was found in 55% of patients with venous outflow disorders, in 65% of patients of group A and only 10% of patients in group G. Empty sella syndrome (ESS) were presented mainly in the patients with endocrinological problems. As a result of our investigation we have determined high level of CSF pressure (18–30 mm Hg) in all patients (Fig. 1a).

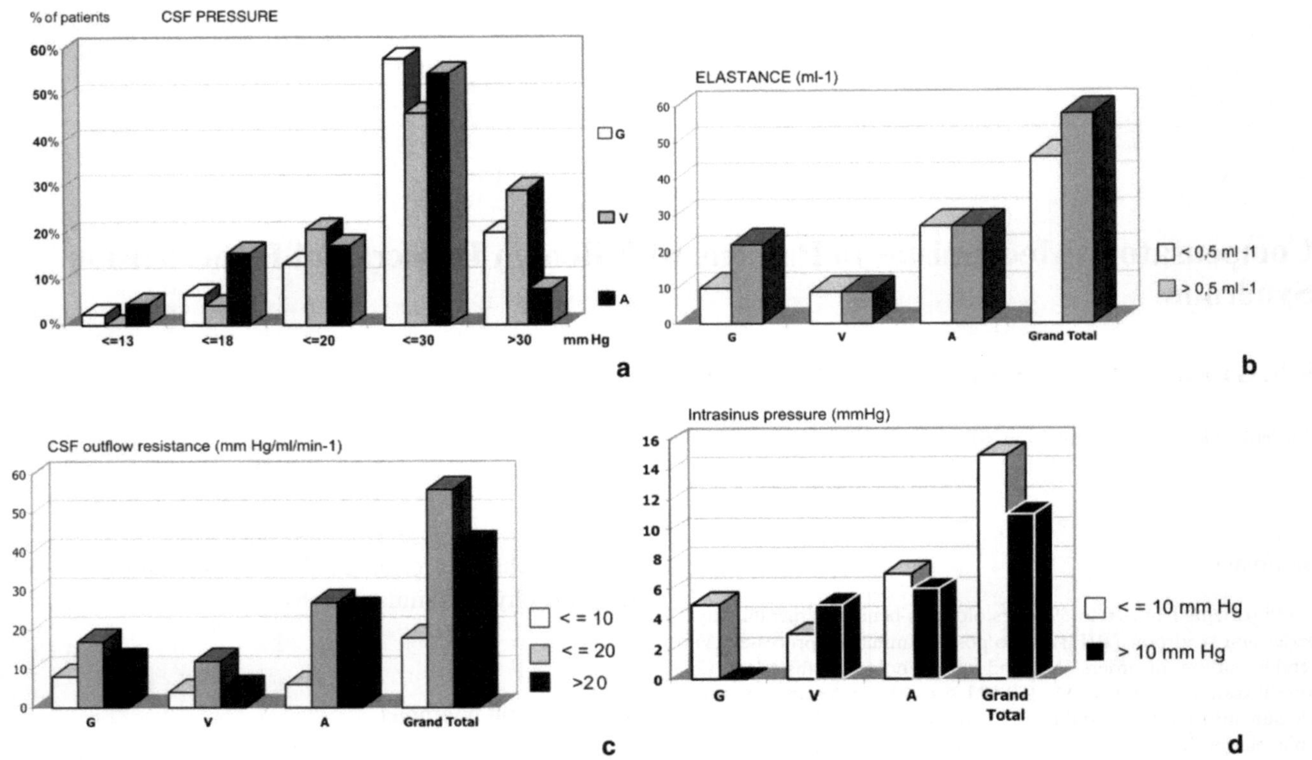

Fig. 1. (a) CSF pressure in the patients with BIH syndrome. (b) Elastance in the patients with BIH syndrome. (c) CSF outflow resistance in the patients with BIH syndrome. (d) Intrasinus pressure in the patients with BIH syndrome

CSF outflow resistance was significantly higher in 85% of the patients [from 20–30 mmHg/(ml/min)], more often (90%) in group A (Fig. 1c). Increasing of elastance more than 0.5 ml^{-1} was identified in 55% of patients. In group G we found high level EL in a half of cases (Fig. 1b). CSF production rate was higher than normal range (up to 0.5 ml/min) in patients with endocrinological disorders. Intrasinus pressure was increased up to 10 mm Hg in patients of groups V and A, and it was in a normal range in the patients of group G (Fig. 1d).

Correlative analysis of the obtained clinical and CSF dynamics data was performed and the main mechanisms of evolution and compensation of BIH syndrome were estimated. In patients from group A disturbances of CSF circulation with high level of R and secondary elevation of EL were common. In patients of this group venous disorders were of secondary nature and appeared in a later period of the disease. In patients from group G we found high level of EL and increased CSF production rate. Increased R in patients of this group seems to be a secondary reaction. The patients from group V showed increasing value of Pis, which correlated to high R and EL.

Discussion

The obtained data confirm functional interrelation between CSF system and venous outflow system. It is well known that adequate venous outflow is possible due to positive pressure gradient between cerebral vein pressure (CVP) and intrasinus pressure [1, 4, 5]. High range of CSF pressure may significantly change these interactions. Increased sinus pressure leads to elevation of CVP and cerebral blood volume (CBV). Under these conditions normal CSF absorption will deteriorate. Increased Pis, R and Pcsf in our study confirm these propositions. These data are well related to the results by P. Janny *et al.* (1981). Elevated CBV was found along with increased EL with PVL on CT in the patients with raised Pcsf, R and Pis. Severe papilloedema may be the consequence of the slow compensatory reactions for increased CBV. In patients with endocrinological disturbances, the rate of CSF production was up to 0,5 ml/min. This may be reflection of elevated CVP.

We suppose these results are in good agreement with Monro-Kellie doctrine in patients with clinical symptoms of severe BIH syndrome. The quick and severe impairment of visual function in patients with venous outflow disorders confirms the hypothesis of a low capacity of compensatory mechanisms of cerebrospinal fluid system. The increased R is a result of venous outflow disorders in the sinuses, bridging veins and cerebral veins, and leads to increased cerebral blood volume in association with periventricular edema. We suppose that an increased EL may be caused not only by the CSF disturbances, but also by the venous outflow disorders. In patients with BIH syndrome the impairment of venous outflow causes the elevation of Pis, R, Po, and is accompanied by an increased EL and CBV.

Finally, we conclude that in patients of group A disturbances of CSF absorption caused the secondary elevation of EL. Venous disorders in group A seems to be of secondary nature and appeared in the latest period of the disease.

In patients from group G we found signs of CSF hyperproduction with high level of EL in association with periventricular lucency. Increased R in patients of this group seems to be a secondary reaction. The patients from group V showed severe early papilloedema, increase of Pis, which correlated to high R and EL. These changes reflect the compensatory mechanisms for stabilizing the cerebrospinal fluid system in intracranial hypertension in patients with venous outflow deterioration.

Main stages of evolution and compensation of hypertension in patients with BIH syndrome were defined. The obtained data may be used in optimizing the therapeutical procedures and establishing the indications for lumboperitoneal shunting.

References

1. Marmorou A, Shulman K, La Lorgese J (1977) Compartmental analysis of compliance and outflow resistance of the cerebrospinal fluid system. J Neurosurg 43: 523–534
2. Malm J, Kristiansen B, Markgren P, Ekstedt J (1992) CSF hydrodynamics in idiopathic intracranial hypertension: a long-term study. Neurology 42: 851–858
3. Portnoy HD, Croisant PD (1976) A practical method for measuring hydrodynamics of cerebrospinal fluid. Surg Neurol 5: 273–277
4. Janny P, Chazal J, Colnet G, Devoize JL, Baretto LL (1981) L hypertension intracranienne benigne. Etude clinique physiopathologique and nosographique. Neurochirurgie 27: 79–88
5. Johnston I, Hawke S, Halmagui M, Teo C (1991) The pseudotumor syndrome: disorders of CSF circulations causing intracranial hypertension without ventriculomegaly. Arch Neurol 48: 740–747

Correspondence: Dr. S. S. Gasparian, Burdenko Neurosurgical Institute, 1231, 4 Tverskaya-Yamskaya, 16, 125047 Moscow Russia.

Acta Neurochir (2002) [Suppl] 81: 35–38

Intracranial Hypertension after Surgery in Patients with Chiari I Malformation and Normal or Moderate Increase in Ventricular Size

M. A. Poca, J. Sahuquillo, J. Ibañez, S. Amorós, F. Arikan, and E. Rubio

Department of Neurosurgery, Vall d'Hebron University Hospitals, Barcelona, Spain

Summary

Objective. To determine ICP changes in patients with Chiari type I malformation after posterior fossa reconstruction (PFR).

Patients and Methods. We continuously monitored ICP before and after PFR in 12 patients with Chiari I malformation and with an Evans' Index below or equal to 0.33. Mean ICP (epidural sensor) and percentage of B waves were calculated 24 hours before surgery and during the first 7 days after surgery.

Results. Mean ICP and percentage of B waves significantly increased after surgery despite a significant increase in the volume of the posterior fossa. The main finding revealed by control CT scans was compression of the quadrigeminal cistern with a reduction in size of the fourth ventricle. In six patients, a small transitory increase in supratentorial ventricular size was found.

Conclusions. A transitory increase in ICP is common after PFR. This increase could be explained by an initial reperfusion phenomena in the cerebellum that provokes a transitory deterioration in CSF dynamics. The effacement of the quadrigeminal cistern and the reduction in size of the fourth ventricle suggests this hypothesis.

Keywords: Chiari I malformation; posterior fossa reconstruction; ICP monitoring; intracranial hypertension.

Introduction

It is well known that patients with Chiari malformation present alterations in CSF dynamics secondary to herniation of the cerebellar tonsils into the upper cervical canal. This herniation produces dissociation of craniospinal pressure [4, 6, 7]. In these patients posterior fossa reconstruction should restore normal CSF circulation at the level of the foramen magnum with a secondary improvement in CSF dynamics. However, patients often present transitory, sometimes severe, headaches in the immediate postoperative period after successful surgery and in some cases compensated hydrocephalus may become active [3, 8]. To date, few studies have investigated the repercussions of craniovertebral decompression on ICP [6]. To determine ICP changes after craniovertebral decompression, we continuously monitored extradural ICP (mean ICP and percentage of B-waves) before and after PFR in 12 patients with Chiari I malformation and with normal or moderate increase in ventricular size.

Patients and Methods

A prospective study was carried out in 12 patients with Chiari I malformation and an Evans' Index below or equal to 0.33 (8 women and 4 men, mean age 40.5 ∀ 11, range 23–58). The Evans' Index was measured as the maximum distance between the frontal horns divided by the maximum inner diameter of the skull, both measured at the same CT scan slice [2]. Four of the 12 patients presented an associated syringomyelia. Clinical findings of the study group are summarised in Table 1.

Posterior fossa reconstruction was performed in all patients. Surgical technique included an extensive suboccipital craniectomy with a wide opening of the foramen magnum and resection of the posterior C1 arch. Next, the dura mater was opened, with preservation of the arachnoid membrane when possible. A wide dural allograft (Tutoplast, Primmer-Vigo, GmbH+Co, Erlangen, Germany) was then implanted and was closed watertight with fibrin adhesive (Tissucol, Immuno, SA, Barcelona, Spain) [3].

In all patients, continuous ICP monitoring was performed with a fiberoptic extradural sensor (LADD Research Industries, Inc., Burlington, Vermont). Mean ICP and percentage of B-waves were calculated both before and after surgery. ICP was monitored for at least 24 hours before PFR. Early postoperative period was considered as the 3 days after surgery and late postoperative period between days 4 and 7. The Kruskal-Wallis test was used in the statistical analysis. Differences were considered significant when $P < 0.05$.

Results

None of the patients died or presented neurological deterioration after PFR. In seven patients transitory headaches appeared for the first time or pre-existing headaches became worse in the early postoperative

Table 1. *Characteristics of Patient Group*

Patient	Age/sex	Evans' index before PFR	Associated syringomyelia	Arachnoid integrity*	Postoperative headaches	Evans' index** after PFR	Quadrigeminal cistern effacement** (control CT)
1	23/f	0.30	yes	yes	no	0.30	yes
2	46/f	0.20	no	yes	no	0.20	yes
3	44/m	0.25	no	yes	yes	0.27	yes
4	34/f	0.24	no	yes	yes	0.28	yes
5	47/f	0.29	no	no (>4 mm)	no	0.29	yes
6	38/f	0.27	no	yes	yes	0.28	yes
7	52/f	0.25	no	no (>4 mm)	yes	0.25	no
8	49/f	0.33	yes	no (>4 mm)	yes	0.35	yes
9	29/m	0.32	no	yes	no	0.31	no
10	25/f	0.26	yes	yes	no	0.26	no
11	58/m	0.30	no	yes	yes	0.32	yes
12	42/m	0.25	yes	no (>4 mm)	yes	0.26	yes

PFR Posterior Fossa Reconstruction, * Small holes in the arachnoid were sealed with bipolar coagulation. ** Control CT scan was performed during the first week after PFR.

period. In five patients these headaches disappeared or diminished in the late postoperative period (Table 1).

Control CT scans showed no surgical complications in any of the patients. A small increase in supratentorial ventricular size was found in six patients and the quadrigeminal cistern was effaced in nine (Table 1). This effacement was associated with a simultaneous reduction in size of the fourth ventricle. Postoperative MRI studies performed 3 months after surgery showed upward migration of the tonsils and formation of an artificial cisterna magna in all patients. Reduction or collapse of syringomyelia was also found in all patients.

After surgery, mean ICP significantly increased in 10 of the 12 patients. Percentage of B-waves significantly increased in all patients, both in the early and in the late postoperative periods (Fig. 1). In 10 patients ICP recordings qualitatively improved at the end of the first week after surgery. High ICP values persisted several months after surgery in three patients and a ventriculoperitoneal shunt was implanted. Detailed ICP recordings of an illustrative case are shown in Fig. 2.

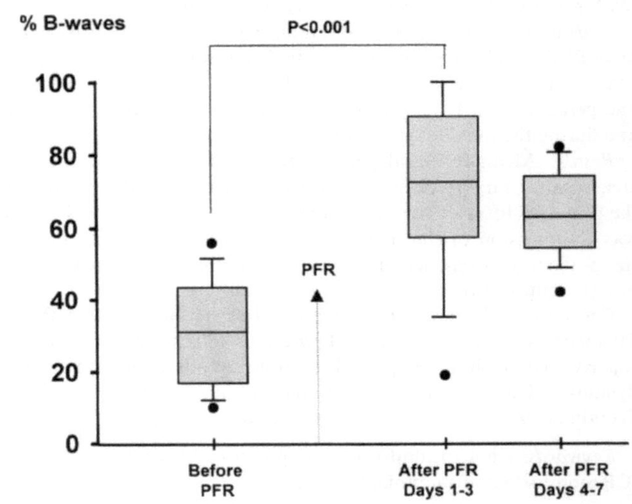

Fig. 1. Figure showing percentage of B-waves before and after posterior fossa reconstruction (*PFR*). Percentage of B-waves significantly increased both in the early (days 1–3) and in the late (days 4–7) postoperative periods compared with presurgical period ($P < 0.001$). Statistical differences between the early and the late postoperative periods were not significant ($P = 0.67$)

Discussion

Chiari I malformation is characterised by impaction of the hindbrain in an abnormally small posterior fossa. This compression obstructs the normal venting of CSF in and out of the craniocervical subarachnoid space, establishing pressure gradients between cranial and spinal compartments [4, 6, 7]. Abnormalities in CSF flow in the foramen magnum have been related to the origin and progression of associated hydrocephalus and/or syringomyelia [5, 7, 8]. Therefore, decompression or enlargement of the posterior fossa to establish normal CSF pathways should be the primary goal of surgical intervention. Successful craniovertebral decompression should be followed by normalisation of ICP recordings, reduction or collapse of syringomyelia, and decrease in ventricular size. In our

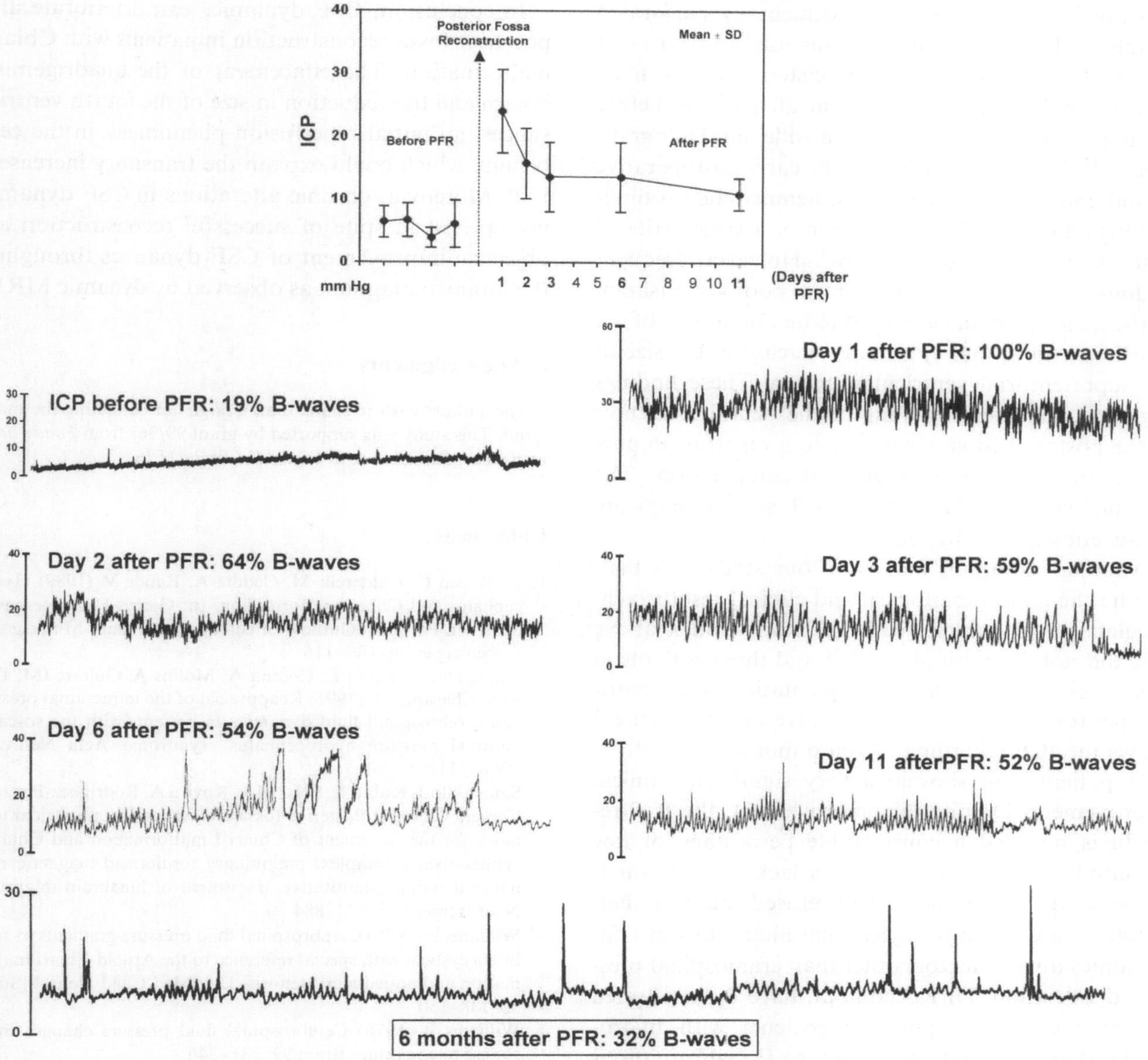

Fig. 2. Samples of ICP recordings obtained in a 58-year-old patient in whom ICP monitoring was performed twice: when posterior fossa reconstruction (*PFR*) was performed and again 6 months later. After PFR percentage and amplitude of B-waves showed a considerable increase. ICP recordings progressively improved in the following days, but low amplitude B-waves persisted 6 months after surgery. X-axis shows temporal evolution of patient. Days marked in bold = days after PFR in which ICP was monitored

experience a reduction or collapse of the syrinx is an almost constant finding, but ventricular dilation is rarely reduced and the hydrocephalus of some patients is even clinically decompensated after surgery [3]. In addition, patients fairly frequently present transitory headaches in the immediate postoperative period after PFR. In the present study ICP not only did not diminish but even showed a transitory increase after PFR. These findings suggest that the pathogenic alterations in CSF dynamics in patients with Chiari malformation involve other factors apart from obstructive ones.

The increase in ICP observed after PFR in all patients in the present study could be attributed to contamination of the CSF by blood or to other surgical problems. However, PFR is an extra-arachnoidal technique [3] which includes opening of the dura mater and preservation of the arachnoid membrane. In patients in whom the arachnoid was accidentally perforated (Table 1), bipolar coagulation was used to try to seal the small holes. A re-expanded cisterna magna filled with clean CSF was observed in all patients before closing the dura watertight with a wide dural allograft. Control CT scans performed in the early postoperative period confirmed the absence of hemorrhagic complications and showed the formation of a large artificial cisterna magna filled with CSF. However, frequent findings in control CT scans were: a) poor visualisation of the quadrigemina cistern, b) reduction in size of the fourth ventricle, and c) a small increase in the size of the supratentorial ventricular system. These findings suggest a transitory swelling of the neural structures of the posterior fossa secondary to a reperfusion phenomenon after craniovertebral decompression. The patients' clinical symptoms and CT scan findings are consistent with this hypothesis.

Another important finding of our study was that, despite the good radiological and clinical results, ventricular size in patients with an Evans' Index above 0.30 did not diminish after PFR and three patients in this series needed posterior implantation of a ventriculoperitoneal shunt. The illustrative case in Figure 2 shows the ICP recording, taken 6 months after PFR, of a patient who showed a very significant clinical improvement. Despite this improvement, the ICP recordings revealed a considerable percentage of low amplitude B-waves. Because of a lack of symptomatology at that time, the patient refused shunt implantation. These findings suggest that alterations in CSF dynamics involve factors other than craniospinal pressure dissociation. Di Rocco *et al.* have demonstrated defective CSF absorption in patients with hydrocephalus associated with Chiari type II malformations [1]. This additional pathogenic mechanism could also be present in patients with ventricular dilatation associated with Chiari I malformation, and could be responsible for the lack of reduction in ventricular size in our patients. Consequently, in our opinion, the treatment of symptomatic patients with hydrocephalus associated with Chiari I malformation should be first directed towards treating hydrocephalus and always before PFR is performed.

In conclusion, CSF dynamics can deteriorate after posterior fossa reconstruction in patients with Chiari I malformation. The effacement of the quadrigeminal cistern and the reduction in size of the fourth ventricle suggest an initial reperfusion phenomena in the cerebellum, which could explain the transitory increase in ICP. Moreover, chronic alterations in CSF dynamics may persist in spite of successful reconstruction and objective improvement of CSF dynamics throughout the foramen magnum as observed by dynamic MRI.

Acknowledgments

The authors wish to thank Gail Craigie for correcting the manuscript. This study was supported by grant 99/968 from *Fondo de Investigación Sanitaria de la Seguridad Social* (FIS).

References

1. Di Rocco C, Calderelli M, Ceddia A, Rende M (1989) Hydrocephalus and Chiari malformation. In: Gjerris F, Borgesen SE, Sorensen PS, (eds) Outflow of cerebrospinal fluid. Munksgaard, Copenhagen, pp 106–116
2. Sahuquillo J, Rubio E, Codina A, Molins A, Guitart JM, Poca MA, Chasampi A (1991) Reappraisal of the intracranial pressure and cerebrospinal fluid dynamics in patients with the so-called "normal pressure hydrocephalus" syndrome. Acta Neurochir (Wien) 112: 50–61
3. Sahuquillo J, Rubio E, Poca MA, Rovira A, Rodriguez-Baeza A, Cervera C (1994) Posterior fossa reconstruction: a surgical technique for the treatment of Chiari I malformation and Chiari I/ syringomyelia complex: preliminary results and magnetic resonance imaging quantitative assessment of hindbrain migration. Neurosurgery 35: 874–884
4. Williams B (1975) Cerebrospinal fluid pressure-gradients in spina bifida cystica, with special reference to the Arnold-Chiari malformation and aqueductal stenosis. Dev Med Child Neurol [Suppl] 35: 138–150
5. Williams B (1976) Cerebrospinal fluid pressure changes in response to coughing. Brain 99: 331–346
6. Williams B (1980) Cough headache due to craniospinal pressure dissociation. Arch Neurol 37: 226–230
7. Williams B (1981) Simultaneous cerebral and spinal fluid pressure recordings. 2. Cerebrospinal dissociation with lesions at the foramen magnum. Acta Neurochir (Wien) 59: 123–142
8. Williams B (1993) Surgery for hindbrain syringomyelia. In: Symon L, Calliauw L, Cohadon F, *et al* (eds) Advances and technical standards in neurosurgery, Springer, Berlin Heidelberg New York Tokyo, pp 107–164

Correspondence: Dra. M. A. Poca, Ferran Puig 70-72, 1-2, 08023 Barcelona, Spain.

Acta Neurochir (2002) [Suppl] 81: 39–41

The Role of Cerebral Blood Flow and Cerebrovascular Reserve Capacity in the Diagnosis of Chronic Hydrocephalus – a PET-Study on 60 Patients

P. Klinge[1], G. Berding[2], T. Brinker[1], M. Schuhmann[1], E. Weckesser[2], W. H. Knapp[2], and M. Samii[1]

[1] Department of Neurosurgery, Medical School Hannover, Germany
[2] Department of Nuclear Medicine, Medical School Hannover, Germany

Summary

Aim. To investigate the clinical value of cerebral blood flow (CBF) and cerebrovascular reserve capacity (CVR) in the management of chronic hydrocephalus.

Global cortical CBF and CVR in 60 patients (66 ± 12 yrs) with chronic hydrocephalus were investigated before, one week (7 d) and 7 months (7 m) after shunting by 15-O-H_2O PET (Siemens ECAT 951/31) at rest and after application of acetazolamide (1 g). After 7 months, clinical outcome was assessed according to Stein and Langfitt and patients were classified into responder (n = 31) and non-responder (n = 29).

Before Surgery, responder had lower blood flow values compared to non responder (36 ± 8 vs. 41 ± 11 ml/100 ml/min; $p = 0.04$), whereas CVR was not different between outcome groups (33 ± 10 vs. $41 \pm 8\%$; $p > 0.05$). After shunting, CVR in non-responder decreased from $41 \pm 8\%$ to $32 \pm 5\%$ (7 d), whereas in responder significant increases ($p < 0.02$) to $55 \pm 46\%$ (7 d) and $54 \pm 31\%$ (7 m) were observed. Regarding early individual changes in CVR, the majority (12/18; 66%) of non-responder had marked decreases in CVR-levels (< 30%), whereas clinical responder considerably improved in CVR (> 30%) in half of patients (7/14).

Measurement of cerebral blood flow in chronic hydrocephalus might substantially contribute to selection of shunt candidates and neurological sequels may be rather related to early regeneration of the hemodynamic reserve.

Keywords: Hydrocephalus; hemodynamic reserve; PET; outcome.

Introduction

Previous SPECT-studies have already shown that mapping of cerebral blood flow might be helpful in prognostication and selection of shunt candidates [6] however, a definitive diagnostic value has not been found [5].

We used ^{15}O-H_2O-PET as a unique modality for performing quantitative studies in diagnosing ischemic conditions [1] to investigate the value of cerebral blood flow (CBF) and cerebrovascular reserve capacity (CVR) measurement in the management of chronic hydrocephalus patients.

Material and Methods

Measurement of global cortical CBF in 60 patients (66 ± 12 yrs) and CVR in 33 patients (67 ± 12 yrs) presenting with clinical and radiological signs of chronic hydrocephalus were investigated before, one week (7 d) and 7 months (7 m) after shunting. Annihilation photons were registered with a PET scanner (Siemens ECAT 951/31). After a bolus injection of 3.7 GBq ^{15}O-H_2O, multiple sequential periods were recorded (12×5 sec, 4×15 sec, 2×30 sec, 2×60 sec). Radial artery blood samples (1 ml) were taken and cerebral blood flow (CBF) was calculated (ml/100 ml/min) using a one-compartment-model (Kety-Schmidt). Corrections for delay and dispersion of input function have been described by Van den Hoff *et al.* [4]. Regions of interest were corresponding to the vascular territories (ACA, MCA and PCA) of both hemispheres based on the atlas of Talairach and Tournoux [3] on a representative slice at the level of the basal ganglia. Cerebrovascular reserve capacity (CVR) was determined after intravenous application of 1 g acetazolamide (DIAMOX®) over 5 min after a time interval of 15 minutes post injection and was determined as the relative difference in CBF of baseline and during stimulation (percent change). All, except one patient that underwent endoscopic ventriculostomy, were treated with a ventriculoperitoneal shunt-system: PUDENZ-SCHULTE®-medium-pressure (n = 25), CODMAN-HAKIM®-programmable (n = 32) and CODMAN-HAKIM® medium-high-range (n = 2). After 7 months, clinical outcome was assessed according to Stein and Langfitt [2] with scores provided for both, mental and gait disturbances. A decrease in the score sum of at least 3 points was regarded as clinical improvement and patients were classified into responder (n = 31) and non-responder (n = 29). Statistical analysis was performed by ANOVA (Fisher's PLSD) and paired or unpaired Student's t-test.

Results

Individual values of global CBF before surgery were varying (38 ± 12 ml/100 ml/min), whereas global

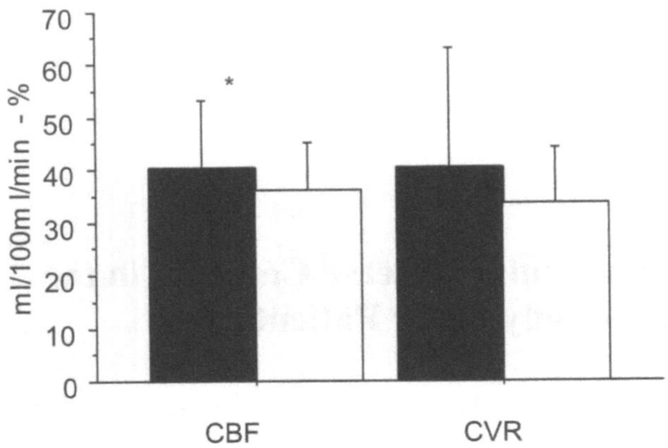

Fig. 1. Preoperative mean values of global CBF (left columns; ml/100 ml/min) and global CVR (right columns; %) in clinical responder (white bars) and non-responder (black bars); asterisks: $p < 0.05$; error bar: 1 SD

CVR was preserved (i.e. >30%) in the majority of patients (26/33).

Before surgery, responder had lower blood flow values than non-responder (36 ± 8 vs. 41 ± 11 ml/100 ml/min; $p = 0.04$) and, although average CVR appeared also lower in responder compared to non-responder (33 ± 10 vs. 41 ± 8%; $p > 0.05$) differences were not significant (Fig. 1).

While after shunting no significant changes in global CBF in both outcome groups were observed, CVR displayed great variations: In non-responder, global CVR decreased after seven days (32 ± 5% vs. 41 ± 8% (pre); $p < 0.05$) and returned to the preoperative level after seven months. In contrast, responder displayed significant increases in CVR already one week after treatment from 33 ± 8 to 58 ± 46% (7 d) and remained at a high level of 57 ± 32% (7 m); $p < 0.02$. Specifically regarding the individual situation of early (7 d) changes in reserve capacity, the majority of non-responder (12/18; 66%) had marked decreases (> 30%) or at least, no significant improvement in CVR levels have occurred (16/18) (Fig. 2). In clinical responder, however, half of patients (7/14) considerably improved in global CVR (> 30%) and compared with non-responder, at least no decreases in global CVR were found with the exception of two patients that had slight reductions of less than 10% (Fisher's exact p-value 0.004) (Fig. 2).

Discussion

Regarding global CBF, clinical responder had significantly lower values than non-responder prior to surgery. After shunt treatment, cerebrovascular reserve capacity displayed most variations and the most relevant result was that early regeneration of the hemodynamic reserve was related to a good prognosis concerning long-term outcome in the individual case. At least no marked deterioration of CVR in clinical improvement should be expected. Thus, early hemodynamic changes may not merely contribute to pathophysiological understanding of neurological sequels to CSF-shunting but, together with measurement of CBF at baseline, may also be helpful in prognostication of long-term outcome and selection of shunt candidates in challenging cases of chronic hydrocephalus syndrome.

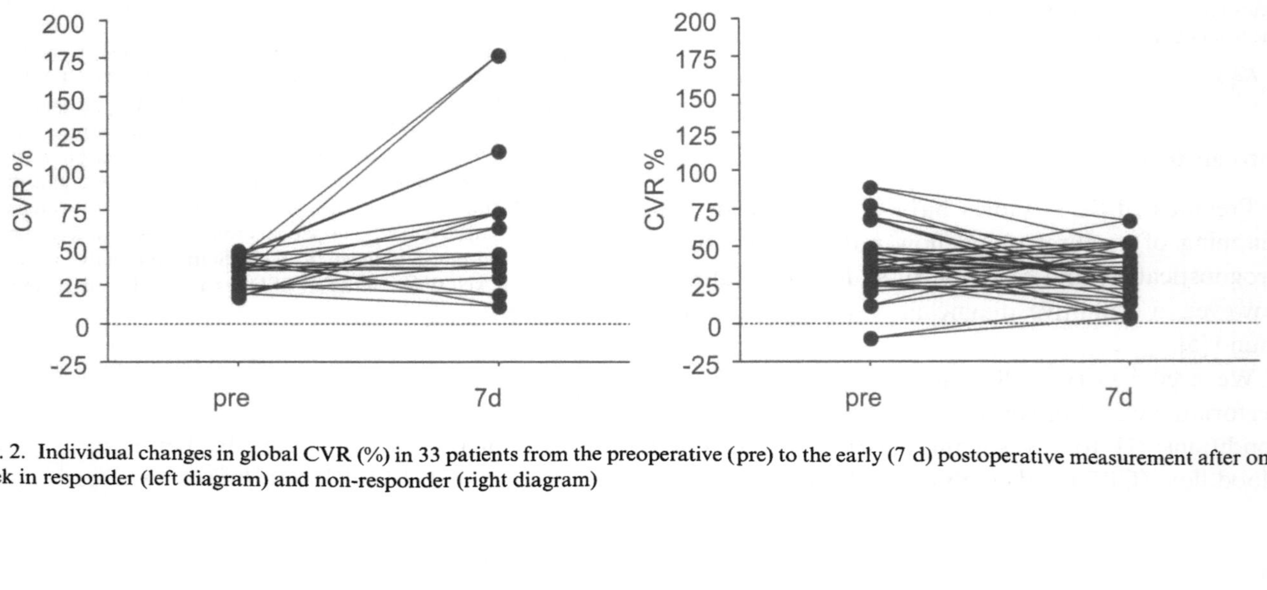

Fig. 2. Individual changes in global CVR (%) in 33 patients from the preoperative (pre) to the early (7 d) postoperative measurement after one week in responder (left diagram) and non-responder (right diagram)

References

1. Broich K, Abass A, Kushner M (1992) Positron Emission Tomography in Cerebrovascular Disorders. Sem Nucl Med 4: 224–232
2. Stein SC, Langfitt TV (1974) Normal pressure hydrocephalus. Predicting results of cerebrospinal fluid shunting. J Neurosurg 41: 463–470
3. Talairach J, Tournoux P (1988) 3-dimensional proportional system; an approach to cerebral imaging. Co-planar stereotaxis atlas of the human brain. Georg Thieme, New York
4. Van den Hoff J, Burchert W, Müller-Schauenburg W *et al* (1993) Accurate local blood flow measurements with dynamic PET: fast determination of input function delay and dispersion by multilinear minimization. J Nucl Med 34: 1770–1777
5. Vanneste JA (1994) Three decades of normal pressure hydrocephalus: are we wiser now? J Neurol Neurosurg Psychiatry 57: 1021–1025
6. Vorstrup S, Christensen J, Gjerris F *et al* (1987) Cerebral blood flow in patients with normal pressure hydrocephalus before and after shunting. J Neurosurg 66: 379–387

Correspondence: Thomas Brinker, M.D. Ph.D., Department of Neurosurgery, Nordstadthospital Hannover, Haltenhoffstraße 41, 30167 Hannover.

Acta Neurochir (2002) [Suppl] 81: 43–45

PET-Studies in Idiopathic Chronic Hydrocephalus Before and after Shunt-Treatment: The Role of Risk Factors for Cerebrovascular Disease (CVD) on Cerebral Hemodynamics

P. Klinge[1], G. Berding[2], T. Brinker[1], M. Schuhmann[1], W. H. Knapp[2], and M. Samii[1]

[1] Department of Neurosurgery, Medical School Hannover, Germany
[2] Department of Nuclear Medicine, Medical School Hannover, Germany

Summary

Aim. To investigate the impact of cerebrovascular risk factors in idiopathic chronic hydrocephalus concerning cerebral hemodynamics and clinical outcome after shunting.

Global cortical cerebral blood flow (CBF) and cerebrovascular reserve capacity (CVR) in 53 patients (67 ± 11 yrs) were determined by 15-0-water-PET studies before and after administration of acetazolamide (1 g) prior (pre), one week (7 d) and seven months (7 m) after shunting. According to the prevalence of vascular risk factors (American subcommittee on reporting standards for cerebrovascular disease) patients were classified into a "low-risk" (n = 27) and "high-risk" (n = 20) group; patients with a history of stroke (n = 6) were separated. After 7 months, clinical outcome was assessed according to Stein and Langfitt.

While CBF in "high-risk" patients prior to surgery was significantly lower in clinical responder compared to non-responder (32 ± 5 vs. 42 ± 15 ml/100 ml/min; $p < 0.05$), CVR was marginal in both outcome groups (< 30%). One week after shunting, CVR in responder of "high-risk" significantly increased (64 ± 30 vs. 31 ± 10% pre; $p < 0.01$). In "low-risk" patients, differences in CVR prior to shunting were found: CVR was lower in clinical responder than in non-responder (36 ± 11 vs. 47 ± 22% pre; $p > 0.05$) and deteriorated in non-responder (29 ± 15% vs. 47 ± 22 pre; $p < 0.02$) one week after shunting.

Different peri-operative characteristics in global CVR regarding clinical response after shunting between both "risk-groups" were observed. Pathophysiological mechanisms upon clinical sequels after shunting in idiopathic hydrocephalus may not be unique.

Keywords: Idiopathic hydrocephalus; cerebrovascular disease; hemodynamics; outcome.

Introduction

The prevalence of risk factors for cerebrovascular disease in idiopathic NPH has been frequently reported [2, 3] and it was even postulated that there were common pathophysiological pathways [3]. However, there is still controversy whether they may be indicative for an unfavourable prognosis after CSF-shunting [2].

We used $^{15}O\text{-}H_2O$-PET together with the administration of acetazolamide for CVR mapping as a powerful modality for performing quantitative studies in cerebrovascular disorders [4] to find out whether the prevalence of vascular risk factors may be related to hemodynamic restoration and neurological sequels after shunt treatment in idiopathic chronic hydrocephalus.

Material and Methods

53 patients (67 ± 11) presenting with clinical and radiological signs (CCT/MRI) of idiopathic chronic hydrocephalus were investigated. Based on the hierarchy of risk factors for cerebrovascular disease (Table 1) patients were classified into a "low-risk" – (n = 27) and "high-risk" – (n = 20) group according to the subcommittee on reporting standards for cerebrovascular disease [1]. Patients with residual symptoms from completed stroke (> 6 months) and/or residual lesions on CCT (n = 6; 7%) were regarded as a separate group. Annihilation photons were registered with a PET scanner (3.7 GBq $^{15}O\text{-}H_2O$; Siemens ECAT 951/31) before (pre), one week (early) and 7 months (late) after shunting. On a representative slice at the level of the basal ganglia global cortical CBF was calculated (ml/100 ml/min) from the time course of tissue and blood activity using a one-compartment-model (Kety-Schmidt). Cerebrovascular reserve capacity was determined after intravenous application of 1 g acetazolamide (DIAMOX®) over 5 min after a time interval of 15 minutes post injection as the relative difference in CBF of baseline and during stimulation (percent change). All patients were treated with a ventriculoperitoneal shunt system (PUDENZ-SCHULTE® medium-pressure-, CODMAN-HAKIM® programmable- or medium-high-(100 ± 10 mmH₂O) valves). After 7 months, clinical outcome was assessed based on the scoring system of Stein and Langfitt [5]. A decrease in the score of at least 3 points was regarded as clinical improvement and patients were classified into responder (n = 27) and non-responder (n = 26). Statistics were based on the paired or unpaired Student's t-test.

Table 1. *Clinical Criteria for "High-Risk" and "Low-Risk" Groups Classification According to the American Subcommittee on Reporting Standards for Cerebrovascular Disease [1]*

"High-risk"	"Low-risk"
Medical treated hypertonus (> 1 drug)	no current clinical hypertonus (easily controlled; no drug)
Cardiac disease (drug-compensated congestive failure/history of myocardial infarction/stable angina and/or dysrhythmia)	cardiac disease (asymptomatic ECG and/or occult MI by ECG)
Juvenile onset diabetes or adult diabetes (insulin controlled)	adult diabetes/no insulin
Tobacco use one pack per day and or abstinence < 1 year	no current tobacco use
Hyperlipidemia (drug controlled)	"mild" hyperlipidemia (no drug)
Vascular occlusive disease and/or carotid stenosis (drug compensated and or surgically treated)	vascular occlusive disease and/or carotid stenosis (asymptomatic, i.e. no drug and no surgical treatment required)
History of TIA's and PRIND's (single episodes; no clinical and radiological residual signs)	no history of TIA's and PRIND's (no CCT-defects)

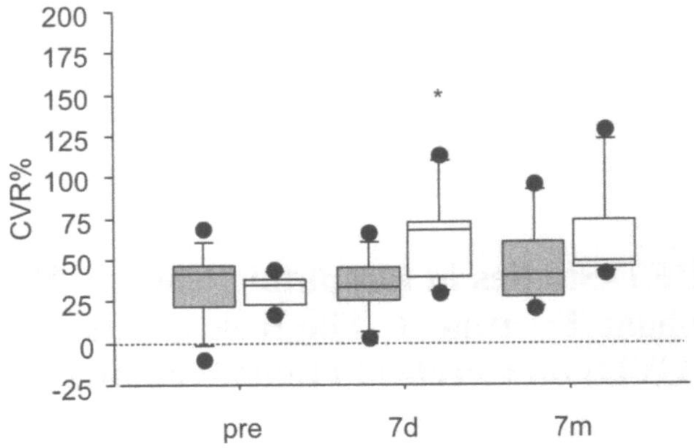

Fig. 1. Box plot of changes of cerebrovascular reserve capacity (CVR%) in responder (white boxes) and non-responder (grey boxes) before (pre), one week (7 d) and seven months (7 m) after shunt treatment in "high-risk" patients; *student's t-; $p < 0.05$

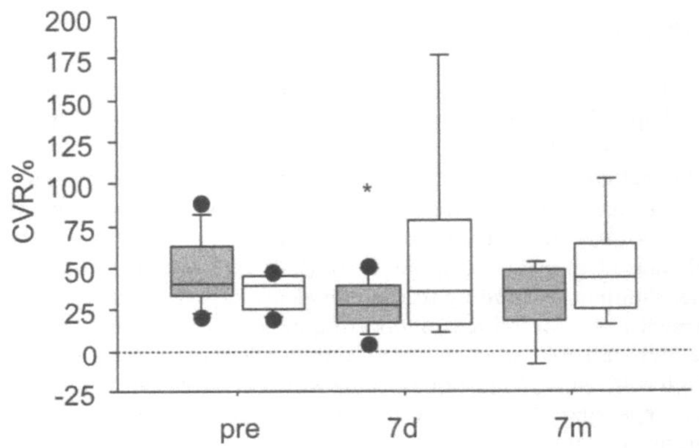

Fig. 2. Box plot of changes of cerebrovascular reserve capacity (CVR%) in responder (white boxes) and non-responder (grey boxes) before (pre), one week (7 d) and seven months (7 m) after shunt treatment in "low-risk"-patients; *student's t-; $p < 0.05$

Results

The distribution of clinical outcome was not different between risk groups; i.e. responder/non-responder: 10/10 in "high-risk" and 16/vs. 11 in "low-risk" ($p = 0.56$; Fisher's exact p). As expected, patients of "high-risk" were significantly older than those of "low-risk" (72 ± 21 vs. 61 ± 13 years; $p < 0.01$), however, age-differences between clinical responder and non-responder within both risk-groups were not found. Regarding global CBF prior to shunting, differences concerning clinical outcome were only observed in "high-risk" patients: responder had significantly lower values than non-responder (32.3 ± 4.6 vs. 42.2 ± 15.5 ml/100 ml/min; $p < 0.05$). After shunting, CBF did not display any variation in patients of "high-" and "low-risk", respectively.

Concerning pre-and postoperative changes in cerebrovascular reserve capacity, risk groups displayed different profiles with respect to shunt response: in "high-risk" patients global CVR before surgery was marginal in both outcome groups (31.5 ± 7.9 in responder and 29.1 ± 30.7% in non-responder), however, in clinical responder CVR significantly increased one week after shunting (64.9 ± 29.5 vs. 31.5 ± 9.7% pre; $p = 0.03$) compared to non responder, that showed no changes in the hemodynamic reserve (Fig. 1). In "low-risk" patients, differences in CVR prior to shunting were found: CVR was lower in clinical responder than in non-responder (36.2 ± 11.3 vs. 46.5 ± 21.8%; $p > 0.05$). While CVR in responder varied one week after shunting, non-responder deteriorated in CVR (29.1 ± 15.2 vs. 46.5 ± 21.8% pre; $p < 0.02$) (Fig. 2). Evaluation of late changes (7 months) did not reveal any differences comparing with the early postoperative measurements. In patients with completed stroke (72 ± 6 years) of at least 6 months history prior to shunt treatment, only one of six individuals definitely improved. Of those, that showed at least an initial response to shunting (5/6), a slight improvement of the hemodynamic reserve seven months after shunting was also observed (61.5 ± 34.4 vs. 42.7 ± 3.8% pre; $p > 0.05$).

Discussion

Most relevant finding in the present study was, that the evidence of risk factors for arteriosclerotic disease in idiopathic hydrocephalus patients was not related to an unfavourable prognosis after treatment, however, with respect to hemodynamical changes, even a dramatic improvement of CVR in "high-risk" patients with shunt response early after treatment was found. The pathophysiological basis might be a restoration from a chronic dilatation of distal resistance vessels with a diminished autoregulatory response as regularly found in cerebrovascular disease [4] in order to counteract the hypotensive situation in the hydrocephalic condition. Thus, disappointing surgical results in a subgroup of patients with cerebrovascular disease [2] may be actually related to a failure in hemodynamical restoration. The observed differences in perioperative CVR profiles further indicate that mechanisms upon clinical symptoms in idiopathic chronic hydrocephalus and its neurological sequels after shunting are not unique.

References

1. Baker JD, Rutherford RB, Bernstein EF *et al* (1988) Suggested standards for reports dealing with cerebrovascular disease. J Vasc Surg 8: 721–729
2. Boon AJW, Tans JT, Delwel EJ *et al* (1999) Dutch Normal-Pressure Hydrocephalus Study: the role of cerebrovascular disease. J Neurosurg 90: 221–226
3. Kraus JK, Regel JP, Vach W *et al* (1996) Vascular risk factors and arteriosclerotic disease in idiopathic normal-pressure hydrocephalus of the elderly. Stroke 27: 24–29
4. Sette G, Baron JC, Mazoyer B, Levasseur M *et al* (1989) Local brain heamodynamics and oxygen metabolism in cerebrovascular disease. Brain 112: 931–951
5. Stein SC, Langfitt TV (1974) Normal pressure hydrocephalus. Predicting results of cerebrospinal fluid shunting. J Neurosurg 41: 463–470

Correspondence: Thomas Brinker, M.D. Ph.D., Department of Neurosurgery, Nordstadthospital Hannover, Haltenhoffstraße 41, 30167 Hannover.

Acta Neurochir (2002) [Suppl] 81: 47–49

Regional Cerebral Blood Flow Profiles of Shunt-Responder in Idiopathic Chronic Hydrocephalus – A 15-O-Water PET-Study

P. Klinge[1], **G. Berding**[2], **T. Brinker**[1], **E. Weckesser**[2], **W. H. Knapp**[2], and **M. Samii**[1]

[1] Department of Neurosurgery, Medical School Hannover, Germany
[2] Department of Nuclear Medicine, Medical School Hannover, Germany

Summary

Aim. To find out if regional characteristics of cerebral blood flow (CBF) and cerebrovascular reserve capacity (CVR) may indicate shunt response in idiopathic chronic hydrocephalus.

11 patients with idiopathic chronic hydrocephalus (65 ± 13 yrs) were followed-up within a year after shunting. Patients were classified into clinical responder (n = 5) and non-responder (n = 6) according to Stein and Langfitt. All patients had measurement of CBF and CVR with dynamic 15-O-water PET (Siemens ECAT 951/31) before and after application of acetazolamide (1 g). Regional differences between outcome groups were analysed with "Statistical Parametric Mapping" (SPM99b; Wellcome Department, London, UK). Group differences were regarded as significant, when uncorrected p-value on voxel and on cluster level were $p < 0.001$ and $p < 0.05$, respectively.

Regarding CBF distribution there was significantly reduced CBF in the frontobasal cortex in responder compared to non-responder (cluster level $p = 0.026$). In CVR, a variety of cortical regions showed significant decreases compared with non-responder: also in frontobasal cortex (on cluster level $p = 0.009$). However, most significant reductions were found in temporodorsal and limbic cortical regions (on cluster level $p < 0.001$).

Preoperative hemodynamics displayed a regional profile of reduced CBF and CVR in patients with shunt improvement. Prospective studies for determining the accuracy of regional blood flow characteristics for outcome prediction are warranted.

Keywords: Hydrocephalus; regional blood flow; PET; outcome.

Introduction

Although assessment of regional blood flow characteristics have been helpful in the pathophysiological understanding of dementia in several degenerating diseases of the brain such as Alzheimer's and Parkinson's disease [3, 6], its clinical value in the diagnosis of chronic hydrocephalus patients is still regarded with suspicion, since metabolic brain mapping with FDG-PET has shown that regional differences in cerebral metabolism were not relevant [2].

We performed quantitative ^{15}O-H_2OPET-studies on cerebral blood flow (CBF) and cerebrovascular reserve capacity (CVR) to find out if regional pattern might be predictive of clinical response after shunting in idiopathic chronic hydrocephalus.

Material and Methods

11 patients with idiopathic chronic hydrocephalus (65 ± 13 yrs) were consecutively followed-up within a year after shunting. All patients were treated with a ventriculoperitoneal shunt system (CODMAN-HAKIM®-programmable or PUDENZ-SCHULTE®-medium-pressure valves). Patients were classified into clinical responder (n = 5) and non-responder (n = 6) according to the classification system of Stein and Langfitt [4] based on the degree of functional disturbances for gait and mental symptoms ranging from 0 (none) to five (no capacity for independent function). Annihilation photons were registered with a PET scanner (Siemens ECAT 951/31) after a bolus injection of 3.7 GBq ^{15}O-H_2O (sequential time periods: 12 × 5 sec, 4 × 15 sec, 2 × 30 sec, 2 × 60 sec). Radial artery blood samples (1 ml) were taken and CBF was calculated (ml/100 ml/min) using a one-compartment-model (Kety-Schmidt). Corrections for delay and dispersion of input function have been described by Van den Hoff *et al.* [5]. Cerebrovascular reserve capacity was determined after application (i.v.) of 1 g acetazolamide (DIAMOX®) over 5 min after a time interval of 15 minutes. Regional differences between outcome groups were analysed with "Statistical Parametric Mapping" (SPM99b; Wellcome Department of Cognitive Neurology, London, UK) using "Compare-populations, two sample t-test". Group differences were regarded as significant when uncorrected p-value on voxel and on cluster level were $p < 0.001$ and $p < 0.05$ (extended threshold at least 6 voxel), respectively.

Table 1. *Selected Regions Displaying Significant Decreases of Cortical Regional CBF (Cerebral Blood Flow) and CVR Cerebrovascular Reserve Capacity) in Shunt-Responder Compared to Non-Responder (Voxel-Level p-Uncorrected < 0.001; Extend Threshold k = 6); CBF and CVR*

Localisation	Brodman area	CBF cluster-level p-uncorrected	CBF voxel-level Z	CVR cluster-level p-corrected	CVR voxel-leve Z
Frontal inferior	47	0.026; k = 204	4.45	0.009; k = 8	4.08
Frontal rostral	8/9	0.142; k = 84	4.42	0.004; k = 6	3.69
Temporal inferior	20/38	0.144, k = 6	4.14	0.021; k = 6	4.39
Temporal dorsal	37	%		0.0001; k = 26	4.07
Cingulum	24/31	0.343; k = 34	3.89	0.001; k = 15	4.23
Parietal	7	%		0.009; k = 8	3.87

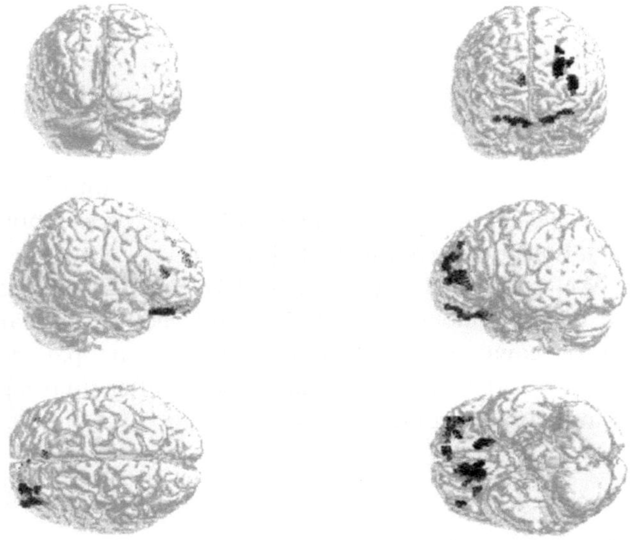

Fig. 1. SPM-projection on MRI surface scans. Shunt responder (see methods) showed significantly lower cerebral blood flow values in areas of the frontal cortex (Brodman area 46 and 47) before surgery

Results

Regarding CBF distribution there was significantly reduced CBF in the frontobasal cortex in responder compared to non-responder (brodman area 46 and 47; cluster level $p = 0.026$); Table 1; Fig. 1.

In CVR, however, a variety of cortical regions displayed significant differences between outcome groups: like in CBF, frontobasal and frontopolar cortex also showed significant reductions when comparing shunt responder with non-responder (brodman area 8, 11, 47; cluster level $p = 0.009$), however, most significan decreases in CVR were observed in temporodorsa (broadman area 37; cluster-level $p < 0.0001$) anc limbic cortical areas (broadman area 31; cluster leve $p < 0.001$); Table 1, Fig. 2.

Regions of increased CBF or CVR in clinical re sponder in comparison to non-responder have no been observed.

Discussion

The present study revealed that CBF reductions spe cifically in frontal cortex were correlated with goo outcome, which is in accordance with previous SPECT studies suggesting a low anterior/posterior ratio i shunt-responsive NPH [1]. In contrast to regiona blood flow, cerebrovascular reserve capacity showed variable pattern of significant reductions in clinica responder compared to non-responder with emphasi on temporal and limbic regions.

These regions, however, were also regarded as path ognomonic to other cerebral degenerating disorder such as dementia of the Alzheimer and Non-Alzheime type [6], a finding, that might be suggestive of a com mon pathway in metabolic and hemodynamica disturbances in dementia of different neurological di eases. Prospective studies for determining the accurac of regional blood flow characteristics for outcome pre diction and differential diagnosis in idiopathic chroni hydrocephalus are warranted.

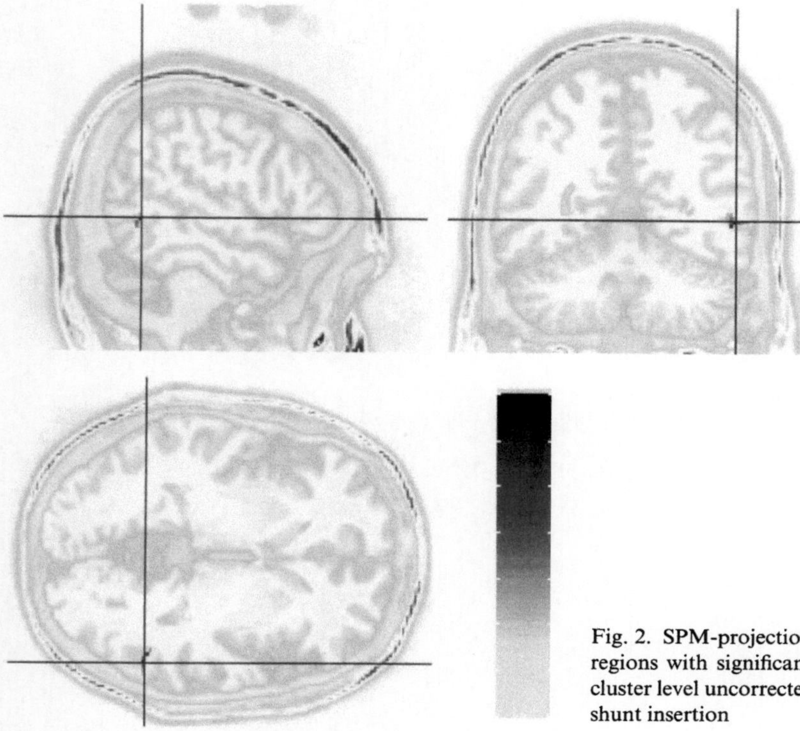

Fig. 2. SPM-projection on axial, coronal and sagittal MRI scans displaying regions with significant reduction of cerebro-vascular reserve capacity (on cluster level uncorrected $p < 0.005$) in patients with clinical response prior to shunt insertion

References

1. Larsson A, Bergh AC, Bilting M *et al* (1994) Regional cerebral blood flow in normal pressure hydrocephalus: diagnostic and prognostic aspects. Eur J Nucl Med 21: 118–123
2. Mazziotta JC, Frackowiak RSJ, Phelps ME (1992) The use of positron emission tomography in the clinical assessment of dementia. Sem Nucl Med 4: 233–246
3. Sawada H, Udaka F, Kameyama M *et al* (1992) SPECT findings in Parkinson's disease associated with dementia. J Neurol Neurosurg Psychiatry 55: 960–963
4. Stein SC, Langfitt TV (1974) Normal pressure hydrocephalus. Predicting results of cerebrospinal fluid shunting. J Neurosurg 41: 463–470
5. Van den Hoff J, Burchert W, Müller-Schauenburg W *et al* (1993) Accurate local blood flow measurements with dynamic PET: fast determination of input function delay and dispersion by multilinear minimisation. J Nucl Med 34: 1770–1777
6. Waldemar G, Bruhn P, Kristensen M *et al* (1994) Heterogeneity of neocortical cerebral blood flow deficits in dementia of the Alzheimer type: a 99 m-Tc-d, 1-HMPAO SPECT study. J Neurol Neurosurg Psychiatry 57: 285–295

Correspondence: Thomas Brinker, M.D., Ph.D., Department of Neurosurgery, Nordstadthospital Hannover, Haltenhoffstraße 41, 30167 Hannover, Germany.

Acta Neurochir (2002) [Suppl] 81: 51–53

Neuropsychological Testing to Improve Surgical Management of Patients with Chronic Hydrocephalus after Shunt Treatment

P. Klinge[1], **N. Rückert**[2], **M. Schuhmann**[1], **L. Dörner**[1], **T. Brinker**[1], and **M. Samii**

[1] Department of Neurosurgery, Medical School and Nordstadt Hospital Hannover, Hannover, Germany
[2] Protestant University of Applied Sciences, Hannover, Germany

Summary

Aim. To find out a practical neuropsychological tool for early and reliable outcome assessment in chronic hydrocephalus.

In 30 patients (65 ± 13 yrs.) 11 neuropsychological tests providing a wide range of psychomotor functions (visual and verbal attention, verbal memory and learning and visuomotor skills) were applied before (pre), one week (early) and 7 months (late) after shunting. After 7 months, clinical outcome was classified according to Stein and Langfitt. Statistics included factor analysis, logistic regression and non-parametric tests.

Visual attention ("Digit-symbol"), verbal recall ("10-words-list") and motor precision ("line-tracing") were the most representative (and practical) tests (orthogonal loads > 0.9). These tests, in contrast to others, revealed significant differences between outcome groups concerning early postoperative changes: responder showed marked improvement in visual attention t-scores (47 ± 8 vs. 41 ± 8 (pre); $p = 0.005$) and motor precision scores (109 ± 26 vs. 149 ± 47 (pre); $p = 0.03$). Non-responder even decreased in verbal recall t-scores early after shunting (35 ± 7 vs. 41 ± 11 (pre); $p = 0.007$). By logistic regression, visual attention was most sensitive indicating shunt-response by early psychometric changes ($p = 0.04$).

Psychomotor deficits in hydrocephalic patients can be represented by a few neuropsychological skills: visual attention, verbal recall and line tracing. Since they showed early post-operative differences regarding long-term response to shunting they may offer a practical and standardised method for reliable follow-up.

Keywords: Hydrocephalus; psychometry; outcome; prognostication.

Introduction

In general, diagnosis and follow-up assessment in chronic hydrocephalus are based on gait- and balance problems that are considered the most important sign in chronic hydrocephalus [1, 2]. Previous studies have shown, that neuropsychological testing improves both, diagnosis and psychomotor follow-up in chronic hydrocephalus patients [2, 3] however most tests were time consuming and generally performed by trained neuropsychologists [6].

The aim of the present study was to create a simple and practical neuropsychological tool for surgical outcome assessment and standardised follow-up in chronic hydrocephalus.

Material and Methods

30 patients (65 ± 13 yrs) with clinical and neuroradiological signs (CCT/MRI) of chronic hydrocephalus (27 idiopathic, 3 aqueduct stenosis) were investigated. The degree of neurological impairment was assessed using the classification system of Stein and Langfitt based on functional grounds for mental and motor disabilities [5]. Additionally, epidural ICP-monitoring (>48 hours) and CSF-dynamic-testing (Rout and PVI) were preformed. Almost all patients were treated by ventriculoperitoneal shunting (CODMAN-MEDOS®-programmable-, n = 21 and medium high-range-valve (100 ± 10 mmH_2O), n = 3; PUDENZ-SCHULTE®-medium-pressure, n = 5) except one by endoscopic vetriculostomy. General clinical improvement after 7 months (long-term outcome) was classified into responder (n = 15) and non-responder (n = 15) if a decrease in the score assigned to Stein and Langfitt of three or more points had occurred.

11 neuropsychological tests providing a wide range of cognitive and psychomotor functions [4]: Auditory attention ("Digit-span"), verbal memory and learning (LURIA "10-words-list"), visual attention ("Digit-symbol"), visuomotor tracking ("number connection"), motor precision ("line-tracing"), motor velocity ("serial dotting") and evaluation of balance and gait [2] were applied before (pre), one week (early) and 7 months (late) after shunting. Raw data were converted into standard scores: t-scores (mean 50 ± 10) and s-scores (SD −3 to +1), respectively. Tests were grouped into mental and motor tests. Statistical procedures included dimensionality testing by factor analysis (orthogonal loads > 0.9 were regarded as representative), logistic regression and non-parametric tests (Wilcoxon-signed-rank and Mann-Whitney-U).

Results

Visual attention ("Digit-symbol"), early verbal recall ("10-words-list") and motor precision ("line-tracing") were the most representative tests (principle

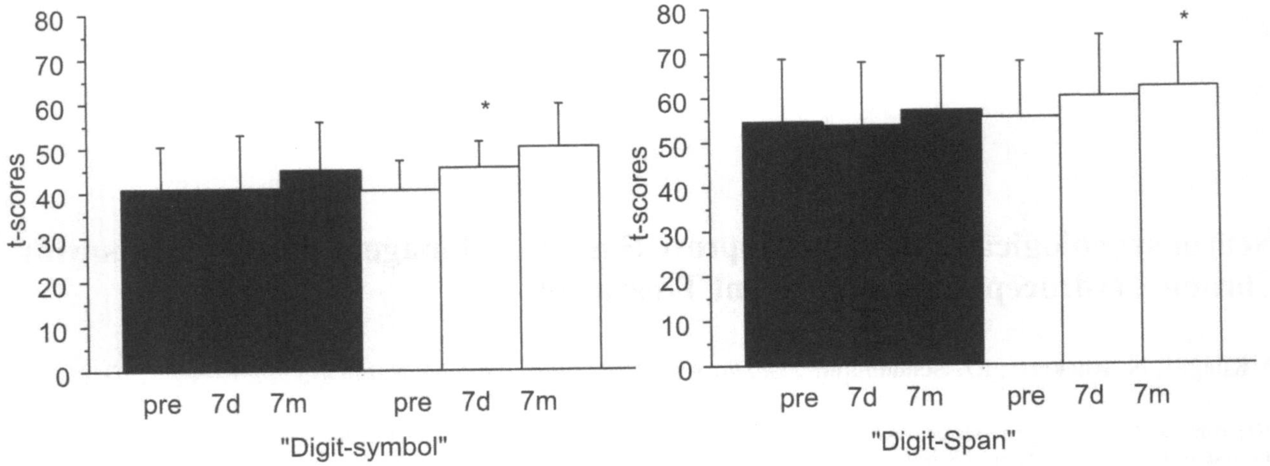

Fig. 1. Visual vs. auditory attention. Mean t-scores (error bar: 1SD) of non-responder (black bars) and responder (white bars) before (pre), one week (7 d) and seven months (7 m) after shunting in visual attention ("Digit-symbol") and auditory attention ("Digit-span"); *p < 0.05

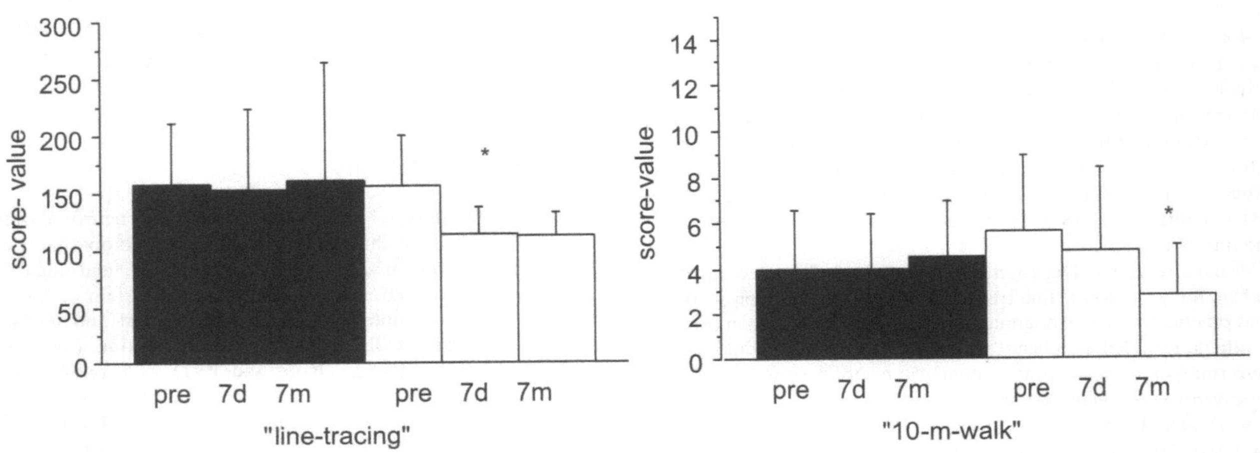

Fig. 2. Motor precision vs. balance. Mean scores (error bar: 1SD) of non-responder (black bars) and responder (white bars) before (pre), one week (7 d) and seven months (7 m) after shunting in motor precision ("line-tracing") and gait profiles ("10-m-walk"); *p < 0.05

component analysis – orthogonal loads > 0.9) among both, mental and motor tests. These tests, in contrast to others, also revealed significant differences between outcome groups concerning early psychometric changes: in mental tests, responder showed marked increases in visual attention (47 ± 8 vs. 41 ± 8 (pre) t-scores; p = 0.004) in comparison to non-responder, that even decreased in verbal recall (35 ± 7 vs. 41 ± 11 (pre) t-scores; p = 0.01) one week after shunting. Auditory attention, however, displayed no early differences between outcome groups, only after seven months improvement in surgical responder was also observed (63 ± 8 vs. 55 ± 12 (pre) t-scores; p = 0.04); Fig. 1.

Regarding motor functions, also in motor precision ("line-tracing") early significant improvement in shunt-responder occurred (109 ± 26 vs. 149 ± 47 (pre) scores; p = 0.003), whereas significant improvement in gait-scores was first found after seven months; Fig. 2. By logistic regression visual attention was the most sensitive test indicating clinical response to shunting by early postoperative psychometric changes (p = 0.04).

Discussion

Psychomotor deficits in hydrocephalic patients can be represented by a few neuropsychological skills: visual attention, verbal recall and motor precision ("line-tracing"). These tests furthermore displayed early postoperative differences regarding response to CSF-shunting, and the "Digit-Symbol", providing a measure of visual (figural) attention, was the most sensitive test indicating late clinical outcome. Surprisingly, also "line tracing", a motor precision task, appeared even more powerful in motor follow-up than classical gait- and balance-evaluation. Since they were all pencil-paper-tests [4], they may not merely offer a more practicable but also a standardised and reliable tool for outcome assessment and improved surgical follow-up management of patients with chronic hydrocephalus after shunt treatment.

References

1. Blomsterwall E, Bilting M, Stephensen H *et al* (1995) Gait abnormality is not the only motor disturbance in normal pressure hydrocephalus. Scand J Rehab Med 27: 205–209
2. Boon AJW, Tans JTJ, Delwel EJ *et al* (1997) Dutch normal pressure hydrocephalus study: baseline characteristics with emphasis on clinical findings. Eur J Neurol 4: 39–47
3. Iddon JL, Pickard JD, Cross JJL *et al* (1999) Specific patterns of cognitive impairment in patients with idiopathic normal pressure hydrocephalus and Alzheimer's disease: a pilot study. J Neurol Neurosurg Psychiatry 67: 723–732
4. Lezak MD (1976) Neuropsychological Assessment. University Press. New York, Oxford
5. Stein SC, Langfitt TW (1974) Normal-pressure hydrocephalus. Predicting the results of cerebrospinal fluid shunting. J Neurosurg 41: 463–467
6. Raftopolous C, Deleval J, Chaski, C *et al* (1994) Cognitive Recovery in Idiopathic Normal Pressure Hydrocephalus: A Prospective Study. Neurosurgery 35: 397–405

Correspondence: Thomas Brinker, M.D., Ph.D., Department of Neurosurgery, Nordstadthospital Hannover, Haltenhoffstraße 41, 30167 Hannover, Germany.

Acta Neurochir (2002) [Suppl] 81: 55–57

Neuropsychological Sequels to Changes in Global Cerebral Blood Flow and Cerebrovascular Reserve Capacity after Shunt Treatment in Chronic Hydrocephalus – A Quantitative PET-Study

P. Klinge[1], N. Rückert[2], M. Schuhmann[1], G. Berding[3], T. Brinker[1], W.-H. Knapp[3], and M. Samii[1]

[1] Departments of Neurosurgery, Medical School and Nordstadt Hospital Hannover, Hannover, Germany
[2] Protestant University of Applied Sciences, Hannover, Germany
[3] Department of Nuclear Medicine, Medical School Hannover, Hannover, Germany

Summary

Aim. To study relationship of neuropsychological deficits in chronic hydrocephalus before and after shunting with dynamics in cerebral blood flow.

In 27 patients (65 ± 13 yrs) with idiopathic chronic hydrocephalus 11 selected neuropsychological tests, providing a wide range of psychomotor functions, were performed before, one week (early) and 7 months (late) after shunting. Parallel global cortical blood flow (CBF) and cerebrovascular reserve capacity (CVR) were determined by dynamic 15-O-water PET studies (Siemens ECAT 951/31) before and after application of acetazolamide (1 g). Test raw data and changes after treatment were compared with global and regional blood flow values by polynomial regression.

No relationship of test profiles with hemodynamics before surgery was found. After one week, improvement of gait was related to an increase in cerebrovascular reserve capacity ($p = 0.05$). After 7 months changes in mental tests were related to changes in hemodynamics: again increases in CVR were significantly related to improvements in visual attention and verbal memory ($p < 0.01$).

Early improvement of hemodynamic reserve was related to improvement in gait, whereas mental improvement was particularly related to increases in global CVR at later periods after shunting. These results indicate that neurological sequels in idiopathic chronic hydrocephalus after shunting may actually depend on consecutive improvement of cerebral hemodynamics.

Keywords: Hydrocephalus; psychometry; cerebral hemodynamics; follow-up.

Introduction

Both experimental and clinical findings have indicated that neurological impairment in chronic hydrocephalus may be related to disturbances in cerebral blood flow [2, 3]. Also, clinical findings showed that in shunt-responsive hydrocephalus increases in global and regional cerebral blood flow have occurred [7].

Using a variety of common neuropsychological tests, providing a wide range of psychometric tasks, we wanted to study, whether psychomotor changes after shunt treatment were related to early and late changes in cerebral hemodynamics of chronic hydrocephalus patients.

Material and Methods

27 patients (65 ± 13 yrs) with clinical and radiological presentation of chronic hydrocephalus were investigated. All patients suffered from psychomental deterioration, motor disturbances, whereas incontinence was variable feature. Almost all patients were treated by ventriculoperitoneal shunting (CODMAN-MEDOS®-programmable, CODMAN-MEDOS®-medium-high (100 ± 10 mm H_2O) and PUDENZ-SCHULTE® medium-pressure valves) except one endoscopic ventriculostomy. Cortical cerebral blood flow (CBF) and cerebrovascular reserve capacity (CVR) were determined by dynamic 15-O-water PET studies (Siemens ECAT 951/31) before and after application of acetazolamide (1 g). Global and regional CBF was calculated (ml/100 ml/min) from the time course of tissue and blood activity using a one-compartment-model (Kety-Schmidt) based on the ROI-technique on a representative slice at the level of the basal ganglia. Regions of interest were manually defined corresponding to the territories of the anterior (ACA), medial (MCA) and posterior cerebral artery (PCA) of both hemispheres. Cerebrovascular reserve capacity (CVR) was determined after application (i.v.) of 1 g acetazolamide (DIAMOX®) over 5 min after a time interval of 15 minutes post injection as the relative difference in CBF of baseline and during stimulation (percent change). Measurement was done one week (early) and seven months (late) after shunt insertion and at parallel intervals, 11 neuropsychological tests providing a wide range of cognitive and psychomotor functions [4] were performed: Auditory attention ("Digit-span"); verbal memory and learning ("Luria 10 words-list"); visual attention ("Digit-symbol"), visuomotor tracking ("number connection"), motor precision ("line-tracing") and psychomotor velocity ("serial dotting") and evaluation of balance- and gait-profiles (10-m-

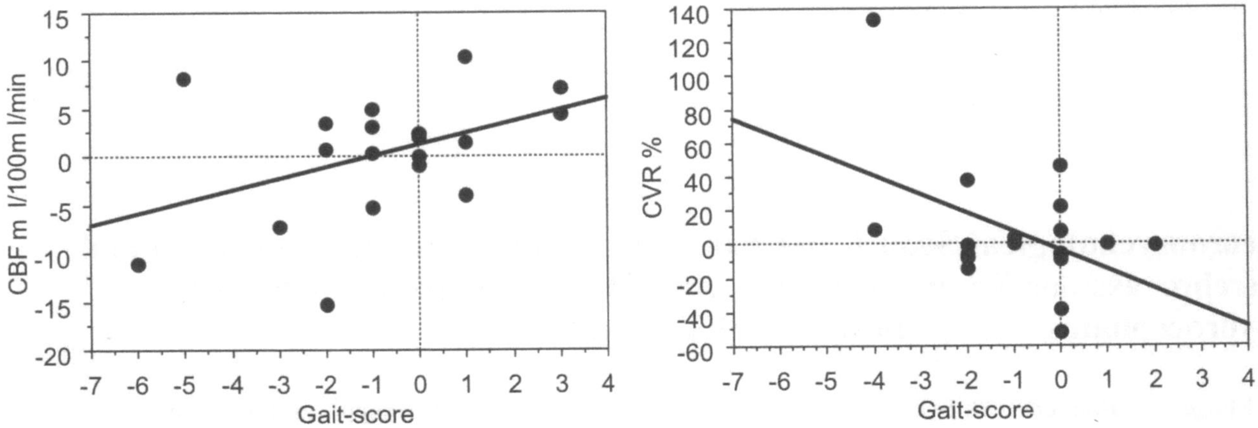

Fig. 1. Regression plot of absolute changes in global cerebral blood flow (ml/100 ml/min; y-axis, left diagram) and cerebrovascular reserve capacity (%; y-axis, right diagram) vs. changes in gait-scores (x-axis) one week after shunt-insertion

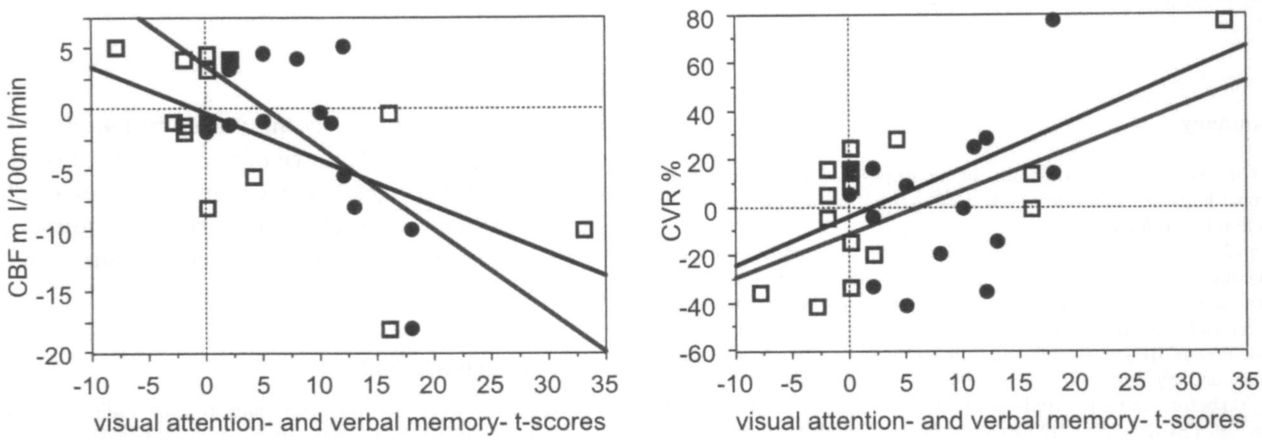

Fig. 2. Regression plots of changes in global cerebral blood flow (left diagram; y-axis) and cerebrovascular reserve capacity (right diagram; y-axis) vs. changes in mental t-scores for visual attention ("Digit-Symbol"; bold line and round spots) and verbal memory ("10 words-list" dashed line and cubic spots) seven months after shunt treatment

walk) [1]. Raw values were converted into standard scores: t-scores (mean 50 ± 10) and s-scores (SD −3 to +1), respectively. Comparison of CBF and CVR before and after surgery with psychometric changes was done by simple linear regression with $p < 0.05$ for linear relationship.

Results

Prior to surgery, no clear relationship of test t-scores with global CBF and CVR as observed. One week after shunt insertion an improvement in gait-profiles, i.e. improvement of step number and walking-time, was related to a decrease in global CBF ($p = 0.05$; $R^2 = 0.175$) and increase in CVR ($p = 0.04$; $R^2 = 0.211$), while cognitive tests displayed no early relationship with hemodynamic changes; Fig. 1.

After 7 months, however, changes in global hemodynamics were related to cognitive improvement: increases in visual attention-("Digit-symbol") and verbal memory-t-scores ("10-words-list") were both found to correlate with decreasing CBF ($R^2 = 0.415$ and $R^2 = 0.383$; $p < 0.01$) and a concomitant increase in global cerebrovascular reserve capacity ($R^2 = 0.20$ and $R^2 = 0.485$; $p = 0.05$ and $p < 0.01$); Fig. 2.

Discussion

The relationship of local blood flow decreases and mental deterioration has already been shown in several degenerative diseases of the brain [5]. In the present study, psychomotor evolution was related to early and late changes in global hemodynamics: a decrease in CBF was observed with a concomitant increase in CVR indicating regeneration of the hemodynamic reserve [6]. The Most relevant finding was that early improvement of hemodynamics was related to motor improvement, whereas cognitive restoration was particularly related to increases in global CVR at later periods after shunting. Thus, the time course of hemodynamic changes mirrors the general evolution of psychomotor improvement after CSF-shunting in chronic hydrocephalus indicating that pathophysiological mechanisms may actually depend on the restoration of cerebrovascular function with consecutive metabolic regeneration.

References

1. Boon AJW, Tans JTJ, Delwel EJ *et al* (1997) Dutch normal pressure hydrocephalus study: baseline characteristics with emphasis on clinical findings. Eur J Neurol 4: 39–47
2. Del Bigio MR, Bruni JE (1988) Changes in periventricular vasculature of rabbit brain following induction of hydrocephalus and after shunting. J Neurosurg 69: 115–120
3. Jellinger K (1976) Neuropathological aspects of dementias resulting from abnormal blood flow and cerebrospinal fluid dynamics. Acta Neurol Belg 76: 83–102
4. Lezak, MD (1976) Neuropsychological Assessment. University Press. New York, Oxford
5. Risberg J, Passant U, Warkentin S *et al* (1993) Regional cerebral blood flow in Frontal lobe Dementia of Non-Alzheimer Type. Dementia 4: 186–187
6. Sette G, Baron JC, Mazoyer B *et al* (1989) Local brain haemodynamics and oxygen metabolism in cerebrovascular disease. Brain 112: 931–951
7. Tamaki N, Kusunoki T, Wakabayashi T *et al* (1984) Cerebral hemodynamics in normal pressure hydrocephalus. J Neurosurg 61: 510–514

Correspondence: Thomas Brinker, M.D. Ph.D., Department of Neurosurgery, Nordstadthospital Hannover, Haltenhoffstraße 41, 30167 Hannover, Germany.

Acta Neurochir (2002) [Suppl] 81: 59–63

Communicating Hydrocephalus: The Biomechanics of Progressive Ventricular Enlargement Revisited

A. Peña[1,2,4], N. G. Harris[1,2,3], M. D. Bolton[4], M. Czosnyka[1,2,3], and J. D. Pickard[1,2,3]

[1] Academic Neurosurgery Unit, University of Cambridge, UK
[2] Wolfson Brain Imaging Centre, University of Cambridge, UK
[3] Cambridge Centre for Brain Repair, University of Cambridge, UK
[4] Department of Engineering, University of Cambridge, UK

Summary

Background. This article investigates the physical mechanisms involved in the chronic ventricular enlargement that accompanies communicating hydrocephalus (CH) – including its normal and low-pressure forms. In particular, it proposes that this phenomenon can be explained by the combined effect of: (*a*) a reversal of interstitial fluid flow in the parenchyma, and (*b*) a reduction in the elastic modulus of the cerebral mantle.

Method. To investigate this hypothesis, these changes have been incorporated into a finite element computer simulation of CH, in which brain tissue is idealized as a sponge-like material. The fluid pressure in the lateral ventricles and the subarachnoid space has been set to 10 mmHg, while the fluid pressure inside the parenchyma has been set to 7.5 mmHg. The elastic moduli of white and gray matter have been set to the reduced values of 1 and 5 kPa, respectively.

Findings. The simulation revealed a substantial ventricular distension (6.5 mm mean outward displacement), which was accompanied by the appearance of stress concentrations in the cerebral mantle.

Interpretation. These results support the notion that a relative reduction in intraparenchymal fluid pressure coupled with low tissue elasticity can produce both a significant ventricular enlargement and periventricular solid stress concentrations.

Keywords: Communicating hydrocephalus; biomechanics; ventricular enlargement.

Introduction

Hydrocephalus presents many paradoxes including the distribution of periventricular tissue damage, association of ventricular dilatation with high blood pressure, specific neuropsychological deficits and lack of correlation in many cases between the size of ventricles, clinical symptoms and the efficacy of a shunt [25]. While it is easy to understand that ventricular distension in non-communicating hydrocephalus (NCH) can be attributed to a transmantle pressure gradient subsequent to obstruction of the aqueduct of Sylvius, it remains an unresolved question why in communicating hydrocephalus (CH) the ventricles continue to dilate despite free communication between ventricles and the subarachnoid space and a normalization of ICP [13].

Several authors have proposed explanations for ventricular enlargement, including: alterations in the viscoelastic properties of brain parenchyma [23, 33], raised mean ICP and intracranial pulse pressure [8], normal tissue stresses [16] and the existence of transmantle pressure gradients [4, 38]. However, none of these studies have been able to convincingly integrate theoretical considerations, drawn usually from continuum mechanics, with experimental and clinical observations.

In this article we propose the hypothesis that the chronic ventricular distension that accompanies CH can be explained by the combined effect of: (*a*) a reversal of interstitial fluid flow into the parenchyma, and (*b*) a reduced tissue elasticity.

Methods

Biomechanics was introduced to the study of hydrocephalus by Hakim *et al.* [14, 15, 16]. In their pioneering work they proposed that brain parenchyma can be regarded as "an open cell sponge made of viscoelastic material". Nagashima *et al.* [22] formalized this concept in terms of the theory of poroelasticity [3], which studies the deformation of porous elastic materials. Since then, the view of brain tissue as a poroelastic material has been used in a number of studies [18, 24, 37]. The deformation mechanics of a poroelastic material is described by Biot's equations. As these equations have no general analytical solution, an approximate or numerical solution needs to be computed using finite element analysis [40]. The anatomical information required to construct the FE mesh for our simulation was obtained from a T2-weighted, horizontally-orientated MR image of a brain from a normal volunteer.

Although the material properties of brain tissue are incompletely defined, experimental evidence suggests that the normal stiffness value of brain tissue is in the range 10 to 100 kPa [12]. In the hydrocephalic brain there is indirect evidence in the form of histological data from experimental models [28–30] and reduced PVI clinical data [6, 10, 36] which suggests that the brain tissue elasticity is reduced. In this study we have assumed isotropic material properties of 1 kPa and 5 kPa for the elastic moduli of white and gray matter, respectively. A Poisson's ratio of 0.30 and an hydraulic conductivity of 10^{-11} m^4 N^{-1} s^{-1} has also been assumed. The fluid pressure in the lateral ventricles and the subarachnoid space has been defined at 10 mmHg, within the normal range of ICP.

While it is generally agreed that there is fluid exchange between the CSF and brain via perivascular spaces, the magnitude and direction of flow remains controversial [26]. Intraventricular dye-injection experiments have demonstrated that the brain parenchyma acts as a CSF sink during hydrocephalus [20] while ventricle perfusion experiments suggest that there is a reversal of transependymal flow of interstitial fluid from CSF to brain [27]. More recently it has been established that perivascular spaces serve as conduits to transport cerebral interstitial fluid (ISF) to both blood and lymph [5]. In order to simulate this behavior, a reduced fluid pressure inside the parenchyma has been defined at 7.5 mmHg. Intra-vascular pressure at different points of the cerebrovascular bed will differ from adjacent interstitial fluid pressure as the result of the interposed compliance of the vascular wall [7]. Therefore in this study interstitial fluid pressure refers to the extracellular space fluid pressure and not to venous pressure.

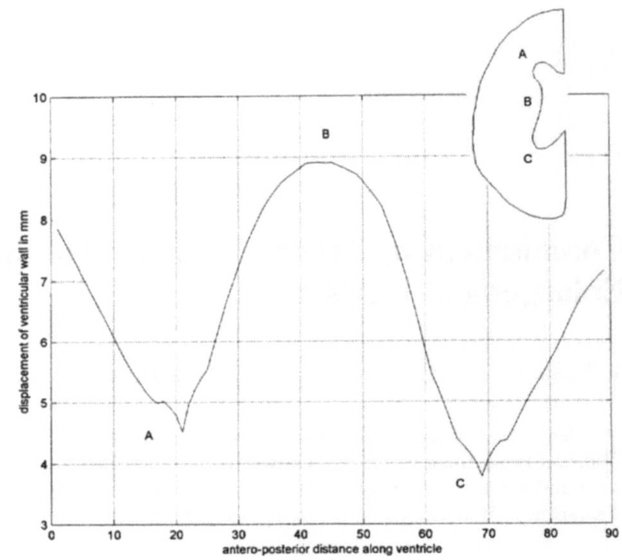

Fig. 1. This graph illustrates the magnitude of the outward displacement of the ventricular surface

Results

In accordance with clinical and experimental observations, the simulation of brain deformation during hydrocephalus, as defined by a sequence of FE meshes demonstrated progressive ventricular expansion. The magnitude of this enlargement at steady-state is illustrated in Fig. 1. The outward movement or displacement of the ventricular wall associated with this distension was heterogeneous along the antero–posterior direction of the ventricle. The maximum displacement occurred in the region of the thalamus with a value of almost 9 mm (Fig. 1, point B). This was followed by displacements of 8 and 9 mm in the anterior and posterior cyngulate gyri, respectively (Fig. 1, points A & C, respectively) and two regions of very small displacements near the anterior and posterior horns (4.5 and 5.0 mm, respectively). The overall mean outward displacement of the ventricles was 6.5 mm.

Discussion

Several studies have emphasized the importance of various physiological mechanisms in the development of chronic ventricular enlargement during CH [4, 8, 16]. Our FE simulation enabled us to investigate the effects of intraparenchymal fluid pressure and tissue elasticity on this process. Our theoretical analysis confirms that realistic alterations in these variables can result in both a significant ventricular enlargement and periventricular solid stress concentrations.

One of the early theories of normal pressure hydrocephalus (NPH) was that of Fishman [9] and Guinane [13] who proposed that it was not the absolute ventricular pressure, but rather the difference between ventricular pressure and the pressure over the cerebral convexity (the so-called transmantle pressure), that was the physiological determinant for ventricular dilatation. However, the existence of such a pressure gradient has been difficult to confirm. For example, Hoff and Barber [17] found an elevated transmantle pressure in three of four hydrocephalic patients and Conner [4] detected a gradient of 0.5 kPa (3.4 cm H_2O) in the cat. However, Shapiro *et al.* [32] failed to measure any pressure gradient. Regardless of these data, the measured values of Conner *et al.* are too small to create any substantial ventricular distention, given that they are is less than 5% of the typical range of the stiffness modulus of brain parenchyma. Hakim *et al.* [16] who also postulated the existence of a transmantle pressure gradient, proposed that one of the laws of mechanics could be applied to the understanding of hydrocephalus: $P = F/A$ where *P*, *F*, and *A* are pressure, force and area, respectively. However, while this reference to Pascal's law enables the computation of changes in pressure, force and area on the *surface* on the brain, it provides no information about the deformation sustained *inside* the parenchyma. Finally, Pang and Altschuser [23] suggested that ventricular enlargement is related to an alteration of the viscoelastic modulus of the brain, secondary to expulsion of extracellular water from the brain parenchyma and to structural changes in brain tissues. However, changes in the mechanical properties of tissue without the presence of a pressure gradient cannot produce ventricular distension.

The theories discussed above provide insufficient explanations for ventricular distension. This is evident if we frame the discussion in terms of the fundamental principle established by Hooke in 1675 on the relationship between deformation and an applied force: $dL/L = (P/A)/E$, where dL is the change in length of the sample, L is the original length of the sample, P is the applied force, A is the cross-sectional area of the sample, and E is a proportionality constant known as Young's modulus [11]. Relative deformation or strain (i.e. dL/L) is directly proportional to an applied stress (i.e. P/A) and inversely proportional to the elasticity modulus (E) of the material. It follows that a substantial deformation of the cerebral mantle may be produced by the *combined* application of an increased pressure gradient together with a reduction in tissue elasticity. The application of this simple principle has

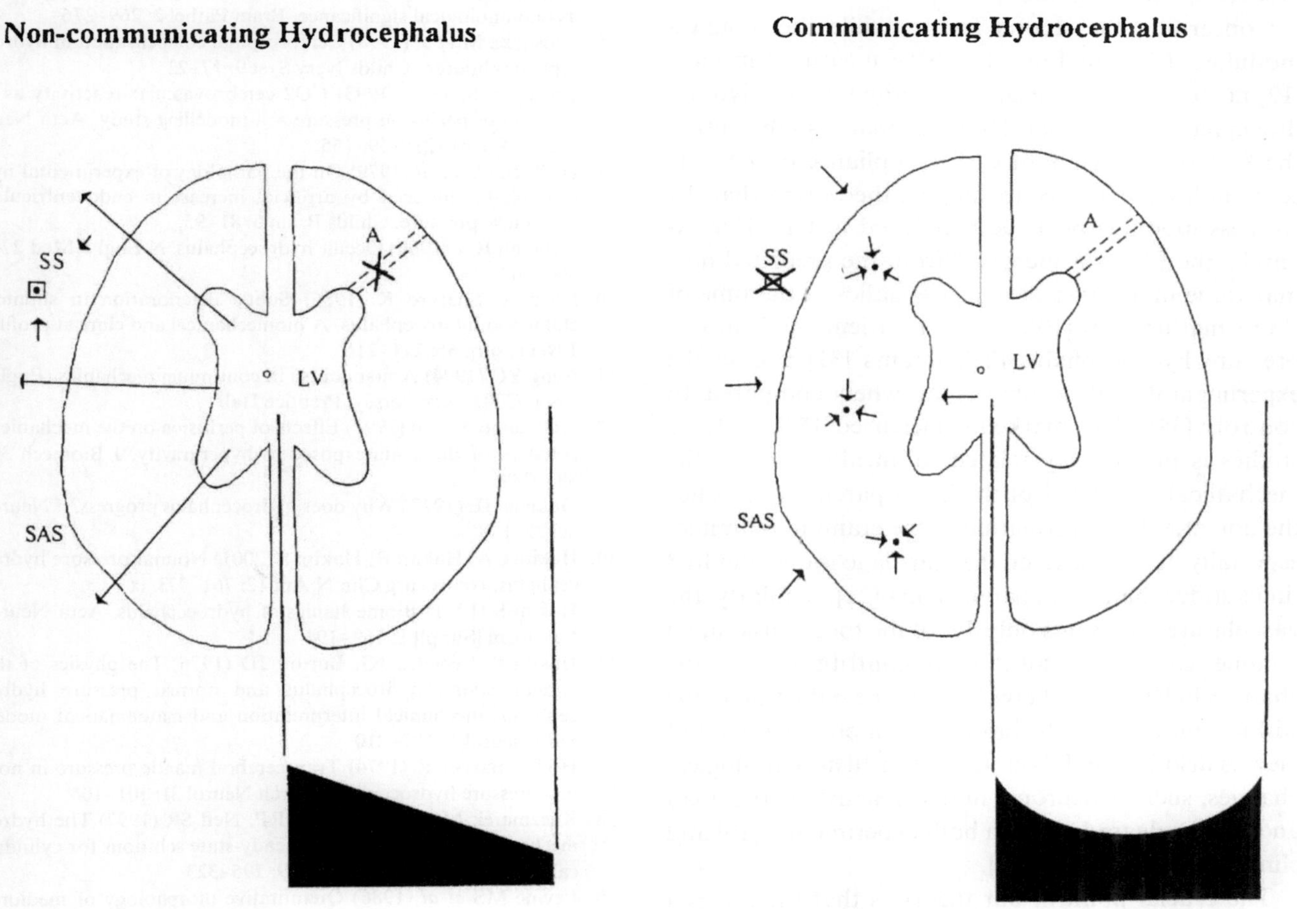

Fig. 2. This diagram illustrates the interaction of the various mechanisms involved in the development of non-communicating (*left*) and communicating (*right*) hydrocephalus. The arrows represent the interstitial CSF flow. The open dot represents sources of CSF. The closed dot represents sinks. The square represents the sagital sinus (*SS*). The cross represents an obstruction to CSF flow. The broken line represents the aqueduct of Sylvius. LV stands for lateral ventricles. SAS for subarachnoid space. In the case of NCH, due to the obstruction of of the aqueduct, a transmantle pressure (shown in black) is established between the LV and the SAS. CSF follows this gradient moving across the parenchyma to be finally absorbed at the SS. In the case of CH, there is no obstruction to the aqueduct but rather at the sagital sinus. An intramantle pressure gradient (shown in black) is produced, as the CSF is absorbed by the parenchyma. In both situations, ventricular distension occurs

led us to formulate the hypothesis that the chronic ventricular distension that accompanies CH can be explained by the combined effects of two factors: (a) a reversal of interstitial fluid flow in the parenchyma with a subsequent absorption of CSF by the tissue, and (b) a low tissue elasticity, brought about by a series of pathological changes.

Concerning the first factor, there is some convincing evidence for transependymal absorption of CSF. Early work on the pathways for CSF absorption postulated an alternative transventricular route [39] and these alternative pathways were demonstrated to be pressure dependent in the experimental hydrocephalic dog [2]. Subsequent studies substantiated the idea of transventricular absorption after demonstrating uptake of label into the parenchyma of various experimental models of hydrocephalus [1, 35].

Concerning the second factor, while the Young's modulus of bovine brain has been measured in vitro [12] no equivalent clinical or experimental in vivo hydrocephalic data exists. However many studies using the PVI as a measure of CSF compliance do provide some indirect evidence to support the notion that the stiffness modulus of tissue is reduced in CH. For example, the PVI was increased from the predicted normal value in a group of hydrocephalics at the time of shunt malfunction [10], in NPH patients [36], in low pressure hydrocephalus [23], infants [31] and in the experimental hydrocephalic cat when compared to controls [34]. The markedly increased PVI in these studies is presumably related to an alteration in the mechanical properties of the brain parenchyma, since the potential for deformation of the cranium is limited, especially in adults, given that cartilage is one hundred times stiffer than brain parenchyma [21]. Similarly, the vasculature represents only 7% of the total intracranial volume so that a substantial contribution to the changes in PVI is unlikely. Finally, the reduction in the stiffness modulus of the brain, from a physical point of view is also inferred from the major histopathological changes, such as neuronal injury, reactive astrocytosis and myelin degradation, in both experimental [19] and clinical hydrocephalus [30].

The crucial point in our theory is that the reversal of CSF transependymal flow implies that the fluid pressure is *smaller* in the parenchyma than in the surrounding CSF spaces. As a consequence of the movement of fluid into the tissue, a pressure gradient is established between the CSF spaces and the cerebral mantle: an *intramantle* pressure gradient.

Acknowledgments

AP is in receipt of a Wellcome Trust Training Fellowship in Mathematical Biology, and NGH of a Merck, Sharp & Dohme Research Fellowship.

References

1. Ahmadi J *et al* (1979) Evidence for transventricular absorption in the hydrocephalic dog. Invest Radiol 14: 432–437
2. Bering EA, Sato O (1963) Hydrocephalus: changes in the formation and absorption of cerebrospinal fluid within th ecerebral ventricles. J Neurosurg 20: 1050–1063
3. Biot MA (1941) General theory of three dimensional consolidation. J Appl Phys 12: 1244–1258
4. Conner ES, Foley L, Black PM (1984) Experimental normal-pressure hydrocephalus is accompanied by increased transmantle pressure. J Neurosurg 61: 322–327
5. Cserr HF, Harling-Berg CJ, Knopf PM (1992) Drainage of brain extracellular fluid into blood and deep cervical lymph and its immunological significance. Brain Pathol 2: 269–276
6. Czosnyka M *et al* (1993) Cerebrospinal compensation in hydrocephalic children. Childs Nerv Syst 9: 17–22
7. Czosnyka M *et al* (1993) CO2 cerebrovascular reactivity as a function of perfusion pressure – a modelling study. Acta Neurochir (Wien) 121: 159–165
8. Di Rocco C *et al* (1979) On the pathology of experimental hydrocephalus induced by artificial increase in endoventricular CSF pulse pressure. Childs Brain 5: 81–95
9. Fishman RA (1966) Occult hydrocephalus. N Engl J Med 274: 466–467
10. Fried A, Shapiro K (1986) Subtle deterioration in shunted childhood hydrocephalus. A biomechanical and clinical profile. J Neurosurg 65: 211–216
11. Fung YC (1994) A first course in continuum mechanics. Englewood Cliffs, New Jersey, Prentice Hall
12. Guillaume A *et al* (1997) Effects of perfusion on the mechanical behavior of the brain-exposed to hypergravity. J Biomech 30: 383–389
13. Guinane JE (1977) Why does hydrocephalus progress? J Neurol Sci 32: 1–8
14. Hakim CA, Hakim R, Hakim S (2001) Normal-pressure hydrocephalus. Neurosurg Clin N Am 12: 761–773, ix
15. Hakim S (1971) Biomechanics of hydrocephalus. Acta Neurol Latinoam [Suppl] 1: 169–194
16. Hakim S, Venegas JG, Burton JD (1976) The physics of the cranial cavity, hydrocephalus and normal pressure hydrocephalus: mechanical interpretation and mathematical model. Surg Neurol 5: 187–210
17. Hoff J, Barber R (1974) Transcerebral mantle pressure in normal pressure hydrocephalus. Arch Neurol 31: 101–105
18. Kaczmarek M, Subramaniam RP, Neff SR (1997) The hydromechanics of hydrocephalus: steady-state solutions for cylindrical geometry. Bull Math Biol 59: 295–323
19. Levine MS *et al* (1986) Quantitative morphology of medium-sized caudate spiny neurons in aged cats. Neurobiol Aging 7: 277–286
20. Miyagami M, Nakamura S, Moriyasu N (1975) [Hydrodynamic of the CSE under experimental occlusion of superior sagittal sinus (author's transl)]. No Shinkei Geka 3: 739–745
21. Mow VC *et al* (1980) Biphasic creep and stress relaxation of articular cartilage in compression? Theory and experiments. J Biomech Eng 102: 73–84

22. Nagashima T *et al* (1987) Biomechanics of hydrocephalus: a new theoretical model. Neurosurgery 21: 898–904
23. Pang D, Altschuler E (1994) Low-pressure hydrocephalic state and viscoelastic alterations in the brain. Neurosurgery 35: 643–655; discussion 655–656
24. Pena A *et al* (1999) Effects of brain ventricular shape on periventricular biomechanics: a finite-element analysis. Neurosurgery 45: 107–116; discussion 116–118
25. Punt CJ (1992) Principles of CSF diversion and alternative treatments. Hydrocephalus. In: Schurr PH, Polkey CE (eds) Oxford University Press, p 139–160
26. Rennels ML *et al* (1985) Evidence for a 'paravascular' fluid circulation in the mammalian central nervous system, provided by the rapid distribution of tracer protein throughout the brain from the subarachnoid space. Brain Res 326: 47–63
27. Rosenberg GA, Saland L, Kyner WT (1983) Pathophysiology of periventricular tissue changes with raised CSF pressure in cats. J Neurosurg 59: 606–611
28. Rubin RC *et al* (1976) Hydrocephalus: III. reconstitution of the cerebral cortical mantle following ventricular shunting. Surg Neurol 5: 179–183
29. Rubin RC *et al* (1976) Hydrocephalus: II. cell number and size, and myelin content of the pre-shunted cerebral cortical mantle. Surg Neurol 5: 115–118
30. Rubin RC *et al* (1976) Hydrocephalus: I. histological and ultrastructural changes in the pre-shunted cortical mantle. Surg Neurol 5: 109–114
31. Shapiro K, Fried A, Marmarou A (1985) Biomechanical and hydrodynamic characterization of the hydrocephalic infant. J Neurosurg 63: 69–75
32. Shapiro K *et al* (1987) Progressive ventricular enlargement in cats in the absence of transmantle pressure gradients. J Neurosurg 67: 88–92
33. Shapiro K, Marmarou A, Shulman K (1982) Abnormal brain biomechanics in the hydrocephalic child. From: concepts in pediatric neurosurgery vol 2. Pediatr Neurosurg 19: 216–222; discussion 223
34. Shapiro K *et al* (1985) Experimental feline hydrocephalus. The role of biomechanical changes in ventricular enlargement in cats. J Neurosurg 63: 82–87
35. Strecker EP *et al* (1973) Cerebrospinal fluid absorption in communicating hydrocephalus. Evaluation of transfer of radioactive albumin from subarachnoid space to plasma. Neurology 23: 854–864
36. Tans JT, Poortvliet DC (1988) Reduction of ventricular size after shunting for normal pressure hydrocephalus related to CSF dynamics before shunting. J Neurol Neurosurg Psychiatry 51: 521–525
37. Tenti G, Drake JM, Sivaloganathan S (2000) Brain biomechanics: mathematical modeling of hydrocephalus. Neurol Res 22: 19–24
38. White DN *et al* (1979) The limitation of pulsatile flow through the acqueduct of Sylvius as a cause of hydrocephalus. J Neurol Sci 42: 11–51
39. Wislocki GB, Putnam TJ (1921) Absorption from the ventricles in experimentally produced internal hydrocephalus. Am J Anatomy 29: 313–316
40. Zienkiewicz OC, Taylor RL (1991) The finite element method. McGraw-Hill

Correspondence: M. Czosnyka, Department of Neurosurgery, Box 167 Addenbrooke's Hospital, Cambridge CB2 2QQ, UK.

Clinical Management of Head Injury

Acta Neurochir (2002) [Suppl] 81: 67–68

Is CPP Therapy Beneficial for all Patients with High ICP?

M. Oertel, D. F. Kelly, J. H. Lee, T. C. Glenn, P. M. Vespa, and N. A. Martin

Division of Neurosurgery, UCLA Medical Center, Los Angeles, CA

Summary

Induced blood pressure elevation has become a popular treatment for intracranial hypertension. However, there remains a concern that in some patients blood pressure elevation will further elevate ICP. This study was conducted to test the hypothesis that increasing MAP decreases ICP. A total of 47 studies were performed on 23 intubated patients with head injury. MAP and SjvO2 were continuously monitored. MAP was raised significantly by 13.8 (5.9) mmHg (t-test; $p < 0.0001$) using phenylephrine infusion. The percent change ICP per mmHg increase in MAP (%ΔICP/mm Hg MAP) was calculated. Pearson correlation coefficient, t-test and logistic regression analysis were used for statistical evaluation. Increasing MAP resulted in a decrease in ICP in 38.3% and in an increase in ICP in 61.7% out of 47 studies. The following characteristics were seen in patients in whom a decrease in ICP was associated with an increase in MAP: High GCS ($r = -0.61$; $p = 0.004$) and low SjvO2 ($\chi^2 = 4.89$; $p = 0.027$). In patients with lower GCS and high SjvO2 an increase in MAP resulted in an increase in ICP. We concluded that in the majority of studies increasing MAP was followed by an increase in ICP. CPP therapy has a selective indication in patients with high GCS, low SjvO2 and increased ICP.

Keywords: CPP Therapy; intracranial hypertension; ICP treatment.

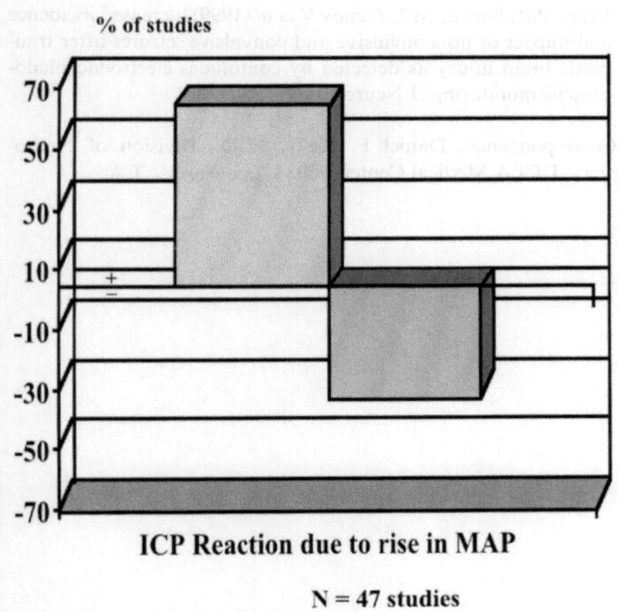

Fig. 1. In the majority of studies (61.7%) an increase in ICP was seen after rising MAP whereas a decrease was rare (38.3% of studies). ■ Increase ICP, ▨ Decrease ICP

Introduction

Over the last decade induced arterial hypertension became popular to decrease elevated intracranial pressure in patients with traumatic brain injury (TBI). This concept is based on the assumption that after TBI the vasoconstrictory cascade is intact. 1. This study was conducted to test the hypothesis that increasing MAP decreases ICP after TBI.

Patients and Methods

A total of 47 studies were performed on 23 intubated patients with head injury (m:f = 4.75:1, age 28.3 ± 11.1 yrs, admission GCS 6 ± 2). All studies were done between day 0–13 postinjury. ICP, MAP and SjvO2 were continuously monitored. MAP was raised significantly by 13.8 ± 5.9 mmHg (t-test; $p < 0.0001$) using phenyl ephrine infusion. The percent change ICP per mmHg increase in MAP (%ΔICP/mm Hg MAP) was calculated. Pearson correlation coefficient, t-test and logistic regression analysis were used for statistical evaluation.

Results

Increasing MAP resulted in a decrease in ICP in 18 (38.3%) and in an increase in ICP in 29 studies (61.7%) out of 47 studies. In the subgroup of studies (21/47) with baseline ICP > 20 mmHg the same ratio was found: ICP increased in 61.9% and decreased in 38.1% of studies. We focused the further investigation on the subgroup of studies with ICP > 20 mm Hg. The following characteristics were seen in patients in whom a decrease in ICP (mean 1.09 ± 1.1%/mm Hg MAP) was associated with an increase in MAP: High GCS ($r = -0.61$; $p = 0.004$) and low SjvO2 ($\chi 2 = 4.89$; $p = 0.027$). In patients with lower GCS and high SjvO2 an increase in MAP resulted in an increase in ICP by 2.4 ± 3.55%/mmHg MAP.

Discussion

Our data shows that after TBI in the majority of cases ICP increases due to increase of MAP. This suggests that the vasoconstrictory cascade is not functioning in the majority of patients.

Over the last decade CPP therapy became a popular treatment for increased ICP. It was shown that outcome after TBI was significantly improved if CPP (= MAP-ICP) was kept over 70 mm Hg [4]. In patients with increased ICP (> 20 mmHg) only an increase in MAP could achieve this goal. The pathophysiological concept is based on the assumption that the vasoconstrictory cascade and pressure autoregulation is intact after TBI. Numerous investigators supported this concept [3, 5, 6]. Indeed, CPP > 70 mmHg seemed to be a critical threshold not only for better outcome but also for a reduction in secondary brain damage, e.g. due to excitatory amino acids or low tissue partial oxigen pressure [6, 7]. However recent investigations have shown that there is no difference in outcome when patients were treated with CPP targeted therapy [2, 3, 6]. Furthermore the hemodynamic response of the brain after TBI seemed to have a phasic time course [1]. Therefore a rigid lower threshold for CPP is questionable for a targeted therapy. Especially in cases with posttraumatic hyperemia an additional increase of MAP could be harmful to the patients.

Our results showed that CPP therapy has an indication in patients with high GCS, low SjvO2. We conclude that in the majority of studies ICP increased by increasing the MAP. We therefore cannot recommend CPP Therapy as a general concept for treating increased ICP.

References

1. Martin NA, Patwardhan RV, Alexander MJ *et al* (1997) Characterization of cerebral hemodynamic phases following severe head trauma: hypoperfusion, hyperemia, and vasospasm. J Neurosurg 87: 9–19
2. Juul N, Morris GF, Marshall SB, Marshall LF (2000) Intracranial hypertension and cerebral perfusion pressure: influence on neurological deterioration and outcome in severe head injury. The Executive Committee of the International Selfotel Trial [see comments]. J Neurosurg 92: 1–6
3. Robertson CS, Valadka AB, Hannay HJ *et al* (1999) Prevention of secondary ischemic insults after severe head injury. Crit Care Med 27: 2086–2095
4. Rosner MJ, Rosner SD, Johnson AH (1995) Cerebral perfusion pressure: management protocol and clinical results [see comments]. J Neurosurg 83: 949–962
5. Stocchetti N, Chieregato A, De Marchi M, Croci M, Benti R, Grimoldi N (1998) High cerebral perfusion pressure improves low values of local brain tissue O2 tension (PtiO2) in focal lesions. Acta Neurochir (Wien) [Suppl] 71: 162–165
6. Unterberg AW, Kiening KL, Härtl R, Bardt T, Sarrafzadeh AS, Lanksch WR (1997) Multimodal monitoring in patients with head injury: evaluation of the effects of treatment on cerebral oxygenation. J Trauma 42: S32–37
7. Vespa PM, Nuwer MR, Nenov V *et al* (1999) Increased incidence and impact of nonconvulsive and convulsive seizures after traumatic brain injury as detected by continuous electroencephalographic monitoring. J Neurosurg 91: 750–760

Correspondence: Daniel F. Kelly, M.D., Division of Neurosurgery, UCLA Medical Center, 90024, Los Angeles, CA.

Acta Neurochir (2002) [Suppl] 81: 69–70

Metabolic Suppressive Therapy as a Treatment for Intracranial Hypertension – Why it Works and when it Fails*

M. Oertel, D. F. Kelly, J. H. Lee, T. C. Glenn, P. M. Vespa, and N. A. Martin

Division of Neurosurgery UCLA Medical Center, Los Angeles

Summary

Thirty years after its first description metabolic suppressive therapy is still controversial in patients with intractable intracranial hypertension. In this study high dose propofol was used to induce metabolic suppression. The effects on intracranial pressure (ICP) and the cerebral metabolic rates for oxygen and glucose ($CMRO_2$ and CMRGlc) are reported. A total of 28 studies were performed on 14 head injured patients. A $Xenon^{133}$ cerebral blood flow (CBF) and a CO_2-reactivity (CO_2R) test were performed prior to induction of metabolic suppression. The following parameters were continuously monitored: EEG, $etCO_2$, $SjvO_2$, ICP, MAP and bilateral MCA flow velocity (V_{MCA}). PCO_2 was obtained before and during propofol-induced EEG burst-suppression in arterial and jugular-venous blood. $CMRO_2$, CMRGlc and Metabolic Ratio ($MR = CMRO_2/CMRGlc$) were calculated. $MR < 0.6$ was defined as relative hyperglycolysis.

ICP decreased by $24.1 \pm 29.0\%$ during burst-suppression. Arterial, jugular-venous and $etCO_2$ also decreased. Multiple regression analysis revealed that CO_2 was the strongest predictor for ICP. Lower baseline ICP and normal CO_2 reactivity were predictors for normal metabolic suppression reactivity. In studies with normal metabolic ratio, ICP reduction was associated with a reduction in $CMRO_2$. In studies with hyperglycolysis, ICP reduction was poor but CMRGlc decreased significantly. In conclusion, intact CO_2R, normal or only moderately elevated ICP and normal MR are predictive of ICP reduction with high dose propofol after head injury.

Keywords: Metabolic suppressive therapy; ICP treatment; hyperglycolysis; traumatic brain injury.

Introduction

Fifteen percent of all head injury patients suffer from intractable intracranial hypertension [3]. In previous reports, the response rate to high dose barbiturate therapy has ranged from approximately 25 to 80% [4]. Even 30 years after Shapiro *et al.* [6] first reported the use of pentobarbital to induce metabolic suppression and hypothermia, this therapy remains controversial mainly because of the potential side effects [7]. This study was conducted to help clarify the pathophysiological mechanism and identify predictors of efficacy of this treatment.

Patients and Methods

A total of 28 TCD-based vasoreactivity studies were performed on 14 intubated TBI patients (m:f = 13:1, age 29 ± 11 years, median GCS on admission 5.5). All studies were done between day 0–13 postinjury. A $Xenon^{133}$ cerebral blood flow (CBF) and a CO_2-reactivity (CO_2R) test were performed prior to induction of metabolic suppression. The following parameters were continuously

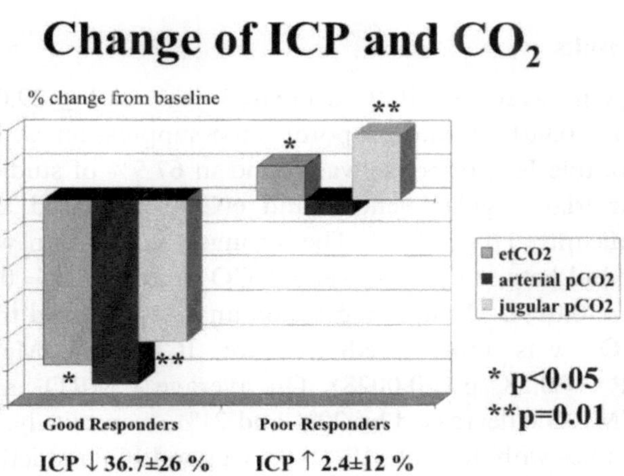

Fig. 1. The total number of studies (n = 28) was divided into favorable (67.9%) and poor (32.1%) responders to metabolic suppressive therapy. On average ICP dereased by 36.7% in the good responding group but increased by 2% in the poor responding group. The ICP decrease was associated with a significant decrease in $etCO_2$ arterial CO_2 and jugular venous CO_2. In comparison to the poor responding group only $\%etCO_2$ and jugular venous $\%CO_2$ were significantly different

* This work was in part supported by a grant from Astra Zeneca Pharmaceuticals.

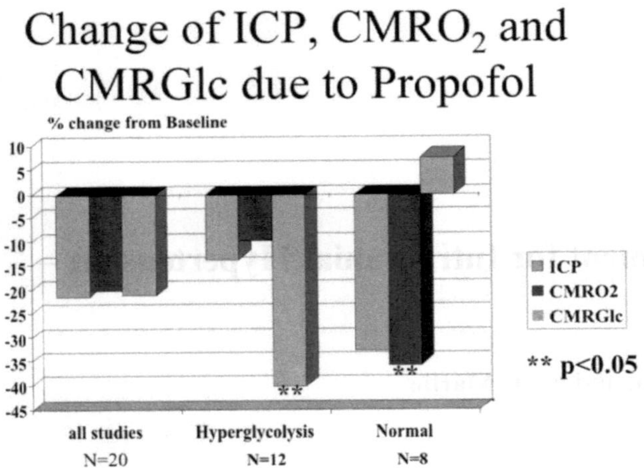

Fig. 2. The change of ICP and its relation to the change of $CMRO_2$ and CMRGlc are shown. A total of 20 studies were included. A good ICP response was associated with a significant decrease in $CMRO_2$. In studies with hyperglycolysis, CMRGlc decreased significantly but ICP showed a poor response

monitored: EEG, $etCO_2$, $SjvO_2$, ICP, MAP and bilateral MCA flow velocity (V_{MCA}). PCO_2 was evaluated before and during propofol-induced EEG burst-suppression (5–10 sec) in arterial and jugular-venous blood. The MAP was kept constant by phenylephrine infusion. Metabolic reactivity (MetR) was calculated (%decrease V_{MCA}-$_{CO_2}$-corrected). $CMRO_2$ and CMRGlc were obtained before and during burst suppression. Metabolic Ratio (MR) was defined by $CMRO_2$\CMRGlc. Hyperglycolysis was defined as MR < 0.6. A favorable ICP response was defined as an ICP < -2 mm Hg. Student's t-test, Pearson regression correlation and multiple regression analysis were performed.

Results

On average, ICP decreased by $24.1 \pm 29.0\%$ ($p < 0.001$) during propofol burst-suppression. A favorable ICP response was found in 67.9% of studies. Arterial, jugular venous and $etCO_2$ decreased significantly ($p < 0.001$). The strongest correlation was found between jugular-venous CO_2 and ICP ($r = 0.6$; $p = 0.011$). Multiple regression analysis revealed that CO_2 was more predictive for ICP than MetR ($R^2 = 0.38$, $p = 0.0028$). On average $CMRO_2$ and CMRGlc decreased by 20% and 21%, respectively. In studies with normal MR (> 0.6) a good ICP reduction was associated with a decrease in $CMRO_2$ ($p = 0.002$). In studies with hyperglycolysis, ICP reduction was poor but a significant decrease in CMRGlc ($p = 0.014$) was observed. A lower baseline ICP ($r = -0.58$; $p < 0.01$) and relatively normal CO_2 reactivity ($r = 0.34$, $p = 0.012$) were predictors for normal MetR.

Discussion

Reduction of ICP with propofol-induced burst suppression correlated most strongly with both systemic and brain CO_2 reduction. Therefore it is postulated that a key mechanism of ICP reduction associated with metabolic suppressive therapy is a decrease in CO_2 production inducing a global "pharmacological hypocapnia". This concept is supported by previous reports from other groups [2, 5]. The association of decrease in $CMRO_2$ and ICP was also reported previously [2]. Hyperglycolysis is seen in the early phase after head injury [1]. Since oxygen metabolism is already decreased in these patients, the pathophysiological meaning of the additional decrease in glucose metabolism is unclear. In conclusion, intact CO_2R appears to be a necessary condition for favorable reduction of ICP due to metabolic suppressive therapy. In addition the absence of hyperglycolysis and normal or only moderately elevated ICP seem to be beneficial for the therapy's success.

References

1. Bergsneider M, Hovda DA, Shalmon E *et al* (1997) Cerebral hyperglycolysis following severe traumatic brain injury in humans: a positron emission tomography study. J Neurosurg 86: 241–251
2. Cormio M, Gopinath SP, Valadka A, Robertson CS (1999) Cerebral hemodynamic effects of pentobarbital coma in head-injured patients. J Neurotrauma 16: 927–936
3. Gudeman SK, Miller JD, Becker DP (1979) Failure of high-dose steroid therapy to influence intracranial pressure in patients with severe head injury. J Neurosurg 51: 301–306
4. Marshall LF, Smith RW, Shapiro HM (1979) The outcome with aggressive treatment in severe head injuries. Part II: acute and chronic barbiturate administration in the management of head injury. J Neurosurg 50: 26–30
5. Nordström CH, Messeter K, Sundbärg G, Schalén W, Werner M, Ryding E (1988) Cerebral blood flow, vasoreactivity, and oxygen consumption during barbiturate therapy in severe traumatic brain lesions. J Neurosurg 68: 424–431
6. Shapiro HM, Wyte SR, Loeser J (1974) Barbiturate-augmented hypothermia for reduction of persistent intracranial hypertension. J Neurosurg 40: 90–100
7. Ward JD, Becker DP, Miller JD *et al* (1985) Failure of prophylactic barbiturate coma in the treatment of severe head injury. J Neurosurg 62: 383–388

Correspondence: Daniel F. Kelly, M.D., Division of Neurosurgery, UCLA Medical Center, 90024, Los Angeles, CA.

Acta Neurochir (2002) [Suppl] 81: 71–72

Can Hyperventilation Improve Cerebral Microcirculation in Patients with High ICP?

M. Oertel, D. F. Kelly, J. H. Lee, T. C. Glenn, P. M. Vespa, and N. A. Martin

Division of Neurosurgery, UCLA Medical Center, Los Angeles, CA

Summary

Gosling's pulsatility index (PI) is generally thought to reflect cerebrovascular resistance. Hyperventilation and increased intracranial pressure (ICP) usually increase PI. In this study, the effect of hyperventilation on PI was assessed in head injured patients with and without elevated ICP. A total of 73 hyperventilation studies were conducted on 20 intubated TBI patients. EtCO2, ICP, MCA flow velocity and MCA PI bilaterally were recorded simultaneously. Hemispheric CO2-Reactivity (hCO2R) was calculated. Only studies with a baseline ICP < 15 or > 30 mm Hg were included for analysis. With hyperventilation pCO2 decreased on average from 33.54.2 to 26.84.8 mmHg. PI increased significantly in patients with baseline ICP < 15 mmHg (11.8%; $p < 0.0001$) but decreased significantly if baseline ICP was >30 mm Hg (12.21%; $p = 0.0013$). High baseline ICP, low initial GCS and impaired hCO2R were associated with the decrease of PI. Hyperventilation unexpectedly reduced PI in patients with high ICP. Because decreased PI suggests decreased CVR, it is postulated that hyperventilation in the setting of raised ICP improves cerebral microcirculation.

Keywords: Transcranial doppler sonography; pusatiliy index; hyperventilation; traumatic brain injury.

Introduction

Gosling's pulsatility index (PI) is known to correlate with cerebrovascular resistance. Elevated ICP and hyperventilation usually increase the PI. During CO2 reactivity studies using continuous bilateral transcranial Doppler monitoring, a phenomenon was observed that has not previously been reported. This report describes the effect of hyperventilation on PI in the setting of elevated ICP.

Patients and Methods

A total of 73 hyperventilation studies were conducted on 20 intubated TBI patients (m:f = 4:1; age 30 ± 11 years, GCS on admission 6 ± 3). All studies were done on postinjury day 0–5. EtCO2, ICP, MCA flow velocity and MCA Pulsatility Index (V_{MCA} systolic – V_{MCA} diastolic/V_{MCA} mean) bilaterally were recorded simultaneously. With hyperventilation pCO2 decreased on average, from 33.5 ± 4.2 to 26.8 ± 4.8 mmHg. Hemispheric CO2-Reactivity (hCO2R) was calculated (change %V_{MCA}/mmHg etCO2). Two study groups were compared: those with baseline ICP < 15 mmHg and those with ICP > 30 mmHg. Logistic regression analysis was used to evaluate the predictors of the these findings.

Results

In a total of 20 studies, baseline ICP was <15 mmHg and in 14 studies baseline ICP was >30 mm Hg. For all studies a statistically significant ($p < 0.005$) decrease was achieved in the following parameters by hyperventilation: ICP, V_{MCA} and etCO2. PI increased significantly in patients with baseline ICP < 15 mmHg (11.8%; $p < 0.0001$) but decreased significantly when baseline ICP was >30 mm Hg (12.21%; $p = 0.0013$). High baseline ICP (likelihood ratio $\chi 2 = 31$; $p < 0.0001$), low initial GCS ($\chi 2 = 15.98$; $p < 0.0001$)

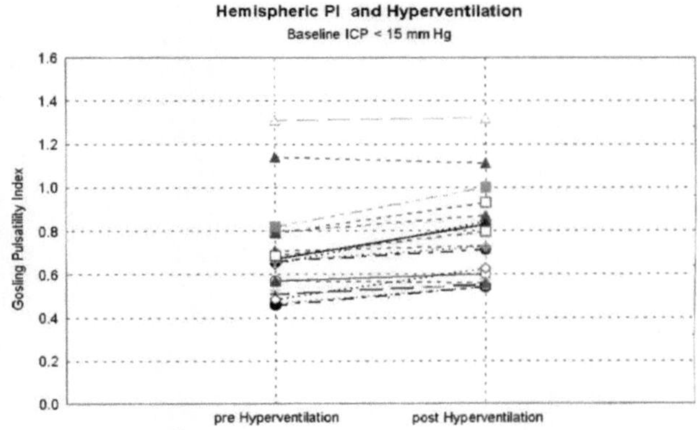

Fig. 1. The pre- and post hyperventilation change of PI is shown in the group of ICP < 15 mm Hg. On average PI increased by 11.8% ($p < 0.0001$). VMCA and ICP decreased by 28.7% and 41.7%, respectively

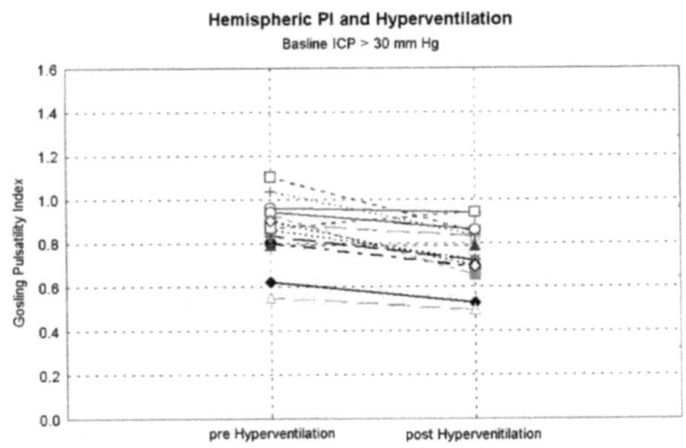

Fig. 2. The pre- and post hyperventilation change of PI in studies with ICP > 30 mm Hg. On average PI decreased by 12.2% ($p = 0.0013$). In this group VMCA and ICP decreased by 13.1% and 37.6%, respectively. The decrease in VMCA was significantly less than in the group ICP < 15 mm Hg ($p = 0.0003$)

and impaired hCO2R ($\chi 2 = 12.044$; $p = 0.0005$) were associated with the decrease of PI.

Discussion

In this study a new pathophysiological phenomenon is described. Hyperventilation decreased Gosling's Pulsatility (PI) index in TBI patients with high ICP, low initial GCS and impaired hCO2R. Transcranial doppler and (PI) [3] are widely used to estimate the cerebral blood flow velocity [1] and cerebrovascular resistance in patients after subarachnoid hemorrhage and TBI [4, 7]. There is general acceptance that increased ICP is associated with increased PI [2, 5]. Hyperventilation is a reliable method to reduce ICP by pial arteriolar vasoconstriction, which is normally reflected by an increase in PI [6]. In this study, in the setting of ICP > 30 mmHg, hyperventilation resulted in a decrease in PI despite a decrease in both mean flow velocity and ICP. However a final answer requires further investigation. At this point, since PI is generally accepted to reflect cerebrovascular resistance, it is postulated that a decrease in PI indicates improved microcirculation as a result of hyperventilation.

References

1. Aaslid R (1992) Cerebral Hemodynamics. In: Newell DW, Aaslid R (eds) Transcranial Doppler. Raven Press, Ltd, New York, pp 49–55
2. Boishardy N, Granry JC, Jacob JP, Houi N, Fournier D, Delhumeau A (1994) Value of transcranial Doppler ultrasonography in the management of severe head injuries. Annales Françaises D'Anesthésie et de Réanimation 13: 172–176
3. Gosling R, King D (1974) Arterial assessment by Doppler shift ultrasound. Proc R Soc Med: 447–449
4. Martin NA, Patwardhan RV, Alexander MJ *et al* (1997) Characterization of cerebral hemodynamic phases following severe head trauma: hypoperfusion, hyperemia, and vasospasm. J Neurosurg 87: 9–19
5. Norelle A, Fischer AQ, Flannery AM (1989) Transcranial Doppler: a noninvasive method to monitor hydrocephalus. J Child Neurol [Suppl] 4: S87–90
6. Ringelstein E, Otis MO (1992) Physiological testing of vasomotor reserve. In: Newell DW, Aaslid R (eds) Transcranial Doppler. Raven Press, Ltd, New York, pp 83–99
7. Steinmeier R, Laumer R, Bondár I, Priem R, Fahlbusch R (1993) Cerebral hemodynamics in subarachnoid hemorrhage evaluated by transcranial Doppler sonography. Part 2. Pulsatility indices: normal reference values and characteristics in subarachnoid hemorrhage. Neurosurgery 33: 10–18, discussion 18–19

Correspondence: Matthias Oertel, M.D., Division of Neurosurgery, UCLA Medical Center, 90024, Los Angeles, CA.

Acta Neurochir (2002) [Suppl] 81: 73–75

Cerebral Perfusion Pressure and Spect in Patients after Craniocerebral Injury with Transtentorial Herniation

M. Smrčka[1], K. Máca[1], V. Juráň[1], M. Vidlák[1], V. Smrčka[1], J. Prášek[2], and R. Gál[3]

[1] Neurosurgical Department, University Hospital Brno, Czech Republic
[2] Nuclear Medicine Department, University Hospital Brno, Czech Republic
[3] Anaesthesiological Department, University Hospital Brno, Czech Republic

Summary

We present a group of 29 consecutive head injured comatose patients with the syndrome of transtentorial herniation. All patients had urgent surgery and then continuous monitoring of ICP, CPP, blood pressure and jugular bulb oximetry was instituted. Two postoperative CT and SPECT examinations were performed in each patient.

15 patients had a normal CPP (>70 mmHg) throughout the postoperative period, 80% of them had a favourable outcome. On the other hand 14 patients had decreased CPP lasting at least one hour and only 36% of them had a favourable outcome ($p < 0,05$). Similar relationships were found comparing GOS in patients with normal and increased ICP (> 20 mmHg) and normal and decreased S_jO_2 (<55%). All but 3 patients had ischaemia on SPECT. Ischaemia improved on the 2nd SPECT in 11 patients and 10 (91%) of them had a favourable outcome. GOS (mean follow up 9 months) is: 12 patients good, 5 moderately disabled, 2 vegetative, 10 died.

We conclude that SPECT is able to disclose even reversible ischaemic changes. In these patients all effort has to be made to keep CPP on normal levels. Improvement in cerebral perfusion is related to a better outcome.

Keywords: Head injury; transtentorial herniation; cerebral perfusion; SPECT.

Introduction

Traumatic transtentorial herniation (temporal conus) due to the acute epidural or subdural haematoma may cause an early death due to the brain stem compression. Even in case of an urgent evacuation of the haematoma, the patient may still die due to the secondary ischaemic brain damage. Transtentorial herniation syndrome consists of a deep coma (usually Glasgow Coma Scale – GCS 3–5), unilateral (or bilateral) mydriasis, hemiparesis and disturbed vital functions [1]. A typical mass effect is usually seen on a CT scan. An early operation may influence the onset of secondary ischaemia, but the most important phase of the treatment of already developed ischaemia is that on the intensive care unit [9]. Complex monitoring of intracranial pressure (ICP), cerebral perfusion pressure (CPP) and jugular bulb oximetry (SjO_2) are important for a rational therapy [2, 4, 5, 8].

Materials and Methods

We have prospectively studied 29 consecutive patients with traumatic transtentorial herniation syndrome, age 16–67, mean age 42,7. 11 patients had epidural, 17 subdural and one patient had intracerebral haematoma. We excluded patients with extensive primary brain damage (gunshot wounds, high velocity injuries) and patients older 70 years of age.

In each patient we performed an urgent operation (evacuation of the haematoma, decompressive craniectomy in six patients), insertion of the parenchymal probe (Codman) for continuous ICP and CPP monitoring (invasive blood pressure from the radial artery) and a jugular bulb probe for a continuous SjO_2 monitoring (Baxter). On the first and fifth postoperative days we performed a CT scan and SPECT to detect perfusion disturbances.

Results

Continuous monitoring showed a pathological ICP (> 20 mmHg for more than one hour) in 10 patients, CPP (< 70 mmHg for more than one hour) in 14 patients, decreased SjO_2 (< 50% for more than one hour) in 12 patients and increased SjO_2 (> 80% for more than one hour) in 6 patients. Patients with pathologies in these monitored parametres had more frequently worse outcome compared to patients with normal monitored values (Fig. 1). The first postoperative CT showed ischaemia in 9 patients, 8 of them died. SPECT, however, showed ischaemia in 26 patients.

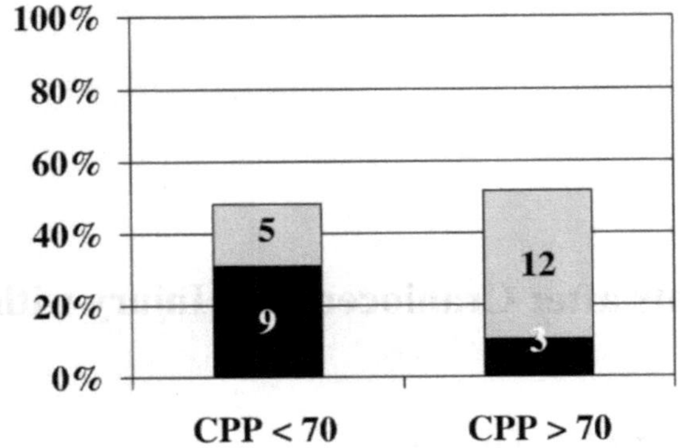

Fig. 1. Cerebral perfusion pressure and GOS. The majority of patients with no pathological CPP values in the posttraumatic course had a favourable outcome (Student's t-test, $p < 0,05$). Similar result was achieved also for other monitored parametres (ICP, SjO_2). □ Favor, ■ Unfavor

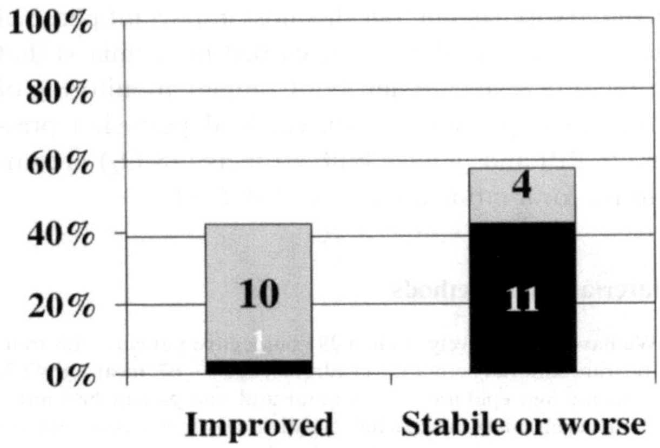

Fig. 2. Ischaemia on the 2nd SPECT and GOS. If the follow up SPECT showed some improvement in perfusion compared to the first SPECT, the result was usually favourable. Three patients with normal perfusion already on the first SPECT are not involved in this graph. □ Favor, ■ Unfavor

Patients with improvement of perfusion on the second SPECT had usually a good outcome (Fig. 2) and they had more commonly normal values of CPP (Fig. 3). In 11 patients we found ischaemia in both SPECT and jugular bulb, in 15 patients only in SPECT and in 2 patients only in the jugular bulb.

The overall results according to Glasgow Outcome Score (mean follow up 9 months) are: good in 12, moderately disabled in 5, vegetative in 2, death in 10.

Discussion

Most of the patients had a disturbed cerebral perfusion and SPECT proved to be very sensitive to detect it. Hypoperfusion was found usually in the brain tissue

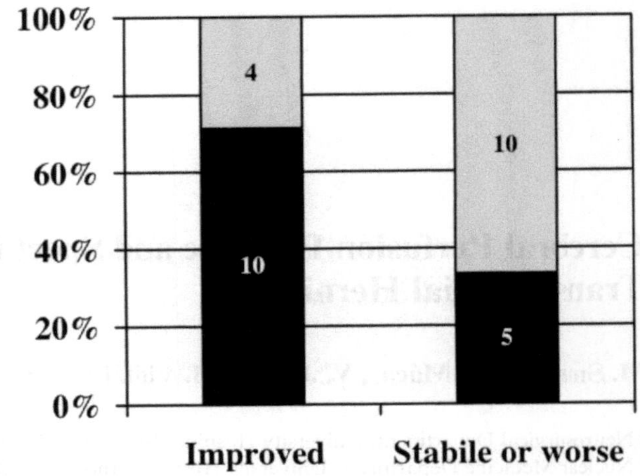

Fig. 3. Ischaemia on SPECT and CPP. Approximately 2/3 of patients with improvement of perfusion on the 2nd SPECT had a normal CPP in the whole posttraumatic course. 2/3 of patients with no improvement in previously disturbed perfusion had CPP < 70 mmHg for at least one hour in the posttraumatic course (Student's t-test, $p < 0,05$). □ CPP below 70, ■ CPP above 70

just close to the previous haematoma, although this was already evacuated. It may be that the pressure of the haematoma caused the collapse of microcirculation in this area. A repeated SPECT showed that in some patients the perfusion disorder may be improved. Most of the patients with improvement on SPECT were patients where CPP could be maintained on the normal levels. Moreover patients who had an improvement of perfusion on the second SPECT had a better outcome than those with worsening or those with a stabile perfusion disorder. 8 out of 9 patients with ischaemia already on the first CT scan on day 1 after the operation died. An early CT visible ischaemia seems to be a bad prognostic sign.

The fact that desaturation periods in the jugular bulb do not correlate well with regional hypoperfusion disclosed by SPECT is not surprising and is known from the literature [4, 8]. The focal changes seen on SPECT could not probably influence the SjO_2 values which reflect the metabolism of the brain in a much more global way.

We do not advertise SPECT to be a routine in management of patients with a very severe head injury. On the other hand its ability to visualize the real ischaemic territories forces us to performe an intensive treatment towards improvement of cerebral perfusion and neuroprotection. The exact location of the tissue which is in the highest risk of secondary brain damage may be used for the placement of the tissue oximetry probe.

References

1. Andrews BT, Pitts LH (1991) Functional recovery after traumatic transtentorial herniation. Neurosurgery 29(2): 227–231
2. Bruzzone P, Dionigi R, Bellinzona G, Imberti R, Stocchetti N (1998) Effect of cerebral perfusion pressure on brain tissue PO2 in patients with severe brain injury. Acta Neurochir (Wien) [Suppl] 71: 111–113
3. Cohen JE, Montero A, Israel ZH (1996) Prognosis and clinical relevance of anisocoria craniotomy latency for epidural hematoma in comatose patients. J Trauma 41(1): 120–122
4. Kiening KL, Unterberg AW, Bardt TF, Schneider GH, Lanksch WR (1996) Monitoring of cerebral oxygenation in patients with severe head injuries: brain tissue PO2 versus jugular vein oxygen saturation. J Neurosurg 85(5): 751–757
5. Miller JI, Cou MW, Capocelli A, Bolognese P, Pan J, Milhorat TH (1998) Continuous intracranial multimodality monitoring comparing local cerebral blood flow, cerebral perfusion pressure, and microvascular resistance. Acta Neurochir (Wien) [Suppl] 71: 82–84
6. Quigley MR, Vidovich D, Cantella D, Wilberger JE, Maroon JC, Diamond D (1997) Defining the limits of survivorship after very severe head injury. J Trauma 42(1): 7–10
7. Sakas DE, Bullock MR, Teasdale GM (1995) One-year outcome following craniotomy for traumatic hematoma in patients with fixed dilated pupils. J Neurosurg 82(6): 961–965
8. Unterberg AW, Kiening KL, Hartl R, Bardt T, Sarrafzadeh AS, Lanksch WR (1997) Multimodal monitoring in patients with head injury: evaluation of the effects of treatment on cerebral oxygenation. J Trauma 42 [Suppl] 5: S32–37
9. Warme PE, Bergstrom R, Persson L (1991) Neurosurgical intensive care improves outcome after severe head injury. Acta Neurochir (Wien) 110(1–2): 57–64
10. Wilberger JE Jr, Harris M, Diamond DL (1991) Acute subdural hematoma: morbidity, mortality and operative timing. J Neurosurg 74(2): 212–218

Correspondence: Ass. Prof. Vladimír Smrčka, M.D., Ph.D., Chairman of the Neurosurgical Department, President of the Czech Neurosurgical Society, University Hospital Brno, Jihlavská 20, 639 00 Brno, Czech Republic.

Correspondence: Martin Smrčka, M.D., Ph.D., Neurochirurgická klinika, FN Brno – Bohunice, Jihlavská 20, 639 00, Brno, Czech Republic.

Acta Neurochir (2002) [Suppl] 81: 77–79

Decompressive Craniectomy Following Traumatic Brain Injury: ICP, CPP and Neurological Outcome

G.-H. Schneider, T. Bardt, W. R. Lanksch, and A. Unterberg

Department of Neurosurgery, Charité, Virchow Med Campus, Humboldt University Berlin, Germany

Summary

Decompressive craniectomy is often the final option in the management of posttraumatic intracranial hypertension. Aim of this study was to investigate the effect of secondary decompression on intracranial pressure (ICP), cerebral perfusion pressure (CPP) and neurological outcome.

62 patients decompressed after severe head injury were included in the retrospective study. Decompression was performed when ICP could not be controlled by non-surgical treatment. Mean age was 36.6 yrs, 77.4% were male. Initial Glasgow Coma Score (GCS) was 6. Outcome was determined 6 months after trauma according to the Glasgow Outcome Scale (GOS) and the functional Barthel-Index (BI).

In the last hour before decompression ICP was 40.5 ± 1.6 mmHg and CPP was 65.3 ± 2.1 mmHg (being maintained, if necesarry, by catecholamines). ICP was significantly reduced to 9.8 ± 1.3 mmHg by surgery and CPP improved to 78.2 ± 2.3 mmHg. 12 hrs following decompression mean ICP rose to 21.6 ± 1.7 mmHg again (CPP: 73.6 ± 1.7 mmHg), but in the following period ICP could be kept below 25 mmHg in the majority of patients. 6 months after trauma 22.5% of the patients had died (except one all these patients were aged more than 50 yrs). 48.4% of patients survived with an unfavourable outcome (GOS 2 + 3), while 29.1% had a favourable outcome (GOS 4 + 5).

Decompressive craniectomy is highly effective to treat otherwise uncontrollable intracranial hypertension and improves CPP. A satisfactory outcome, however, is only achieved under strict consideration of negative predictors (e.g. age).

Keywords: Decompressive craniectomy; intracranial pressure; cerebral perfusion pressure; outcome.

Introduction

Posttraumatic increase of intracranial pressure (ICP) refractory to non-surgical management plays a major role concerning mortality after severe head injury [2]. Decompressive craniectomy as treatment for otherwise uncontrollable intracranial hypertension following brain trauma has experienced a renaissance in the recent years [1, 3, 5, 7]. Despite a fast and safe relief from high ICP, secondary decompressive surgery is still discussed controversely concerning indication and outcome [3], as often survivors of such posttraumatic increases of ICP are left in a vegetative state or stay severely disabled [4]. This study, therefore, was conducted to assess the efficacy of decompressive surgery in treatment of posttraumatic intracranial pressure and cerebral perfusion pressure (CPP) as well as its effect on neurological outcome.

Materials and Methods

Patients Characteristics

From 1994 to 1999 sixty-two severely head injured patients – 48 male and 14 female – with a mean age of 36.6 ± 2.5 yrs ranging from 4 to 74 yrs treated by secondary decompression were included in the retrospective analysis. Glasgow Coma Score (GCS) on admission to the hospital was 6.2 ± 0.5. Monitoring of patients comprised intracranial pressure (n = 56), mean arterial pressure and the resulting cerebral perfusion pressure. Non-surgical management of intracranial pressure consisted of head elevation, sedation, moderate hyperventilation, mannitol and barbiturate coma, which were used according to AANS guidelines. Decompressive craniectomy was performed 82 ± 10 hrs, i.e. 3 to 4 days following trauma. In 51 patients decompression was unilateral, in 11 cases bilateral surgery was necessary.

Indications and Operative Procedure

If non-surgical treatment of intracranial hypertension failed to control ICP, that is if ICP exceeded 40 mmHg in adults or 25 mmHg in children and no otherwise surgically treatable mass lesion was found on CT scan, decompressive craniectomy was indicated. Additionally, decompressive surgery was considered in patients who deteriorated neurologically: worsening of Glasgow Coma Score and/or development of a dilated pupil unresponsive to light. Patients with deleterious primary brain damage with a persisting GCS of 3 and/or bilaterally fixed and dilated pupils were not decompressed.

For the operative procedure a large fronto-temporo-parietal curvilinear skin incision was used and a bone flap with a longitudinal diameter of at least 12 cm was removed either unilaterally or bilaterally either in the same operation or consecutively depending on the lesions and clinical course of patients. Care was taken to carry the removal of bone down to the temporal base to ensure lateral decompression of temporal lobes. The superior sagittal sinus was left covered by bone to avoid complications concerning the sinus. Additionally, a dural enlargement was performed, opening the dura diagonally from front to back with further perpendicular incisions and watertight placement of a large dural graft as to gain sufficient space for the swollen brain. The removed bone flaps were stored frozen under sterile conditions. Mean time to reimplantation in survivors was 3 months.

Six months after trauma outcome was determined according to the Glasgow Outcome Scale (GOS) and the functional Barthel-Index (BI).

Results

Intracranial pressure and cerebral perfusion pressure one hour before as well as one hour and 12 hrs after decompressive surgery are illustrated by boxplots in Fig. 1. Decompressive craniectomy leads to a fast and significant reduction of ICP from 40.5 ± 1.6 to 9.8 ± 1.3 mmHg ($p < 0.01$) in the first hour after surgery. 12 hrs later, however, ICP increased to 21.6 ± 1.7 mmHg again making further non-surgical treatment of ICP – even barbiturates – necessary. In seven patients (11.3%) ICP increased above 30 mmHg despite decompressive surgery and conservative treatment. Decompressive surgery improved cerebral perfusion pressure from 65.3 ± 2.1 to 78.2 ± 2.3 mmHg (73.6 ± 1.7 mmHg 12 hrs after surgery).

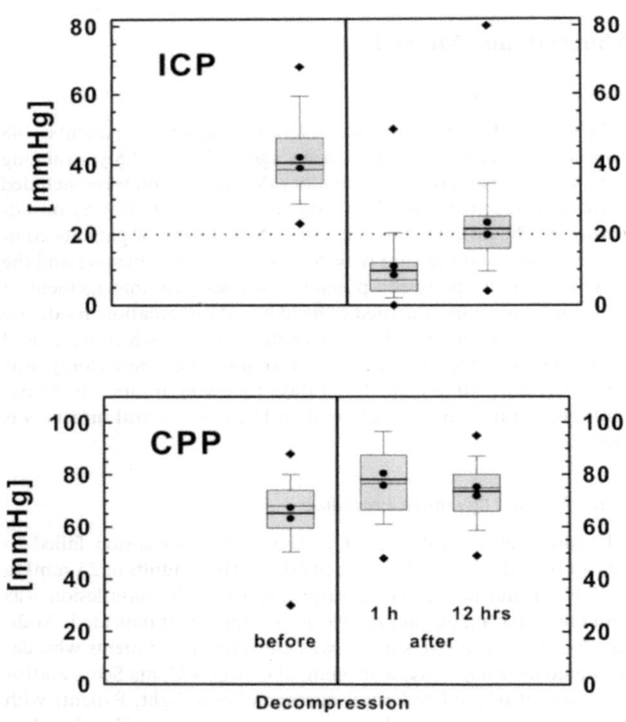

Fig. 1. Boxplots showing reduction of ICP and improval of CPP after decompressive surgery. (The thick black line in the box is mean, the thin black line gives median, dots are ±SEM and diamonds show min and max)

Table 1 demonstrates the distribution of unfavourable (GOS 1–3) vs. favourable outcome (GOS 4 + 5) against different age-groups. Nearly all patients younger than 30 yrs (91.6%) survived the trauma. With the exception of three patients aged more than 50 yrs a favourable recovery was only found in patients younger than 40 yrs (24.2% of all patients). Above the age of 50 (n = 20) the proportion of unfavourable outcomes (85%) was clearly leading. There was no significant correlation of the functional Barthel-Index (activities of daily life, ranging from 0 as worst to 100 points as best). The best functional outcome with 90 or more points in BI were found under the age of 40 yrs.

Table 2 summarizes the six month outcome after surgical decompression for posttraumatic hypertension as assessed by the Glasgow outcome scale. Of a total of 62 patients 14 died. Mortality thus was 22.5%. 14% were left in a vegetative state by the trauma and 34% survived severely disabled. Taken together 70.9% had an unfavourable outcome. 28 patients achieved a GOS of 4 or 5 resulting in a favourable outcome in 29%.

Table 1. *Distribution of Outcome (6 month GOS) vs. Age-Groups Following Decompressive Craniectomy for Uncontrollable Posttraumatic Intracranial Hypertension*

GOS	Unfavourable	Unfavourable	Unfavourable	Favourable	Favourable
	1	2	3	4	5
Age 0–30 yrs	2	6	9	6	1
31–40 yrs	2	–	3	5	3
41–50 yrs	–	2	3	–	–
>50 yrs	10	1	6	3	–

GOS 1 Death, *GOS 2* vegetative state, *GOS 3* severe disability, *GOS 4* moderate disability, *GOS 5* good recovery.

Table 2. *Survey of Outcome 6 Months after Trauma as Assessed by GOS*

GOS	1	2	3	4	5
No. of Patients	14	9	21	14	4
%	22.5	14.5	33.9	22.6	6.5
Mean age	52.3	27.4	34.1	34.9	30

Discussion

Decompressive craniectomy for the treatment of otherwise uncontrollable intracranial hypertension has been known for a long time [6]. It is regarded as a second-tier therapy for posttraumatic treatment-refractory increases of ICP according to the current European and American guidelines for treatment of head injury (European Brain Injury Consortium, 1995 and AANS, 1996) like barbiturate coma, forced hyperventilation and mild hypothermia. Despite being used in a lot of hospitals, secondary decompressive surgery has been controversely discussed concerning indication and outcome, because controlled studies were lacking in the last decades. In 1997 Polin published a case-controlled retrospective analysis by matching surgically decompressed patients with conservatively treated control patients taken from the Traumatic Coma Data Bank and demonstrated that the outcome of operated patients was significantly better compared to control patients and that patients fared better when they were younger than 17 yrs [5]. A recent prospective study of Kleist-Welch Guerra reported the outcome of 57 patients who underwent decompressive craniectomy for over 20 years [3]. They used strict guidelines for indication of decompression. In case of progressive treatment-refractory intracranial hypertension correlated with clinical deterioration only patients to the upper age limit of 50 yrs were craniectomized. During different periods of the study patients aged above 40 yrs or initially even patients older than 30 yrs were not included in the study. Additionally, patients with primary fatal brain damage and bilaterally fixed and dilated pupils were excluded. Mortality was 19% and a favourable outcome (GOS 4 + 5) was seen in 58% of the patients, while severe disability occurred in 11% and 9% were left in a vegetative state 12 months after the trauma [3].

Our data confirm that surgical decompression is a fast and safe measure to control otherwise untreatable intracranial hypertension and to reduce posttraumatic mortality. However, in contrast to the study of Kleist-Welch Guerra the proportion of unfavourable outcome is higher (70.9% GOS 1–3) in our findings. The difference in results may be explained when one looks at the different distribution of age in both studies. The mean age of each outcome group in our study was significantly higher – 19 patients (30.6%) were older than 50 yrs (as compared to an average age of 23 yrs). This underlines that the use of decompressive surgery in patients older than 50 yrs may significantly reduce the proportion of a favourable outcome. In respect to the quality of life of a patient surviving severe head injury and the socioeconomic consequences of the functional outcome it is therefore very important to strictly consider negative predictors like age in order to achieve a satisfactory outcome.

References

1. Gower DJ, Lee KS, McWhorther JM (1988) Role of subtemproal decompression in severe closed head injury. Neurosurgery 23: 417–422
2. Juul N, Morris GF, Marshall SB *et al* (2000) Intracranial hypertension and cerebral perfusion pressure: influence on neurological deterioration and outcome in severe head injury. The Executive Committee of the International Selfotel Trial. J Neurosurg 92: 1–6
3. Kleist-Welch Guerra W, Gaab MR, Dietz H *et al* (1999) Surgical decompression for traumatic brain swelling: indications and results. J Neurosurg 90: 187–196
4. Marshall LF, Gautille T, Klauber MR *et al* (1991) The outcome of severe closed head injury. J Neurosurg 75: S28–S36
5. Polin RS, Shaffrey ME, Bogaev CA *et al* (1997) Decompressive bifrontal craniectomy in the treatment of severe refractory posttraumatic cerebral edema. Neurosurgery 41: 84–94
6. Spiller WG, Frazier CH (1906) Cerebral Decompression. Palliative operations in the treatment of tumors in the brain, based on the observation of fourteen cases. JAMA 47: 679–683
7. Yamakami I, Yamaura A (1993) Effects of decompressive craniectomy on regional cerebral blood flow in severe head trauma patients. Neurol Med Chir 33: 616–620

Correspondence: Dr. Gerd-Helge Schneider, Department of Neurosurgery, Charité, Campus Virchow-Klinikum, Augustenburger Platz 1, D-13353 Berlin, Germany.

Acta Neurochir (2002) [Suppl] 81: 81–82

Evolving Lesions in Traumatic Subarachnoid Hemorrhage: Prospective Study of 110 Patients with Emphasis on the Role of ICP Monitoring

F. Servadei[1], V. Antonelli[1], G. Giuliani[1], E. Fainardi[2], A. Chieregato[3], and L. Targa[3]

[1] Department of Neurosurgery, WHO Neurotrauma Collaborating Center, Ospedale M. Bufalini, Cesena, Italy
[2] Department of Neuroradiology, WHO Neurotrauma Collaborating Center, Ospedale M. Bufalini, Cesena, Italy
[3] Department of Intensive Care Unit, WHO Neurotrauma Collaborating Center, Ospedale M. Bufalini, Cesena, Italy

Summary

We have consecutively studied 110 patients with traumatic subarachnoid hemorrhage (tSAH) on the first Computed Tomography (CT) scan (obtained in each case within 3 hours from injury). The only exclusion criteria were brain death on admission, and severe hypotension due to extracranial injuries. All CTs were reviewed by one of us and the "worst" CT examination was determined. We defined the worst CT examination as that showing the most extensive degree of parenchymal-associated damage. Intracranial pressure was monitored in 25 severely head injured patients. Seventy-four patients (66%) showed an evolution from the initial CT scan (worst CT not corresponding to the admission CT). The outcome was favorable in 53 cases (73%) of patients with evolving lesions and in 32 cases (89%) with non evolving lesion. In the 25 severely head injured patients, Intra-cranial Pressure (ICP) monitoring (in combination with scheduled repeat CT scan) was helpful to identify the timing of the worst parenchymal damage and of surgery in those patients with an initial normal intracranial pressure in spite of an evolving lesion.

Keywords: Traumatic subarachnoid hemorrage; evolving lesions; ICP monitoring; brain contusions.

Introduction

Posttraumatic intracranial lesions may evolve over time. Early (within 3 hours of injury) CT underestimate the ultimate size of parenchymal contusions. Patients with an admission CT showing traumatic subarachnoid hemorrhage (tSAH) are probably at higher risk of evolution [7]. Aim of this study was to identify, in a series of patients with tSAH, those where the "worst" CT scan did not correspond to the admission CT. We also related the timing of the worst CT with the course of ICP monitoring in a sub-population of severely head injured patients.

Material and Methods

From 1/1/97 to 31/1/99 we consecutively admitted 110 patients with tSAH on the first CT scan (obtained in each case within 3 hours from injury). The only exclusion criteria were brain death on admission, and severe hypotension due to extracranial injuries. The patients were prospectively submitted to several CT examinations (within 12 hours from injury and on day two; other CT examinations were scheduled according to clinical and radiological findings). In severely head injured patients an extra CT was obtained in the case of ICP raise (> 25 mmHg) or CPP decrease (< 70 mmHg). All CTs were reviewed by one of us (E.F.) and the "worst" CT examination was determined. We defined the worst CT examination as that showing the most extensive degree of parenchymal-associated damage. Intracranial pressure possibly by intraventricular catheter was monitored in 25 severely head injured patients. Outcome was consistently assessed at least at six months after injury according to the Glasgow Outcome Scale dichotomized (favorable-unfavorable).

Results

Our material consisted of 110 cases with tSAH on admission. There were 79 males (72%), mean age was 48 years (from 12 to 84 years). Admission GCS was 3–8 (severe head injuries) in 31 (28%) patients, 9–13 (moderate h.i.) in 38 (34%), 14–15 (mild h.i.) in 41 (38%). Seventy-four patients (66%) showed an evolution from the initial CT scan (worst CT not corresponding to the admission CT). When we related presence of evolving damage to the GCS scoring, an evolution of parenchymal damage occurred in 23 cases (56%) of mild injuries, in 31 cases (81%) of moderate injuries and in 20 cases (63%) of severe injuries. The outcome was favorable in 53 cases (73%) of patients with evolving lesions and in 32 cases (89%) of patients with non evolving lesions. We then reviewed the relationships between ICP monitoring and the appearance of the worst CT scan. In 10 patients the worst CT corresponded to the first CT scan: ICP monitoring was used as therapeutic guide. In 5 cases (20%) an ICP raise corresponded with the identification of the worst examination. In the remaining 10 cases (40%) the worst CT examination was identified by a scheduled CT scan. ICP monitoring in those cases was helpful for "subsequent" surgical indications. Four of these cases were in fact submitted to surgical procedures according to late ICP increase, which occurred hours/days after the identification of the worst CT.

Discussion

TSAH is a frequent finding after head injury, about 40% of moderate and severe head injury patients in the Traumatic Coma Data Bank [2] and in the European Brain Injury Consortium [6] data collections. Both studies showed significantly worse outcomes in the patients admitted with tSAH. The reasons for these bad outcomes are poorly understood. The presence of vasospasm in tSAH patients, especially if hemodynamically significant [4], has a documented impact on outcome [8]. However, its incidence has been demonstrated to be low in comparison with aneurysmal SAH [3]. We have shown how the vast majority of patients with tSAH on an admission CT will present parenchymal damage evolution on follow-up CT examinations. The presence of tSAH on admission was also found significant in predicting evolving parenchymal damage in a series of 206 patients with acute subdural hematomas [7]. This finding may contribute to the worse prognosis of tSAH patients. In the case of traumatic intracerebral hematomas/contusions, ICP monitoring alone is inadequate to follow hematoma evolution. In a series of 30 patients with an initial low pressure, 5 cases deteriorated because of clinical or CT signs of evolution which were not detected by ICP monitoring [1]. Therefore a combination of ICP recordings and repeat CT scanning seems to be helpful in the detection of lesions that evolve [5], as in our cases. We have also used ICP monitoring as a guide for "subsequent" surgical indications in patients with a normal ICP at the time of the worst anatomical damage, but with a late ICP increase [9].

References

1. Bullock R, Golek J, Blake G (1989) Traumatic intracerebral hematoma-Which patients should undergo surgical evacuation? CT scan features and ICP monitoring as a basis for decision making. Surg Neurol 32: 181–187
2. Eisenberg HM, Gary HE Jr, Aldrich EF *et al* (1990) Initial CT findings in 753 patients with severe head injuries: A report from the NIH traumatic coma data bank. Neurosurgery 5: 566–569
3. Fukuda T, Masamichi H, Hiroshi (1998) Does traumatic subarachnoid hemorrhage caused by diffuse brain injury cause delayed ischemic brain damage? Neurosurgery 43: 1040–1049
4. Lee JH, Martin A, Alsina G, McArtur DL, Zuacha K, Hovda DA, Becker DP (1997) Hemodynamically significant vasospasm and outcome after head injury: a prospective study. J Neurosurg 87: 221–233
5. Marshall LF: Comment to Servadei *et al* (1995) Neurosurgery 37: 907
6. Murray GD, Teasdale GM, Braakman R *et al* (1999) The European brain injury consortium survey of head injuries. Acta Neurochir (Wien) 141: 223–236
7. Servadei F, Nasi MT, Giuliani G, Cremonin AM, Cenni P, Zappi D, Taylor GS (2000) CT prognostic factors in acute subdural haematomas: the value of the worst CT scan. Br J Neurosurg 14: 110–116
8. Taneda M, Kataoka K, Fumiharu A, Asai T, Sakata I (1996) Traumatic subarachnoid hemorrhage as a predictable indicator of delayed ischemic symptoms. J Neurosurg 84: 762–768
9. Unterberg A, Kiening K, Schmiedek P, Lanksch W (1993) Long term observation of ICP pressure after severe head injury. The phenomenon of secondary raise of intracranial pressure. Neurosurgery 32: 17–24

Correspondence: Dr. Franco Servadei, Neurosurgical Unit, WHO Neurotrauma Collaborating Center, Ospedale M. Bufalini, 47023 Cesena, Italy.

Acta Neurochir (2002) [Suppl] 81: 83–84

Effect of Early Induction of Hypothermia on Severe Head Injury

S. Hayashi, S. Inao, M. Takayasu, Y. Kajita, J. Ishiyama, T. Harada, and **J. Yoshida**

Department of Neurosurgery, Nagoya University, Postgraduate School of Medicine, Nagoya, Japan

Summary

Although therapeutic hypothermia for patients with head injury has improved the outcome, the results in the most severe cases (GCS 3–6) have not been satisfactory so far. We induced hypothermia in head injury patients within 3 hours after the trauma, and compared the outcome of the treatment without hypothermia. Fourteen patients with GCS less than 6 were entered into this study (age range 13 to 58, mean 27.0 years). Seven of them were treated by hypothermia and 6 by the conventional method. The patients undergoing hypothermia were cooled to 34 °C within 3 hours after injury, kept at 32–34 °C for 48 hours, and then rewarmed.

The outcome was evaluated at 6 months post-trauma, and the results were compared in the two groups. Therapeutic hypothermia dramatically suppressed brain swelling on CT in 3 of 7 patients. Four patients including these 3 showed a favorable outcome (good or moderate disability) and 3 died in the hypothermia group. In the conventional treatment group, only 1 patient was moderately disabled and 6 exhibited an unfavorable outcome (severely disabled, vegetative, or death). Early induction of hypothermia can improve the outcome in patients with severe head injury by reducing the severe brain swelling.

Keywords: Brain edema; hypothermia; outcome; severe head injury.

Introduction

Many reports stressed the use of therapeutic hypothermia for severely head-injured patients to improve the outcome. However, especially patients with a GCS score of 3 or 4 do not benefit from therapeutic hypothermia [3]. The specific effects of hypothermia include reducing cerebral ischemia, edema, and tissue injury and preserving the blood brain barrier, all of which are thought to be crucial components of many severe head injuries [3]. The concept of the therapeutic window in treatment of cerebral infarction is well established, and the mechanisms of cellular injury after head injury are reported to be very similar to ischemia-induced damage [4]. As with ischemic injury, we thought the early induction of hypothermia could bring more beneficial effects and improve the outcome especially in patients with the most severe head injuries.

Materials and Methods

Fourteen patients with closed head injuries with a score of 3 to 6 on the Glasgow Coma Scale were admitted to our emergency center from April 1998 through March 2000. According to our criteria, 7 patients were excluded for hypotension (less than 90 mmHg of systolic pressure) in three cases, and advanced age (over 60 years) in 4 cases. Seven patients who met our criteria were assigned to the hypothermia group. Seven patients (five males and two females) ranged in age from 19 to 30 years (mean 23.4 years). Their post-resuscitation GCS ranged from 3 to 6, with mean GCS of 4.

In the emergency room, they were initially intubated under deep sedation with thiamylal sodium. We cooled patients to 34 °C using nasogastric lavage with iced water, achieving induction of hypothermia to 34 °C within 3 hours after trauma in all cases. Emergent evacuation of subdural hematoma was performed in three cases and ventriculostomy in four cases. Their temperature was kept at 34 °C during the procedure. Patients had received continuous infusions of a paralytic drug (vecuronium bromide, 4 mg/hour) and intravenous sedation (midazolam, 10 mg/hour) until rewarming was completed. Core temperature was controlled by surface cooling. A consecutive head CT scan was performed every day for one week after admission to evaluate the effect of hypothermia on the intracranial condition. The arterial pressure and PaCO2 were controlled to within the physiological range by adequate treatment. Neither corticosteroids nor barbiturates were used during the therapeutic hypothermia. The desired core temperature of 32 or 34 °C was sustained for approximately 48 hours, patients were then slowly rewarmed (approximately 1 °C/day).

To compare the clinical outcome between the hypothermia group and non-hypothermia group, we retrospectively investigated the patients who were not treated by hypothermia from April 1996 through March 1998, a time when we did not perform therapeutic hypothermia. As a result, 6 patients who met our criteria were assigned to the non-hypothermia group. These 6 patients (four males and two females) ranged in age from 13 to 49 years, with the mean age of 28 years. Their post-resuscitation GCS ranged from 3 to 6, with a mean GCS of 4.8. The neurologic outcome 6 months after injury was scored according to the Glasgow Outcome Scale in both groups.

Results

Four patients showed good recovery and 3 died in the hypothermia group. However, all 7 patients excluded from the hypothermia group died. In the hypothermia group, 5 patients had a GCS score of 4, 3 of them had a good recovery and 2 died. In the non-hypothermia group, only two patients were moderately disabled and four others exhibited an unfavorable outcome (severely disabled, vegetative, or death).

CT taken daily for initial 7 days after introducing hypothermia demonstrated dramatic suppression of brain swelling. Especially in 3 patients who suffered from acute subdural hematoma, brain swelling that would otherwise be fatal in many cases was dramatically suppressed.

Discussion

A patient with an initial GCS of 3 or 4 does not benefit from hypothermia [3]. However, in our preliminary trial of early induction of hypothermia, 3 of 5 patients with an initial GCS score of 4 showed good recovery 6 months after trauma. These 3 patients suffered from acute subdural hematoma with hemispheric swelling reduced by the hypothermia. Cerebral hemispheric swelling was associated with a high mortality rate and uncontrollable intracranial hypertension [1]. It remains controversial that surgical evacuation within 4 hours or external decompression could improve outcome in patients with acute subdural hematoma. High ICP usually is fatal in patients with acute subdural hematoma [5]. Our experience of early induction of hypothermia resulted in good suppression of brain swelling on serial CT scan and showed a relatively good outcome compared to the non-hypothermic group. The mechanism of the beneficial effect on brain swelling is thought to be that the early induction of hypothermia prevents the progression of secondary damage including brain edema or swelling in its early stage [2] [4]. The duration between induction of hypothermia and the onset of trauma may influence the resulting outcome.

References

1. Lobato RD, Sarabia R, Cordobes F *et al* (1988) Posttraumatic cerebral hemispherics welling. J Neurosurg 68: 417–423
2. Marmarou A, Barzo P, Fatouros P *et al* (1997) Traumatic brain swelling in head injured patients: Brain edema of vascular engorgement. Acta Neurochir [suppl] 70: 68–70
3. Marion DW, Penrod LE, Kelsey S *et al* (1997) Treatment of traumatic brain injury with moderate hypothermia. N Engl J Med 336: 540–546
4. Teasdale GM, Graham DI (1998) Craniocerebral trauma: protection and retrieval of the neuronal population after injury. Neurosurgery 43: 723–738
5. Wilberger JE, Harris M, Diamod DL (1991) Acute subdural hematoma: morbidity, mortality, and operative timing. J Neurosurg 74: 212–218

Correspondence: Dr. S. Hayashi, Department of Neurosurgery, Nagoya University, Postgraduate School of Medicine, 65 Tsurumai, Showa, Nagoya 466-8550, Japan.

Acta Neurochir (2002) [Suppl] 81: 85–87

Significance of Temperature Difference Between Cerebral Cortex and Axilla in Patients Under Hypothermia Management*

D.-S. Yoo, D.-S. Kim, C.-K. Park, K.-S. Cho, P.-W. Huh, and **J.-K. Kang**

Department of Neurosurgery, Uijongbu St. Mary's Hospital, The Catholic University of Korea, College of Medicine, Seoul, Korea

Summary

It is believed that the brain temperature is about 1 °C higher than the other peripheral temperature. But the result has been mostly obtained in normothermia patients. The objective of this study was to evaluate whether the brain temperature is still higher than the axillary one in the hypothermia patients.

Sixty-three patients who underwent craniotomy with implantation of the thermal diffusion thermometer were included in this study. Fifty-four patients were in normothermia and nine patients were managed with mild to moderate hypothermia (about 32 °C). The temperature of the cerebral cortex and axilla was measured simultaneously every 2 hours. 1900 paired sample data were collected and analyzed.

The temperature difference between the cerebral cortex and the axilla was 1.04 ± 0.67 °C in normothermia patients and 0.91 ± 0.84 °C in hypothermic patients. The temperature difference has no statistical significance between the two groups (unpaired t-test, $P > 0.05$).

Our results demonstrate that the brain temperature in the patients under hypothermia management appears to be still about 1 °C higher than the axilla throughout the study period almost in the same fashion as in normothermia patients.

Keywords: Temperature difference; brain temperature; axillary temperature; hypothermia.

Introduction

Recent laboratory results have indicated that the ischemic brain is very sensitive to minor variations in temperature. That has created new interest in hypothermia and brain temperature. Optimal use of hypothermia as a therapeutic tool requires a method of monitoring brain temperature accurately [5]. There is, however, very little information available regarding human intracerebral temperature and its relation to body core temperature during the hypothermia management.

This study particularly addresses the question of whether the temperature difference between the brain and axilla can routinely be used for estimating the hypothermia brain temperature.

* This study was supported by grant from of Korea Health 21 R&D Project, Ministry of Health & Welfare, Republic of Korea. (HMP-00-CN-01-0018)

Materials and Methods

Between May 1998 and January 2000, sixty-three patients who underwent craniotomy with implantation of the thermal diffusion flowmetry sensor (SABER 2000; Flowtornics, Phonics, USA) were included in this study. There were 25 males and 38 females with a mean age of 45.9 years (range 6–80 years). The brain temperature was monitored by thermal diffusion flowmetry and axillary temperature was monitored by digitalized mercury thermometer. The influence of local heat production from the pathologic lesions may mislead the brain temperature. The thermal diffusion flowmetry sensor was placed on the opposite side or far from the pathologic lesion site according to the operation methods (Fig. 1). Mild to moderate hypothermia management was applied to patients with increased intracranial pressure by using the cold water blanket (Mditherm II; Gaymar Ind., NY). Paired data of the brain and axillary temperature were saved every 2 hours, simultaneously. Normothermia group is defined as an axillary temperature ranging from 36.5 °C to 38.3 °C and hypothermia group is defined as an axillary temperature ranging from 32 °C to 36 °C.

All data are presented as mean ± standard deviation. Comparisons between data groups were computed using unpaired t-test. Statistical significance was defined as a probability value of less than 0.05.

Results

1539 paired data from 54 normothermia patients and 361 paired data from 9 hypothermia patients were analyzed. In the normothermia group, the mean brain temperature was 37.8 ± 1.69 °C and mean axillary temperature was 36.9 ± 0.52 °C. In the hypothermia

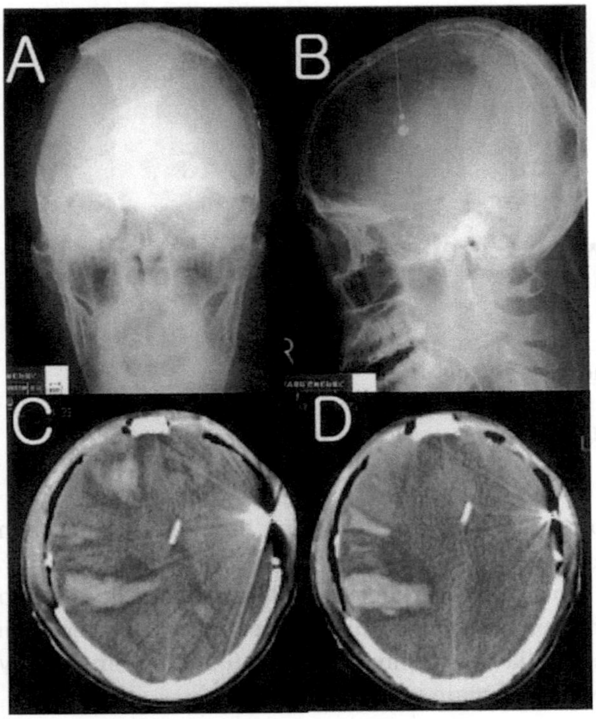

Fig. 1. Illustration of brain temperature monitoring. (A and B) Post-operative plain skull radiography shows metallic sensor shadow which was placed at the left fronto-parietal region. (C and D) Post-operative brain CT scan shows metallic artifact at the opposite side of pathologic lesion

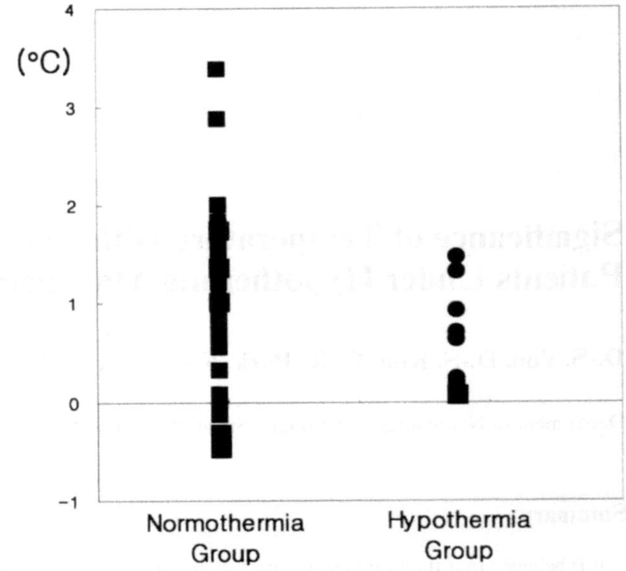

Fig. 2. Temperature differences between the brain and axilla in normothermia and hypothermia groups

group, the mean brain temperature was 35.8 ± 1.21 °C and mean axillary temperature was 34.7 ± 1.40 °C. The temperature difference between the brain and the axilla was 1.04 ± 0.67 °C in normothermia patients and 0.91 ± 0.84 °C in hypothermic patients (Fig. 2). As a result, there is no statistical significance between the two groups (unpaired t-test, $P > 0.05$).

Discussion

A surge of interest in brain temperature has recently followed reports by several groups that the ischemic brain is very sensitive to minor (2–3 °C) changes in temperature. Using different animal models, researchers have shown that mild hypothermia is protective during and immediately after an ischemic insult [5]. Also recent clinical trials reported that hypothermia could improve the neurologic outcome of head trauma patients, [1]. When a patient is managed with hypothermia therapy, the clinician needs an effective temperature modulating equipment and an accurate brain temperature monitoring device. Unfortunately, not in all clinical situations such monitoring device is available and even though, the accuracy of such devices can be troublesome.

According to previous reports, the brain temperature is 0.4–1.1 °C higher than the other body temperature in normothermia patients [2, 4]. Other studies about brain temperature in a specific case reported that the temperature difference was decreased during the barbiturate coma therapy and was increased in the state of seizure [6, 7]. Some studies reported that the difference (brain and other body temperature) was greater at temperatures outside the normal temperature range (brain temperature over 38 °C, under 36 °C) [3]. But there is no report available regarding the degree of temperature difference between the human intracerebral temperature and its relation to other body temperature during hypothermia circumstance. Considering the physiological response to hypothermia, peripheral vessels will be constricted and the temperature difference between the brain and other body temperature will be increased.

Our study shows that the brain temperature in the patients under mild to moderate hypothermia management appears to be still about 1 °C higher than the axilla throughout the study period a result which is almost the same in normothermia patients. The purpose of brain temperature monitoring is now an issue of discussion because this study shows that the axillary temperature can be used to estimate brain temperature during hypothermia management, which is about 1 °C higher than axillary temperature.

References

1. Bullock MR, Lyeth BG, Muizelaar JP (1999) Current status of neuroprotection trial for traumatic brain injury: Lessons from animal models and clinical studies. Neurosurgery 45: 207–220
2. Haaland K, Steen PA, Thoresen M (1996) Cerebral, tympanic and colonic thermometry in the piglet. Report Fertil Dev 8: 125–128
3. Henker RA, Brown SD, Marion DW (1998) Comparison of brain temperature with bladder and rectal temperatures in adults with severe head injury. Neurosurgery 42: 1071–1075
4. Kiley JP, Eldrige FL, Millhorn DE (1984) Brain, blood and rectal temperature during whole body cooling. Comp Biochem Physiol A 79: 631–634
5. Mellergard P, Nordstrom CH (1991) Intracerebral temperature in neurosurgical patients. Neurosurgery 28: 709–713
6. Petrova EV (1999) Thermal interhemispheric asymmetry of the brain in rats in a cataleptic state. Zh Vyssh Nerv Deiat Im I P Pavlova 49: 338–344
7. Rumana CS, Gopinath SP, Uzura M, Valadka AB, Robertson CS (1998) Brain temperature exceeds systemic temperature in head-injured patients. Crit Care Med 26: 562–567

Correspondence: Dal-Soo Kim, M.D., Department of Neurosurgery, Uijongbu St. Mary's Hospital 65-1, Kumoh-dong, Uijongbu-city, Korea 480-130.

Acta Neurochir (2002) [Suppl] 81: 89–91

ICP is Lower During Propofol Anaesthesia Compared to Isoflurane and Sevoflurane

K. D. Petersen[1], U. Landsfeldt[1], G. E. Cold[1], C. B. Pedersen[2], S. Mau[2], J. Hauerberg[3], and P. Holst[3]

[1] Department of Anaesthesia and Neurosurgery, Aarhus University Hospital, Denmark
[2] Department of Anaesthesia and Neurosurgery, Rigshospitalet, Denmark
[3] Department of Anaesthesia and Neurosurgery, Glostrup Hospital, Denmark

Summary

Objectives. Propofol is a cerebral vasoconstrictor while inhalation anaesthetics like isoflurane and sevoflurane act as cerebral vasodilators in both animal and human studies. This difference of action upon cerebral vessels might implicate a lower ICP during propofol anaesthesia. Cerebral metabolism is decreased by all three anaesthetics. In a prospective, randomised multicenter study ICP was compared during anaesthesia with propofol, isoflurane and sevoflurane.

Methods. 117 patients subjected to elective craniotomy for supratentorial tumour. Propofol: N = 41; isoflurane: N = 38; sevoflurane: N = 38. Nitrous oxide was omitted and all anaesthetics were supplemented with a continuous infusion of fentanyl. ICP was measured subdurally after removal of the bone flap. MABP, CPP, PCO2, AVDO2, rectal temperature, tumour size and midline shift were registered too. Statistics: Kruskal-Wallis Variance on Ranks. All values in medians with range. $P < 0.05$ was considered significant.

Results. ICP (mmHg): propofol 7 (−1–20), isoflurane 12 (1–29), sevoflurane 11 (2–32). ICP was significantly lower in the propofol group compared to the isofluane and sevoflurane groups. CPP (mmHg): propofol 80 (45–104), isoflurane 60 (32–84), sevoflurane 63 (44–77). CPP was significantly higher in the propofol group compared to the isoflurane and sevoflurane groups. AVDO2 (mmol/l): propofol 3.1 (0.9–5.1), isoflurane 2.5 (1.1–4.5), sevoflurane 2.6 (0.8–4.1). AVDO2 was significantly higher in the propofol group compared to the isoflurane and sevoflurane groups. No significant differences in PCO2, rectal temperature, tumour size and midline shift were found.

Conclusions. Subdural ICP is significantly lower during propofol anaesthesia compared to isoflurane and sevoflurane anaesthesia. CPP and AVDO2 are significantly higher during propofol anaesthesia compared to isoflurane and sevoflurane anaesthesia.

Keywords: Intracranial pressure, propofol, isoflurane and sevoflurane.

Introduction

The influence of anaesthetics upon cerebral hemodynamics and intracranial pressure (ICP) have been investigated thoroughly in experimental and clinical studies without clear-cut answer to what anaesthetic is most suitable in the clinical setting. Nevertheless, the general concept has been that intravenous anaesthetics are to be preferred for volatile agents. Todd *et al.* [5] measured epidural ICP through the burr hole in patients undergoing craniotomy for cerebral supratentorial tumours, and found that ICP did not differ significantly between three anaesthetic techniques including isoflurane/nitrous oxide, nitrous oxide/fentanyl and propofol/fentanyl. Consequently, the argument that intravenous anaesthetics regarding ICP are to be prefer red for inhalation agents seems to fail. Since 1995 we routinely have used subdural ICP measurement before opening of the dura. With this technique we found that at ICP levels < 7 mm Hg, opening of dura was never accompanied by brain prolapse, but at ICP levels exceeding 10 mm Hg brain prolapse occurred with high probability. These thresholds were found to be independent of pathophysiology (subarachnoid haemorrhage, supratentorial cerebral tumours) and choice of anaesthetic technique (propofol/fentanyl contra isoflurane/nitrous oxide), and indicate that the occurrence of cerebral swelling/herniation after opening of the dura with high probability can be predicted, Cold *et al.* [2, 3]. In a preliminary non-randomised study we found that ICP in patients submitted to craniotomy for cerebral supratentorial tumours was significantly lower during propofol/fentanyl anaesthesia compared with isoflurane/nitrous oxide and sevoflurane anaesthesia [1]. In the present randomised, open labelled study, subdural ICP was measured in patients scheduled for elective craniotomy for supratentorial tumours. Patients were allocated to either propofol/fentanyl, isoflurane/fentanyl or sevoflurane/fentanyl anaesthesia. Subdural ICP was measured before opening of the dura.

Materials and Methods

Patients subjected to elective craniotomy for cerebral supratentorial tumours were included. The ages of the patients ranged from 18 to 70 years. All patients had a cerebral CT/MRI scanning preoperatively and a diagnosis of cerebral tumour with shift of the midline ≤ 10 mm. The investigation was a Danish multicenter study with three participating hospitals and the patients were enrolled between March 1998 and December 1999. The Local Ethics Committee approved the protocol. The patients were premedicated with diazepam 0.15–0.20 mg/kg orally one hour before induction of anaesthesia. If preoperative steroid and anticonvulsant treatment was instituted, it was given together with diazepam. The patients were randomised to one of three anaesthetic groups: propofol/fentanyl, isoflurane/fentanyl or sevoflurane/fentanyl. The patients were randomised in blocks of 21 in sealed, numbered envelopes with seven envelopes for each anaesthetic group.

Group 1: Propofol/fentanyl supplemented with oxygen/air, F_iO_2 0.5–0.6. Anaesthesia was induced with fentanyl 4 µg/kg and propofol 1–2 mg/kg given over 1 minute. Lidocaine 1 mg/kg was administered over 1 minute followed by muscular relaxation by atracurium 0.5 mg/kg. Maintenance of anaesthesia with infusions of propofol 6–10 mg/kg/h and fentanyl 2–4 µg/kg/h. Controlled ventilation was applied and P_aCO_2 was targeted between 4.0–4.5 kPa. Bupivacaine 0.25% with epinephrine was used for infiltration of the scalp.

Group 2: Isoflurane/fentanyl supplemented with oxygen/air, F_iO_2 0.5–0.6. Anaesthesia was induced with fentanyl 2 µg/kg and propofol 1–2 mg/kg given over 1 minute. Lidocaine 1 mg/kg was administered over 1 minute followed by muscular relaxation by atracurium 0.5 mg/kg. Maintenance of anaesthesia with isoflurane 1–2 MAC and fentanyl 2 µg/kg/h and then treated as group 1.

Group 3: Sevoflurane/fentanyl treated similarly as outlined for group 2.

ICP, MABP and $AVDO_2$ Measurements

In accordance with recent studies ICP was measured subdurally after removal of the bone flap by an intravenous cannula, 22 G/0.8 mm (Venflon®) connected to a standard, commercial saline-filled polyethylene catheter and pressure transducer without a continuous flush of saline [1]. Mean arterial blood pressure (MABP) was measured continuously in the radial artery. Cerebral perfusion pressure (CPP) was calculated as the difference between MABP and ICP. P_aO_2, P_aCO_2, rectal temperature and haemoglobin concentration were measured. A jugular bulb catheter was inserted and arteriovenous difference of oxygen content ($AVDO_2$) was calculated. Pathohistological diagnosis, tumour localization, midline shift and tumour size (largest area seen on CT/MRI scan) were registered as well.

Kruskal-Wallis One Way Analysis of Variance on Ranks was used for statistical analysis of non-Normal distributed data. One-Way ANOVA was used for analysis of Normal distributed data.

Results

117 patients were included in the study. 41 patients were allocated to the propofol group, 38 to the isoflurane and the sevoflurane groups respectively. Demographic and radiological data are presented in Table 1. No significant differences between groups were disclosed as regards gender, age, weight, height, midline shift, and tumour size. Localization of tumours, and histopathological findings did not differ between groups (not shown).

Clinical results are shown in Table 2. P_aCO_2 and rectal temperature were not significantly different between the groups. ICP was significantly lower in the propofol group (7 mm Hg) compared to isoflurane (12 mm Hg) and sevoflurane (11 mm Hg). MABP was significantly higher in the propofol compared with the isoflurane group and the sevoflurane group. As a consequence CPP was significantly higher in the propofol group, 80 mm Hg compared to isoflurane 60 mm Hg and sevoflurane 63 mm Hg. $AVDO_2$ was significantly higher for the propofol group, 3.1 mmol/l versus 2.5 mmol/l for isoflurane and 2.6 mmol/l for sevoflurane.

Table 1. *Demographic and Radiological Data*

	Propofol N = 41	Isoflurane N = 38	Sevoflurane N = 38
Sex (male/female)	20/21	16/22	20/18
Age (years)	57 (20–70)	56 (33–70)	55 (22–70)
Height (cm)	170 (147–186)	170 (162–190)	170 (154–186)
Weight (kg)	74 (48–108)	70 (50–106)	75 (45–115)
Midline shift (mm)	4.0 (0.0–20.0)	4.0 (0.0–10.0)	4.5 (0.0–10.0)
Tumour size (cm^2)	11.8 (2.3–86.4)	11.8 (3.1–94.3)	12.6 (2.4–86.4)

Table 2. *Clinical Results*

	Propofol N = 41	Isoflurane N = 38	Sevoflurane N = 38
ICP (mm Hg)	7 (−1–20)	12* (1–29)	11* (2–32)
MABP (mm Hg)	85.0 (57–116)	71.0* (59–97)	76.5* (55–100)
CPP (mm Hg)	80 (45–104)	60* (32–84)	63* (44–77)
P_aCO_2 (kPa)	4.5 (4.1–5.6)	4.5 (3.9–5.7)	4.8 (3.9–5.5)
Temperature (°C)	35.9 (34.7–36.7)	36.0 (34.6–37.1)	36.0 (34.4–37.1)
$AVDO_2$ (mmol/l)	3.1 (0.9–5.1)	2.5* (1.1–4.5)	2.6* (0.8–4.1)

Medians are indicated with range.
* Indicate $P < 0.05$ compared with propofol.

Discussion

We have demonstrated a significantly lower ICP and higher CPP during propofol/fentanyl anaesthesia compared to isoflurane/fentanyl and sevoflurane/fentanyl anaesthesia in a uniform group of patients with cerebral supratentorial tumours. In a comparative trial of three anaesthetics in a similar group of patients no differences in ICP were disclosed, but like in the present study, CPP and MABP were significantly lower in the isoflurane/N_2O group compared to patients anaesthetised with propofol/fentanyl [5]. In the same study ICP was found to be 12 mm Hg (mean) in patients allocated to propofol. In our study we found ICP to be 7 mm Hg (median) during propofol anaesthesia. The reason for this discrepancy is probably a difference in methodology of ICP measurement. Todd *et al.* measured ICP through the first burr hole in their study. In the present study ICP was measured after removal of the bone flap. The removal of the bone flap hypothetically exerts a certain degree of intracranial decompression. Recently, in a non-published study of 28 patients subjected to craniotomy, we found a difference of 5 mm Hg in subdural ICP measured through the first burr hole and after removal of the bone flap; ICP decreased from 13.5 mm Hg to 8.5 mm Hg (medians).

Our results indicate that inhalation agents exert a lower $AVDO_2$ compared with propofol. This is in accordance with the concept that inhalation agents compared with propofol exert a more intense cerebral vasodilatation, suggesting that CBV (cerebral blood volume) and ICP are increased [6]. In traumatic brain injury CPP above 60 mm Hg is important to avoid neurological deterioration [4]. In the present study all three anaesthetic techniques fulfilled this goal. Whether a CPP threshold of 60 mm Hg can be applied to elective surgery for supratentorial tumours is unknown. In our study CPP was significantly higher in the propofol group. We believe that a relatively high CPP might prevent the development of cerebral ischaemia in regions where retractors are applied. In this respect the present study indicate that propofol is to be preferred for inhalation agents.

Conclusion

In a randomised clinical multicenter study subdural ICP was compared with three different anaesthetic techniques in patients with supratentorial tumours. ICP was significantly lower and CPP significantly higher during propofol/fentanyl anaesthesia compared to isoflurane/fentanyl and sevoflurane/fentanyl anaesthesia. Additionally, $AVDO_2$ was significantly lower during anaesthesia with isoflurane/fentanyl and sevoflurane/fentanyl.

References

1. Bundgaard H, Cold GE (1997) Acta Anaesthesiol Scand [Suppl] 110: 195
2. Bundgaard H, Landsfeldt U, Cold GE (1998) Acta Neurochir (Wien) [Suppl] 71: 276–278
3. Cold GE, Tange M, Jensen TM, Ottesen S (1996) Br J Neurosurg 10: 69–75
4. Juul N, Morris GF, Marshall SB, Marshall LF (2000) J Neurosurg 92: 1–6
5. Todd MM, Warner DS, Sokoll MD *et al* (1993) Anesthesiology 78: 1005–1020
6. Todd MM, Weeks J (1996) J Neurosurg Anesthesiol 8: 296–303

Correspondence: Georg Emil Cold, M.D., Ph.D., Dept. of Anaesthesia, Aarhus University Hospital, Aarhus Kommunehospital, Norrebrogade 44, building 10, 7'th floor, Denmark.

Acta Neurochir (2002) [Suppl] 81: 93–97

Effects of Positive End-Expiratory Pressure on Intracranial Pressure and Cerebral Perfusion Pressure

W. Videtta, F. Villarejo, M. Cohen, G. Domeniconi, R. Santa Cruz, O. Pinillos, F. Rios, and B. Maskin

From the ICU, Hospital Nacional¨Prof. A. Posadas¨, University of Buenos Aires, Haedo, Argentina

Summary

The effect of positive end-expiratory pressure (PEEP) on intracranial pressure (ICP) and cerebral perfusion pressure (CPP) has been reported by several investigators, without any consensus being reached. Acute neurological and neurosurgical patients suffer intracranial hypertension and acute lung injury with hypoxemia. Since PEEP may improve hypoxemia but elevate ICP and decrease CPP, it is important to determine the influence of varying levels of PEEP on ICP and CPP. The aim of the study was to investigate the changes in ICP and CPP associated with different levels of PEEP. Twenty patients requiring ICP monitoring and mechanical ventilation were enrolled. Patients had severe head injury (n = 10), spontaneous intracerebral haemorrhage (n = 5), and subarachnoid haemorrhage (n = 5). PEEP was raised from 5 (basal) to 15 cm H_2O in steps of 5 cm H_2O. After at least 10 minutes of each new PEEP setting, ICP and CPP were measured. PEEP at 10 and 15 cm H_2O produced a significant ($p < 0.05$) increase in intracranial pressure 11.6 ± 5.6 and 14.6 ± 6.28 mm Hg, respectively; no significant ($p = 0.819$) change occurred in CPP.

Keywords: Intracranial pressure; positive end-expiratory pressure; cerebral perfusion pressure; acute lung injury.

Introduction

Under circumstances of acute brain injury, monitoring ICP and CPP becomes a critical determinant of cerebral blood flow. Patients suffering severe traumatic brain injury (sTBI), spontaneous intracerebral haemorrhage (sICH) and subarachnoid haemorrhage (SAH) may raise ICP, which increases risk of herniation. When CPP falls too low, cerebral ischemia or infarction can occur. Low cerebral perfusion pressure (< 60 mm Hg) represents ischemic tendency. ICP and CPP are variables semi-independent [16]. These patients have a relative risk of secondary cerebral injury as determined by the primary injury process and coexisting systemic injuries, like hypoxemia. Acute lung injury (ALI) is a recognized complication of severe traumatic brain injury [20, 29, 31], SAH and ICH. This can be caused by acute injuries to the central nervous system (CNS) [22] or by coexisting systemic injuries. Acute lung injury is characterized by severe hypoxemia, defined as $PaO_2/F_IO_2 < 300$. An array of conditions common in patients with intracranial injury [3] seem to share the final common pathway of the so-called adult respiratory syndrome (ARDS). The hypoxemia result from low functional residual capacity (FRC), mismatch between ventilation/perfusion and increased pulmonary shunt [5, 11, 18]. The respiratory management of these patients requires adequate oxygenation by using mechanical ventilation (MV). Positive end-expiratory pressure (PEEP) is an effective mean of improving hypoxemia [14, 25]. PEEP increases FRC [8, 19] and decreases pulmonary shunt without necessitating an increase in the inspired oxygen concentration (F_IO_2) into a potentially toxic range [14, 18, 25, 26]. While improving arterial oxygenation, PEEP can reduce cardiac output and blood pressure [15]. PEEP impedes thoracic venous flow, increases central venous pressure, and might also increase ICP. These side effects of PEEP [4, 14, 26] could potentially produce critical reductions and elevations in CPP and ICP, respectively. The relationship of PEEP therapy on ICP and CPP has been of considerable interest to many investigators [3, 7, 9, 11, 30]. Thus, a considerable effort has been made for investigating repeatedly in human [1, 3, 5, 9, 11, 21, 30] and animal experiments [2, 10, 12, 18], with different designs, to understand the interplay between PEEP and the physiologic dynamics relating to cardiac, pulmonary and CNS. Sometimes, the results of the studies are contradictory [6, 10] and conclusions unclear [5]. To predict the potential impact of using PEEP on ICP, MAP, CPP, PaO_2, static lung compliance (SLC) in any particular situation is critical. The aim of the study was to investigate the changes in ICP and CPP associated with changes in PEEP.

Materials and Methods

All neurological and neurosurgical patients who received mechanical ventilation (MV) and ICP monitoring simultaneously as part of the routine management were eligible for inclusion in the study. Inclusion criteria were: (1) acute neurological or neurosurgical disorder that required ICP monitoring, (2) need of MV, at least 24 hours, (3) hemodynamic stability (without inotropic drugs requirements in the last 30 minutes), (4) stable mean arterial pressure (MAP) in the last 30 minutes, (5) stable ICP measures (with variations of 3 mmHg in the last 30 minutes, prior to initiation of measure), and (6) normal rectal temperature in the last 30 minutes prior first measure. Exclusion criteria were: (1) age < 14, > 80 years old, (2) bulluos lung disease, (3) pneumothorax, (4) pregnancy, and (5) refusal of consent. All patients were admitted to the ICU between August 1999 and February 2000. Twenty-four patients were eligible for inclusion in the study. Twenty patients completed the study. Ten of these patients had suffered severe traumatic brain injury, five subarachnoid haemorrhage, and five spontaneous intracerebral haemorrhage. After the etabablishment of an adequate airway, mechanical ventilation, and appropriate support of vital functions, the patients were examined neurologically and classified according to Glasgow Coma Scale (GCS) [32]. The patients' diagnoses were established by computed tomographic (CT) scanning cerebral angiography, or magnetic resonance images (MRI), as indicated. When appropriate, surgical treatment was done. Patients were ventilated using Pruritan Bennett, series 740 and 7200 (Pruritan Bennett Corporation, Carlsbad, CA, USA), Infrasonic Adult Star 2000 (Infrasonic CS, INC., San Diego, CA, USA), and Siemens SV 900 (Siemens – Elema, Solna, Sweden). All patients received mechanical ventilation, using volume control ventilation. The attending physician set F_iO_2, PEEP and respiratory rate. Continuous monitoring of ICP was performed routinely. Intracranial pressure was measured with a parenchyma fiberoptic catheter Camino™ (V420, Camino Medical Products, San Diego, Ca, USA). Blood pressure measurements were obtained from a radial catheter Angiocath™ 16 ga 2 in (Becton Dickinson Vascular Access, Sandy, Utah, USA) connected to a pressure transducer connected to a Critikon™ (Dinamap Plus, Vital Signs Monitor, Tampa, FL, USA.) monitor or with a non-invasive blood pressure cuff applied to the upper arm (1846 SX, Dinamap, Tampa, FL, USA) connected to a Critikon™ (Dinamap Plus, Vital Signs Monitor, Tampa, FL, USA.) if there was no arterial catheter in place. External chest leads were placed for routine monitoring of the electrocardiogram. Cerebral perfusion pressure was calculated as mean arterial pressure (mm Hg) minus intracranial pressure (mm Hg). A value of ≤ 60 mm Hg was considered to represent a significant decrease in CPP. The patients were nursed in the 30° head-up position and the neck in the midline position. Analgesia, sedation and muscle relaxation were achieved using fentanyl, midazolam and vencoronium bromide [27], respectively, and maintained with the same doses of fentanyl, midazolam, and vencoronium bromide administered intravenously by an infusion pump. Inotropic drugs, dopamine and nor adrenaline were administered intravenously using an infusion pump. The administration of inotropic drugs was maintained with the same doses during overall study.

Baseline measurements (PEEP = 5 cm H_2O) of intracranial pressure, MAP, CPP, static lung compliance, arterial blood gases were obtained and recordered. APACHE II (Acute Physiology and Chronic Health Evaluation) [13] at the time of the admission and the Glasgow Coma Scale (GCS) [32] were calculated. The degree of lung injury was assessed employing the score described by Murray *et al.* [23]. The PEEP value used was equal to the one the patient had been exposed before the study. Arterial blood gases were measured before the study and used to calculate the PaO_2/F_iO_2 ratio. Chest radiography was obtained bedside, using a portable machine in the morning and was interpreted by a staff intensivist. Static lung compliance was determined at each level of PEEP. Static lung compliance was calculated as tidal volume (ml)/end-expiratory pressure (cm H_2O) minus level of PEEP (cm H_2O). A value of 30 ml/cm H_2O or less was considered to represent significantly decreased lung compliance.

During the study, all patients were exposed to PEEP settings of 5, 10, and 15 cm H_2O. PEEP was raised in steps of 5 cm H_2O. The measurements were done bedside and after the patient was hemodynamically stabilized and intracranial pressure under control. The trial was discontinued if the patient demonstrated: (1) CPP < 60 mm Hg, (2) ICP > 30 mm Hg, (3) clinical neurological deterioration, (4) hemodynamic instability, (5) myocardial infarction within 12 weeks of the study, (6) increase of pressure plateau > 35 cm H_2O, (7) $SaPO_2 < 90\%$, and (8) suspicion of pneumothorax. After at least 10 minutes at each PEEP setting, the hemodynamic parameters, the ventilatory parameters, intracranial pressure, and cerebral perfusion pressure were recorded. This amount or period of time is believed to be sufficient for the cardiovascular effects of PEEP to become manifest [24, 28]. After the study, the ventilation parameters were resumed in all patients.

The data were analysed, using analysis of variance (ANOVA) or the non-parametric test of Kruskal-Wallis. The statistical analyses were performed using the software Statisca, version 5.1/97 (Stat-Soft Co, Tulsa, OK) and the statistical package True Epistat, version 5.0 (Windows 95). Intracranial pressure, cerebral perfusion pressure, mean arterial pressure, static lung compliance, Injury lung score, $PaCO_2$, PaO_2, $SaPO_2$ data were analysed at PEEP of 10 and 15 cm H_2O and compared with PEEP = 5 cm H_2O. Correlation test "r" of Pearson was used for correlation of variables. All data are expressed as mean $\pm$ SD. A $p < 0.05$ was considered statistically significant. This research protocol was approved by the Hospital National "Prof. A. Posadas" affiliated to Buenos Aires University, and Research and Ethics Committees, and written informed consent from either the patient's relatives or the next-of-kin of patients was obtained in the study.

Results

Twenty patients were included in the study, fifteen men and five women. The mean age was 36.3 $\pm$ 18.5 years, range: 14–74 y. Ten of these patients had suffered sTBI, five sICH and 5 SAH. Mean Apache II score was 16.9 $\pm$ 10.3, mean GCS was 7.62 $\pm$ 2.83, and mean MAP was 99.3 $\pm$ 15.8 mm Hg. The other variables of the study population are described in Table 1. Parenchymal fiberoptic catheter had been placed in 20 patients. All patients showed radiological evidence of lung injury and improved oxygenation with PEEP at 5 cm H_2O.

Table 1. *Study Population. Baseline Measurements, PEEP = 5 cm H_2O*

	Mean ± SD – (Median)
Age (years)	36.3 ± 18.5 (34)
Gender (M/F)	15:5
APACHE II	16.9 ± 10.3 (14.5)
GCS	7.62 ± 2.83 (7.5)
LIS	1.77 ± 0.71 (1.75)
RT (°C)	37.8 ± 0.74 (37.6)
HR (beats/min)	105.5 ± 18.4 (107.5)
MAP (mmHg)	99.3 ± 15.8 (97)
ICP (mmHg)	10.1 ± 6.13 (8.5)
CPP (mmHg)	89.6 ± 15.5 (85.5)
PaO_2 (mmHg)	101.2 ± 37.7 (100)
$PaCO_2$ (mmHg)	34.9 ± 6.42 (32.5)
V_t (liters)	0.61 ± 0.09 (0.6)
RR (breaths/min)	15.3 ± 3.21 (16)
SLC (ml/cm H_2O)	49.5 ± 43.3 (35.5)
DLC (ml/cm H_2O)	30.6 ± 26.0 (24)

APACHE Acute Physiology and Chronic Health Evaluation; *GCS* Glasgow Coma Scale; *LIS* Lung Injury Score; *RT* rectal temperature; *HR* hearth rate; *MAP* mean arterial pressure; *ICP* intracranial pressure; *CPP* cerebral perfusion pressure; V_t tidal volume; *RR* respiratory rate; *SLC* static lung compliance; *DLC* dynamic lung compliance.

ICP ranged from 2 to 27 mm Hg, at different PEEP levels. The ICP values at different setting of PEEP were: 10.1 ± 6.13 mm Hg at 5 cm H_2O; 11.6 ± 5.6 mm Hg at 10 cm H_2O; 14.6 ± 6.28 mm Hg at 15 cm H_2O. PEEP increments at 10 and 15 cm H_2O significantly increased intracracranial pressure, $p < 0.049$ (ANOVA). Only two patients had intracranial hypertension (ICP ≥ 20 mm Hg), 20 and 25 mm Hg and corresponding CPP values: 79 and 120 mm Hg, at PEEP = 5 cm H_2O. During the study, in the first patient ICP decreased to 17 and 16 mm Hg and corresponding CPP values: 75 and 82 mm Hg, at PEEP = 10 and 15 cm H_2O. In the other one, ICP remained at high values of 24 and 25 mm Hg and corresponding CPP values increased to 121 and 132 mm Hg, at PEEP = 10 and 15 cm H_2O. During PEEP application, three of eighteen patients with normal intracranial pressure at PEEP = 5 cm H_2O raised ICP to 20, 25, and 25 mm Hg with corresponding CPP values: 88, 86, and 87 mm Hg at PEEP = 15 cm H_2O.

The range of cerebral perfusion pressure was 60 to 132 mm Hg and did not decrease to <60 mm Hg in any patient at any level of PEEP. CPP values at different PEEP levels were: 89.6 ± 15.5, 86.4 ± 16.4, and 87.7 ± 19.5 mm Hg. No significant difference ($p = 0.819$ (ANOVA)), was noted in cerebral perfusion pressure at any PEEP level.

The SLC values at different PEEP levels were: 49.5 ± 43.3 mm Hg at 5 cm H_2O, 49.9 ± 34.4 mm Hg at 10 cm H_2O, and 42.5 ± 20.0 mm Hg at 15 cm H_2O, $p = 0.825$ (NS) (Test Kruskal-Wallis); and corresponding $PaCO_2$ values: 34.9 ± 6.42 mm Hg, 36.2 ± 5.65 mm Hg, and 38.0 ± 11.8 mm Hg, $p = 0.466$ (ANOVA).

Discussion

Our results show that in neurological and neurosurgical patients, application of PEEP at 10 or 15 cm H_2O increased intracranial pressure significantly, with no significant change on cerebral perfusion pressure. All the patients but two in this series had normal intracranial pressure with PEEP at 5 cm H_2O. Patients with raised ICP (range: 20–27 mm Hg) at PEEP level of 5 cm H_2O did not decrease CPP at any level of PEEP (with CPP > 60 mm Hg; range: 75–132 mm Hg). The SLC and the $PaCO_2$ were similar in both patients with values between 16–30 ml/cm H_2O, and 39–49 mm Hg, respectively. We cannot explain why ICP raised in these patients. In contrast, three patients with normal ICP at PEEP = 5 cm H_2O, and patients with SLC > 45 ml/cm H_2O (range: 46.6–69.2 ml/cm H_2O) and $PaCO_2$ between 31–53 mm Hg, increased ICP at PEEP = 15 cm H_2O with CPP > 60 mm Hg. This fact, in part may be explained by normal SLC and elevated $PaCO_2$. The use of PEEP in neurocritical patients is controversial [30]. PEEP improves PaO_2 by increasing FRC. In our study, Lung Injury Scores were mild to moderate (1.77 ± 0.71), as indicated by the Murray scores [23]. We believe that our results are partially affected by the transmission of PEEP applied to the airway to the intrathoracic

Table 2. *Effects of Different PEEP Levels on ICP and CPPP*

	PEEP = 5 cm H_2O	PEEP = 10 cm H_2O	PEEP = 15 cm H_2O	p (ANOVA)
ICP mmHg	10.1 ± 6.13	11.6 ± 5.60	14.6 ± 6.28	$P < 0.049$
CPP mmHg	89.6 ± 15.5	86.4 ± 16.4	87.7 ± 19.5	$p = 0.819$

vasculature, then to the intracranial compartment. McGuire *et al.* [21] concluded that their results were independent from noncompliant lungs and that the PEEP was transmitted to the intrathoracic vasculature. These results can be explained in part by the fact that Lung Injury Scores were mild to moderate, as we found out. As Cooper *et al.* [9] pointed out, it is important to note that only a group of variables considered together may contribute to a significant increase in ICP. PEEP alters many variables simultaneously so that change in one variable is virtually always either offset or amplified by changes in other variables. Like other series [1, 3, 9, 11, 17, 21, 30], we confirm that PEEP can increase ICP, depending on the patient's baseline hemodynamic and ventilatory status and the effect of PEEP on MAP, CPP, $PaCO_2$, $SaPO_2$, PaO_2, intraabdominal pressure, patient's position and the interplay between these factors. We agree with McGuire [21], that when assessing the effects of PEEP on ICP, CPP must be used as an index too, in addition to ICP. Like other authors [9, 21] who examined the effects of increase with PEEP on ICP and CPP, our results achieved statistical significance at PEEP levels of 10 and 15 cm H_2O. We cannot conclude that this finding is clinically important. We found no statically significant change in CPP, which was ≥ 60 mmHg. Thus, the changes in CPP were of dubious clinical importance. There was no increase in ICP in two patients with elevated baseline ICP, the group of greatest clinical concern. Cooper *et al.* [9] has shown similar results in eight patients. Perhaps the adverse effects of PEEP on ICP seen in other studies depended on the various factors discussed previously. We conclude that the use of PEEP at 10 and 15 cm H_2O produces significant increase in ICP without clinical relevance. We found no statiscally significant decrease in cerebral perfusion pressure. We propose that presently ICP and CPP monitoring are necessary aspects of the management of neurocritical patients who require mechanical ventilation with positive end-expiratory pressure.

References

1. Abbushi W, Herkt G, Speckner E *et al* (1980) Beeinflussung des Hirndruckes bei Patienten mit Schädel-Hirn-Trauma durch PEEP-Beatmung und Oberkörper-Hochlagerung. Anaesthesist 29: 521–524
2. Aidinis SJ, Lafferty J, Shapiro HM (1976) Intracranial responses to PEEP. Anesthesiology 45: 275–286
3. Apuzzo ML, Weiss MH, Petersons V *et al* (1977) Effect of positive end expiratory pressure ventilation on intracranial pressure in man. J Neurosurg 46: 275–286
4. Asbaugh DG, Bigelow DB, Petty TL *et al* (1967) Acute Respiratory disease in adults. Lancet 2: 319–323
5. Burchiel KJ, Steege TD, Wyler AR (1981) Intracranial pressure changes in brain-injured patients requiring positive end-expiratory pressure ventilation. Neurosurgery 8: 443–449
6. Chapin JC, Downs JB, Douglas ME *et al* (1979) Lung expansion, airway pressure transmission, and positive end-expiratory pressure. Arch Surg 114: 1193–1197
7. Cooper KR, Boswell PA (1983) Reduced functional residual capacity and abnormal oxygenation in patients with severe head injury. Chest 84: 29–35
8. Cooper KR, Boswell PA (1983) Accurate measurement of functional capacity and oxygen consumption of patients on mechanical ventilation. Anaesth Intensive Care 11: 151–157
9. Cooper KR, Boswell PA, Choi C (1985) Safe use of PEEP in patients with severe head injury. J Neurosurg 63: 552–555
10. Cotev S, Paul WL, Ruiz BC *et al* (1981) Positive end-expiratory pressure (PEEP) and cerebrospinal fluid pressure during normal and elevated intracranial pressure in dogs. Intensive Care Med 7: 187–191
11. Frost EAM (1977) Effect of positive end-expiratory pressure on intracranial pressure and compliance in brain-injured patients. J Neurosurg 48: 689–703
12. Huseby JS, Pavlin EG, Butler J (1978) Effect of positive end-expiratory pressure on intracranial pressure in dogs. J Appl Physiol 44: 25–27
13. Knaus WA, Draper EA, Wagner DP *et al* (1985) APACHE II: A severity of disease classification system. Crit Care Med 13: 818–829
14. Kirby RR, Perry JC, Calderwood HW *et al* (1975) Cardiorespiratory effects of high positive end-expiratory pressure. Anesthesiology 43(50): 533–539
15. Koehler RC, Michael JR (1985) Transmission of intrathoracic pressure to intracranial pressure. Clin Crit Care 1: 212–214
16. Lang EW, Chesnut RM (1995) Intracranial pressure and cerebral perfusion pressure in severe head injury. New Horizons 3(3): 400–409
17. Lodrini S, Montolivo M, Pluchino F *et al* (1979) Positive end expiratory pressure in supine and sitting positions: Its effect on intrathoracic and intracranial pressures. Neurosurgery 24: 873–877
18. Luce JM, Huseby JS, Kirk W *et al* (1982) A Starling resistor regulates cerebral outflow in dogs. J Appl Physiol 53: 1496–1503
19. Lutch JS, Murray JF (1972) Continuous positive-pressure ventilation: effects on systemic oxygen transport and tissue oxygenation 76: 193–202
20. Marshall LF, Becker DP, Bowers SA *et al* (1983) The National Traumatic coma Data Bank. Part 1: Design, purpose, goals and results. J Neurosurg 59: 276–284
21. McGuire G, Crossley D, Richards J *et al* (1997) Effects of varying levels of positive end-expiratory pressure on intracranial pressure and cerebral perfusion pressure. Crit Care Med 25(6): 1059–1062
22. Miller JD, Butterworth JF, Gudeman SK *et al* (1981) Further experience in the management of severe head injury. J Neurosurg 54: 289–299
23. Murray JF, Mattay MA, Luce JM *et al* (1988) An expanded definition of the adult distress syndrome. Am Rev Respir Dis 138: 720–723
24. Perschau RA, Pepine CJ, Nichols WW *et al* (1979) Instantaneous blood low responses to PEEP with spontaneous ventilation. Circulation 59: 1312–1318
25. Powers SR Jr (1974) The use of positive end-expiratory pressure for respiratory support. Surg Clin North Am 54: 1125–1136

26. Powers SR Jr, Mannal R, Neclerio M *et al* (1973) Physiologic consequences of positive end-expiratory pressure (PEEP) ventilation. Ann Surg 178: 265–272
27. Prielipp RC, Coursin DB (1995) Sedative and neuromuscular blocking drug use in critically ill patients with head injuries. New Horizons 3(3): 456–468
28. Rose DM, Downs JR, Henan TJ (1981) Temporal response of FRC and oxygen changes in PEEP ventilation. Crit Care Med 9: 79–82
29. Schumacker PT, Rhodes GR, Newell JC *et al* (1979) Ventilation-perfusion imbalance after head trauma. Am Rev Resp Dis 119: 33–43
30. Shapiro HM, Marshall LF (1978) Intracranial pressure responses to PEEP in head-injured patients. J Trauma 18: 254–256
31. Sinha RP, Ducker TB, Perot PL Jr (1973) Arterial oxygenation: findings and its significance in central nervous system trauma patients. JAMA 224: 1258–1260
32. Teasdale G, Jennett B (1974) Assessment of coma and impaired consciousness. A practical scale. Lancet 2: 81–84

Correspondence: Walter Videtta, M.D., Güemes 2292, 1722 Merlo, Argentina.

Acta Neurochir (2002) [Suppl] 81: 99–101

The Safety of the Open Lung Approach in Neurosurgical Patients

S. Wolf, L. Schürer, H. A. Trost, and C. B. Lumenta

Department of Neurosurgery, Academic Hospital Munich-Bogenhausen, Technical University of Munich, München, Germany

Summary

A recent randomized controlled trial in patients with ARDS showed the beneficial effect of mechanical ventilation according to the so called *Open Lung Approach*, consisting of low tidal volumes and elevated PEEP settings after performing recruiting maneuvers. However, neurosurgical patients were excluded from this and other ARDS trials due to concerns of intracranial deterioration.

In this report, we present the clinical data of eleven patients with known intracranial pathology and concomitant ARDS which was treated according to the Open Lung concept.

The mean oxygenation index (p_aO_2/F_iO_2) increased from 132 ± 88 to 325 ± 64 measured 24 hours after initiation of Open Lung ventilation ($p < 0.001$). Mean PEEP level after the first recruiting maneuver was 14.9 ± 3.2 mmHg. Comparison of mean and peak ICP values over 24 hours of time before and after the first recruitment maneuver revealed a non-significant decline in ICP despite a moderate increase in mean p_aCO_2. Although two patients needed additional ICP treatment, no patient had to be withdrawn from Open Lung ventilation.

In our series, Open Lung ventilation in neurosurgical patients with ARDS was a safe method to improve oxygenation. Careful ICP monitoring provided, there is no reason to withhold this modern ARDS treatment in the neurosurgical intensive care unit.

Keywords: Mechanical ventilation; Open Lung; ICP; oxygenation.

Introduction

Modern respiratory management in ARDS tries to avoid additional damage from the mechanical ventilation itself, the so-called *ventilator induced lung injury*. Nowadays evidence is increasing that peak inspiratory pressure in mechanical should be kept below 30 mmHg (to avoid barotrauma) and several studies addressed the deletious impact of high tidal volumes (termed volutrauma) [10, 12]. To optimize oxygenation and to protect a patient with ARDS from additional damage, Lachmann proposed in an editorial in *Intensive Care Medicine* to "open up the lung and keep the lung open" [6]. Key issues of this concept were the frequent use of short inflation periods on temporary high pressure level to reopen collapsed alveoli (recruiting maneuvers), ventilation with elevated PEEP levels to avoid collapse of lung parenchyma and the use of low tidal volumes to avoid overdistension of the lung. In a recent randomized controlled trial the superiority in terms of survival of this *Open Lung Approach* was shown [1]. However, neurosurgical patients were excluded from this and other ARDS trials due to the potential risk of deterioration of intracranial pressure. Up to now, respiratory management in many neurosurgical centers still avoids PEEP levels above 5 mmHg.

Material and Methods

We report the clinical course of eleven patients with known intracranial pathology and concomitant acute lung injury. Primary neurosurgical diagnosis was traumatic brain injury (3 patients), aneurysmal subarachnoid hemorrhage (3 patients), intracranial hemorrhage (3 patients), cerebellar infarction (1 patient) and frontal meningeoma (1 patient). The diagnosis of acute lung injury was established according to the ARDS consensus conference definition [3].

All patients were mechanically ventilated (Puritan Bennett PB 7200) and analgosedated with Fentanyl/Midazolam. ICP monitoring, either via ventriculostomy or with an intraparenchymal device, was present in all patients. In four patients, ICP data was collected with multimodal monitoring devices (GMS, Kiel, Germany and/or Hellige-Marquette, Freiburg, Germany) with a sampling rate of 1 per minute. The ICP data from the other seven patients was extracted retrospectively from the records. For each patient, a mean value per hour was calculated and taken for statistical analysis.

Respiratory Management: Chest x-ray and bronchoscopy were performed as necessary, at least once before onset of Open Lung ventilation. An additional thoracic CT scan to exclude ventral pneumothorax was performed in three patients. Recruitment maneuvers consisted of elevating the PEEP level at least 5 cmH_2O higher than the previous setting. Then a short period of two to three breath cycles with an inspiratory pressure of 40 mmHg above PEEP was applied and instantly decreased to a maximum of 15 mmHg, with respect to a tidal volume of maximal 6 ml/kg ideal body weight. All patients received pressure controlled ventilation with an initial I:E ratio of

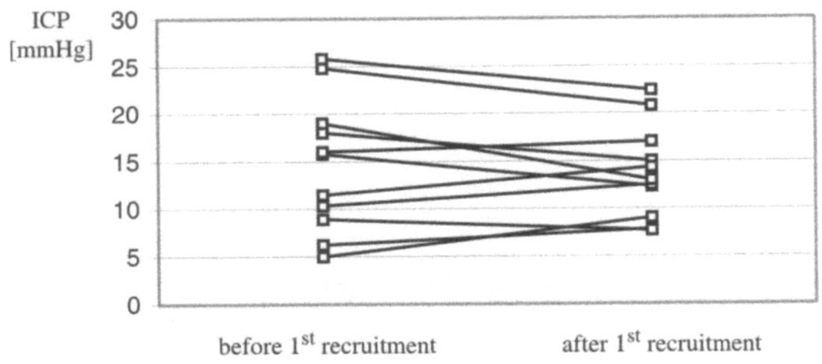

Fig. 1. Mean ICP values 24 hours before and after first recruitment

1 : 1, which was then adapted to gain an auto PEEP of 2–3 mmHg. Initial starting respiratory frequency was 15 per minute. We performed frequent blood gas analysis and tried at first to adjust the F_iO_2 to 0.4 and then to reduce the PEEP level in steps of 2 cmH_2O. If derecruitment occurred (notable in a decline of p_aO_2 and/or pulmonary static compliance), another recruiting maneuver was performed and PEEP level was adjusted 2 cmH_2O higher than the last PEEP setting.

Results

In all patients, an improvement of oxygenation after initiation of ventilation according to the Open Lung Approach was noticed. The mean oxygenation index (p_aO_2/F_iO_2) increased from 132 ± 88 to 325 ± 64 measured 24 hours after the first recruitment maneuver ($p < 0.001$). The F_iO_2 necessary to provide a P_aO_2 around 100 mmHg decreased from 0.73 ± 0.21 to 0.39 ± 0.06 after 24 hours ($p < 0.001$). The p_aCO_2 increased from 37.0 ± 5.4 mmHg to 40.6 ± 4.4 mmHg 24 hours later. Mean PEEP level after the onset of Open Lung ventilation was 14.9 ± 2.7 mmHg (range: 10–19 mmHg). The first recruiting maneuver had to be repeated due to derecruitment in 5 patients. Complications as tension pneumothorax due to a recruitment maneuver did not occur.

Comparing mean as well as peak ICP values in the last 24 hours before the first recruitment maneuver with mean respectively peak ICP value in the next 24 hours, a slight but insignificant decrease was noticed (14.8 ± 8.1 mmHg vs. 13.7 ± 6.4 mmHg mean ICP, n.s., resp. 18.6 ± 11.2 mmHg vs. 18.1 ± 7.4 mmHg peak ICP, n.s.). Patients with lower mean ICP values tended to increase, while patients with higher mean ICP values were more likely to decrease in mean ICP values (Fig. 1). Two patients with an initial ICP value below 20 mmHg needed additional ICP treatment, which consisted of additional mannitol in one patient and deepening of analgosedation in another. Other ICP rises attributable to initiation of Open Lung ventilation were not noticed. No patient had to be withdrawn from Open Lung ventilation due to an increase in ICP.

Discussion

Low tidal volume ventilation and the Open Lung Approach are the first ways of mechanical ventilation proven in randomized controlled trials in achieving a better survival in patients with acute lung injury or ARDS. However, up to now in the literature on ARDS in neurosurgical patients no experience with Open Lung ventilation is reported; only casual reports exist on low tidal volume ventilation [11]. The experience with elevated PEEP level concepts in neurosurgical patients is controversial. The most frequent findings over the last three decades are that elevated PEEP levels may lead to a moderate ICP increase in patients with previously normal ICP, while in patients with already high ICP no further increase is found [2, 4, 7]. Our data supports this observation. Even permissive hypercapnia may be well tolerated in neurosurgical patients if applied gradually [11].

Table 1. *Oxygenation Values and ICP Data*

	Before first recruitment	After first recruitment	Significance
F_iO_2[mmHg]	73 ± 20	39 ± 6	$p < 0.001$
P_aO_2/F_iO_2	132 ± 88	325 ± 64	$p < 0.001$
P_aCO_2 [mmHg]	37.0 ± 5.4	40.6 ± 4.4	$p = 0.006$
ICP mean [mmHg]	14.8 ± 8.1	13.7 ± 6.4	n.s.
ICP peak [mmHg]	18.6 ± 11.2 mmHg	18.1 ± 7.4	n.s

Oxygenation values and ICP data 24 hours before and after first recruitment (mean $\pm$ SEM). Oxygenation data is given as values directly before initiation of Open Lung ventilation and 24 hours later; ICP data is given as 24-hour time course before and after initiation of Open Lung ventilation.

Two recent studies showed that low tidal volume ventilation leads to a decreased systemic release of proinflammatory cytocines [10, 12], which are elevated in neurosurgical patients with unfavourable outcome [8, 9]. The observed decrease in mean ICP data, which is a major factor relevant for outcome in brain injured patients [5], may therefore possibly be explained by a diminished inflammatory process due to a decreased liberation of proinflammatory cytokines during Open Lung ventilation.

Although lacking of a control group, the presented data shows the feasibility of the Open Lung Approach in neurosurgical patients with concomitant lung injury. There is no reason to routinely exclude patients with intracranial lesions from Open Lung ventilation. In our opinion, the potential risk of intracranial deterioration seems far lower than the achievable benefit of improved oxygenation with Open Lung ventilation. However, the existing data does not support to apply this ventilator strategy without concern in neurosurgical patients. Careful monitoring of pulmonary function, hemodynamic parameters and ICP is mandatory.

References

1. Amato MB, Barbas CS, Medeiros DM *et al* (1998) Effect of a protective-ventilation strategy on mortality in the acute respiratory distress syndrome. N Engl J Med 338: 347–354
2. Apuzzo LJ, Wiess MH, Petersons V *et al* (1977) Effect of positive end expiratory pressure ventilation on intracranial pressure in man. J Neurosurg 46: 227–232
3. Artigas A, Bernard GR, Carlet J *et al* (1998) The American-European Consensus Conference on ARDS, part 2. Ventilatory, pharmacologic, supportive therapy, study design strategies and issues related to recovery and remodeling. Intensive Care Med 24: 378–398
4. Cooper KR, Boswell PA, Choi SC (1985) Safe use of PEEP in patients with severe head injury. J Neurosurg 63: 552–555
5. Juul N, Morris GF, Marshall SB *et al* (2000) Intracranial hypertension and cerebral perfusion pressure influence on neurological deterioration and outcome in severe head injury. J Neurosurg 92: 1–6
6. Lachmann B (1992) Open Up the Lung and keep the lung open. Intensive Care Med 18: 319–321
7. McGuire G, Crossley D, Richards J *et al* (1997) Effects of varying levels of positive end-expiratory pressure on intracranial pressure and cerebral perfusion pressure. Crit Care Med 25: 1059–1062
8. McKeating EG, Andrews PJ, Signorini DF *et al* (1997) Transcranial cytokine gradients in patients requiring intensive care after acute brain injury. Br J Anaesth 78: 520–523
9. Osuka K, Suzuki Y, Tanazawa T *et al* (1998) Interleukin-6 and development of vasospasm after subarachnoid haemorrhage. Acta Neurochir (Wien) 140: 943–951
10. Ranieri M, Suter M, Tortorella, C *et al* (1999) Effect of mechanical ventilation on inflammatory mediators in patients with acute respiratory distress syndrome: a randomized controlled trial. JAMA 282: 54–61
11. Tasker RC, Peters MJ (1998) Combined lung injury, meningitis and cerebral edema: how permissive can hypercapnia be? Int Care Med 24: 616–619
12. The Acute Respiratory Distress Syndrome Network (2000) Ventilation with lower tidal volumes as compared with traditional tidal volumes for acute lung injury and the acute respiratory distress syndrome. N Engl J Med 342: 1301–1308

Correspondence: Dr. S. Wolf, Department of Neurosurgery, Academic Hospital Munich-Bogenhausen, Technical University of Munich, München, Germany.

Acta Neurochir (2002) [Suppl] 81: 103–105

Optimizing Cerebral Perfusion Pressure During Fiberoptic Bronchoscopy in Severe Head Injury: Effect of Hyperventilation

I. J. Previgliano[1], P. I. Ripoll[1], G. Chiappero[1], F. Galíndez[2], L. Germani[2], D. H. González[1], N. Ferrari[1], A. Hlavnicka[1], and C. Purvis[3]

[1] ICU Hospital Fernández and Antártida Private Hospital, University del Salvador, Argentina
[2] Respiratory Medicine Antártida Private Hospital, Argentina
[3] Neurosurgery Resident Hospital Fernández, Argentina

Summary

The aim of this study was to evaluate if Hyperventilation (HV) could avoid the Intracranial Pressure (ICP) peak that occurs during Fiberoptic Bronchoscopy (FB) in severely head injured patients. A Cerebral Perfusion Pressure (CPP) > 75 mmHg was maintained in 34 patients, with a subgroup randomized to receive controlled HV during FB. Measurements were done before the procedure, during maximum ICP values and 30 minutes after FB. The HV group had minor ICP values after FB, without differences in CPP and ICP peak values.

Keywords: Fiberoptic bronchoscopy; head injury; hyperventilation.

Introduction

Several hemodynamic changes can occur while Fiberoptic Bronchoscopy (FB) is performed in head injured patients. One of the most important is the peak of Intracranial Pressure (ICP) that frequently occurs during the procedure. Even though there are some papers that ensure that FB is a safe procedure [1, 8, 9], none of them have analyzed all the cerebral and non cerebral variables that play a role in that setting. In previous investigations we found out that optimizing Cerebral Perfusion Pressure (CPP) during FB can minimize cerebral hemodynamic changes. We hypothized that hyperventilation (HV) during FB could avoid or buffer the ICP peak during the placement of the bronchoscope.

Material and Methods

Setting: Intensive Care Unit at University affiliated, private (Antártida) and public (Fernández) Hospitals.

Study design: multicentre, prospective, controlled, randomized trial.

Inclusion criteria: severe closed head injury defined as Glasgow Coma Scale (GCS) < 8 after cardio-respiratory resuscitation; FB indicated for Bronchoalveolar Lavage (BAL) or athelectasis resolution.

Interventions: All patients were intubated and mechanically ventilated and had an ICP monitoring device (Camino Laboratories, San Diego, Calif), arterial oxygen pulse saturometry (SpO2) and arterial and central venous lines. Patients allocated to the HV group also had end-tidal carbon dioxide (ETCO2) monitor (Novametrix), as well as a near-infrared cortical oxygen saturation (rSO2) monitor (Somanetics, Invos 3000, Troy, Mi). All of them were sedated with midazolam, under analgesia with morphine and paralyzed with pancuronium bromide. None of the patients received steroids. All patients had hemoglobin levels between 9.5 and 12 mg%. FB was performed using a bronchoscope (Pentax FB 15 A 5,0 mm external diameter) through a swivel adapter.

All patients were ventilated according to Meduri's recommendations for FB.

CPP was calculated as the difference between MAP and ICP. Patients were randomly assigned to a CPP management (CPP group) or to CPP plus HV (HV group). For both groups a CPP > 75 mmHg was tried to be achieved with fluids and inotropic drugs. In addition, HV group's hemodynamics was intended to be optimized to: a) ETCO2 (< 30 mmHg) and b) rSO2 55–75%, which was achieved by means of augmenting respiratory rate. After FB the ventilator was set to basal parameters.

Measured parameters: mean arterial pressure (MAP), ICP, CPP, ETCO2, arterial carbon dioxide (PCO2), SpO2, rSO2, respiratory and cardiac rate. All these parameters were recorded at the beginning of the FB (B), at the maximum ICP value during FB (Mx), and at 30 minutes after FB (A), except PCO2 that was recorded B & A in the CPP group and before HV (BB), B & A in the HV group. rSO2 values were recorded BB, B, Mx and A only in the HV group. The ICP gradients (Δ) were calculated from (B-Mx) and (B-A).

Statistical analysis: Student's t test for difference of means.

Results

Since January 1st 1998 to January 31st 1999, 34 patients were enrolled. Sixteen belonged to the CPP group and 18 to the HV group.

Table 1. *Demographic Characteristics*

	CPP Group (n = 16)	HV Group (n = 18)
Age	39 ± 12	39 ± 22
Male	15 (94%)	15 (83%)
Female	1 (6%)	3 (17%)

Table 2. *Hemodynamic Values*

	CPP Group	HV Group
MAP (B)	101 ± 15	104 ± 20
MAP (Mx)	120 ± 22	113 ± 22
MAP (A)	107 ± 31	98 ± 18
CPP (B)	83 ± 18	90 ± 18
CPP (Mx)	80 ± 26	83 ± 22
CPP (A)	78 ± 26	84 ± 18
ICP (B)	18 ± 9	14 ± 10
ICP (Mx)	40 ± 24	30 ± 12
ICP (A)	30 ± 15	14 ± 6

Table 3. *PCO2 and rSO2 Values for each Group of Patients*

	CPP Group	HV Group
PCO_2 (BB)		33 ± 6
PCO_2 (B)	35 ± 6	27 ± 3
PCO_2 (A)	41 ± 7	31 ± 4
rSO_2 (B)		70 ± 6
rSO_2 (Mx)		72 ± 11
rSO_2 (A)		73 ± 7

Table 4. *Δ ICP Values for each Group of Patients*

	CPP Group	HV Group
ΔICP (BMx)	−16 ± 9	−20 ± 16
ΔICP (B-A)	−11 ± 11	6 ± 16

Their demographic characteristics are shown in Table 1. There were no substantial differences among both groups.

Hemodynamic values are shown in Table 2, PCO2 and rSO2 values in Table 3 and ICP in Table 4, with mean values and standard deviations. Statistical differences (two tails) were found for PCO2 B ($p < 0.01$) and A ($p < 0.01$) minor in HV group, ICP A ($p < 0.01$) minor in HV group, Δ ICP (B-A) (p 0.01) minor in HV group.

Discussion

Regarding previous papers [9], we didn't have episodes of arterial hypotension along the complete procedure. This is a considerable difference, taking into account that in-hospital hypotension has proved to worsen neurological outcome [5–6]. The key for this finding is the active management of MAP with fluids and inotropic agents [10, 12], which differs from the classic protocols of fluid restriction, but is in accordance with the recently published Guidelines for the Management of Severe Head Injury [4]. CPP accompanied the changes in MAP at all different moments of the FB, as it occurs in Keving's paper [8], revealing that autoregulation was conserved. Mean CPP values in this paper are in accordance with our findings.

The ICP peak developed during FB has no explanation. All the patients were properly sedated, under analgesia and neuromuscular blockade. They had no cough reflex and they also couldn't perform a Valsalva maneuver. One explanation given by Peerless *et al.* [1] is that a decrease in the cross-sectional area of the endotracheal tube (ETT) occurs when a bronchoscope is placed for FB generating an increase on the intrinsic positive end expiratory pressure. In their study, they didn't find a correlation between ETT size and increase of ICP, and neither do us. In that study they neither measured PCO2 nor ETCO2 and left the question open if the raises in ICP could be attributed to increased levels of CO2. Our results, measuring ETCO2, showed no correlation with ICP because they were in the normal range. On the other hand, none have shown that the modifications on the cross-sectional area of the airway by FB could generate changes in the air dead space; so the relationship between ETCO2 and PCO2 should remain unchanged.

One possible explanation can be found in Rosner's vasodilatory and vasoconstrictory cascades [11–12], but the CPP levels were in the range of autoregulation as is evident by the raises in MAP that followed raises in ICP.

Even though patients in the HV group had minor absolute ICP values after the procedure and in Δ ICP B-A, there were no statistical differences in CPP, MAP, peak ICP (Mx) values, and in Δ ICP B-Mx. The ICP peak during FB could not be abolished either by optimizing CPP or by HV.

Taking into account Bouma's papers [2–3] assuring that HV is harmful in the management of head injured patients, our results show that HV has no role in preventing the ICP peak during FB. We conclude that mantaining a CPP above 75 mmHg during FB is enough to make it a safe procedure, since no changes are shown with HV.

References

1. Bajwa MK, Henein S, Kamholz SL (1993) Fiberoptic bronchoscopy in the presence of Space-occupying Intracranial Lesions. Chest 104: 101–103
2. Bouma GJ, Muizelaar JP, Choi SC, Newlon PG, Young HF (1991) Cerebral circulation and metabolism after severe traumatic brain injury: the elusive role of ischemia. J Neurosurg 75: 685–693
3. Bouma GJ, Muizelaar JP (1995) Cerebral blood flow in severe clinical head injury. New Horiz 3: 384–394
4. Bullock R, Chesnut R, Clifton G *et al* (1996) In Brain trauma foundation (ed) Guidelines for the management of severe head injury. Brain Trauma Foundation, New York
5. Chesnut RM, Marshall SB, Piek J *et al* (1993) Early and late systemic hypotension as a frequent and fundamental source of cerebral ischemia following severe brain injury in the Traumatic Coma Data Bank. Acta Neurochir (Wien) [Suppl] 59: 121–126
6. Chesnut RM (1997) Avoidance of hypotension: conditio sine qua non of successful severe head-injury management. J Trauma 42: S4–S9
7. Kerwin AJ, Croce MA, Timmons SD, Maxwell RA, Malhotra AK, Fabian TC (2000) Effects of fiberoptic bronchoscopy on intracranial pressure in patients with brain injury: a prospective clinical study. J Trauma 48: 878–882
8. Lee TS (1994) Fiberoptic bronchoscopy and intracranial pressure. Chest 107: 1909
9. Peerless JR, Snow N, Likavec MJ, Pinchak AC, Malangoni MA (1995) The effect of fiberoptic bronchoscopy on cerebral hemodynamics in patients with severe head injury. Chest 108: 962–965
10. Previgliano I, Ceraso D, Rozas MC, Ferrari N, Vidiella E (1997) Cerebral perfusion pressure management in head injury. Crit Rev Neurosurg 7: 36–44
11. Rosner MJ (1993) Pathophysiology and management of increased intracranial pressure. In: Andrews BT (ed) Neurosurgical intensive care. McGraw Hill, San Francisco, pp 57–112
12. Rosner MJ, Rosner SD, Johnson AH (1995) Cerebral perfusion pressure: management protocol and clinical results. J Neurosurg 83: 949–962

Correspondence: Ignacio J. Previgliano, Virrey Loreto 2676 7°, 1426 Buenos Aires, Argentina.

Assessment of Cerebrovascular Reactivity

Acta Neurochir (2002) [Suppl] 81: 109–111

ICP and CBF Regulation: Effect of the Decompressive Craniectomy

A. Carmelo[1], **A. Ficola**[2], **M. L. Fravolini**[2], **M. La Cava**[2], **G. Maira**[1], **A. Mangiola**[1], and **E. Marchese**[1]

[1] Institute of Neurosurgery, Catholic University, Rome, Italy
[2] Institute of Electronics, University of Perugia, Italy

Summary

The view of the intracranial system as a rigid and closed box has been criticised by many authors who take into account the possibility of a certain degree of elastic bulk accommodation, mainly in the spinal sac.

In nine patients, who underwent decompressive craniectomy for treatment of life-threatening intracranial hypertension, when the clinical conditions improved, just before cranioplasty, the blood flow velocities at middle cerebral artery (MCA) and at superior sagittal sinus (SSS) level were simultaneously recorded. The measurements were repeated after cranioplasty.

The blood flow velocity recorded from SSS in craniectomized patients appeared flat, without evident pulsation; after cranioplasty a clear-cut pulsatile wave became again evident.

The disappearance of a pulsatile shape in the blood flow velocity recorded from the SSS when the intracranial system was "open" and the reappearance of a pulsatile blood flow waveform after the "closure" of the skull confirm that the venous bed acts as a bulk compensatory system in order to maintain the intracranial volume absolutely constant.

Keywords: Intracranial system; CBF velocity; decompressive craniectomy.

Introduction

Most authors conceive the cerebrospinal space as an elastic system able to expand or reduce in order to damp changes in its volume, as those related to arterial input [1] or those artificially induced by fluid injection or withdrawal [2, 3]. This volume buffering-capacity, in the opinion of the authors, is mainly located at the spinal level where the dura is not enclosed within a "rigid" container like the skull. Shapiro *et al.* [5] clearly demonstrated the great importance of the dural envelopes not depending on the integrity of the skull, in determining the "stiffness" of the intracranial system, so re-proposing a more strict interpretation of the Monro-Kellie doctrine. Intracranial system, i.e. an incompressible organ contained within a stiff envelope, has to keep absolutely constant its internal volume in order to maintain an adequate perfusion. In such a system any change in volume, however small, if not immediately and totally compensated, will cause an increase in the outflow resistance potentially able to determine a vicious circle eventually leading to the disastrous condition of cerebral circulatory arrest (so-called "brain tamponade"). This is also true for the physiological volume perturbations associated with the arterial inflow during each cardiac cycle: in our opinion they must be instantaneously compensated by venous outflow modifications. Cerebrospinal fluid (CSF), surrounding basal arteries and bridging veins, acts as a hydraulic piston, moved from arterial vasodilation to compress the distal collapsible part of cerebral veins. By means of this mechanism, an amount of blood exactly equivalent to the arterial volume displacement associated to cerebral blood inflow is expelled from the intracranial system, so maintaining absolutely constant the intracranial volume. Since the crucial point of this hypothesis is represented by the closure of the intracranial system to atmosphere, we planned a clinical-experimental study in order to evaluate the occurring haemodynamic changes following the removal of the skull and the enlargement of the dura mater (so-called "decompressive craniectomy").

Materials and Methods

Nine patients, who underwent decompressive craniectomy for the treatment of a life-threatening condition of an otherwise untreatable intracranial hypertension, are the object of this study.

When the ICP was definitively under control and the brain protrusion through the skull window disappeared, we planned the closure of the intracranial system. Just before this last surgical proce-

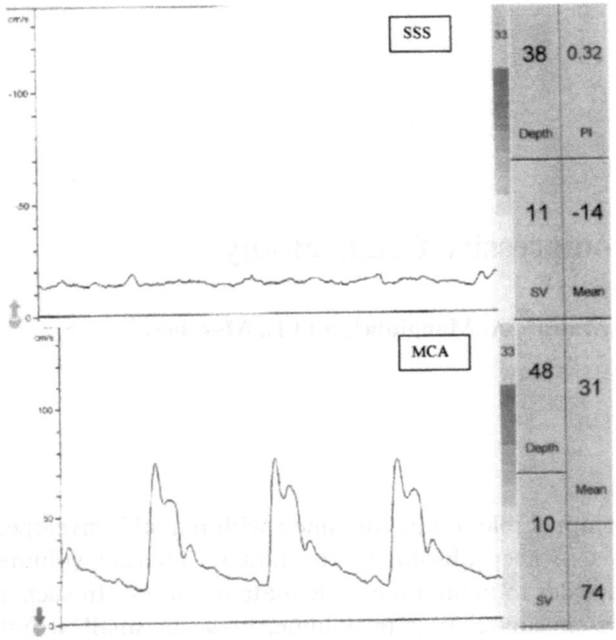

Fig. 1. Blood flow velocity recordings from SSS (upper trace) and MCA (lower trace) in a patient with decompressive craniectomy and dural enlargement

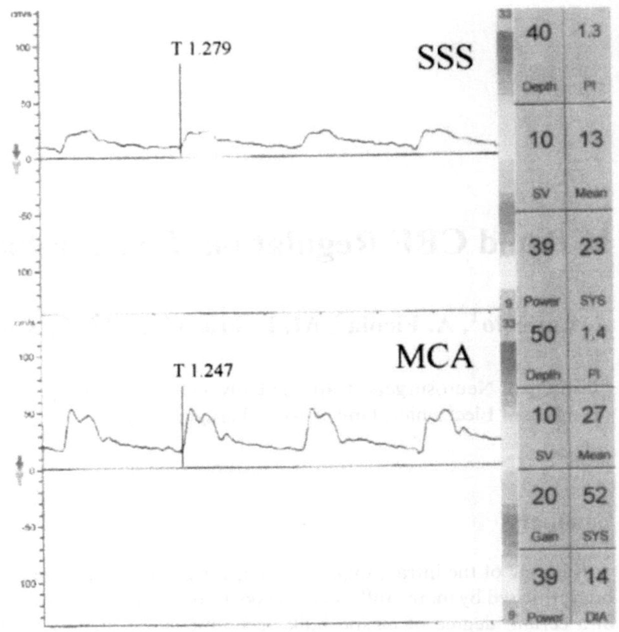

Fig. 2. Simultaneous blood flow velocity recordings from SSS (upper trace) and MCA (lower trace) in the same patient of figure 1 after cranioplasty. The delay between arterial and venous blood flow velocity was 32 msec

dure, the blood flow velocities at MCA and at SSS level were simultaneously recorded by means of two 5 MHz transcranial probes (Nicolet Pioneer System, Nicolet Biomedical, Madison Wi). Particular care was put in positioning the probe on the SSS, in order to be able to reproduce, after the cranioplasty, the same orientation for a correct insonation of the vascular structure. To this aim, at closure of the skull, a little window (utilising, eventually, a pre-existing burr-hole) was made in the operculum. Blood flow velocity recordings were repeated after cranioplasty with the same modalities as before.

Results

In craniectomized patients, when the intracranial system was open, the blood flow velocity wave at SSS level appeared flat, without any clear evidence of a pulsatile shape. On the contrary, the MCA blood flow velocity waveform was similar to that observed in normal subjects (Fig. 1).

In all patients, after the cranioplasty, a clear-cut blood flow velocity pulsatile wave was observed at SSS level. This waveform was synchronous with that recorded at MCA level, the delay ranging between 30 and 40 msec (Fig. 2).

Discussion

The disappearance of a pulsatile shape in the blood flow velocity recorded from the SSS when the intracranial system is "open" and the reappearance of a pulsatile blood flow waveform after the "closure" of the skull seem to confirm that, in normal conditions at least, the venous bed acts as a bulk compensatory mechanism in order to maintain the intracranial volume absolutely constant.

In other words, when the intracranial system is open, the cerebral blood volume increase, due to the arterial input inflow, is compensated by the brain expansion to the atmosphere and no CSF mediated cuff-compression on the veins is determined by the arterial dilatation: no pulsatile shape of blood flow velocity is observed at SSS level. The closure of the intracranial system restores the above-mentioned hydraulic mechanism.

The second finding shown in this study concerns the delay between arterial and venous blood flow velocity. Even if we assume a pulse propagation rate of 5 m/sec (the highest propagation rate at aortic level) and consider the length of the cerebral vascular tree in humans (from 60 to 80 cm; not the total length, obviously, but the shortest distance between the arterial inlet and the venous outlet), the very short delays we recorded in our clinical observations are more in agreement with an extravascular transmission through CSF pathways (shorter distance: shorter delay) rather than with an intravascular transmission through the cerebral vasculature (longer distance: longer delay).

In conclusion, both findings reported here agree with our above mentioned hypothesis regarding the hydraulic mechanism regulating the intracranial volume and the cerebral perfusion, and reaffirm the validity of the old Monro-Kellie doctrine. Futhermore, a source of the CSF pulse pressure from the venous bed instead of the arterial one [4] can no longer be sustained.

References

1. Avezaat CJJ, van Eijndhoven JHM, Wyper DJ (1979) Cerebrospinal fluid pulse pressure and intracranial volume-pressure relationships. J Neurol Neurosurg Psych 42: 687–700
2. Marmarou A (1973) A theoretical model and experimental evaluation of the cerebrospinal system. Thesis, Drexel University
3. Miller JD, Pickard JD (1974) Intracranial volume-pressure studies in patients with head injury. Injury 5: 265–269
4. Portnoy HD, Chopp M, Branch C (1983) Hydraulic model of myogenic autoregulation and the cerebrovascular bed: the effects of altering systemic arterial pressure. Neurosurgery 13: 482–498
5. Shapiro K, Fried A, Takei F, Kohm I (1985) Effects of the dura opening on neural axis pressure-volume relationships and CSF dynamics. J Neurosurg 63: 76–81

Correspondence: Anile Carmelo, M.D., Institute of Neurosurgery, Catholic University, Largo "A. Gemelli" 8, 00168 Roma, Italy.

Acta Neurochir (2002) [Suppl] 81: 113–116

ICP and CBF Regulation: A new Hypothesis to Explain the "Windkessel" Phenomenon

A. Carmelo[1], A. Ficola[2], M. L. Fravolini[2], M. La Cava[2], G. Maira[1], and A. Mangiola[1]

[1] Institute of Neurosurgery, Catholic University, Rome, Italy
[2] Institute of Electronics, University of Perugia, Italy

Summary

The brain tamponade represents the final condition of a progressive intracranial pressure (ICP) increase up to values close to arterial blood pressure (BP) producing a reverberating flow pattern in the cerebral arteries with no net flow. This finding implies intracranial volume changes, therefore a full application of the Monro-Kellie doctrine is impossible. To resolve this contradiction, in eight pigs a reversible condition of brain tamponade was produced by infusing saline into a cerebral ventricle. The following parameters were measured: BP in the common carotid artery, ICP by the same needle utilised for the infusion, arterial and venous blood flow velocity (BFV) at, respectively, internal carotid artery (ICA) and sagittal sinus (SS) site by ultrasound technique.

When ICP approached carotid BP values, reverberating BFV waves both at ICA and SS site were simultaneously observed. The arterial and venous reverberating waves appeared to be almost exactly superimposable, with a delay of about 40 msec. This synchronism between the pulsatile arterial and venous BFV indicates that the residual pulsation, still occurring at the arterial proximal level, is compensated by a passive compression-distension of the SS with no blood volume (that is net flow) crossing the intracranial vasculature.

Keywords: Brain tamponade; windkessel phenomenon; cerebral blood flow velocity.

Introduction

It is known that an increase in ICP above 40 mmHg may produce a reduction in cerebral blood flow (CBF) up to intracranial blood circulation arrest (the so-called "brain tamponade") when ICP approaches arterial BP [3]. This phenomenon is explained by the so-called "vasodilatory cascade" [5], that is a progressive increase in the intracranial blood volume due, initially, to the arterial-arteriolar vasodilation and, subsequently, to the venous engorgement caused by bridging veins compression [6] at site of "lacunae laterales". The obstacle to venous outflow determines in a closed intracranial system, the stop of the arterial inflow too. In this condition a reverberating flow pattern in the cerebral arteries, both at extracranial and intracranial level, with no net flow, has been already demonstrated. In the opinion of many authors the reverberating flow occurs because "... the blood column in the large brain-supplying arteries does not completely stop but oscillates due to elasticity of the arterial wall ... This so-called stroke volume reflects a corresponding *volume change* in the distal vasculature ..." [4]. This condition is regarded as an ideal "windkessel" (air-chamber) model, that is a *compliant* system in which flow is proportional to pressure. This statement, however, does not take into consideration that in a closed and "rigid" system, like the intracranial system, there is no "physical" space to allow the changes in arterial blood volume provoked by the arterial "elastic" oscillations. Indeed, even if we assume that in normal conditions small intracranial volume changes can be damped by cerebrospinal fluid (CSF) displacement into the spinal sac, no CSF passage through occipital foramen may happen in brain tamponade condition.

To resolve this contradiction we studied the following experimental model.

Materials and Methods

In eight domestic pigs (all female) weighing between 20 and 25 kg, an experimental reversible condition of intracranial hypertension was produced by infusing saline into a lateral ventricle until ICP approached carotid BP ("brain tamponade" condition). The animals were tranquilized with 5 mg/kg ketamine, paralysed with 0.4 mg/kg pancuronium bromide and mechanically ventilated with a gas mixture of 0.5–1% halothane, 50% N_2O, and the remainder oxygen. The respiration of the animals was adjusted to yield a $PaCO_2$ of about 35 mmHg and a PaO_2 of more than 100 mmHg.

ICP was measured through the same 18 G epidural needle utilised for the infusion; carotid BP through a 16 G catheter inserted into the right common carotid artery in the neck. CBF velocities were simultaneously measured by utilising two ultrasound 8- and 4-MHz continuous wave probes located intracranially at the SS and at the left ICA level through two adequately tailored skull windows positioned, respectively, in the posterior part of the middle vertex and in the left temporal bone. The anatomy of the intracranial cerebral arterial and venous system in pig is quite similar to that found in man; the SS, in particular, drains exclusively from cortical and bridging veins to systemic circulation.

The integrity of the skull was reconstituted with dental acrylic cement.

All signals were continuously recorded both on chart and on magnetic tape for delayed automatically data processing and storage utilising a self-developed software based on the Fourier's frequency analysis.

Saline was infused at a progressively increasing rate, starting from 12 ml/hr, until a condition of "brain tamponade" was reached as documented by the observation of a reverberating blood flow velocity wave pattern both at ICA and SS level with a mean value of zero. This condition was maintained for 15 min in four animals, 30 min in three and 60 min in the last one. At the end of the infusion the experimental observation was prolonged until intracranial and haemodynamic variables returned to basal values.

Results

In basal conditions the CBF mean velocities at SS and at ICA level ranged, respectively, from 8 to 12 and from 18 to 22 cm/sec. At both sites, furthermore, a typical pulsatile pattern synchronous with ICP pulsation was clearly evident. Saline infusion provoked, together with ICP increase, a progressive modification in arterial and venous CBF velocities. When ICP values approached carotid BP levels, BFV reverberating waves were simultaneously observed at ICA and SS sites so indicating a "brain tamponade" condition (Fig. 1).

Utilising delayed computerised data processing, the arterial and venous reverberating waves appear to be almost exactly superimposable with a delay, between arterial and venous waves, of about 40 msec.

In all the animals, at the end of the intraventricular infusion, ICP progressively decreased to initial values followed by arterial and venous BFV recovery to basal conditions.

Discussion

Starling [7] empirically documented the first observation concerning a pulsatile venous outflow at SS site synchronous with the arterial pulsation at the beginning of twentieth century. This finding, however, was subsequently so disregarded that the most widely accepted theoretical models of intracranial system considered the venous cerebral outflow as continuous, not pulsatile. On the basis of this incorrect assumption, the intracranial system was conceived as an elastic system able to expand or reduce in order to damp changes in its volume, as those related to arterial input or those artificially induced by fluid injection or withdrawal. Our previous experimental studies [2] and others' clinical observations [1] have, recently confirmed the former observation, re-stating the concept of an intracranial system at fixed and absolutely constant volume.

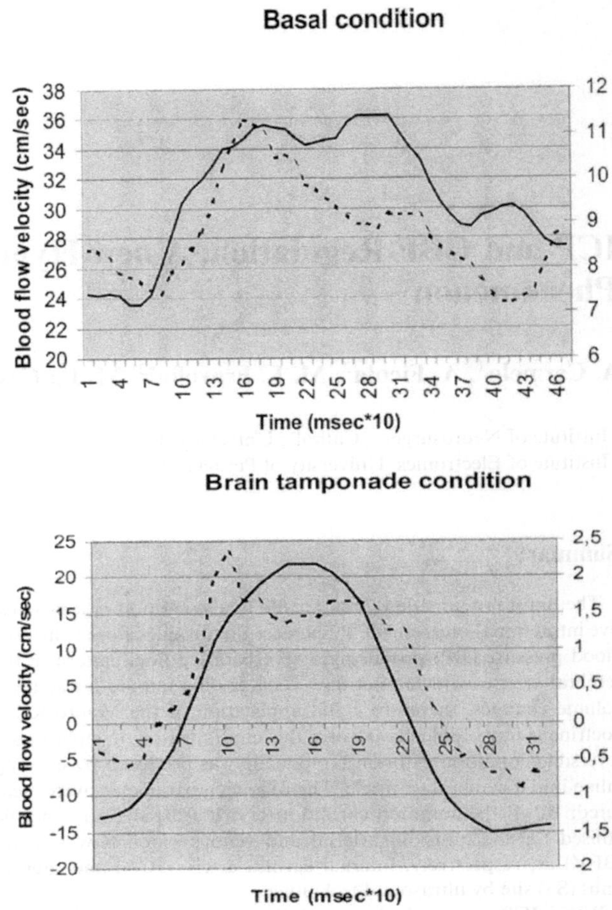

Fig. 1. Example of simultaneous recordings of ICA and SS blood flow velocity reverberating waves in brain tamponade condition: the delay between arterial and venous wave for each cardiac cycle is of about 40 msec. — ICA; ---- SS

Following this concept, in such a system the arterial inflow volume perturbations must be instantaneously compensated by venous outflow modifications. In a normal perfused brain, the CSF surrounding basal arteries and bridging veins acts as a hydraulic piston, moved from arterial vasodilation and compressing the distal collapsible part of cerebral veins. By means of

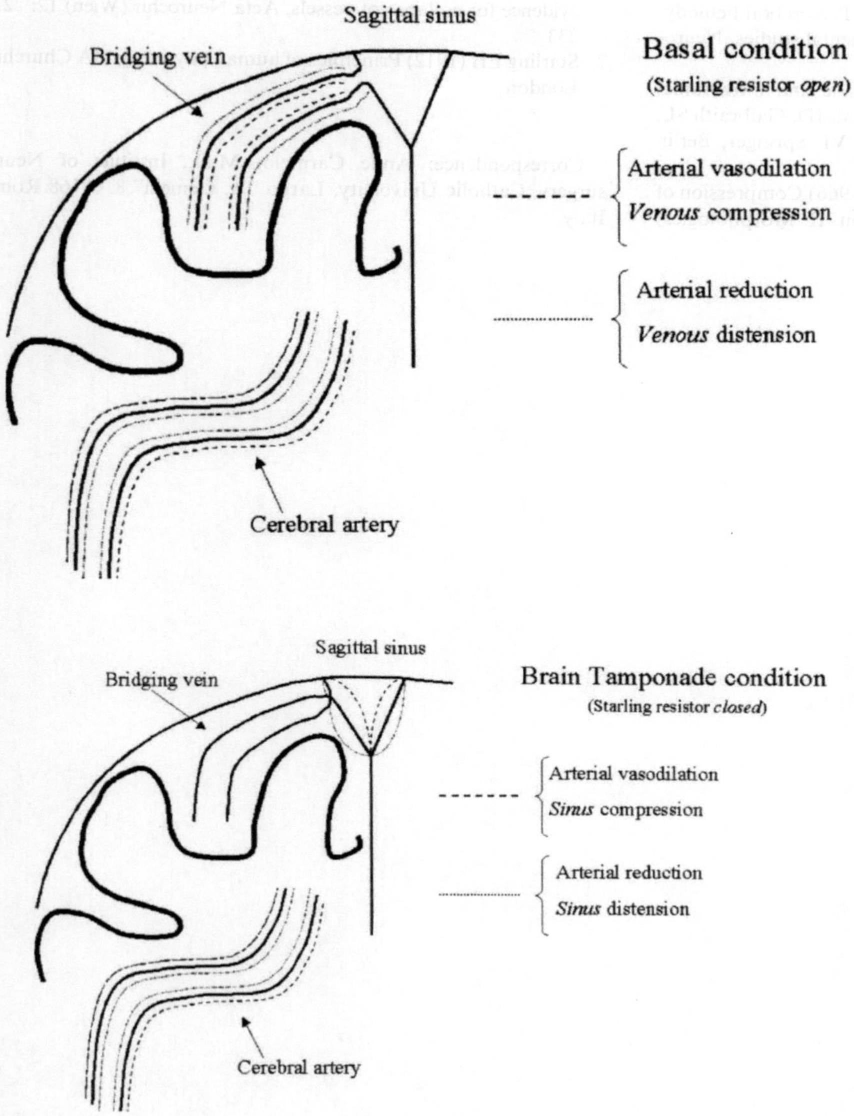

Fig. 2. The graphic illustrates the hydraulic mechanism underlying the simultaneous occurrence of reverberating waves both at arterial and venous (*SS*) site in "brain tamponade" condition (see text for full explanation)

this mechanism, an amount of blood exactly equivalent to the arterial volume displacement associated to cerebral blood inflow is expelled from the intracranial system, so maintaining absolutely constant the intracranial volume.

In a "brain tamponade" condition, when the volume buffering capacity of the venous bed is exhausted, the arterial pulsation is compensated by the passive oscillations of the SS walls (Fig. 2) with no blood volume (that is net flow) crossing the intracranial vasculature.

References

1. Aaslid R, Newell DW, Stooss R, Sorteberg W, Lindegaard K-F (1991) Assessment of cerebral autoregulation dynamics from simultaneous arterial and venous transcranial doppler recordings in humans. Stroke 22: 1148–1154
2. Anile C, Rinaldi A, Mangiola A, Amante P, Palma P, Maira G, Della Corte F, Calimici R and Ferraresi A (1993) Biomechanical regulation of cerebral blood flow. In: Avezaat CJJ, van Eijndhoven JHM, Maas AIR and Tans JThJ (eds) Intracranial pressure VIII. Springer, Berlin Heidelberg New York Tokyo, pp 265–268
3. Hassler W, Steinmetz H, Pirschel J (1989) Transcranial doppler study of intracranial circulatory arrest. J Neurosurg 71: 195–201

4. Lindegaard K-F, Grip A, Nornes H (1980) Precerebral hemodynamics in brain tamponade. Part 2: experimental studies. Neurochirurgia (Stuttg) 23: 187–196
5. Rosner MJ (1986) The vasodilatory cascade and intracranial pressure. In: Miller JD, Teasdale GM, Rowan JD, Galbraith SL, Mendelow AD (eds) Intracranial pressure VI. Springer, Berlin Heidelberg New York Tokyo, pp 137–141
6. Shapiro HM, Langfitt TW, Weinstein JD (1966) Compression of cerebral vessels by intracranial hypertension. II. Morphological evidence for collapse of vessels. Acta Neurochir (Wien) 12: 223–233
7. Starling EH (1912) Principles of human physiology. JA Churchill, London

Correspondence: Anile Carmelo, M.D., Institute of Neurosurgery, Catholic University, Largo "A. Gemelli" 8, 00168 Roma, Italy.

Acta Neurochir (2002) [Suppl] 81: 117–119

Clinical Significance of Cerebral Autoregulation

M. Czosnyka[1], P. Smielewski[2], S. Piechnik[1], and J. D. Pickard[1]

[1] Academic Neurosurgical Unit, Addenbrooke's Hospital, Cambridge, UK
[2] Wolfson Brain Imaging Centre, University of Cambridge, UK

Summary

Objectives. Disturbed cerebral autoregulation is believed to be associated with an unfavourable outcome following head injury. Previously, using ICP monitoring and transcranial Doppler ultrasonography, we investigated whether cerebral response to spontaneous variations in arterial pressure (ABP) or cerebral perfusion pressure (CPP) provide reliable information on cerebral autoregulatory reserve. In the present study we have correlated these methods with clinical findings.

Methods. 188 head injured sedated and ventilated patients were studied daily. Waveforms of intracranial pressure (ICP), arterial pressure and transcranial Doppler flow velocity (FV) were captured over a half to two hour periods. Time averaged mean flow velocity (FV) and CPP were resolved. The correlation coefficient indices between FV and CPP (Mx) and between ICP and ABP (PRx) were calculated over 3 minutes epochs, and averaged for each investigation.

Results. The relationship between indices of outoregulation and outcome (favourable-unfavourable) was significant and stronger than the association between admission GCS and outcome. With rigorously maintained CPP-oriented therapy relationship between CPP and outcome became non-significant. Mortality in patients with consistently disturbed autoregulation ranged 47%, while in patients with good autoregulation mortality was 11% (difference: $p < 0.0001$).

Conclusions. Positive values of indices of autoregulation, expressing positive association between slow waves of CPP and blood flow velocity or ABP and ICP, indicate disturbed autoregulation. These indices correlate with unfavourable outcome following head injury and should be used to guide intensive therapy.

Keywords: Head injury; transcranial Doppler; autoregulation; outcome.

Introduction

Factors determining outcome following head injury are still poorly identified [1, 2]. Traditionally, admission GCS, age, brain imaging were listed as strong predictors of outcome, but inclusion of other factors as ICP, CPP, pre-defined secondary insults, brain oxygentaion, etc., was problematic.

Methods

188 head-injured, sedated and ventilated patients were studied daily. Waveforms of intracranial pressure (ICP), arterial pressure and transcranial Doppler flow velocity (FV) were captured over periods ranging from half to two hour. Time averaged mean flow velocity (FV) and CPP were resolved. The correlation coefficients between FV and CPP (Mx) and between ABP and ICP (PRx) were calculated over 3 minutes epochs, and time-averaged for each investigation [3, 4].

Results

31% of patients had a good outcome, 21% were moderately disabled, 20% severely disabled, 3% (5 patients) were in persistent vegetative state and 25% died following their head injury.

For patients with favorable (good outcome and moderate disability) and unfavorable outcomes (severe disability, persistent vegetative state and dead) the studied variables were averaged and compared (Table 1). Patients with favorable outcome had better admission Glasgow Coma Score, had lower ICP and better autoregulation (lower values of Mx and PRx).

Rank correlation coefficients between GOS and the analyzed parameters were calculated and are listed in descending order of absolute R values. Worse outcome was associated with worse admission worse autoregulation Mx ($R = -0.2592$; $p < 0.0001$), worse pressure-reactivity index PRx ($R = 0.278$; $p < 0.0001$), higher intracranial pressure ($R = -0.195$; $p < 0.01$), worse GCS ($R = -0.18$; $p < 0.014$).

Correlations between outcome, CPP, ABP and FV did not reach statistical significance. Analysis of outcome was used to establish a threshold value for Mx (calculated as the value of Mx where the descriptor of the Kruskal-Wallis test reaches its maximum). A value

Table 1. *Mean (Standard Deviation) or Median Values of the Analyzed Parameters in Patients who Attained Favorable and Unfavorable Outcome Following Head Injury*

	Favorable	Unfavorable	P value (Mann-Whitney test)
GCS (medians)	4	6	$P < 0.0018$
Mx	−0.06 (0.26)	0.15 (0.31)	$P < 0.00002$
PRx	0.038 (0.26)	0.20 (0.34)	$P < 0.0008$
ABP [mm Hg]	88 (12)	91.3 (14)	$P = 0.15$
ICP [mm Hg]	17.0 (8.9)	23.0 (13)	$P < 0.007$
CPP [mm Hg]	71 (14.5)	68 (17.9)	$P = 0.26$
FV [cm/s]	63 (26)	60 (25)	$P = 0.33$
Age [years]	27	32	$P = 0.08$

FV Mean, flow velocity; *Mx* Mean Index of autoregulation; *ICP* intracranial pressure; *ABP* mean arterial blood pressure; *GOS* Glagow Outcome Score, *CPP* cerebral perfusion pressure.

of 0.23 was found (descriptor of the Kruskal-Wallis test: 17.7) indicating disturbed autoregulation associated with unfavorable outcome for values above this threshold and adequate autoregulation contributing to good outcome below this value.

Similar critical value for the PRx was 0.31 (Kruskal-Wallis test 19.8).

Analysis of outcome for patients with average disturbed and preserved autoregulation (Mx above and below the 0.23 threshold value) shows significant differences in all outcome groups (see Fig. 2) with the exception of persistent vegetative state but there were only 5 patients in this outcome group.

Mortality in patients with consistently disturbed autoregulation ranged 47%, while in patients with good autoregulation mortality was 11% (difference: $p < 0.0001$).

Correlation between PRx and Mx indices was significant ($R = 0.57$; $p < 0.00001$).

Discussion

Good correlation between autoregulation and outcome following head injury suggests that self-regulation of CBF is indeed a powerful brain protective mechanism.

Analysis of slow waves in TCD and CPP (Mx index) and ICP-ABP (PRx) index provides similar but not identical information. Indices therefore should be always considered together, and not as one substituting

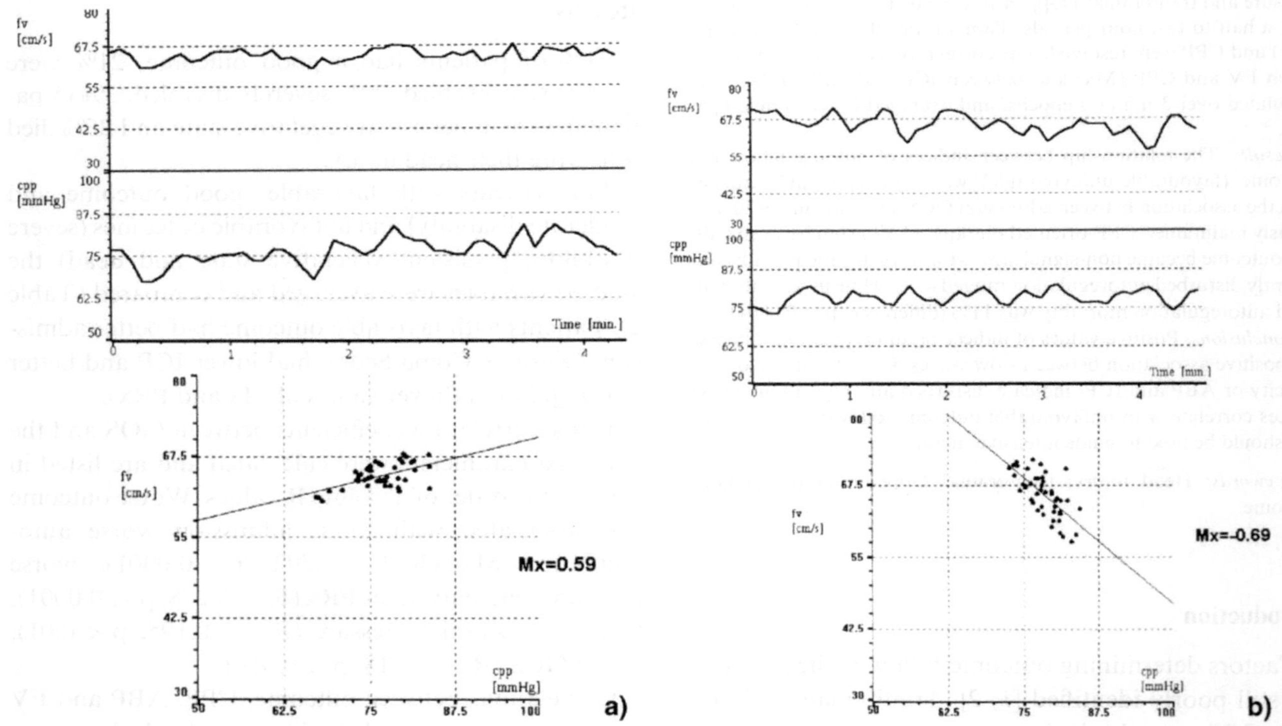

Fig. 1. Example of regression analysis of slow waves of CPP and Flow Velocity (*FV*), which explains interpretation of Mx as a correlation coefficient between CPP and FV from the shown limited time window. (a) On day 2 regression had a positive slope indicating disturbed autoregulation (CPP of 70 mmHg). (b) On next day CPP had increased to above 80 mmHg and Mx decreased to negative values, indicating good autoregulation

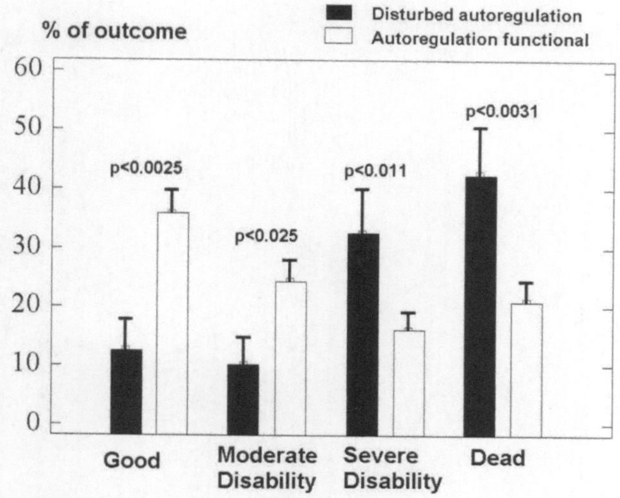

Fig. 2. Distribution of outcome in patients above (black) and below (white) threshold for averaged Mx (0.23). Difference in percentage in outcome in distinctive Glasgow Outcome Scale classes are given above bars. Standard error values are indicated

another. Very different modalities are taken into account for their calculation. Further studies are needed to identify possible clinical situations when PRx and Mx indices differ.

Both indices are suitable for continuous monitoring of cerebral circulation. It will be probably possible to use them to guide intensive therapy, but further prospective clinical studies are needed.

References

1. Bouma GJ, Muizelaar JP (1995) Cerebral blood flow in severe clinical head injury. New Horizons 3: 384–394
2. Cold GE, Jensen FT (1978) Cerebral autoregulation in unconscious patients with brain injury. Acta Anaesthesiol Scand 22: 270–280
3. Czosnyka M, Smielewski P, Kirkpatrick P, Menon DK, Pickard JD (1996) Monitoring of cerebral autoregulation in head-injured patients. Stroke 27: 829–834
4. Czosnyka M, Smielewski P, Kirkpatrick P, Laing RJ, Menon D, Pickard JD (1997) Continuous assessment of the cerebral vasomotor reactivity in head injury. Neurosurgery 41: 11–19

Correspondence: M. Czosnyka, Department of Neurosurgery, Box 167 Addenbrooke's Hospital, Cambridge CB2 2QQ, UK.

Acta Neurochir (2002) [Suppl] 81: 121–124

Routine Utilization of the Transient Hyperaemic Response Test after Aneurysmal Subarachnoid Haemorrhage*

T. Rätsep, J. Eelmäe, and T. Asser

Department of Neurology and Neurosurgery, University of Tartu, Estonia

Summary

In order to explore the applicability of daily cerebral autoregulation monitoring through routine utilization of the transient hyperaemic response (THR) test in patients after aneurysmal subarachnoid haemorrhage (SAH), we performed THR tests daily in 50 consecutive patients with verified SAH.

Out of 1167 studies, the test results were acceptable during 954 procedures (81.5%). 310 negative (32.5%; range 0.75–1.099; mean 1.03) and 644 positive (67.5%; range 1.10–1.77; mean 1.19) test results were obtained. Multiple logistic regression analysis revealed that the registration of negative THR in a middle cerebral artery (MCA) during the period of critical care was related to the patients' poor clinical grade (p-0.02) and Fisher CT-grade (p-0.04) on admission, to the development of vasospasm (p-0.003) and to the detection of ipsilateral intracerebral haemorrhage and/or cerebral infarction (p-0.01). The frequent registration of negative THR tests (negative results in >30% of all the tests in an MCA) was independently related to the detection of ipsilateral intracerebral haemorrhage and/or cerebral infarction (p-0.0001).

THR tests provide information about intracranial alterations and can be safely performed as a routine monitoring tool after SAH.

Keywords: Aneurysmal subarachnoid haemorrhage; cerebral autoregulation; transcranial Doppler; transient hyperaemic response.

Introduction

Defective cerebral autoregulation (CA) after aneurysmal subarachnoid haemorrhage (SAH) enhances vulnerability of the brain to secondary cerebral insults. Regular assessment of autoregulatory reserve could be useful especially in circumstances where it is critical to maintain cerebral perfusion. Several methods have been developed to evaluate CA, yet data about monitoring of CA in daily routine has remained insufficient.

The transient hyperaemic response (THR) test was introduced by Giller in 1991 [4] and later evaluated by a number of researchers [2, 6–8]. The test evaluates hyperaemic response of middle cerebral artery (MCA) blood flow velocity following brief carotid compression and is considered as a simple method to indicate intact or deranged autoregulation. As the THR test is noninvasive and easy to perform at the bedside, it could be suitable for regular assessment of CA in diverse clinical situations. Our study was aimed at exploring the applicability of daily CA monitoring by performing routine THR tests in patients with SAH.

Materials and Methods

The study was comprised of 50 consecutive patients (36 female and 14 male; age 25–82 years, mean 56 years) with verified aneurysmal SAH, treated at the Department of Neurosurgery at the University Hospital of Tartu, Estonia from Dec 1998 to March 2000. All patients were admitted during the acute phase of the disease (78% within 48 hours of the suspected bleed), the diagnosis of SAH was confirmed by computed tomography (CT) and aneurysm location was assessed using digital subtraction angiography (in two patients an aneurysm was revealed during emergency evacuation of intracerebral haemorrhage). The patients' clinical conditions on admission were assessed by means of the World Federation of Neurological Surgeons (WFNS) scale [1]. Initial CT scans were evaluated according to modified Fisher's CT-grading system [3] as follows: CT grade I – thin diffuse or localized blood layers; CT grade II – thick blood layers in at least 2 of the 4 subarachnoid compartments (Sylvian fissures, cortical surface, basal cisterns, frontal interhemispheric space); and CT grade III – thick blood layers in at least 3 of the 4 subarachnoid compartments. Acute hydrocephalus was defined as a bicaudate index above the upper limits for age [10]. Vasospasm was diagnosed according to transcranial Doppler (TCD) mean blood flow velocity (FV) values (FV > 120 cm/s in MCA and Lindegaard index [5] of >3). Consecutive CT scans were performed in all patients and all intracerebral haemorrhages (ICH) and cerebral infarctions (CI) were registered. All patients were treated at neurointensive care unit and the aneurysms were clipped in 47 patients. Ventricular

* This study was supported by grant No. 4333 from the Estonian Science Foundation.

drainage was used in patients with significant ventricular enlargement. All patients received Nimodipin. HHH-therapy was initiated if vasospasm had been diagnosed.

TCD examinations (MultiDop X, DWL, Ueberlingen, Germany) and THR tests in MCAs were performed daily starting from the first day after admission with a 2 MHz handheld probe. THR test results were calculated according to standard formulas [4, 7]. The heart cycle just preceding carotid compression was used to measure baseline systolic FV. Systolic FV during carotid compression was calculated as the average systolic FV from the first two heart cycles after the compression. Systolic FV during hyperaemia was calculated as the average systolic FV from the second and the third heart cycles after the release of the compression. The criteria for accepting THR tests included: 1) a sudden decrease in FV at the onset of compression; 2) stable Doppler signal during compression; 3) compression duration of ≥5 seconds; 4) compression ratios > 30%; 5) no significant response from baroreceptors. THR values above or equal to 1.10 were considered to indicate positive response and intact CA, while values below 1.10 were interpreted as negative response and impaired CA. A negative THR test was repeated at interval of >2 minutes and only the average value of the two tests was recorded for further analysis. For the purpose of statistical analysis, the examined vessels were dichotomized according to detection of negative THR tests (yes/no) and according to frequency of registration of negative THR tests (frequent/no or rare) during the surveillance period. The frequent registration of negative THR tests was defined as negative results in >30% of all the tests in a MCA during the monitoring period. TCD examinations which were consistent with cerebral circulatory arrest were excluded from the study.

Multiple logistic regression analysis (both forward and backward models) was applied to explore the relations between the disease characteristics (WFNS grade, Fisher CT-score, vasospasm, hydrocephalus, detection of ICH/CI) and THR test results in the examined arteries (SAS software, version 6.12, SAS Institute, Cary, North Carolina, USA). A p-value < 0.05 was considered statistically significant.

Results

The patients' clinical and CT characteristics and location of ruptured aneurysms are presented in Table 1.

1167 TCD studies were performed on 50 patients during 2–17 days (mean 12 days) after ictus and THR tests were considered acceptable during 954 procedures (81.7%). THR tests were non-acceptable in 213 cases (18.3%) with the following reasons for failure to carry out the tests: 1) difficulties to perform adequate carotid compression (113 cases; 53%); 2) increased psychomotor activity of the patients (81 cases; 38%); 3) inadequate bone windows (11 cases; 5%); 4) neck pain at carotid compression (8 cases; 4%). THR tests were always acceptable in 50 MCAs (50%). Data about the 7 vessels (7%) where the tests were always non-acceptable was excluded from further analysis. No complications occurred as the result of THR tests.

310 negative (32.5%; range 0.75–1.099; mean 1.03) and 644 positive (67.5%; range 1.10–1.77; mean 1.19) test results were obtained. More (>30%) negative THR tests were recorded in the first three days and from 7 to 14 days after ictus (Fig. 1) and in patients with impaired consciousness according to Glasgow Coma Scale [9] scores (Fig. 2). Negative tests were detected in 70 MCAs (75%). All the studies were positive in 23 (25%) and negative in 6 (6,5%) MCAs. Frequent negative THR tests were detected in 44 MCAs (47%).

With use of multiple logistic regression, 4 factors (initial WFNS grade > 2 and Fisher CT-grade ≥ 2, development of vasospasm and detection of ipsilateral

Table 1. *Characteristics of 50 Patients with SAH*

Characteristic		N	(%)
Aneurysm location			
	MCA	17	(34%)
	AcomA	17	(34%)
	ICA	7	(14%)
	ACA	3	(6%)
	BA	3	(6%)
	other	3	(6%)
WFNS grade			
	1	26	(52%)
	2	8	(16%)
	3	2	(4%)
	4	7	(14%)
	5	7	(14%)
Fisher CT-grade			
	1	18	(36%)
	2	18	(36%)
	3	14	(28%)
Hydrocephalus		16	(32%)
Vasospasm		34	(68%)
Cerebral infarction and/or intracerebral haemorrhage		34	(68%)

N Number of patients; *AcomA* anterior communicating artery; *MCA* middle cerebral artery; *ICA* internal carotid artery; *ACA* anterior cerebral artery; *BA* basilar artery; *WFNS* World Federation of Neurological Surgeons.

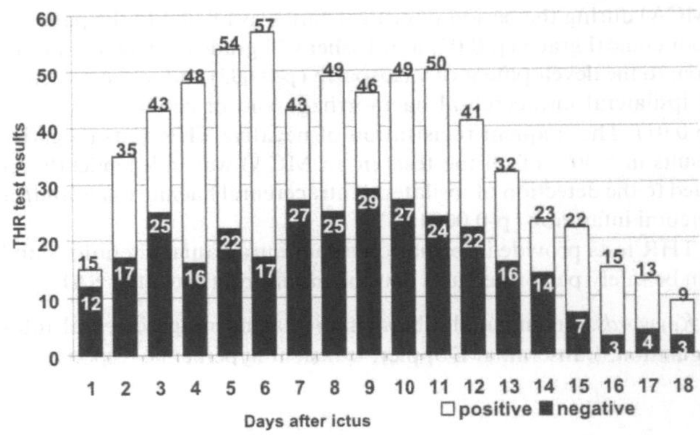

Fig. 1. Bar graph depicting the THR test results in different days after ictus. Note. The day of ictus has been registered as the zero day

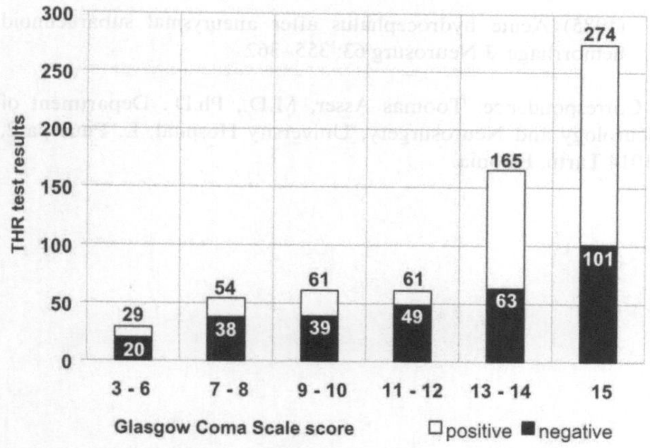

Fig. 2. Bar graph depicting the THR test results in patients with different level of consciousness according to Glasgow Coma Scale score

Table 2. *Factors Related to Registration and Frequent Registration of Negative THR Tests in the Examined Arteries by Multiple Logistic Regression Analysis*

Factors related to registration of negative THR tests in a MCA

Factor	only positive THR tests (N = 23)	negative THR tests (N = 70)	odds ratio	confidence intervals 95%	p-value
WFNS grade > 2	3	27	6.45	1.34–31.01	0.02
Fisher CT-grade ≥ 2	10	51	3.60	1.03–12.56	0.04
Vasospasm	5	44	7.94	2.00–31.44	0.003
Ipsilateral ICH/CI	2	38	8.49	1.66–43.35	0.01

Factors related to frequent registration of negative THR tests in a MCA

Factor	rare negative/ all positive THR tests (N = 49)	frequent negative THR tests (N = 44)	odds ratio	confidence intervals 95%	p-value
Ipsilateral ICH/CI	10	30	8.36	3.26–21.41	0.0001

Values are numbers of examined MCAs. *THR* Transient hyperaemic response; *MCA* middle cerebral artery; *WFNS* World Federation of Neurological Surgeons; *ICH/CI* intracerebral haemorrhage and/or cerebral infarction.

ICH/CI) were found to be independently associated with detection of negative THR in a MCA during the period of critical care (Table 2). Only detection of ipsilateral ICH/CI was independently related to the frequent registration of negative THR tests in a MCA (Table 2).

Discussion

The main objective of this study was to describe regular CA evaluation with THR tests during the period of critical care after SAH.

We succeeded in performing acceptable THR tests during 81.7% of the routine daily TCD examinations in patients with SAH. Regardless of the failure to carry out about 18% of the tests, the detection of negative test results was significantly associated with the disease characteristics. Although there has been considerable interest in bringing CA testing into clinical routine, technical difficulties and remarkable differences in patients' clinical conditions in conjunction with the potential danger from manipulations of arterial blood pressure have precluded daily utilization of the majority of CA tests after SAH. Our study indicates that the THR test is a simple method for repeated measurements and is exceptionally suitable for routine CA assessment in patients with SAH.

We conclude that daily monitoring of CA is safely executable with THR tests and, by providing information about intracranial alterations, could be useful in the management of SAH. However, the relevance of THR test results in certain clinical situations remains a subject for further studies.

References

1. Anonymous (1988) Report of World Federation of Neurological Surgeons Committee on a Universal Subarachnoid Hemorrhage Grading Scale. J Neurosurg 68: 985–986
2. Czosnyka M, Pickard J, Whitehouse H, Piechnik S (1992) The hyperaemic response to a transient reduction in cerebral perfusion pressure. A modelling study. Acta Neurochir (Wien) 115: 90–97
3. Fisher CM, Kistler JP, Davis JM (1980) Relation of cerebral vasospasm to subarachnoid hemorrhage visualized by computerized tomographic scanning. Neurosurgery 6: 1–9
4. Giller CA (1991) A bedside test for cerebral autoregulation using transcranial Doppler ultrasound. Acta Neurochir (Wien) 108: 7–14
5. Lindegaard KF, Nornes H, Bakke SJ, Sorteberg W, Nakstad P (1988) Cerebral vasospasm after subarachnoid haemorrhage investigated by means of transcranial Doppler ultrasound. Acta Neurochir (Wien) [Suppl] 42: 81–84
6. Smielewski P, Czosnyka M, Iyer V, Piechnik S, Whitehouse H, Pickard J (1995) Computerised transient hyperaemic response test – a method for the assessment of cerebral autoregulation. Ultrasound Med Biol 21: 599–611
7. Smielewski P, Czosnyka M, Kirkpatrick P, McEroy H, Rutkowska H, Pickard JD (1996) Assessment of cerebral autoregulation using carotid artery compression. Stroke 27: 2197–2203

8. Smielewski P, Czosnyka M, Kirkpatrick P, Pickard JD (1997) Evaluation of the transient hyperemic response test in head-injured patients. J Neurosurg 86: 773–778
9. Teasdale G, Jennett B (1974) Assessment of coma and impaired consciousness. A practical scale. Lancet 2: 81–84
10. van Gijn J, Hijdra A, Wijdicks EF, Vermeulen M, van Crevel H (1985) Acute hydrocephalus after aneurysmal subarachnoid hemorrhage. J Neurosurg 63: 355–362

Correspondence: Toomas Asser, M.D., Ph.D., Department of Neurology and Neurosurgery, University Hospital, L. Puusepa 2, 51014 Tartu, Estonia.

Acta Neurochir (2002) [Suppl] 81: 125–127

Is Transcranial Doppler Ultrasonography (TCD) Good Enough in Determining CO_2 Reactivity and Pressure Autoregulation in Head-Injured Patients?

S. C. P. Ng[1], W. S. Poon[1], M. T. V. Chan[2], J. M. K. Lam[1], and W. W. M. Lam[3]

[1] Neurosurgical Unit, Department of Surgery, The Chinese University of Hong Kong, Shatin, New Territories, Hong Kong
[2] Department of Anaesthesia and Intensive Care, The Chinese University of Hong Kong, Shatin, New Territories, Hong Kong
[3] Department of Diagnostic Radiology & Organ Imaging Prince of Wales Hospital, The Chinese University of Hong Kong, Shatin, New Territories, Hong Kong

Summary

Disturbance of cerebral haemodynamic status, cerebral vasoreactivity (CVR) to carbon dioxide (CO_2) and pressure autoregulatory response (PAR) have been shown to be associated with severity of head injury and to correlate with neurological condition and clinical outcome. Information regarding impaired CVR and/or lost PAR has been shown to be of prognostic value in treating head-injured patients. The classic method of evaluating cerebral haemodynamic status requires an invasive measurement of cerebral blood flow (CBF) such as the technique of Kety and Schmidt or by the ^{133}Xe inhalation method. Transcranial Doppler ultrasonography (TCD) is a simple and non-invasive method for its assessment. In this study, cerebral haemodynamic status as determined by TCD was compared with that of stable xenon-enhanced cerebral blood flow (XeCBF) which is generally regarded as a gold standard in CBF measurement with minimal complication, suggesting that employing CO_2 and blood pressure challenge with TCD measurement to assess the CVR and PAR in head-injured patients, provides a relatively less invasive method and can be repeated at least daily to assess the cerebrovascular autoregulatory reserve.

Keywords: Cerebral vasoreactivity; pressure autoregulatory response; cerebral blood flow; blood flow velocity.

Introduction

Cerebral vasoreactivity (CVR) to carbon dioxide (CO_2) and pressure autoregulatory response (PAR) are two important criteria in determining cerebral haemodynamic status [1]. Cerebral vasodilatation and vasoconstriction in response to arterial hypercapnia or hypocapnia defines the CVR and is vital to intracranial pressure management. PAR is a physiological compensatory response that permits constant cerebral blood flow (CBF) to be maintained despite changes in cerebral perfusion pressure (CPP). Impairments in PAR will render the brain more susceptible to systemic insults. These two mechanisms have been shown to be affected after head injury and correlated with neurological condition and clinical outcome. In addition, haemodynamic status may vary with time as patients deteriorate or recover. Although direct measurement of CBF to CO_2 and/or blood pressure alteration will be more accurate in assessing the autoregulatory status, the methods are cumbersome and measurements would only be reliable during stable haemodynamic states. Therefore, it is necessary to have a simple, reliable method for the assessment of cerebral haemodynamic status in head-injured patients.

Transcranial Doppler ultrasonography (TCD) provides a noninvasive measurement of blood flow velocity (BFV) in the basal brain arteries. It has been shown to give accurate indication of changes in CBF. In this study, TCD was employed to determine the CVR and PAR and compare with that of using stable xenon-enhanced cerebral blood flow (XeCBF) measurement, which is considered as the gold standard in CBF measurement [2].

Materials and Methods

Fourteen patients (11 males and 3 females, mean age: 44.2 ± 16.9 years) with moderate to severe head injury defined as admission post-resuscitation Glasgow Come Scale (GCS) score less than or equal to 12 (median GCS: 6.5 points) were included in this study. After surgical treatment, all patients were managed by a standard protocol including artificial ventilation with sedation and muscle paralysis.

The studies were performed within 24 hours after admission and repeated on day 3 and between day 5 and 7. During each study, BFV in both middle cerebral arteries (MCA) were measured continuously by TCD. In each XeCBF measurement, a mixture of 30% stable xe-

Table 1. *Table Showing the Mean, Standard Deviation (S.D.) and Range of Cerebral Blood Flow (CBF), Blood Flow Velocity (BFV) at Middle Cerebral Artery (MCA) Territories and Two CVR and PAR Ratios Determined Using Stable Xenon-Enhanced Cerebral Blood Flow (XeCBF) and Transcranial Doppler Ultrasonography (TCD)*

	Mean	S.D.	Range
CBF (ml/100 g/min)	53.6	22.6	12.8–119.0
BFV (cm/s)	74.4	26.8	29.0–145.0
CVR ratio (%/mmHg $EtCO_2$)			
– by XeCBF	2.9	11.5	−4.4–43.7
– by TCD	2.3	2.6	−2.4–27.1
PAR ratio (%/mmHg mean ABP)			
– by XeCBF	0.8	2.1	−2.8–12.0
– by TCD	0.9	1.9	−2.0–11.7

non and 40% oxygen was administered for 4.5 minutes and 24 enhanced axial brain scans were obtained. The regions of interest in XeCBF measurement were both MCA territories.

Both XeCBF and TCD measurements were performed throughout three stages. (1) Baseline measurement: end-tidal CO_2 ($EtCO_2$) was maintained at a level of moderate hypocapnia of between 23 to 26 mmHg by moderate hyperventilation without any changes in arterial blood pressure (ABP). (2) CVR test (CO_2 challenge): baseline $EtCO_2$ was raised by reduced ventilation to normocapnia level for at least 6 mmHg. The CVR ratio was defined as the percentage change in CBF (using XeCBF) or BFV (using TCD) per unit change in mmHg of $EtCO_2$. (3) PAR test (ABP challenge): normoventilation was kept and induced a 20 to 25% increase in baseline mean ABP. The BFV ratio was defined as the percentage change in CBF (using XeCBF) or BFV (using TCD) per unit increase in mmHg of mean ABP.

Preserved CVR was defined as more than 1% change in CBF (by XeCBF) and BFV (by TCD) per mmHg end-tidal CO_2 and intact PAR was defined as less than 1% change in CBF and BFV per mmHg mean ABP change.

Results

Fourteen ventilated head-injured patients underwent 32 pairs of CVR and PAR tests. MCA CBF and BFV were 53.6 ± 22.6 ml/100 g/min and 74.4 ± 26.8 cm/s respectively (correlation coefficient [r] = 0.49, $p < 0.0005$). Table 1 summarizes the findings of studied parameters.

Figure 1 shows the scatter plot of CVR ratios measured by TCD and XeCBF. The r-value of detecting changes in BFV measured by TCD after CO_2 challenge versus changes in CBF determined by XeCBF was 0.34, whereas the PAR ratios determined using the two measurements correlated well with a higher significance (Fig. 2, $r = 0.73$). Table 2 (a) shows the 2 by 2 tables for evaluating sensitivity and specificity of using TCD in detecting preserved and impaired CVR of 70.5% and 50.0%; and 76.2% and 59.1% for detecting intact and lost PAR using TCD against gold standard CBF measurement (Table 2 (b)). The predictive values of a positive and a negative test using TCD against XeCBF in the two tests were equal to 75.6% and 43.5%, and 76.2% and 59.1% respectively.

Discussion

Blood flow velocity is proportional to CBF and inversely related to cross-sectional area of the blood vessel being studied. If the caliber of the isolated artery remains unchanged, flow velocity is a function of CBF. As MCA carries about 80% of the blood flow volume received by the cerebral hemisphere, it is suggested that MCA velocity measurements give accurate indications of changes in CBF. The results of this study suggested blood flow velocity measurement using TCD, coupled with CO_2 and blood pressure challenge is reliable for accessing cerebral haemodynamic status. In our group of ventilated patients with moderate to severe head injury, correlation in pressure is stronger in comparison to cerebral vasoreactivity.

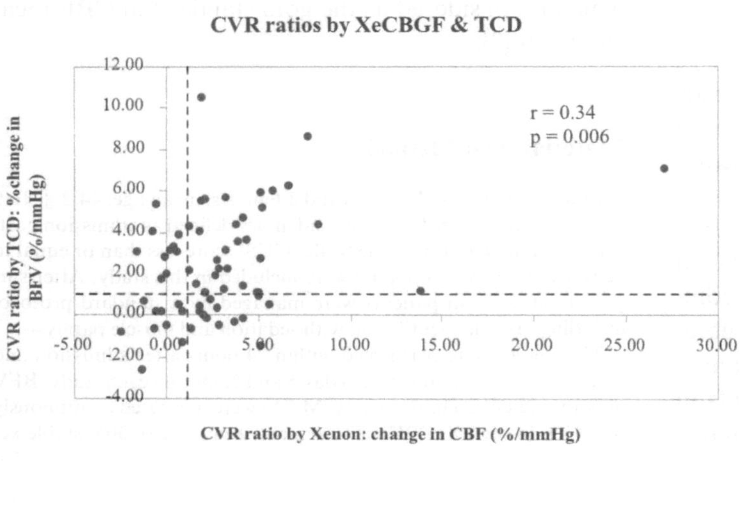

Fig. 1. Graph plotting the cerebral vasoreactivity (*CVR*) ratio using transcranial Doppler ultrasonography (*TCD*) measurement versus that of using stable xenon-enhanced cerebral blood flow measurement (*XeCBF*). The horizontal and vertical dotted lines represent the CVR ratio cut-off point of 1% per unit change in end-tidal carbon dioxide concentration (*$EtCO_2$*)

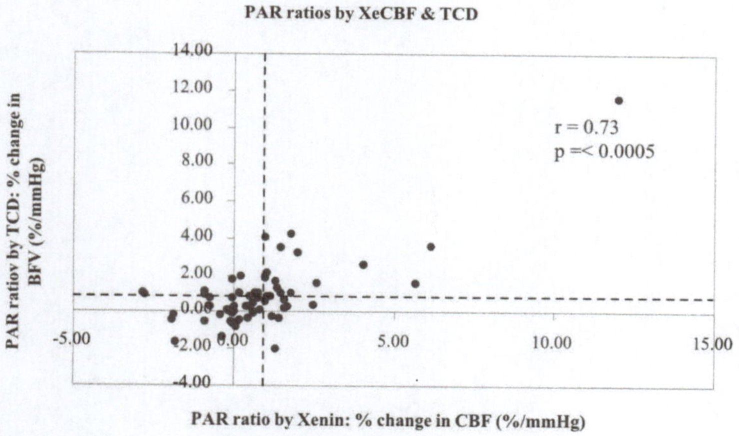

Fig. 2. Graph Plotting the Pressure Autoregulatory Response (PAR) Ratio Using Transcranial Doppler Ultrasonography (TCD) Measurement Versus that of Using Stable Xenon-Enhanced Cerebral Blood Flow Measurement (XeCBF). The horizontal and Vertical Dotted Lines Represent the PAR Ratio Cut-Off Point of 1% per Unit Change in Mean Arterial Blood Pressure (ABP)

Table 2. *(a) and (b) are 2 by 2 Tables for Evaluating Sensitivity, Specificity and Predictive Values of the Cerebral Vasoreactivity (CVR) Test and Pressure Autoregulatory Response (PAR) Test Using Transcranial Doppler Ultrasonography (TCD) Versus Results of Using the Gold Standard: Stable Xenon-Enhanced Cerebral Blood Flow (XeCBF) Measurement*

(a) By TCD	CVR Test (by XeCBF) Preserved	Impaired	(b) By TCD	PAR Test (by XeCBF) Intact	Lost
Preserved	31	10	Intact	32	9
Impaired	13	10	Lost	10	13
Sensitivity		70.5%	Sensitivity		76.2%
Specificity		50.0%	Specificity		59.1%
Predictive value (+)		75.6%	Predictive value (+)		76.2%
Predictive value (−)		43.5%	Predictive value (−)		59.1%

References

1. Endvolesen EM, Jensen FT (19978) Autoregulation and CO_2 responses of cerebral blood flow in patients with acute severe head injury. J Neurosurg 48: 689–703
2. Marion DW and Bouma GJ (1991) The use of stable xeono-enhanced computer tomographic studies of cerebral blood flow to define changes in cerebral carbon dioxide vasoresponsivity caused by a severe head injury. Neurosurgery 29: 869–873

Correspondence: Wai Poon, Neurosurgical Unit, Department of Surgery, Prince of Wales Hospital, The Chinese University of Hong Kong, Shatin, N.T., Hong Kong.

Acta Neurochir (2002) [Suppl] 81: 129–132

Comparison Between two Static Autoregulation Evaluation Methods

C. Puppo[1,2], **L. López**[1], **H. Panzardo**[2], **E. Caragna**[2], **P. Mesa**[2], and **A. Biestro**[1,2]

[1] Centro de Tratamiento Intensivo, Hospital de Clínicas, Montevideo, Uruguay
[2] Unidad Neuroquirúrgica, IMPASA, Montevideo, Uruguay

Summary

Cerebral static autoregulation (AR) was evaluated at bedside in 14 severely head injured patients. 16 investigations were performed. Cerebral perfusion pressure (CPP) was increased by infusing vasopressors during one hour, and registered every 2–5 minutes. CBF was simultaneously estimated by: 1) middle cerebral artery mean flow velocity (FV) monitoring with Transcranial Doppler (TDC), and 2) the reciprocal of arteriovenous oxygen content difference, calculated from basal and hypertensive arterial and jugular bulb blood samples. AR assessment: For TCD results, linear regression method was used, studying two pairs of variables: a) %FV-CPP (the regression slope was the main AR value adopted) and b) % cerebrovascular resistance (CVR)-%CPP. For the AVDO2 method, autoregulation was considered preserved if estimated $\%\Delta CBF/\Delta PPE < 1\%/\text{mm Hg}$. TCD method clearly defined three groups. Group 1 and 2 (8 and 5 investigations) were considered as two grades of preserved AR, and the third one (3 cases) as impaired AR. $AVDO_2$ method: 12 studies were evaluated. 10 showed preserved AR, and 2 impaired AR. There was coincidence of results from both methods in 10 out of 12 studies. (0.83).

Keywords: Cerebral autoregulation; cerebral blood flow velocity; arterio-venous oxygen content difference; severe head injury.

Introduction

The purpose of this study was to evaluate static autoregulation (AR) at bedside using two different methods for estimating cerebral blood flow. CPP was increased and CBF was simultaneously evaluated by: 1) middle cerebral artery mean flow velocity (FV) assessed with transcranial Doppler ultrasonography monitoring (TCD), and 2) the reciprocal of arterio-venous oxygen content difference ($1/AVDO_2$).

Materials and Methods

Fourteen severely head injured patients, with a mean age of 37 years, (range 16–63), 10 males, 4 females, were studied between day 2 and 8 after injury (mean, 4.5 days).

The average Glasgow Coma Score (GCS) during the study ranged between 3 and 8 (mean 6). All patients were admitted to the ICU, intubated and mechanically ventilated.

Intracranial hypertension was treated by means of unspecific and specific measures. Unspecific measures included mechanical ventilation, analgesia, sedation and neuromuscular blockade. Specific measures included hyperventilation, mannitol, indomethacin, barbiturates and moderate hypothermia. Eight out of 14 underwent surgical evacuation of mass lesions. According to the Traumatic Coma Data Bank classification, 4 patients were included in the diffuse injury II category, 2 cases in the diffuse injury III, and 8 patients in the evacuated mass lesion subgroup (V).

Outcome was classified as favorable (good and moderate disability): 7 patients, and unfavorable (severe disability, persistent vegetative state, or death): 7 patients.

Invasive mean arterial blood pressure (MABP) and intracranial pressure (ICP) measurements were made. Cerebral perfusion pressure (CPP) was calculated according to the formula: $CPP = MABP - ICP$. A catheter was inserted at the jugular bulb (usually right) through the internal jugular vein. X-ray verification of the correct placement was obtained. Oxygen saturation was measured from jugular bulb and arterial blood gas samples. Blood oxygen content (CaO_2 and CjO_2) (ml/dl) were calculated as: hemoglobin concentration (g/dl) $\times$ 1.34 $\times$ saturation fraction + 0,0031 $\times$ pO2 (mm Hg). $AVDO_2$ was calculated according to the formula: $AVDO_2 = CaO_2. - CjO_2$.

A 2 MHz pulsed Doppler ultrasonography probe was adjusted by means of a headband to the temporal window after finding the middle cerebral artery optimal signal in order to continuously measure FV and pulsatility index (PI). An EME TC2-64 b ultrasonograph was used. Mean arterial pressure was slowly increased during 60–90 minutes, by means of a vasopressor infusion, (methoxamine or phenilephrine in 10 cases) trying to obtain a minimum of 20 mm Hg change. Every 2–5 minutes, simultaneous PAM, ICP, CPP, FV, and PI values were obtained. Estimated cerebrovascular resistances (CVR) were calculated according to the formula $CVR = CPP/FV$. Between 8 and 38 sets of values (mean 18) were obtained for each patient. Arterial and jugular bulb blood samples were obtained at time 0, 30 and 60 minutes, and $AVDO_2$ and simultaneous CPP were calculated. The 2 $AVDO_2$ values which corresponded to the greatest change in CPP (ΔCPP) were used for calculations. Other variables which could change cerebral blood flow were mantained constant (oxigenation, ventilation, hematocrit, temperature).

Sixteen investigations were performed (one of the patients was studied three times, in three different conditions: 1) hyperventilated –

Table 1. *Results of 1/AVDO$_2$ Method*

Patient number	CPP$_b$ (mmHg)	ΔCPP (mmHg)	DAVO$_2$ b-h (ml/dl)	% ΔCBF/ mmHg	AR
1-indom	96	19	4.20–4.01	.24	P
7	75	84	7.15–6.11	ne	ne
1-hyperv	92	13	0.94–4.71	−6.16	I
4	92	31	3.47–3.25	.22	P
10	103	9	3.49–3.69	ne	ne
2	78	32	6.67–5.89	.42	P
11	69	38	5.80–4.29	.93	P
8	79	10	3.62–3.64	−.05	P
9	88	33	7.15–6.25	.44	P
6	94	3	3.50–3.19	ne	ne
14	86	17	2.64–3.03	−.76	P
3	86	46	2.83–2.75	.06	P
5	87	31	1.62–1.33	.71	P
1-nothing	65	19	6.24–3.53	4.04	I
13	83	31	2.47–3.21	−.75	P
12	87	6	4.77–5.78	ne	ne

Values for the metabolic method, CPP-basal and delta CPP-; DAVO$_2$-basal and hypertensive values- and percentual changes of estimated cerebral blood flow per mmHg change in CPP. (%Δ1/DAVO$_2$/mmHg). *P* Preserved AR; *I* Impaired AR; *ne* not evaluable.

pCO2 30-, 2) with indomethacin, normoventilated, and 3) without indomethacin and normoventilated – pCO2 38-

Assessment of classification criteria:

A) With Transcranial Doppler method, a correlation-regression method was adopted to quantify the relationship between two pairs of variables: 1) FV-CPP and 2) CVR-%CPP. FV and CVR were expressed as a percentage of their mean values. Linear regression slopes were adopted as AR indices Correlation coefficients and their significance were also evaluated.

B) For the metabolic method, only two sets of values were used for each patient (basal and hypertensive). If we accept that CMRO$_2$ is constant during the test, then AVDO$_2$ changes will reflect inverse changes in CBF [6, 7]. The percentual change in CBF (1/AVDO$_2$) relative to the basal value, was calculated with the formula: %1/AVDO$_2$ = ((1/AVDO$_2$h − 1/AVDO$_2$b)/1/AVDO$_2$b)·100. AR has been previously classified by other investigators as preserved if the % change in measured or estimated CBF (1/AVDO2) was lower than 20%, for a CPP change greater than 20%. [4, 7]. Here, the change in 1/AVDO2 was related to the exact change in CPP, and so 1/AVDO2 values < *1% per 1 mm Hg change in CPP* were classified as preserved AR, and greater absolute values were classified as impaired AR [5].

Results

1) AVDO$_2$ method (Table 1): 4 studies were not evaluated (ne) because of ΔCPP < 10 mm Hg. 12 studies were evaluated. 10 cases (0.83) showed preserved (P) AR, and 2 impaired (I) AR (Fig. 1). 8 cases were in the hyperemic range defined as AVDO$_2$ <4 ml/dl during both measurements, and two more cases changed from the hyperemic to the nonhyperemic range – and viceversa – (between 4 and 9 ml/dl) during the study.

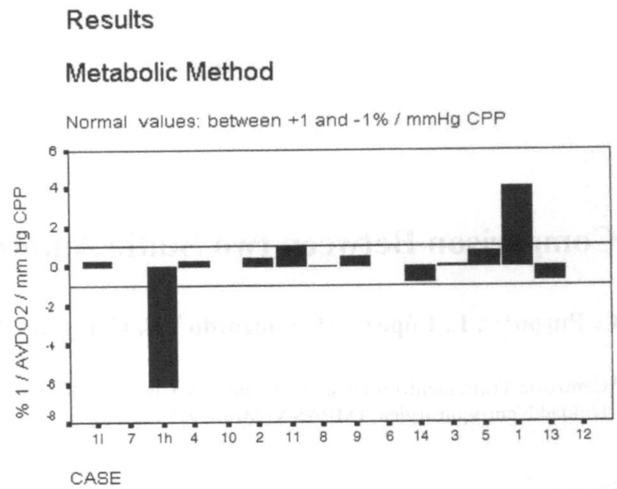

Fig. 1. Bars of individual values of each investigation with the metabolic method. Note that four studies were not evaluated because a low ΔCPP; 8 investigations showed a value between +1 and −1, and in two cases values were far out from the limits

2) TCD method (Table 2): No cases were discarded, as all CPP changes were acceptable.

Group 1: Preserved AR. (Eight studies): Regression slope of %FV/CPP < 0.4, absence of correlation and significance. High correlation and significance (p lower than 0.000) were found for this same group when %CVR-CPP was analyzed, with values of slope greater than 0.7.

Group 2: (Five cases) Intermediate AR. Slope 1 between 0.4 and 0.6, slope 2 between 0.4 and 0.6, intermediate correlation and significance. Group 3 (Three cases): Slope 1 greater than 0.90, excellent correlation and significance; slope 2 < 0.4, no correlation nor significance. Comparison of three groups is shown in Table 3. After comparing with the results of the AVDO$_2$ method, groups 1 and 2 were included as preserved AR (different grades of AR), making a proportion of 0.81 (0.50 + 0.31) of preserved AR for TCD method. The AR values found for both TCD methods (slopes 1 and 2) showed an excellent reciprocal correlation. (r = −0.97, significance 0.001). When TCD results were assessed in the 12 cases evaluated by the metabolic method, 10 out of 12 showed preserved AR, that is: 0.83. Comparison: (comparing the 12 cases left) When we considered TCD group 1 and 2 as preserved AR, both methods showed coincidence of preserved

Table 2. *Results of Correlation-Regression Between %FV-CPP (1) and %CVR-CP (2)*

Patient number	N	CPP (mmHg)	CBFV (cm/sec)	Slope 1	r 1	Sign 1	Slope 2	r 2	Sign 2
1 indometh.	13	96–127	60–72	–.21	.27	.375 ns	1.29	.84	.000**
7	14	61–84	34–44	.07	.08	.779 ns	.93	.81	.000**
1 hyperv.	13	92–113	54–62	.12	.17	.576 ns	.85	.76	.000**
4	26	73–140	52–72	.17	.36	.068 ns	.87	.86	.000**
10	25	78–117	98–118	.24	.59	.002**	.78	.93	.000**
2	13	78–114	54–69	.25	.34	.253 ns	.77	.70	.000**
11	24	66–107	46–64	.29	.38	.056 ns	.78	.81	.000**
8	11	60–89	78–92	.31	.65	.032*	.78	.94	.000**
9	13	84–127	24–36	.48	.63	.020*	.49	.63	.022*
6	12	82–124	64–86	.49	.64	.026*	.51	.63	.028*
14	38	75–121	42–56	.49	.74	.000**	.54	.78	.000**
3	13	86–132	28–46	.51	.6	.047*	.38	.39	.184 ns
5	8	87–118	110–132	.53	.92	.001**	.45	.89	.003**
1 nothing	14	51–92	54–90	.92	.9	.006**	.35	.44	.115 ns
13	29	69–115	44–86	.92	.73	.000**	.15	.19	.337 ns
12	25	77–128	87–93	.93	.94	.000**	.09	.25	.235 ns

Values for TCD method. *N* Number of measurements; CPP-basal and hypertensive- , FV-basal and hypertensive- regression slope between %FV and CPP (slope 1) between %CVR and %CPP (slope 2), Pearson correlation coefficients (r1 and r2) and significances. Notice that only two cases show velocities greater than 100 cm/sec, which could signify hyperemia. (we do not have values of Lindegaard index.)

Table 3. *Comparison of Three TCD Groups*

Group	1	2	3
slope 1	0.16**	0.50**	0.92
r 1	0.29*	0.70	0.79
slope 2	0.88**	0.47	0.19
R 2	0.83	0.66*	0.29

Mean values of the correlation regression for the three groups differentiated by the TCD method and its comparison. Statistic significance is shown as * for $p < 0.05$ and ** for $p < 0.001$.

AR in 9 out of 10, and of impaired AR in 1 out of two. There was coincidence of results in 10 out of 12 studies. (proportion of coincidence: 0.83) (IP: 0.19) (Fig. 2)

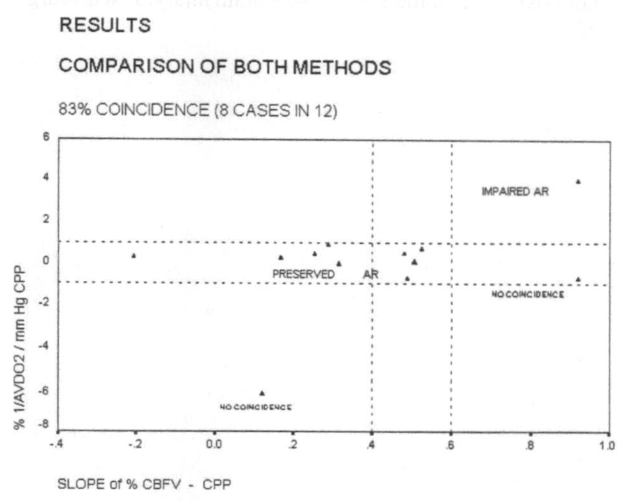

Fig. 2. Comparison of both methods: The %FV-CPP regression slopes are seen on the x-axis. The values of the best autoregulators, intermediate group, and non-autoregulators are separated by two vertical lines: 0.4 and 0.6. The results of the metabolic method are plotted on the y-axis, with AR-preserved values between reference lines (+1 and –1). The comparison between both methods show how groups one and two of the TCD method (slope < 0.6) are almost entirely within the range of preserved AR found with the $1/AVDO_2$ method

Discussion

The literature shows considerable diversity in classification criteria [2, 5, 8]. Transcranial Doppler has been frequently used in this field. One has to accept that MCA diameter does not change during the study in order to be able to interpret relative FV changes as CBF changes. This method showed different grades of AR. The lack of correlation of FV and CPP in the group with preserved AR shows that flow in these cases is independent of pressure. CVR, shows a good correlation with CPP, and explains the abscence of blood flow change. On the contrary, when FV is pressure passive (group 3), correlation and significance are high, and CVR is maintained unchanged. An intermediate group was found, that was identified as preserved AR when simultaneously evaluated by the metabolic method.

The metabolic method has taken into account the CPP change in order to improve its accuracy [5]. We found two cases of values greater than 1% change. A positive one, and a negative one. The latter could signify that flow has diminished instead of increased. This could be explained by a CPP increase in a non-compliant, non autoregulating brain causing vasodilatation and ICP increase and effective CPP decrease, leading to a diminished blood flow [4, 5].

Both methods of evaluation of cerebral autoregulation can be used to evaluate cerebral AR at the bedside, rendering similar results. Anyhow, more numbers are still needed.

References

1. Chan KH, Miller JD, Dearden NM, Andrews PJD, Midgley S (1992) The effect of changes in cerebral perfusion pressure upon middle cerebral artery blood flow velocity and jugular bulb venous oxygen saturation after severe brain injury. J Neurosurg 77: 55–61
2. Czosnyka M, Guazzo E, Iyer V, Kirkpatrick, Smielewski P, Whitehouse H, Pickard JD (1994) Testing of cerebral autoregulation in head injury by waveform analysis of blood flow velocity and cerebral perfusion pressure. Acta Neurochir (Wien) [Suppl] 60: 468–471
3. Czosnyka M, Smielewski P, Kirkpatrick P, Menon DK, Pickard JD (1996) Monitoring of cerebral autoregulation in head-injured patients. Stroke 27: 1829–1834
4. Enevoldsen EM, Jensen FT (1978)Autoregulation and CO2 responses of cerebral blood flow in patients with severe head injury. J Neurosurg 48: 698–702
5. Panerai RB (1998) Assessment of cerebral pressure autoregulation in humans – a review of measurement methods. Physiol Meas 19: 305–338
6. Robertson CS, Narayan RK, Gokaslan ZL, Pahwa R, Grossman RG, Caram P *et al* (1989) Cerebral arteriovenous oxygen difference as an estimate of cerebral blood flow in comatose patients. J Neurosurg 70: 222–230
7. Sahuquillo J, Rodríguez-Baeza A, Baguena M, Reina F, Campos L, Rubio E (1995) Autorregulación cerebral: conceptos fisiopatológicos y metodología para su valoración en el paciente neurotraumatizado. Medicina Intensiva 20: 69–78
8. Tiecks FP, Lam AM, Aaslid R, Newell DW (1995) Comparison of static and dynamic cerebral autoregulation measurements. Stroke 26: 1014–1019

Correspondence: Dra. Corina Puppo Leyenda Patria 2968/001 Montevideo CP 11300 Uruguay.

Acta Neurochir (2002) [Suppl] 81: 133–134

Asymmetry of Cerebral Autoregulation Following Head Injury

E. A. Schmidt, M. Czosnyka, P. Smielewski, S. K. Piechnik, and J. D. Pickard

Academic Neurosurgical Unit, Addenbrooke's Hospital, Cambridge, UK & Wolfson Brain Imaging Centre, University of Cambridge, UK

Summary

Objectives. To investigate asymmetry of cerebra autoregulation in head-injured patients with lateral brain contusions.

Methods. Sixty five patients were admitted to Addenbrooke's Hospital suffering from head injuries with mean Glasgow Coma Score 6 (range 3 to 10). The patients were paralysed, sedated and ventilated to achieve mild hypocapnia. Intracranial pressure (ICP), arterial pressure (ABP) were monitored directly. The left and right Middle Cerebral Arteries were insonated daily and flow velocity (FV) was recorded. Correlation coefficients between slow waves in cerebral perfusion pressure (CPP) and FV were calculated for every 3 minute period. Positive value of Mx denotes a positive association between waves in FV and CPP, therefore deranged autoregulation. Zero or slightly negative value of Mx denotes a good autoregulatory capacity. In each patient all CT scans were reviewed to assess a dominant side of brain contusion and a level of brain compression.

Results. The side-to-side difference in FV, pulsatility indices or critical closing pressures, did not correlate with the side of contusion or midline shift. In contrary, the side-to-side difference in Mx indices were significantly ($p < 0.05$) worse at a side of contusion and at the side of brain expansion in patients presenting with a midline shift ($p < 0.05$). Of those patients who died in hospital, significantly more presented within meaningful (ABS(Mx) > 0.2) asymmetry in cerebral autoregulation (40% versus 12%; $p < 0.05$).

Conclusions. Side-to-side difference in cerebral hemodynamic reserve of injured brain is a predictor of fatal outcome following head injury and correlates with the side of contusion or brain expansion.

Keywords: Head injury; symmetry; autoregulation.

Introduction

Left- and right-side cerebral autoregulatory responses are symmetrical in healthy volunteers. In contrast, in patients with carotid artery stenotic disease, the asymmetry in carbon dioxide reactivity or response to acetozolamide is reported to correlate with the side on which the cerebral hemodynamic deficit is greater. Our aim was to investigate whether a similar asymmetrical pattern can be found in head-injured patients with lateral brain contusions.

Method

Sixty five patients were admitted to Addenbrooke's Hospital suffering from head injuries with mean Glasgow Coma Score 6 (range 3 to 10). The patients were paralysed, sedated and ventilated to achieve mild hypocapnia. Intracranial pressure (ICP) was monitored continuously microtransducer inserted intraparenchymally. Arterial pressure (ABP) was monitored directly. The left and right Middle Cerebral Arteries were insonated daily for a period from 20 minutes to 2 hours and maximal flow velocity (FV) was recorded. Time averaged values of ICP, ABP, cerebral perfusion pressure (CPP = ABP − ICP) were calculated using waveform time integration for 10 seconds intervals. Pearson's correlation coefficients between 36 consecutive samples of averaged CPP and FV were calculated for every 6 minute period. This coefficient, called Mx index characterises the association between slow waves (period from 20 sec to 2 min) in FV and CPP. It has been previously demonstrated to describe cerebral pressure autoregulation [1]. Positive value of Mx denotes a positive association between waves in FV and CPP, and therefore poor autoregulation. Zero or slightly negative value of Mx denotes a good autoregulatory capacity. In each patient all CT scans were reviewed to assess a dominant side of brain contusion and a level of brain compression.

Results

The side-to-side difference in averaged transcranial Doppler flow velocity, pulsatility indices or critical closing pressures, did not correlate with the side of contusion or midline shift. In contrast, the side-to-side difference in pressure autoregulatory indices were significantly ($p < 0.05$) worse on the side of contusion and on the side of brain expansion in patients presenting with a midline shift ($p < 0.05$) – see Figure 1a,b.

Of those patients who died in hospital, significantly more presented with marked (absolute value of left-to-right difference in Mx more 0.2) asymmetry in cerebral autoregulation ($p < 0.05$) – see Fig. 1c. Side-to-side difference in autoregulation was not correlated with mean ICP nor with CT-based pattern of brain oedema.

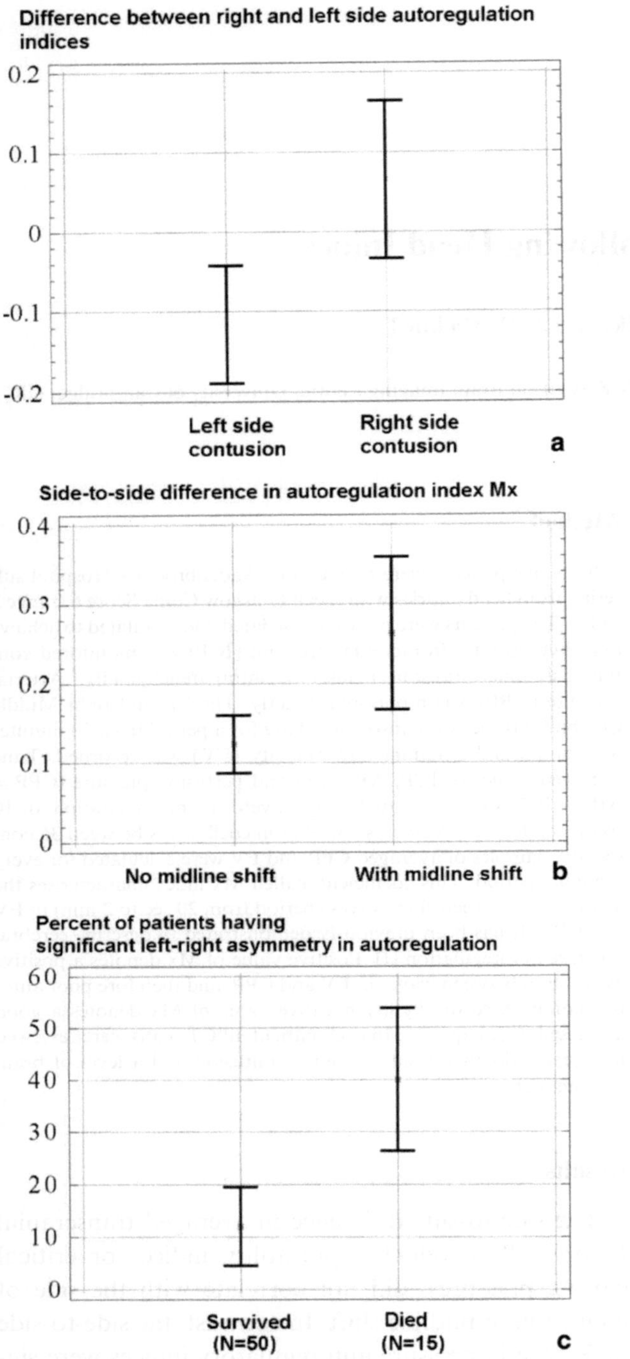

Fig. 1. Autoregulation was significantly worse ($p < 0.05$) at the side of contusion (a). It was significantly less symmetrical in patients with midline shift (b). Significantly more patients died in hospital with remarkable averaged asymmetry in autoregulation (c)

Conclusion

The side-to-side difference in the cerebral hemodynamic reserve of injured brain can be efficiently assessed using left and right autoregulatory indices, based on the analysis of spontaneous slow waves seen in cerebral perfusion pressure and blood flow velocity. This difference is a strong predictor of fatal outcome following head injury.

Reference

1. Czosnyka M, Smielewski P, Kirkpatrick P, Menon DK, Pickard JD (1996) Monitoring of cerebral autoregulation in head-injured patients. Stroke 27: 829–834

Correspondence: Marek Czosnyka, Academic Neurosurgical Unit, Box 167, Addenbrooke's Hospital, Cambridge CB2 2QQ, UK.

Acta Neurochir (2002) [Suppl] 81: 135–137

Oscillations in the Near-Infrared Signal in Patients with Severe Head Injury

O. S. K. Cheng, S. Prowse, and A. J. Strong

Department of Neurosurgery, Kings College London, London, UK

Summary

Objective. To use a non-invasive system, near infrared spectroscopy (NIRS) to detect oscillations in cerebral blood oxygenation in intensive care patients with severe traumatic brain injury.

Materials and Methods. 9 patients (7 male, 2 female) with a GCS < 8 were monitored in the intensive care units at King's College Hospital and the Royal London Hospital. A CCD-based spectrometer was coupled to the patient's forehead with one excitation and one detection optode. Spectra in the range of approximately 600–800 nm were collected at intervals of 2–4 seconds (subject to signal strength) and a curve-fitting algorithm applied, thus extracting time series data for oxyhaemoglobin (HbO), deoxyhaemoglobin (Hb) and cytochrome-c-oxidase (Cyt-c). The oxyhaemoglobin data was subjected to Fast Fourier Transform analysis.

Results. In all nine patients, unequivocal oscillations in the HbO signal were observed. The frequencies of these oscillations were at: 0.013–0.042 Hz (0.78–2.5 cycles min^{-1}), 0.11 Hz (6.7 cycles min^{-1}) and 0.19–0.28 Hz (12–16 cycles min^{-1}).

Conclusions. The presence of oscillations at 0.013–0.033 Hz, 0.11 Hz and 0.19–0.28 Hz are compatible with B-waves, vasomotion and respiratory cycles (respectively). However, due to the unknown contribution of the scalp to the NIR signal this data must be interpreted with care. Further work is required in order to investigate this.

Keywords: Near infrared spectroscopy (NIRS); oscillations.

Introduction

Spontaneous cyclic fluctuations in cerebral oxygen supply that are independent of cardiac and respiratory cycles have been postulated to arise from vasomotor activity in the cerebral microcirculation. Thus detection and understanding these cyclic fluctuations may help head injury management by providing information on cerebral vasoreactivity.

Cyclic fluctuations in the cerebral blood flow velocity (CBFV) have been described in head-injured patients and normal subjects using Laser Doppler Flow (LDF) techniques. The frequency of these fluctuations ranged from 0.5 to 6 cycles min^{-1} [1, 4].

Previous groups using near infrared spectroscopy (NIRS) have demonstrated fluctuations in the cerebral haemoglobin oxygenation state in healthy adult brains [2]. Cyclic fluctuations have also been reported in studies using NIRS to detect changes in cerebral blood volume in healthy infants [5].

We report here the presence of oscillations in the NIRS signal in patients suffering severe head injury and subarachnoid haemorrhage (SAH).

Materials and Methods

9 patients (7 male, 2 female) with a GCS < 8 were monitored in the intensive care units at King's College Hospital and the Royal London Hospital. Inclusion criteria required that selected patients were sedated (because the NIRS was very sensitive to movement artifact), intubated and artificially ventilated. The NIRS system consisted of a back-thinned CCD detector system (John Wright, U.K.) in combination with a spectrograph (Instruments SA, USA) and a xenon light source (Fibre Optic Illuminator Model 77501. Oriel, USA). Light was delivered to the scalp and collected by optodes of 3 mm in diameter. Optodes were held normal to the scalp, thus eliminating any loss of light resulting from use of prisms. The optodes were placed at an interoptode distance of 3.5 cm on the hemisphere ipsilateral to the injury, 2 cm above the supraorbital ridge and 2 cm away from the midline. The changes in optical density were measured between 600–800 nm. The sampling frequency ranged from 0.5–0.25 Hz depending on the strength of the signal sample from each patient. A curve-fitting algorithm based on a modified version of the Beer-Lambert law [3] was applied, thus extracting time series data for oxyhaemoglobin (HbO), deoxyhaemoglobin (Hb) and cytochrome-c-oxidase (Cyt-c). Patients were monitored continuously, in 2 hour periods interleaved with nursing care procedures, for up to 24 hours.

All nursing events that were likely to cause a signal change or an artifact, (for example: neuro-observations, endotracheal suction and physiotherapy) were documented during each session.

The HbO data was subjected to Fast Fourier Transform (FFT) analysis in order to characterise the oscillations. Artifactual data arising from nursing events were removed from the NIRS data, and FFT spectra for the HbO signals were computed (using the 'Timestat' programme) for sets of 512 and 1024 data points.

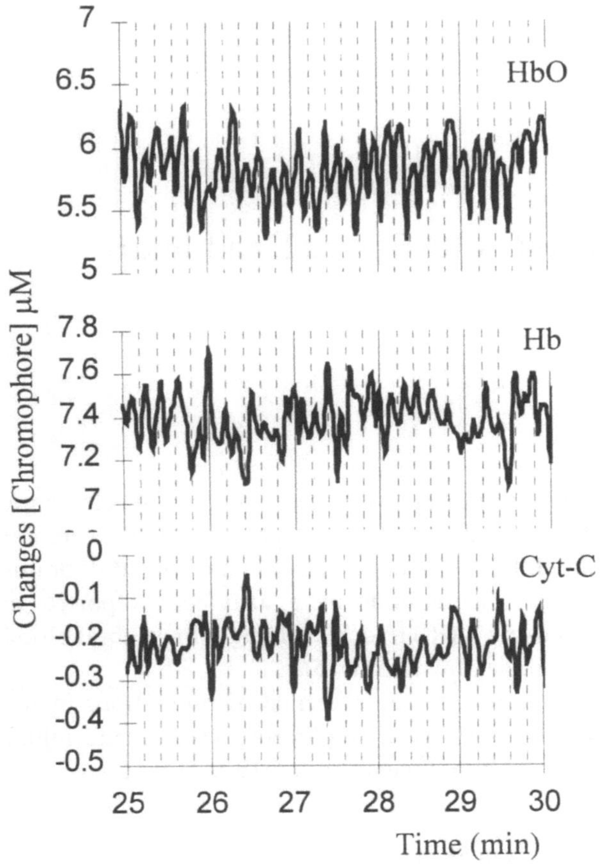

Fig. 1. Graphic display of near-infrared spectroscopy (relative changes in concentration of oxidised cytochrome-c-oxidase [Cyt c], deoxygenated haemoglobin [Hb] and oxygenated haemoglobin [HbO] over time). The figure shows a 5 minute sequence of data monitored from a 24-year old woman with severe headinjury. Oscillations of the [HbO] and [Hb] signals are synchronous with each other, but not with [Cyt C]

Results

Oscillations in the NIRS signal were found in all the patients monitored. The oscillations in the HbO and Hb time series were in synchrony with one another but not with the Cyt-c time series. An example of these oscillations is seen in Fig. 1. Although only 5 minutes of data from one patient is shown in Fig. 1, clear oscillations in the NIRS time series were present in all the patients. FFT was carried out on the HbO signal to ascertain the frequencies of the cyclic oscillations (Fig. 2). In accordance with Niquist's theory, the frequencies of the data obtained by FFT analysis could be split into three ranges. Low frequency oscillations between 0.013 Hz–0.042 Hz (0.78–2.5 cycles min^{-1}) and 0.011 Hz (6.7 cpm) were observed in 6 and 2 patients respectively. Oscillations at a slightly higher frequency 0.19–0.28 Hz (12–16 cycles min^{-1}) were observed in one patient (Table 1).

Discussion

Oscillations in the HbO signal were present in all of the patients monitored. FFT analysis was performed on the HbO signal. The predominant frequencies detected in this study are similar to oscillations reported in CBFV in head-injured patients and normal subjects: 0.5 to 2 cycles min^{-1} [1, 4], approximately 6 cycles min^{-1} [1] and approximately 15 cycles min^{-1} [4]. The slightly higher frequency oscillations in the HbO signal of 12–16 cycles min^{-1} are likely be of respiratory origin. However, the lower frequencies in the range of

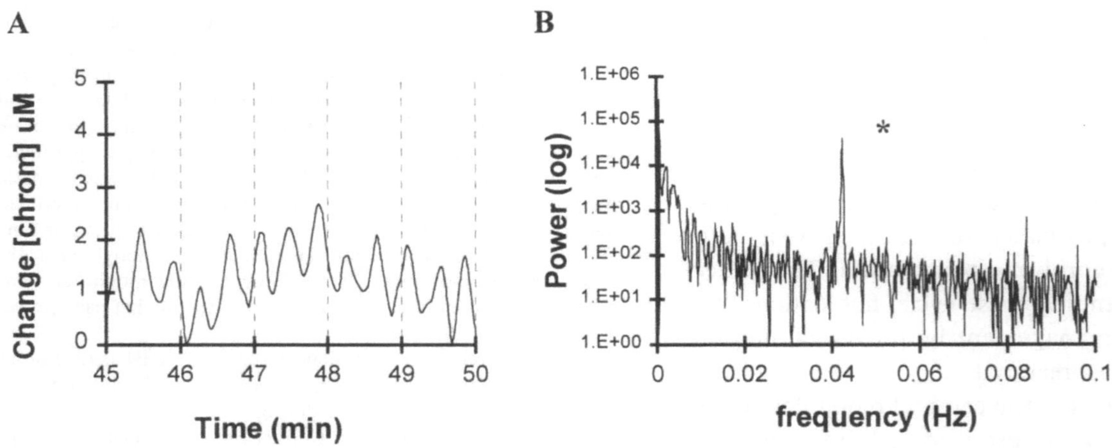

Fig. 2. A representative NIRS dataset showing the relative changes of [HbO] and their corresponding FFT spectra computed for 1024 data points. The [HbO] waveform showed oscillations of 2.5 cycles min^{-1}. The FFT spectragraph confirmed the frequency seen in the [HbO] waveform. A dominant frequency was present at 0.042 Hz (asterisk). The sampling frequency used to collect the data was 0.25 Hz

Table 1. *Summary of the HbO Oscillations Present in the Patients Monitored. Frequencies Determined by Fast Fourier Transform (FFT) Analysis*

[HbO] Oscillations		No. of patients oscillations present in
Frequency (Hz)	Cycles min^{-1}	
0.013–0.042	0.75–2.5	6
0.011	6.7	2
0.19–0.28	12–16	1

0.78–2.5 cycles min^{-1} and 6.7 cycles min^{-1} are likely to be independent of respiratory and cardiac cycles. Oscillations in the range of 0.78–2.5 cycles min^{-1} lie in the same frequency range as B-waves. It has been suggested that the oscillations in the CBFV at 6 cycles min^{-1} are attributable to vasomotion. Therefore it is also possible that the oscillations seen in this study at the similar frequency of 6.7 cycles min^{-1} may also be due to vasomotion present in the cerebral microcirculation.

The patients were monitored using an interoptode distance of 3.5 cm. The scalp circulation is likely to contribute to signals recorded under these conditions, thus oscillations in the scalp circulation may be a possible source of the cyclic fluctuations seen in the NIRS signal. Preliminary studies (J. Nottage, MSc Thesis, Insitute of Psychiatry) appear to discount this possibility: a comparison by subtraction of the NIRS signal obtained at an interoptode distance of 3.5 cm with one of 1.0 cm (a distance that probes predominantly the scalp circulation) demonstrated the presence of waveforms not present in the 1.0 cm signal.

Cyclic fluctuations in the NIRS signal have been demonstrated in the normal human brain in the resting state [2]. These oscillations (0.6–5 cpm) have been attributed to spontaneous neuronal activity.

In conclusion, we have demonstrated cyclic fluctuations in the NIRS signal recorded from patients with HI and SAH, and propose that these oscillations arise from the brain. Future work should seek to confirm this, and to determine whether these oscillations present in traumatic brain injuries share similar amplitudes and frequencies with oscillations present in the normal healthy brain, and whether oscillations vary with different patterns of brain injuries.

Acknowledgment

We thank the National Lottery Charities Board (MC 006189) for their support for this work.

References

1. Diehl RR, Diel B, Sitzer M, Hennerici M (1991) Spontaneous oscillations in cerebral blood flow velocity in normal humans and in patients with carotid artery disease. Neurosci Lett 245: 147–150
2. Hoshi Y, Kosaka S, Xie Y, Kohri S, Tamura M (1998) Relationship between fluctuations in the cerebral haemoglobin oxygenation state and neuronal activity under resting conditions in man. Neurosci Lett 127: 5–8
3. Matcher SJ, Elwell CE, Cooper CE, Cope M, Delpy DT (1995) Performance of several published tissue near infrared spectroscopy algorithms. Anal Biochem 227: 54–68
4. Newell DW, Aaslid R, Stooss R, Reulen HJ (1992) The relationship of blood flow velocity fluctuations to intracranial pressure B waves. J Neurosurg 76: 415–421
5. Urlesberger B, Trip K, Ruchti JJ, Kerbl R, Reiterer F, Müller W (1998) Quantification of cyclical fluctuations in cerebral blood volume in healthy infants. Neuroped 29: 209–211

Correspondence: Professor A. J. Strong, Department of Neurosurgery, King's College Hospital, London. SE5 9RS.

Acta Neurochir (2002) [Suppl] 81: 139–142

Slow Rhythmic Oscillations in Intracranial CSF and Blood Flow: Registered by MRI

C. Strik, U. Klose, C. Kiefer, and **W. Grodd**

Section of Experimental MR of the CNS, Department of Neuroradiology, University of Tuebingen, Germany

Summary

Since Lundberg first described slow oscillations as so called B-waves during ICP-monitoring, similar oscillations have been found in various physiological systems. Thus, the detection of slow waves in intracranial CSF- and blood-flow with MR-techniques seemed very likely. We examined the interventricular CSF-flow and cerebral blood flow of 11 healthy volunteers with dynamic echo-planar imaging by simultaneous registration of respiration and peripheral pulse. The spectral analysis was restricted to slow waves, which were divided into B-waves (0.008–0.05 Hz), Mayer- or C-waves (0.05–0.15 Hz) and respiration-related waves (0.15–0.6 Hz). In the CSF, the integrated amplitude of B-waves accounted for 18.2%, Mayer- or C-waves for 26.9% and respiration-related waves for 55.0%. Proportional values were recorded in the artery and peripheral pulse. In the venous sinus, a higher percentage of B- and Mayer-/C-waves and a lower percentage of respiration related waves were found. In conclusion, with MR-EPI technique, slow rhythmic oscillations in the cerebral blood- and CSF-flow can be analysed non-invasively and independently from the cardiac cycle. The comparable distribution of slow waves in the pulse, arteries and CSF may reflect an origin in autoregulation, whereas divergent patterns like in the incompressible venous sinus may be of a passive origin.

Keywords: CSF-flow; oscillations; MRI.

Introduction

Ever since dynamic CSF-measurements with MR-techniques have been performed, it has been known that the CSF flow is pulsatile [2], depends on the heart cycle and by this on cerebral blood flow. Due to the close relationship between arterial blood pressure (MAP), cerebral perfusion pressure (CPP) and intracranial pressure (ICP) (expressed as ICP = MAP − CPP) and their dependence of cerebral blood flow we expected slow oscillations in the CSF like in arterial blood pressure [4, 8, 9], cerebral blood flow [3] and intracranial pressure [7]. To test this hypothesis we used an echo-planar imaging technique and analysed the frequency pattern of the CSF in the aqueduct of sylvii and of the cerebral blood flow in a great artery and the sagittal sinus.

Material and Methods

We examined 11 healthy volunteers (5 females, 6 males) in the age from 7 to 37 years (mean 28 years). The measurements were performed with a 1.5 T whole body scanner (Vision, Siemens, Erlangen, Germany) in a circular polarised head coil with echo-planar technique (FOV 120 mm, TE 43 ms, TR 156 ms, flip angle 90 degree, matrix 64 × 64, slice thickness 3 mm). In a T2-weighted midsagittal image, a slice was positioned perpendicular to the aqueduct. With 3072 acquisitions, the measurement took 8 minutes and was well tolerated by the volunteers. The heart beat (registered with a pulse oximeter) and the respiration rate (with a respiration belt) were recorded simultaneously during the MRI-measurement. Data recording and analysing were performed as described previously [6].

A signal variation map was generated in which variations in signal intensity in the aqueduct, the basilar artery and the sinus sagittalis superior were displayed. The CSF, arterial and venous MRI-signal were assessed together with recordings from the pulse oximeter and respiration belt in the time domain.

For frequency analysis, the signal levels of the original data from single pixels were centred to zero by subtracting the mean value of the data and filtered by a Hanning function before performing the Fourier transformation (FT). The integral for three different oscillations was calculated for the CSF, artery and vein as well as the heart rate variability.

We divided the whole registered spectrum into three different slow frequencies: the frequency of i) 0.008 to 0.05 Hz, ii) 0.05 to 0.15 Hz and iii) the respiration. The power of this spectra were described as the integral of each frequency range with mean values and SD-deviation calculated as percentage.

Results

Figure 1 shows the time domain and Fig. 2 the corresponding spectral analysis in a 7 year old boy. The time domain analysis shows divergent variations of the

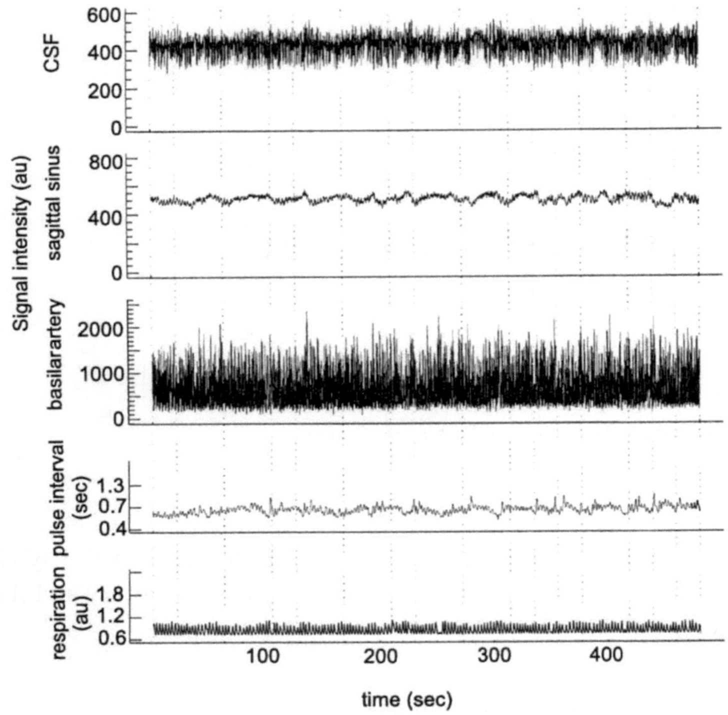

Fig. 1. Signal variation of CSF-flow, blood flow in sagittal sinus and basilar artery, peripheral pulse interval and respiration curve of a 7 year old healthy volunteer

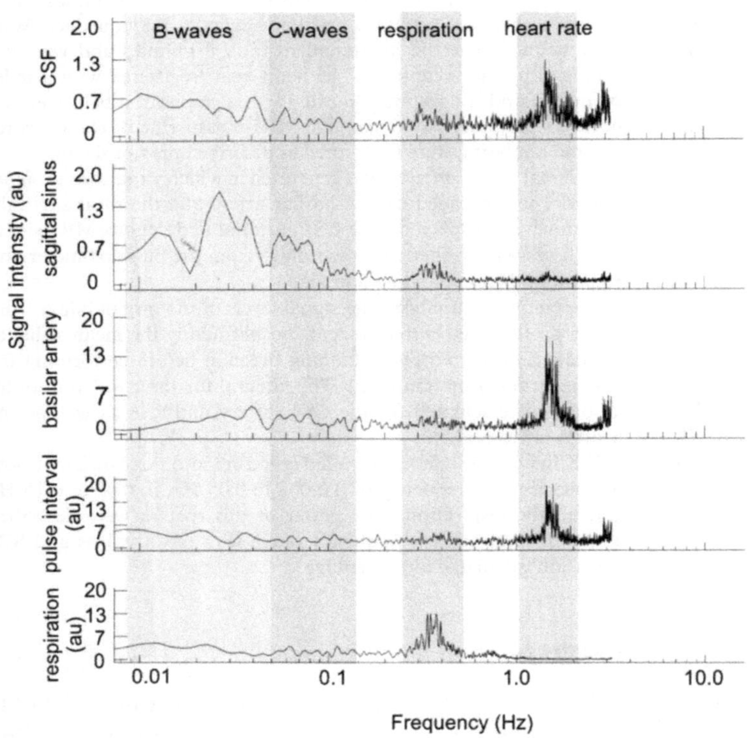

Fig. 2. Corresponding Fourier-Transformation with slow waves, marked as B-wave, C-wave and respiration

signal intensity in CSF, arterial and venous blood flow. The fast variation of the heart cycle is clearly visible in CSF- and blood flow, whereas slower waves are only detectable in the venous blood flow and heart rate variability. In spectral analysis, a peak of the B-waves is demonstrated in CSF, arterial and – more pronounced – in the venous blood flow. Mayer-/C-waves are more prominent in the venous blood flow than in CSF- or arterial blood flow. But the respiration related frequencies are more prominent in CSF flow than in cerebral blood flow.

In the CSF, integrated amplitude of B-waves accounted for a mean of 18.2% ± 5.8 (SD), Mayer-/C-waves for 26.9 ± 10.8% and respiration-related waves for 55.0 ± 12.6% of slow waves. Proportional values were recorded in the artery (17.2 ± 6.8% of B-waves, 30.0 ± 9.7% of Mayer-/C-waves and 54.2 ± 14.6% of respiration related waves) and the pulse (15.8 ± 4.4% – 30.6 ± 8.5% – 53.3 ± 12.4%).

In the venous sinus, however, a higher percentage of B-waves (35.5 ± 11.5%) and Mayer-/C-waves (42.6 ± 11.5%), along with a lower percentage of respiration related waves (22.0 ± 6.1%), were found.

Discussion

Variations in intracranial pressure were described first by Lundberg [7]. He distinguished between A-, B- and C-waves. Other than A-waves, B-waves (0.008–0.05 Hz = 0.5–3/min) and C-waves (0.05–0.15 Hz = 3–9/min) have a wavelength which can be registered within a few minutes. The success of non-invasive registration with MRI of these slow waves depends not only on their regular occurrence, but also requires a real-time measurement technique with long registration period. Echo-planar imaging is a qualitative measurement technique with a high time resolution, which allows the registration of such slow oscillations independently of the cardiac cycle. In healthy volunteers, we found slow waves in the B-wave frequency as well as in the Mayer- or C-wave range with a small amplitude in the interventricular CSF-flow. We conclude that CSF-waves also in the Mayer-frequency range (4–9/min) are not primarily pathologic, as originally claimed [5]. We could find these waves also in the blood flow of the basilar artery in similar amounts as in CSF and peripheral heart rate variability. In the sagittal sinus, these slow blood flow waves are much more pronounced, due to a higher amplitude. The intraventricular CSF-flow therefore is first of all dependent on arterial cerebral blood flow, while the venous outflow seems to have only a minor influence under physiological resting conditions. This may change in elevated intracranial pressure with reduced cerebral compliance where the venous, especially spinal venous system, plays a major role in the regulation of intracranial compliance. Further studies of patients with raised intracranial pressure may therefore reveal different patterns of slow waves in venous blood flow and CSF flow.

The origin of these slow waves is not fully understood. One pacemaker is assumed to be located in the rostral medulla for equivalent slow blood pressure waves. In as much as CSF flow has no pump of its own and cerebral blood flow shows equivalent waves, we assume that oscillations of cerebral blood flow are responsible for these CSF-oscillations. For the venous blood flow in the incompressible dura we assume a passive effect from the pial venous system, where the existence of an active vasomotor tone is known [1].

In conclusion, echo-planar imaging is a real time technique with a high time resolution, which allows the registration of slow waves along with high frequencies. By the use of Fourier-Transformation, we found small amplitude waves in the CSF in the range of B- and C-waves and respiration, as well as in the arterial cerebral blood flow and in the peripheral heart rate variability in healthy volunteers. With time-domain analysis, these slow waves could be also demonstrated in the dural vein.

References

1. Auer LM (1984) Venous-neurogenic regulation of cerebral blood volume. Adv Neurosurg 12: 281–287
2. Bergstrand G, Nordell B, Stahlberg F, Ericsson A, Bergstrom M, Hemmingsson A, Sperber G, Thuomas KA, Jung B (1986) Cerebrospinal fluid flow studied with gated magnetic resonance imaging during the various parts of the cardiac cycle. Acta Radiol [Suppl] (Stockh) 369: 490–491
3. Fasano VA (1988) Intraoperative Use of Laser Doppler in the Study of Cerebral Microvascular Circulation. Acta Neurochir (Wien) 95: 40–48
4. Hering E (1869) Über den Einfluss der Atmung auf den Kreislauf I. Über Atembewegungen des Gefässsystems. Sitzb d mathem-naturw Cl (Wien) 60: 829–856
5. Kjällquist A, Lundberg N, Ponten U (1961) Respiratory and cardiovascular changes during rapid spontaneous variations of ventricular fluid pressure in patients with intracranial hypertension. Acta Neurol Scand 40: 291–317
6. Klose U, Strik C, Kiefer C, Grodd W (2000) Detection of a Relation Between Respiration and CSF Pulsation With Echoplanar Technique. J Magn Res Imaging 11: 438–444
7. Lundberg N (1960) Continuous recording and control of ventricular fluid pressure in neurosurgical practice. Acta Psych Neurol Scand [Suppl] 36: 149

8. Mayer S (1876) Studien zur Physiologie des Herzens und der Blutgefässe. Sitzb d mathem-naturw Cl (Wien) 74: 281–307
9. Traube L (1865) Ueber periodische Tätigkeits-Aeusserungen des vasomotorischen und Hemmungs-Nervenzentrums. Centralbl med Wiss (Berlin) 3: 881–885

Correspondence: Prof. Dr. Dipl. Biol. Wolfgang Grodd, Section of Experimental MR of the CNS, Department of Neuroradiology, University of Tuebingen, Hoppe-Seyler Str. 3, D-72076 Tuebingen, Germany.

Acta Neurochir (2002) [Suppl] 81: 143–145

Cyclic Variation of Cerebral Pial Arteriolar Diameter Synchronized with Positive–Pressure Inhalation

M. L. Daley[1], S. Han[1], and C. W. Leffler[2]

[1] Department of Electrical and Computer Engineering, The University of Memphis, Memphis, TN
[2] Departments of Physiology and Pediatrics, University of Tennessee Health Science Center, Memphis, TN

Summary

Laboratory observations have noted that during normocapnia and intact vascular tone, changes in the intracranial pressure (ICP) and arterial blood pressure (ABP) recordings are not similar. The purpose of the present study was to determine whether: 1) the diameter of cerebral pial arterioles synchronously increases during positive pressure inhalation and decreases during the expiration phase of ventilation; and 2) the variation in arteriolar diameter is greater when vascular tone is intact than when arterioles are maximally dilated. Severe hypercapnia was induced by prolonged ventilation with gas mixture of 20% O2, 10% CO2, and 70% N2 in 8 piglets. S-VHS recordings of 3600X magnification of nine pial arterioles were obtained during conditions of normal vascular tone and severe hypercapnia and digitally analyzed by an image-averaging method. Variation of the amplitude of arteriolar diameter over the ventilation cycle was computed and found to synchronously increase during positive pressure inhalation and to decrease to a steady state baseline during passive expiration. Mean amplitude of variation in diameter ($\pm$S.D.) during normal tone and hypercapnia was computed as 1.63 ($\pm$0.693) μm and 1.012 ($\pm$0.869) μm respectively and found to be significantly greater during the condition of normal vascular tone than during hypercapnia ($p < .006$). These results suggest that a cyclic variation of arteriolar blood volume is one causal factor related to the low frequency variation of the baseline of ICP associated with positive pressure ventilation.

Keywords: ICP; positive-pressure ventilation; pial arteriolar diameter.

Introduction

Previously reported laboratory observations have noted that during normocapnia and intact vascular tone, changes of ICP and ABP recordings are not similar [1, 2, 4]. However, during severe hypercapnia and maximal vascular dilation, the changes in these two pressure recordings become proportional to one another and strongly correlated [1, 2, 4]. From these observations we have developed the hypothesis that when cerebrovascular tone is intact, compression of the cerebral capillary bed and numerous localized sites within the venous drainage network occurs during positive pressure inhalation. The compressional effect on the cerebral vasculature progressively reduces as tone is lost. Thus as a consequence of positive pressure ventilation, cerebral arteriolar diameter should cyclically change during ventilation, increasing during the positive pressure phase of inhalation and decreasing during the passive expiration phase of ventilation. The purpose of the present study was to test this hypothesis by examining whether: 1) the diameter of cerebral pial arterioles synchronously increases during positive pressure inhalation and decreases during the expiration phase of ventilation; and 2) the variation in arteriolar diameter is greater when vascular tone is intact than when arterioles are maximally dilated.

Materials and Methods

Using an approved protocol from the U.T. and U.M. Animal Care and Utilization Committees and procedures similar to those previously described [3], nine α-chloralose anesthetized piglets ranging in weight from 2 to 4 kg were used in this study. Severe hypercapnia was induced by prolonged ventilation with gas mixture of 20% O2, 10% CO2, and 70% N2 in four piglets.

S-VHS recordings of 3600X magnified of five pial arterioles were obtained during conditions of normal vascular tone and severe hypercapnia. Taped images were digitally captured at a rate of 15 frames per sec. Matlab (Matlab Inc., Natick, MA) image processing software was used to develop an image-averaging algorithm. Specifically, for each frame, brain movement and diameter were visually identified and extracted. A threshold for brain movement was used to trigger signal averaging to obtain the time-average frame-by-frame brain movement and diameter change. To further reduce the noise, a four frame moving average was also employed. The amplitude of the variation in diameter over the ventilation cycle was computed as the difference between peak-diameter during inhalation and mean diameter.

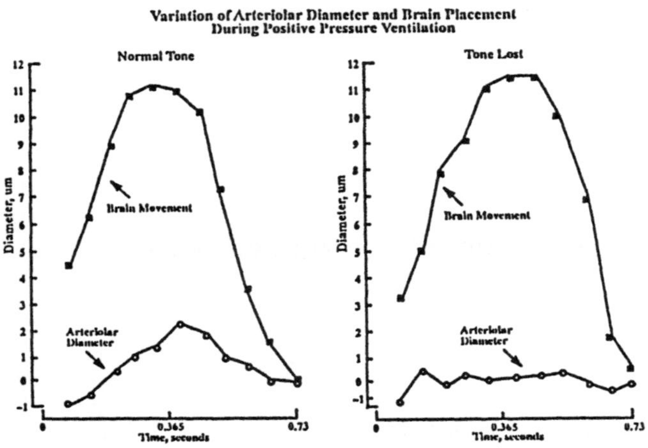

Fig. 1. Variation of Cerebral Arteriolar Diameter and Brain Placement During Positive Pressure Inhalation. Threshold displacement of the brain was used to trigger time-averaged displacement of brain movement and variation of arteriolar diameter during late inhalation and the onset of expiration. Averaging began about midway in the inhalation phase of ventilation and lasted 0.73 sec. Closed and open circles respectively represent mean brain displacement and mean amplitude of arteriolar diameter computed from twenty-two ventilation cycles. Standard error of each mean is within the plotted symbol. The pattern of brain movement is similar for the conditions of normal and lost vascular tone. However, during normal tone the variation of the amplitude of arteriolar diameter peaked during inhalation at approximately 3 μm and decreased during passive expiration. In contrast, during lost tone, the variation of the amplitude of arteriolar diameter remained relatively constant during averaging time

Results

During positive pressure ventilation the brain will generally undergo cyclic movement of about 10–15 μm. In particular, during a proportion of the inhalation phase the brain will slowly start to move and at the onset of expiration the brain will rapidly move back to the baseline position during expiration. An example of such brain movement and the corresponding variation of arteriolar diameter over a portion of the inhalation and expiration phase of ventilation are shown (see Fig. 1). For this example the threshold of brain movement occurred approximately in the middle of the inhalation phase of ventilation. The pattern of brain movement was similar for the conditions of normal and lost vascular tone. In contrast, variation of pial arteriolar diameter was different for these conditions. During normal tone the arteriolar diameter increased steadily by approximately 3 μm during inhalation and then decreased at the onset of expiration. However, during maximal dilation the arteriolar diameter appears to have increased slightly during inhalation. A summary of the change in diameter for the nine arteriolar sites for the conditions of normal tone and maximal dilation is given in Table 1 below. Mean amplitude of variation in diameter (±S.D.) during normal tone and hypercapnia was computed as 1.63 (±0.693) μm and 1.012 (±0.869) μm respectively. Furthermore, the amplitude of diameter-variation was significantly greater during the condition of normal vascular tone than during hypercapnia ($p < .006$).

Discussion

Previously reported laboratory observations have noted that during normocapnia and intact vascular tone, changes of intracranial pressure (ICP) and arterial pressure (ABP) recordings are not similar [1, 2, 4]. However, during severe hypercapnia and maximal vascular dilation, the changes in these two pressure recordings become proportional to one another and strongly correlated [1, 2, 4]. In order to make these consistent laboratory findings described above clinically useful, an understanding of the mechanism(s)

Table 1.

Normal tone					Lost tone				
Animal	Max.	Min.	st. div.	Diff.	Animal	Max.	Min.	st. div.	Diff.
53096	1.67	−0.61	0.98	2.28	53096	0.26	−0.48	0.39	0.73
478	1.44	0.31	0.52	1.12	478	1.96	0.85	0.80	1.11
485	1.38	−0.25	0.70	1.63	485	1.15	0.66	0.79	0.49
485	3.1	−0.29	0.82	3.38	485	2.6	−0.78	0.71	3.38
51200	−0.53	−1.7	0.38	1.19	51200	−0.50	−1.0	0.35	0.54
51900	0.89	−0.52	0.52	1.41	51900	0.48	−0.57	0.51	1.04
52600	0.58	−0.79	0.43	1.37	52600	0.74	−0.26	0.66	0.99
60200	0.03	−0.4	0.47	0.43	60200	−0.38	−0.67	0.62	0.29
60900	1.04	−0.81	0.53	1.85	60900	0.33	−0.19	0.58	0.52

that underlie the increasing correlation between the ICP and ABP recordings with increasing cerebral dilation must be determined. The cyclic variation of intrathoracic pressure during positive pressure ventilation is considered a major causal factor of the corresponding synchronized variation of ICP [3]. Cyclic variation of cerebral pial arteriolar diameter synchronized with ventilation occurs. The amplitude of the variation of pial arteriolar diameter is significantly greater during normal tone than during severe hypercapnia. These results suggest that a cyclic variation of arteriolar blood volume is a causal factor related to the synchronous low frequency variation of the baseline of intracranial pressure observed with positive pressure ventilation.

References

1. Daley ML, Pasupathy H, Griffith M, Robertson JT, Leffler CW (1995) Detection of loss of cerebral vascular tone by correlation of arterial and intracranial pressure signals. IEEE Transactions on Biomedical Engineering 42: 420–424
2. Daley ML, Leffler CW (1998) Correlation coefficient between ICP and arterial pressure: a gauge of cerebral vascular dilation Acta Neurochur (Wien) [Suppl] 71: 285–288
3. Hammer J, Alberti E, Hoyer S, Wiedemann K (1977) Influence of systemic and cerebral vascular factors on the cerebrospinal fluid pulse waves. J Neurosurgery 46: 336–345
4. Portnoy HD, Chopp M, Branch M, Shannon MB (1982) Cerebrospinal fluid pulse waveform as an indicator of cerebral autoregulation. J Neurosurgery 56: 666–678

Correspondence: Michael L. Daley, Ph.D., The University of Memphis, Electrical and Computer Engineering, Campus Box 526574, Memphis, TN 38152.

Acta Neurochir (2002) [Suppl] 81: 147–150

Spectral Characteristics of B-Waves and Other low-Frequency Activity

M. L. Daley[1], R. L. Pasley[1], M. Connolly[1], S. D. Timmons[2], J. Angel[3], G. Stidham[4], and C. W. Leffler[5]

[1] Department of Electrical and Computer Engineering, The University of Memphis, Memphis, TN
[2] Department of Neurosurgery, University of Tennessee Health Science Center, Memphis, TN
[3] Department of Anesthesiology, University of Tennessee Health Science Center, Memphis, TN
[4] Department of Pediatrics, University of Tennessee Health Science Center, Memphis, TN
[5] Departments of Physiology and Pediatrics, University of Tennessee Health Science Center, Memphis, TN

Summary

Low frequency oscillations of intracranial pressure (ICP) between 0.5 to 2.0 cycles/min have been termed B-waves. While such low frequency activity may be generated by cerebral vasomotor activity, activity in the B-wave band may also be related to other causes. The objective of this study is to: 1) describe the low frequency characteristics of ICP and arterial blood pressure (ABP) recordings with a mathematical model based on ventilator-induced intrathoracic pressure (ITP) modulation of arterial blood pressure; and 2) use the model to eliminate low frequency activity within the B-wave range unrelated to vasomotor activity. The model describes the frequency locations of spectra associated with ventilation about both the principal and first harmonic cardiac frequency to within 1% error. Spectra within the B-wave range harmonically related to the ventilator frequency were classified as caused by patient-ventilator interaction. Of 11 patients with severe head-injury, 64% (7/11) demonstrated B-wave activity, and 4 patients demonstrated the activity solely in the ICP recording. Variation of heart rate did not correspond to the occurrence of B-waves. The proposed model describes the low frequency spectra found within ABP and ICP recordings and can be used to eliminate spectra with the B-wave range related to ventilation.

Keywords: Intracranial pressure; B-waves.

Introduction

Four decades ago, Lundberg described slow rhythmic oscillations of ICP in the frequency range of 0.5 to 2.0 cycles/min that he termed B-waves [3]. He suggested in such cases changes in the concentration of arterial CO_2 may result in changes of cerebral blood volume that generate the ICP waves [3]. More recently, Newell and his colleagues demonstrated the occurrence of B-waves corresponding to Doppler derived middle cerebral artery velocity (MCAV) waves [4]. They suggested that B-waves in both healthy subjects and patients with head-injury were the result of vasomotor waves [4]. However, variation of cardic output has also been implicated in the generation of low frequency activity within the B-wave range [2]. The objective of this study is to: 1) describe the low frequency spectral characteristics of ICP and ABP recordings; and 2) use the model to classify and eliminate low frequency activity within the B-wave range unrelated to vasomotor activity.

Materials and Methods

The protocol for this study was reviewed and approved by the Institutional Review Board of the University of Tennessee. Eleven patients, 7 females and 4 males, with an age range of 3–29 yrs. (mean age (± S.D.) 11.7 (± 8.7) yrs) and with initial Glasgow coma scale ranging from 3 to 6 were studied. Pressure recordings were sampled at 250 Hz and artifact screening was accomplished by an updated defined criteria [1]. Calculation of the power spectrum of ABP and ICP 8.74 minute-digitized recordings was done with commercially available DADiSP software. Prior to the spectral computation, the mean of each time series was removed, and a Hamming window was applied. The proposed linear modulation model is based on the assumption that changes of ITP during ventilation cyclically compress the systemic vasculature. The resultant changes of ABP are linearly transmitted to ICP through small cyclic changes of cerebral blood volume. In the model, recorded ABP, $a_r(t)$, is expressed as the product of ITP, p(t), times a(t), the unmodulated ABP. Thus, recorded ABP, $a_r(t)$, is expressed as:

$$a_r(t) = p(t) \cdot a(t) \quad (1)$$

where ITP and unmodulated ABP are approximated respectively as:

$$p(t) = p_0 + p_1 \cos(2 \cdot \pi \cdot f_v \cdot t) + p_2 \cos(4 \cdot \pi \cdot f_v \cdot t) \quad (2a)$$

$$a(t) = a_0 + a_1 \cos(2 \cdot \pi \cdot f_c \cdot t) + a_2 \cos(4 \cdot \pi \cdot f_c \cdot t) \quad (2b)$$

with f_v and f_c respectively representing the principal ventilator and

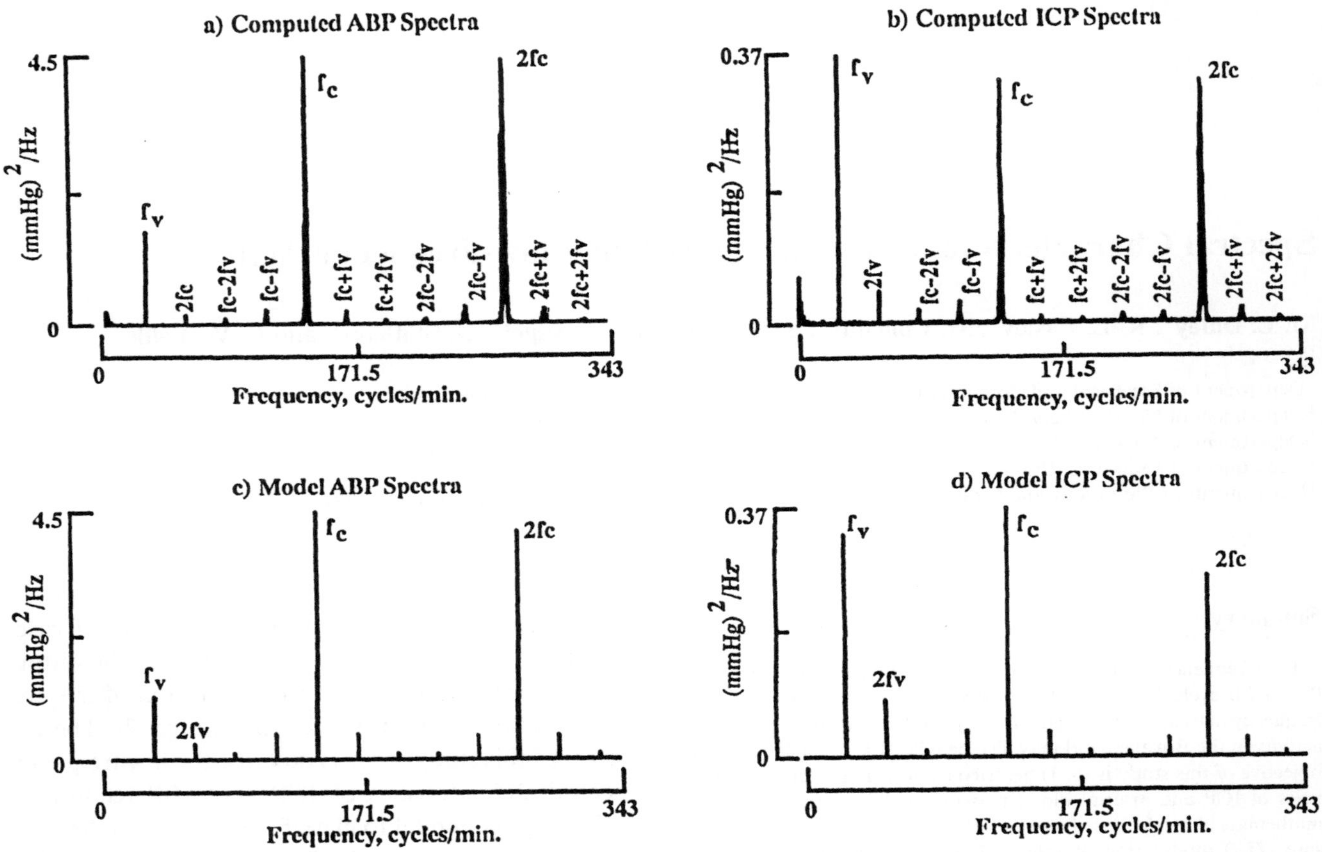

Fig. 1. Computed and Model Generated Power Spectrums (a) Computed ABP Spectrum. (b) Computed ICP Spectrum. The narrow spectra peaks contained in the computed spectrums indicate that both heart-rate and ventilation rate remained relatively constant during the monitoring period. Spectral side-bands related to ventilation are evident about the principal cardiac frequency, fc, and its first harmonic, 2fc. (c) Model ABP Spectra; and (d) Model ICP Spectra. The model predicts the location of the spectral side-bands about fc and 2fc related to the frequency of ventilation

cardiac frequencies and the arbitrary constants and constrained as $p_0 > p_1 > p_2$ and $a_0 > a_1 > a_2$. The Fourier transform of the above equation is expressed as:

$$A_r(f) = P(f) * A(f) \quad (3)$$

the convolution of the respective transformed functions [5]. The criterion for the location of spectra was the presence of a peak at least five times above the average noise of the spectrum.

Results

Computed ICP and ABP power spectrums and spectrums generated by the math model are shown (see Fig. 1). The computed spectrums contain peaks at the ventilator frequency, fv (27 cycles/min), and its first harmonic, 2fv (54 cycles/min), and at the cardiac frequency, fc (151 cycles/min), and its first harmonic, 2fc (302 cycles/min). The corresponding spectrums predicted by the model are also shown (see Fig. 1c,d). Given the principal cardiac and ventilator frequencies and first harmonics, the model generates a spectral line at specific modulation frequencies. For the eleven patients, the model predicted the frequency location of the side-bands about both the principal and first harmonic cardiac spectra with an average error of less than 1% for each side-band location and a grand mean error ($\pm$SD) of (n = 88, +0.56, ($\pm$1.4) cycles/min and (n = 88, 0.57 ($\pm$1.5) cycles/min for ICP and ABP respectively. Furthermore, during monitoring, one patient episodically interacted with the ventilator; as a result both the ABP and ICP recordings contained waves synchronized with mechanical ventilation. The computed spectrums contained sub-harmonic spectral peaks at 1/5 the ventilator frequency. Because these ventilator-related spectra were assumed to reflect corresponding periodic changes of ITP, they were incorporated into the model for this patient. The modified

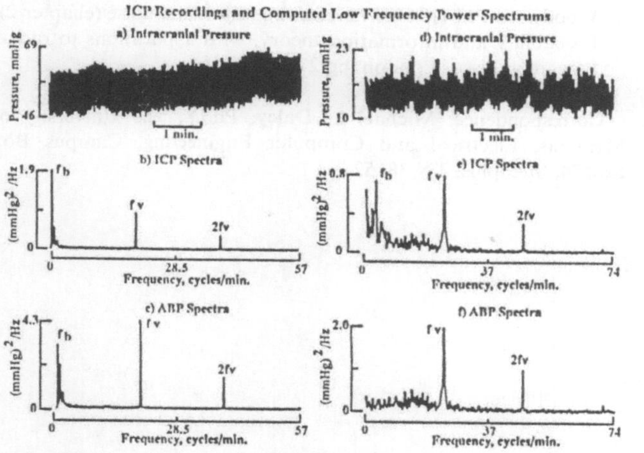

Fig. 2. ICP Recordings and Computed ICP and ABP Spectrums (a) ICP Recording. (b) Computed ICP Spectrum. (c) Computed ICP Spectrum. Both ICP and ABP spectrums contain frequency activity in the B-wave range. (d) ICP Recording. (e) Computed ICP Spectrum. (f) Computed ICP Spectrum. Only ICP spectrum contains salient spectral peaks in the B-wave frequency range

model accurately predicted the 10 locations of higher frequencies associated with the fundamental cardiac frequency with mean error ($\pm$SD) of -0.108 (± 0.06) cycles/min and -0.001 (± 0.023) cycles/min for the ABP and ICP recordings. Seven patients (64%) demonstrated evidence of the occurrence of B-waves. An example of an ICP recording, the computed ICP and ABP spectrums both containing activity in B-wave range is shown (see Fig. 2a,b,c). Fifty-four percent (4/7) of the seven patients exhibited B-wave activity solely within the ICP recording. An example of such an ICP recording and corresponding computed spectrums is shown (see Fig. 2d,e,f). To investigate the possibility that variation of heart rate may be related to B-wave activity, a comparison of heart-rate activity during recording periods with and without the occurrence of B-waves was done. In all cases, heart rate variation was synchronous with the ventilation cycle, maintaining a relatively constant rate and transiently decreasing approximately 2–3 beats/min at the onset of expiration. Variation of heart rate was not related to the occurrence of B-waves.

Discussion

Because of the periodic nature of both the ABP and ITP recordings, the low frequency segments of computed spectrums from all patients contained salient peaks at multiples of the principal cardiac and ventilator frequencies (see Fig. 1). Spectral peaks are also evident about the principal cardiac frequency and first harmonic are at locations of $\pm$fv, and $\pm$2fv (see Fig. 1). Furthermore, because the model is based on the multiplication of two periodic functions, the resultant power spectrum will exhibit side-bands at fixed modulation frequencies as shown (see Fig. 1). The proposed model predicts the frequency locations of the spectral side-bands about the principal cardiac frequency and its harmonic to within a 1% error for all patients. Further support for the validity of the proposed model was obtained from computed spectrums derived from pressure recordings taken during a period in which a patient synchronously interacted with the ventilator. For this case the patient actively expired about every 2.5 ventilation cycles. Based on the assumption that ITP remained high during periods of active expiration, the modified model accurately predicted the frequency location of the side-bands to within a 1% error.

Variation of heart-rate was similar in all patients and was not related to the occurrence of a B-wave. Three patients demonstrated spectral peaks in the B-wave range in computed power spectrums obtained from both the ICP and ABP recordings similar to those shown (see Fig. 2a,b,c). This group contained the only patient who did not recoveryfrom injury (see Fig. 2a,b,c). Four patients demonstrated spectral peaks in the B-wave range only in the computed spectrum obtained from the ICP recording similar to the example given in Fig. 2e,f,g. The absence of corresponding spectral peaks in the B-wave range of the computed ABP power spectrums suggest that variations of cardiac output were not a factor in the generation of the B-wave. From their study on Doppler derived middle cerebral artery velocity waves, Newell and his colleagues have suggested that B-waves in the ICP recording are a secondary effect of vasomotor waves that are produced by fluctuations of cerebral blood flow [2]. Such a mechanism would also produce the spectral characteristics demonstrated by this group of four patients.

References

1. Daley ML, Gallo AE, Mauch W (1986) Analysis of the intracranial pressure pulsation associated with the cardiac cycle. Innovation Et Tech. En Biologie Et Medicine 7: 537–544
2. Hashimoto M, Higashi S, Kogure Y, Fujii H, Tokuda K, Ito H, Yamamoto S (1989) Respiratory and cardiovascular oscillations during B-waves. In: Hoff JT, Betz Al (eds) Intracranial pressure VII. Springer, Berlin Heidelberg New York Tokyo, pp 217–219

3. Lundberg N (1960) Continuous recording and control of ventricular fluid pressure in neurosurgical practice. Acta Psych Neurol Scand [Suppl] 36: 1–193
4. Newell DW, Aaslid R, Stooss R, Reulen HJ (1992) The relationship of blood flow velocity fluctuations to intracranial pressure B waves. J Neurosurgery 76: 415–421
5. Woodward PM (1967) Waveform analysis and noise (chapter 2). Probability and information theory, with applications to radar. Pergamon Press, London, pp 27–33

Correspondence: Michael L. Daley, Ph.D., The University of Memphis, Electrical and Computer Engineering, Campus Box 526574, Memphis, TN 38152.

Acta Neurochir (2002) [Suppl] 81: 151–153

Variation of Proposed Correlation Indices of Cerebrovascular Reactivity with Change of Arteriolar Diameter

M. L. Daley[1], **M. Pourcyous**[2], **A. Willis**[3], and **C. W. Leffler**[3]

[1] Department of Electrical and Computer Engineering, The University of Memphis, Memphis, TN
[2] Departments of Pediatrics, Obstetrics/Gyn., and Physiology, University of Tennessee Health Science Center, Memphis, TN
[3] Departments of Physiology and Pediatrics, University of Tennessee Health Science Center, Memphis, TN

Summary

The purpose of this study was to examine the relationship between proposed correlation indices of cerebrovascular reserve and corresponding changes of cerebrovascular reserve as measured by changes of pial arteriolar diameter. Mild and severe physiologic challenge was produced in piglets by appropriate ventilation with foreign gas mixture and altered alveolar ventilation. Intracranial pressure (ICP), arterial blood pressure (ABP), and video micrometer recordings of pial arteriolar diameter were made. Serial values of ICP and ABP were used to compute the Correlation Coefficient index (Corrx) and the Pressure Reactivity Index (PrX). For the 10 mild physiologic challenge experiments, correlations between percent change index (%ΔCorrx and %ΔPrX) and percent change of pial arteriolar diameter (%Δdia.) induced by mild challenges ($n = 40$) were 0.51 ($p < .005$) and 0.097 (p n.s.) respectively. For 8 asphyxia experiments, serial values with respect to time of the correlation indices were correlated with %Δdia. obtained before, during induction and recovery. The grand mean ($n = 8$) correlation values (±S.D.) of the Corrx and PrX were 0.76 (±0.18, $p < .025$) and 0.21 (±0.38, p n.s.) respectively. In contrast to the PrX index, changes of the Corrx index significantly correlated with changes of pial arteriolar diameter. However, Corrx and PrX were simultaneously high only during a state of maximum dilation. These findings suggest that sudden salient increases of the Corrx and PrX indices induced by physiologic challenge are indicative of vigorous dilatory response of the cerebral arterioles and loss of cerebrovascular reserve.

Keywords: Intracranial pressure; reactivity indices.

Introduction

Recently, two numerical indices, the Corrx and PrX, derived from correlation of features of the ICP and ABP have been proposed as continuous means of evaluating aspects of cerebrovascular reserve in patients with severe traumatic brain injury. The Corrx index is based on independent laboratory observations that during normal cerebral vascular tone the ICP and ABP recordings are not similar [3, 5]. In contrast, during deep hypercapnia and maximal vascular dilation, when the brain has lost the ability to autoregulate, these pressure signals are similar [3, 5]. The PrX index is numerically derived from the correlation of the low frequency characteristics of the ICP and ABP recordings and designed to continuously monitor slow spontaneous waves in ICP and ABP [2]. This index is based on epidemiologic clinical observations which indicated that a sustained high value during the first 2 days following injury was indicative of an unfavorable outcome [2].

The purpose of the present study was to examine changes of the proposed correlation indices of cerebrovascular reserve and corresponding changes of cerebrovascular reserve as measured by changes of pial arteriolar diameter induced by mild and severe physiologic challenge.

Materials and Methods

Using an approved protocol from the institutional review boards involved and similar to those procedures previously described [2], 18 α-chloralose anesthetized piglets ranging in weight from 2 to 4 kg were used in this study. In each piglet a cranial window was placed and video micrometer recordings were made as described previously [3]. A fluid-filled catheter inserted in either the brachial artery or femoral artery was used to record ABP, and ICP was recorded using a Camino transducer placed in the parenchyma. Two groups of piglets were studied. In one group ($n = 10$), ventilation with foreign gas mixtures and altered alveolar ventilation were used to manipulate $PaCO_2$ and PaO_2 and induce mild physiologic challenge. In the other group ($n = 8$), asphyxia was induced by prolonged ventilation with 10% O_2, 10% CO_2, and 80% N_2 gas mixture. Respiratory support and the gas mixture were manipulated to maintain the systemic arterial blood pressure (ABP) above 35 mmHg and the heart-rate between 50 and 80 beats/min [6].

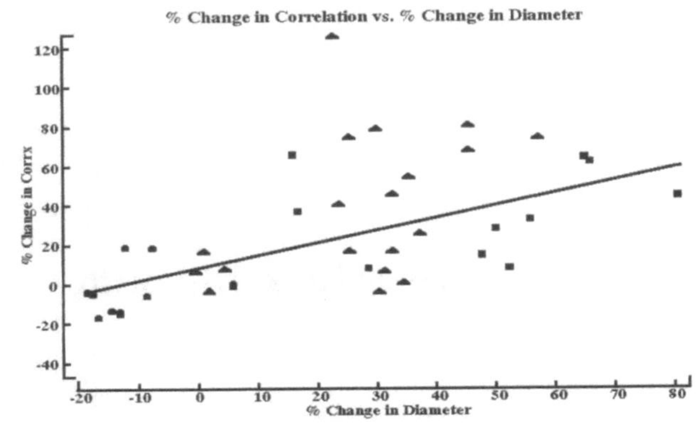

Fig. 1. Percent Change in Proposed Index versus Percent Change in Diameter: a) %ΔCorrx versus %Δdia. Each plotted point represents the maximum average change in a set of 3 arterioles during mild challenge to either an increased $PaCO_2$ (solid squares), a decreased $PaCO_2$ (solid circles), or a decreased PaO_2 (solid triangles) in arterial blood. The regression line has slope and intercept parameters of 0.68 and 8.94% respectively. The correlation between %ΔCorrx and %Δdia. was 0.51 ($n = 40$, $p < .005$). Paired values of %PrX and %Δdia. were highly variable with a correlation of 0.095 (p n.s.) and not plotted

Pressure recordings were sampled at 250 Hz, and artifact screening was accomplished by an updated defined criteria [6]. Using procedures previously described, both the Corrx [3] and the PrX [2] were derived from the digitized recordings using commercially available DADiSP software. For each experiment, 3–5 pial arterioles ranging in diameter from 35 um to 110 um were selected, and the diameter was recorded at two-minute intervals.

Results

For the 10 mild challenge experiments, average changes of PaCO2 (±S.D.) and PaO2 (±S.D.) to increased CO2, decreased CO2, and decreased O2 were: a) 30.2 (±16.7) mmHg and −11.1 (±13) mmHg; b) −15.5 (±3.1) mmHg and 20.7 (±10) mmHg; and c) 0.56 (±3.9) mmHg and −58.0 (±22) mmHg respectively. The values of %ΔCorrx and %ΔPrX and percent change of pial arteriolar diameter (%Δdia.) induced by mild challenges ($n = 40$) were determined. Correlation values for these relationships were 0.51 ($p < .005$) and 0.097 (p n.s.) respectively. Because of the high variablility of %PrX, only values of %ΔCorrx versus %Δdia. are shown (see Fig. 1). For the eight asphyxia experiments, serial values with respect to time of the proposed indices were determined. Typically, the induction of asphyxia produced a 30% to 40% increase in diameter corresponding to a 65% to 75% decrease in the average value of arteriolar resistance (see Fig. 2). Each index was paired with the corresponding value of %Δdia. obtained before, during

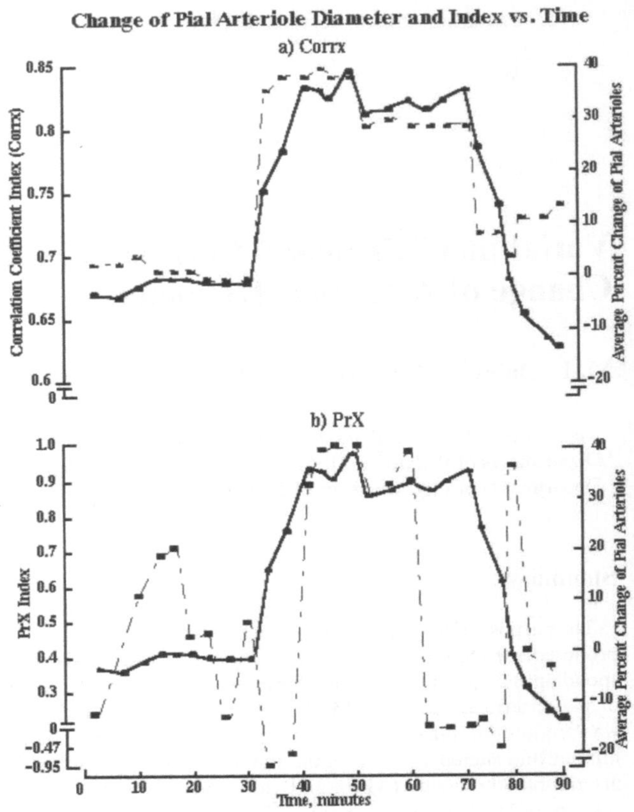

Fig. 2. Example of Serial Values of Proposed Index (Corrx or PrX) and %Δdia. Before, During, and Following Induction of Asphyxia (a) Corrx values (x symbol) and %Δdia. (solid circle) plotted on intervals of 3.33 minutes. (b) PrX values (solid squares) and %Δdia. (solid circle) plotted on intervals of 3.33 minutes. Each plotted %Δdia. value represents the average change in diameter of three arterioles measured every two minutes. Asphyxia induced at 30 minutes and stopped at 70 minutes. Generally, both Corrx and PrX were simultaneously above 0.8 within the first six minutes following induction of asphyxia. Correlation values of Corrx and PrX with %Δdia. were 0.834 ($p < .005$, $n = 28$) and 0.154 (p n.s., $n = 28$) respectively

induction and recovery. The grand mean ($n = 8$) correlation values (±S.D.) for the Corrx and PrX indices were 0.76 (± 0.18, $p < .025$) and 0.21 (± 0.38, p n.s.) respectively. In all cases when both indices were only simultaneously above 0.8 only during asphyxia.

Discussion

For the set of ten mild challenge experiments, it is not surprising that %ΔCorrx was significantly correlated with %Δdia. and %ΔPrX was not (see Fig. 1). The design of the Corrx index is based on laboratory observations that the more similar the ICP and ABP recordings are the more dilated the vasculature [3, 5].

On the other hand, the design of the PrX is based on epidemiological clinical observations and is thought to assess low frequency vasomotor activity [2]. Thus, while mild constrictive or dilatory challenges would be expected to induce corresponding decreases and increases of Corrx, such challenges may not be sufficient to provoke low frequency vasomotor activity in healthy piglets without brain trauma. For the set of eight asphyxia experiments, the strong correlation between Corrx and %Δdia. was expected; however, the lack of a consistent change in PrX was not (see Fig. 2). Within the first six minutes of induction of asphyxia, both the Corrx and PrX indices were simultaneously high, generally above a value of 0.9. But unlike the Corrx index, the PrX generally failed to maintain a consistently high response and became variable during asphyxia. Here again, the lack of consistently high value of PrX may reflect the physiological differences between the laboratory model and the pathophysiology of human traumatic brain injury. However, the lack of a consistent response of the PrX to mild and severe physiological challenge could reflect numerical artifact. While employing a five second moving average effectively produces a low pass filtering of the ICP and ABP recordings, using averages at 5 sec intervals results in down-sampling at a rate of 0.2 Hz or 1.2 cycles/min, and numerical aliasing could become a significant factor.

The Corrx and PrX indices relate to laboratory and clinical work done by others using systems analysis approaches to examine the relationship between ICP and ABP. Chopp and Portnoy have noted that the coherence function is similar to a cross-correlation function in the frequency domain [1]. Furthermore, they found that like the Corrx, the coherence function approached unity at each frequency during severe hypercapnia and maximum dilation [1]. From a spectral analysis of clinical recordings, Piper and his colleagues suggested that the near unity transmission of the cardiac ABP frequency harmonics to the ICP spectrum may indicate reduced cerebrovascular tone.

The results of this experiment demonstrate that Corrx index follows changes of arteriolar diameter and thus reflects changes of cerebrovascular reserve. Furthermore, when both the PrX and Corrx are simultaneously approaching unity, cerebrovascular reserve is likely lost.

References

1. Chopp M, Portnoy HD (1980) Systems analysis of intracranial pressure. J Neurosurg 53: 516–527
2. Czosnyka M, Smielewski P, Kirkpatrick P, Laing R, Menon D, Pickard JD (1997) Continuous assessment of the cerebral vasomotor reactivity in head injury. Neurosurgery 41: 11–19
3. Daley ML, Leffler CW (1998) Correlation coefficient between ICP and arterial pressure: a gauge of cerebral vascular dilation. Acta Neurochir (Wien) [Suppl] 71: 285–288
4. Piper IR, Miller JD, Dearden NM, Leggate JRS, Robertson I (1990) Systems analysis of cerebrovascular pressure transmission: an observational study in head-injury patients. J Neurosurg 73: 871–880
5. Portnoy HD, Chopp M, Branch M, Shannon MB (1982) Cerebrospinal fluid pulse waveform as an indicator of cerebral autoregulation. J Neurosurgery 56: 666–678
6. Pourcyrous M, Parfenova H, Bada HS, Kornes SB, Leffler CW (1997) Changes in cerebral cyclic nucleotides and cerebral blood flow during prolonged asyphyxia and recovery in newborn pigs. Pediatric Res 41: 617–623

Correspondence: Michael L. Daley, Ph.D., The University of Memphis, Electrical and Computer Engineering, Campus Box 526574, Memphis, TN 38152.

Acta Neurochir (2002) [Suppl] 81: 155–157

Use of Resistance-Area Product Derived from Doppler MCA Velocity to Estimate the Range of Active Cerebrovascular Regulation

M. L. Daley[1], **C. W. Leffler**[2], **S. Jackson**[3], and **I. Piper**[3]

[1] Department of Electrical and Computer Engineering, The University of Memphis, Memphis, TN
[2] Departments of Physiology and Pediatrics, University of Tennessee Health Science Center, Memphis, TN
[3] Institute of Neurological Sciences, Glasgow, Scotland

Summary

The purpose of the present study was to explore the development of a method to estimate the range of active cerebrovascular regulation using resistance-area product (RAP) derived from transcranial Doppler ultrasound recordings of middle cerebral artery blood velocity (MCAV) obtained before and after physiologic challenge.

Intracranial pressure (ICP), arterial blood pressure (ABP), and MCAV were monitored on 9 patients before and after challenges with either Noradrenlin or CO2 inhalation. One patient was monitored at 24, 48, 72, and 96 hrs. For each cardiac cycle a value of RAP was computed from the inverse of the slope of the regression line of paired values of aligned MCAV and ABP recordings. Mean values of percent change of difference of RAP (%ΔRAP) versus change of cerebral perfusion pressure (CPP) were computed. Theoretical values of %ΔRAP were derived from reported lab values of percent change diameter of arterioles versus ABP. Of the nine patients, 22% (2/9) demonstrated either impaired dilation and/or constriction. Furthermore, the correlation between theoretical and experimental values of %ΔRAP and CPP ($n = 34$) was strong ($r = .86$, $p < .005$). The serially-monitored patient failed to dilate during all CO2 challenges and to fully constrict to the Noradrenlin challenge at 72 hrs. %ΔRAP associated with corresponding changes of CPP may have value as a clinical method to estimate the range of active cerebrovascular regulation.

Keywords: Pressure regulation; middle cerebral artery blood velocity.

Introduction

Knowledge of the continuous status of pressure autoregulation could be used to devise targeted therapies for patients with severe head injury [2]. Previously, in order to evaluate the status of autoregulation, others have used inert tracer methods to evaluate change in cerebral blood flow from physiologic challenge [1, 4]. Indirect methods have been reported which attempt to derive information on the state of autoregulation through an analysis of the ABP and ICP recordings [3, 5]. While such methods may indicate whether the cerebrovascular bed is dilated, they fail to distinguish whether the state of dilation is due to active or impaired autoregulatory mechanisms. The purpose of the present study was to explore the development of a method to estimate the range of active cerebrovascular regulation using resistance-area product (RAP) derived from transcranial Doppler ultrasound recordings of middle cerebral artery blood velocity (MCAV) obtained before and after physiologic challenge.

Materials and Methods

The study design and patient consent form were reviewed and approved by the local Ethics committee of Southern General Hospital, Glasgow. Nine patients (8 males and 1 female) were recruited into the study. Age ranged from 15–49 years with mean (±S.D.) of 28.9 (±12.9) yrs. Admission Glasgow Coma Scale ranged from 3–12 with mean (±S.D.) of 6.2 (±2.7). Admission CT-Scans showed the primary diagnosis as diffuse injury in 3 patients, subdural haematoma in 2 patients, and unilateral or bilateral contusion in 4 patients. ICP was measured using the Camino intraparenchymal probe. Bilateral MCA TCD velocity (MCA) was monitored using a SciMed QVL Doppler system. All recordings were obtained within 48 hrs of injury and sampled at 250 Hz before, during and after physiologic challenges, applied in random order. Patients were sedated (morphine, midazolam, propofol) and ventilated according to a standardized protocol. $PaCO_2$ was increased by 1 kPa by adding known concentrations of CO_2 in the inspired gas mixture. ABP was increased by 25% from pre-challenge levels by intravenous infusion of noradrenalin (.05 ug/kg/min). Arterial blood samples were taken before, during and after each challenge.

Numerical Methods: Using commercially available DADiSP software, digitized recordings of ABP and MCAV were analyzed to obtain the resistance-area product parameter following a procedure which accounts for changes in critical closing pressure (CCP) described by others [3, 5]. Briefly, the RAP parameter was obtained as follows. For each cardiac cycle, the MCVA and ABP waveforms were aligned, and the regression line between MCAV and ABP was determined as:

$$\text{MCAV} = (\text{slope})^{*}\text{ABP} + (\text{intercept}). \qquad (1)$$

Parameter values derived from aligned cardiac cycles of MCAV and ABP with a correlation value of less than 0.7 were not considered for analysis. From eqn. (1), the RAP value and CCP are expressed as RAP = (1/slope) and CCP = (intercept/slope). Percent change in RAP due to physiologic challenge was calculated as:

$$\%\Delta\text{RAP} = 100^{*}(\text{RAP}_{\text{challenge}} - \text{RAP}_{\text{baseline}})/(\text{RAP}_{\text{baseline}}). \qquad (2)$$

To compute the theoretical relationship between %ΔRAP and cerebral perfusion pressure (CPP), the relationship between change in arteriolar diameter in the range of 30–185 um to mean arterial pressure was extrapolated from published laboratory data (6) as:

$$r_{\text{challenge}} = r_{\text{baseline}} - (0.004)(\Delta\text{CPP})(r_{\text{baseline}}) \qquad (3)$$

where $r_{\text{challenge}}$ and r_{baseline} represent the extrapolated radius of arteriole during challenge and baseline conditions respectively. Change in CPP was computed on the assumption that ICP remains approximately constant during the theoretical challenge and therefore change of ABP represents change in CPP in eqn. (1) above. Finally, to account for a possible change in the area of middle cerebral artery during the challenge a graded linear change in the cross-sectional area of the MCA up to ±10% for a change of CPP at ±40 mmHg was also assumed. Thus, the theoretical expression for %ΔRAP is expressed as:

$$\%\Delta\text{RAP} = 100^{*}((r_{\text{baseline}}/r_{\text{challenge}})^{4}(A_{\text{challenge}}/A_{\text{baseline}}) - 1) \qquad (4)$$

where $A_{\text{challenge}}$ and A_{baseline} represent the area of the middle cerebral artery during challenge and baseline.

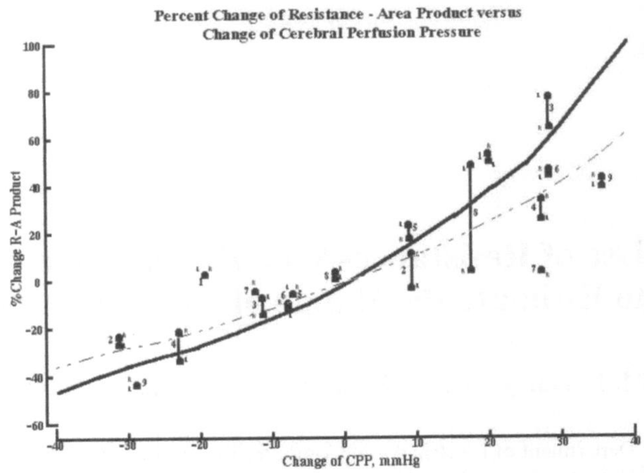

Fig. 1. Percent Change of Resistance-Area Product versus Change of Cerebral Perfusion Pressure. Each plotted point represents the mean %RAP for left (L) and right (R) hemispheres. Number of samples for computation of mean value varies from 68 to 260. For all values the computed standard error falls within the solid circle. Dash line represents theoretical %ΔRAP value computed with a linear change of MCA area limited to 10% for a 40 mmHg change of CPP, and solid line represents computation without possible MCA area adjustment. Patient #7 exhibited a −1.3% change to the noradrenalin challenge and decreased slightly by −2.8% to the CO_2 challenge that produced a 12.5 mmHg change of CPP. Also, Patient #1 apparently failed to dilate during challenge with CO_2 but demonstrated a more than adequate constrictive response when challenged with noradrenalin

Results

Mean values of %ΔRAP and standard deviations were plotted with respect to the corresponding change of CPP associated with the physiologic challenge (see Fig. 1). The solid and dash lines represent the theoretical %ΔRAP without and with MCA area adjustment. For one patient (#7), MCAV recordings were available only from the right MCA. The correlation between theoretical and experimental values of %ΔRAP and CPP (n = 34) was strong ($r = .86$, $p < .005$). Of the nine patients, 22% (2/9) demonstrated either impaired dilation and/or constriction. Specifically, for one patient (#7) the %ΔRAP did not increase during the challenge with noradrenalin and decreased slightly by −2.8% during challenge with CO_2 that resulted in a decrease of CPP by 12.5 mmHg and increase of ICP of 14 mmHg. Another patient (#1) demonstrated a %ΔRAP change of +2.9% during a CO_2 challenge that resulted in a 19 mmHg decrease in CPP. For the single serially-monitored patient, values of %ΔRAP versus change of CPP during challenge are plotted (see Fig. 2). The correlation was also strong ($r = .78$, $n = 18$, $p < .005$). However, apparently this patient consistently failed to fully dilate during all CO2 challenges

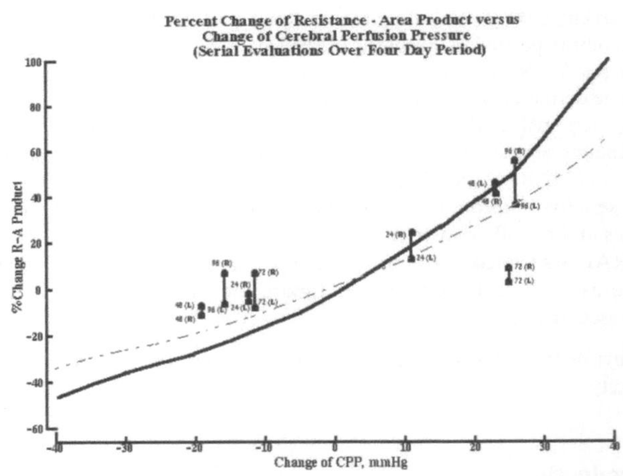

Fig. 2. Serial Evaluations of %ΔRAP versus Change of Cerebral Perfusion Pressure over a Four Day Period. Each plotted point represents the mean %ΔRAP versus change of CPP taken at 24, 48, 72, and 96 hrs. For all values the computed standard error falls within the solid circle. Number of samples for computation of mean varies from 68 to 260. Dash line represents theoretical %ΔRAP value computed with a linear change of MCA area limited to 10% for a 40 mmHg change of CPP, and solid line represents computation without possible MCA area adjustment. During the four day monitoring period, this patient consistently exhibited a weak dilatory response and apparently failed to constrict to the noradrenalin challenge taken at 72 hrs

and to fully constrict during challenge with noradrenalin at 72 hrs.

Discussion

Because during a passive pressure regulation changes of flow are approximately proportional to changes of CPP and resistance remains relatively constant, contributions to %ΔRAP should be approximately zero outside the range of active regulation. Thus, the %ΔRAP index only measures the active change of resistance produced by the physiologic challenge and reflects only the active range over which regulation occurred during the challenge. A value near zero or in the opposite of expectation can be classified as inappropriate. As measured by %ΔRAP, most patients demonstrated an appropriate response when physiologically challenged with only 22% failing to do so. Specifically, one patient demonstrated a decreased value of %ΔRAP of −1.3% to a noradrenalin challenge, and the other patient exhibited an increase of 2.9% during a CO_2 challenge. Also, the one patient who was serially monitored generally demonstrated an adequate increase in %ΔRAP to noradrenalin challenge except at the 72 hr. assessment and a consistently weak response indicative of passive pressure regulation for all CO_2 challenges.

These preliminary results suggest that %ΔRAP associated with corresponding changes of CPP may have value as a clinical method to estimate the range of active cerebrovascular regulation.

References

1. Bouma GJ, Muizelaar P, Bandoh K, Marmarou A (1992) Blood pressure and intracranial pressure-volume dynamics in severe head-injury: relationship with cerebral blood flow. J Neurosurg 77: 15–19
2. Chesnut RM (1996) Treating raised intracranial pressure in head injury. In: Narayan RK, Wilberger JE, Polvishock JT (eds) Neurotrauma. McGraw-Hill, New York
3. Dawson SL, Panerai RB, Potter JF (1999) Critical closing pressure explains cerebral hemodynamics during the Valsava maneuver. J Applied Physiol 86(2): 675–680
4. Enevoldsen EM, Jensen FT (1978) Autoregulation and CO_2 responses of cerebral blood flow in patients with acute severe head injury. J Neurosurgery 48: 689–703
5. Kontos H, Wei EP, Navari RM, Levasseur JE, Rosenblum WI, Patterson JL (1978) Responses of cerebral arteries and arterioles to acute hypotension and hypertension. Am J Physiol 234(4): H371–H383
6. Panerai RB, Coughtrey H, Rennie JM, Evans DH (1993) A model of the instantaneous pressure-velocity relationships of the neonatal cerebral circulation. Physiol Meas 14: 411–418

Correspondence: Michael L. Daley, Ph.D., The University of Memphis, Electrical and Computer Engineering, Campus Box 526574, Memphis, TN 38152.

ICP Analysis

Acta Neurochir (2002) [Suppl] 81: 161–162

Online Analysis of Intracranial Pressure Waves

M. Walter[1], **M. Kiefer**[2], **S. Leonhardt**[1], **W. I. Steudel**[2], and **R. Isermann**[1]

[1] Institute of Automatic Control, Darmstadt University of Technology, Darmstadt, Germany
[2] Department of Neurosurgery, Saarland University, Homburg/Saar, Germany

Summary

Brain pressure waves, particularly B-waves, as they were described by Lundberg contain valuable diagnostic information about the patient's status. So far, this information cannot be used on a daily routine basis because manual analysis of the recorded ICP data is very time consuming. Furthermore, the analysis is only retrospective, after incidents of interest occurred. To overcome these drawbacks, an automated B-wave detection system has been developed. Using a direct spectral estimation method (so called ARMA approach) the most significant spectral components and their amplitudes in the ICP signal are identified. The frequency with the biggest amplitude inside the B-wave band is a reliable indicator of B-wave activity and can be displayed on-line on a bedside computer.

Keywords: ICP; intracranial pressure waves; online analysis; B-waves.

Introduction

The intracranial volume may be subdivided into three compartments (brain tissue, CSF and blood) and is connected to the ICP via a pressure-volume relationship. While the volume of CSF and tissue may be viewed as constant in a short time range, changes in intracranial blood volume account for the faster periodical changes of the ICP. They may either be caused by an increased arterial inflow of blood, changes in the vasomotoric tension, or a decreased venous outflow. Lundberg [3] categorised these pressure waves regarding their shape and frequency (see Fig. 1). A-waves or plateau waves are incidents of a strongly elevated ICP and a duration up to 20 minutes. P-waves are caused by the pulsating inflow of arterial blood and are thus linked to the heart rate. B-waves have frequencies in the range of 0.5 to 2 per minute. Their shape is differing widely. Some follow a sinusoidal pattern, others are sawtooth like. The amplitude of the pressure waves is connected directly to the magnitude of the change in volume and the pressure volume characteristic. Their occurrence and amplitude may support the neurosurgeon in assessment of the patient's status [2].

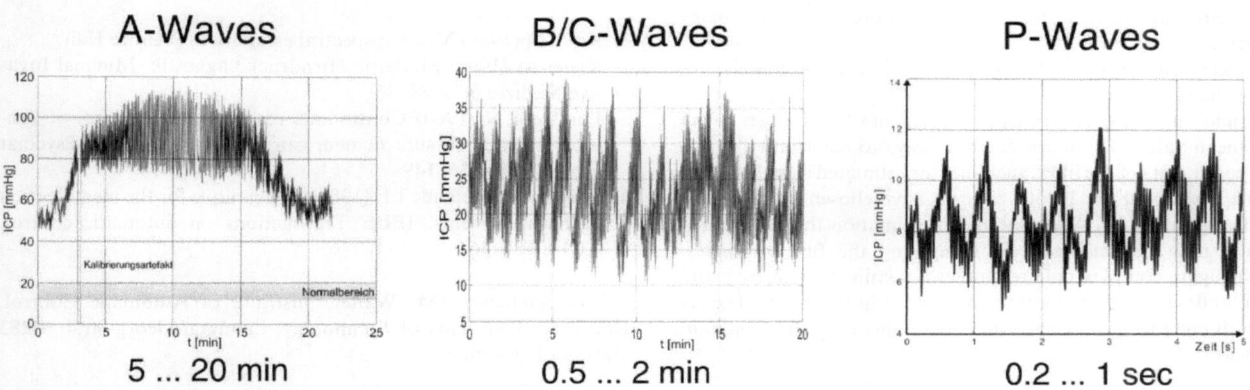

Fig. 1. Intracranial Pressure Waves

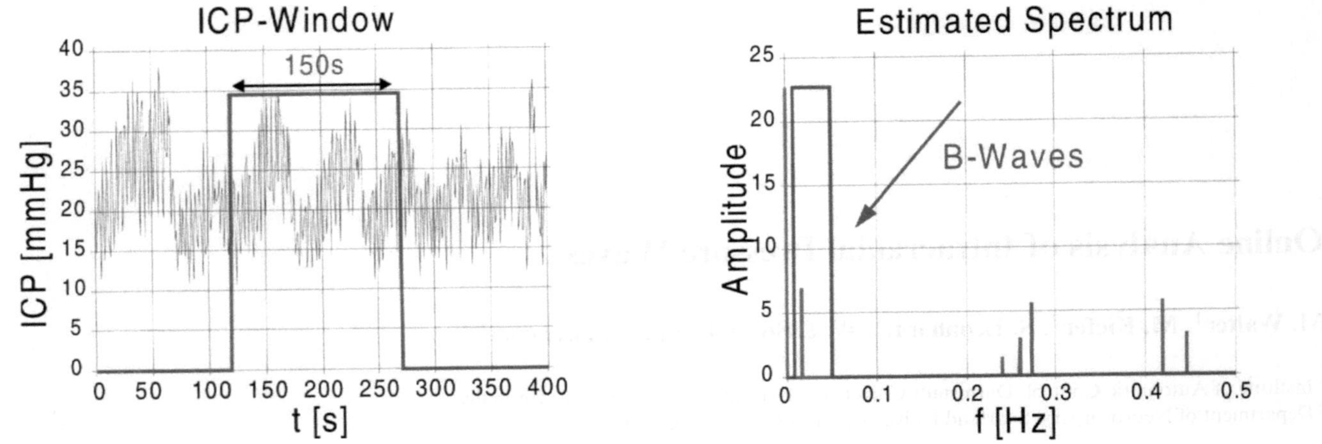

Fig. 2. Analysis window and computed B-wave indicator

Methods

As periodical changes in the ICP are to be detected, it is obvious to apply a frequency analysis. Normally this is done using a Fourier transformation. As we use data sampled at 1 sample/sec, the discrete form of the fourier transformation has to be used. Unfortunately there are certain drawbacks when using the Fourier transformation, which makes it unsuitable in the given context.

- Due to the discrete frequency distribution, a maximum error in amplitude of 36% may be encountered.
- For precise estimation of the frequencies and amplitudes at least four full cycles should be inside the analysis window. Given a minimum frequency of 0.5/min, the analysis window would be 8 minutes long (or 480 samples).
- Often there are only a few consecutive B-waves contained in the ICP. These inconsistencies lead to big errors in the frequency distribution.
- A steady increase in the mean value leads also to big errors in the frequency distribution.
- B-waves are often instationary both in amplitude and frequency. The time between consecutive waves is not constant and the amplitude is changing.
- A change in the signals noise components may also be misinterpreted.

To overcome these problems we used a different approach to frequency analysis: the direct spectral estimation or so called ARMA method. Most signals as in this case contain only a few dominant frequencies.

Its z transform resembles a filter of order 2 n whose impulse response is the estimated ICP signal.

If we add another order we can even account for changes in the signals mean value. There are different ways to determine the unknown parameters of the filter, such that the estimated signal is a best fit to the real signal [1]. In our case we have chosen the Steiglitz-McBride algorithm [4]. After parameter estimation the back transformation may be performed in computing the function poles. Each conjugate complex pole resembles a dominant frequency and the amplitude is given by the function residue in this point. The result is a discrete frequency spectrum containing only the dominant frequencies.

In order to identify B-waves a B-wave band is defined between 0.0083 Hz and 0.05 Hz. The B-wave activity is represented by the largest amplitude inside this band. With each new sample the 150 sample analysis window is shifted and the B-wave indicator computed (see Fig. 2).

Results and Conclusions

So far the algorithm has been tested on 150 offline datasets and the results were compared with the manual analysis of an experienced neurosurgeon. We found a good correlation between computer and human analysis. In a next step we integrated the algorithm in an on-line data acquisition environment, so the B-wave activity can now be displayed on a bedside computer system. It is now possible to value wave activity in correlation with other clinical patient data on a daily routine basis.

References

1. Kay SM (1988) Modern spectral estimation. Prentice Hall
2. Kiefer M (1995) Moderne Hirndruckdiagnostik. Minimal Invasive Medizin 6(2): 78–86
3. Lundberg N (1960) Continuous recording and control of ventricular fluid pressure in neurosurgical practice. Acta Psychiat Scand [Suppl] 36: 149
4. Steiglitz K, McBride LE (1980) A technique for the identification of linear systems. IEEE Transactions on automatic control. AC10: 461–464

Correspondence: M. Walter, Institute of Automatic Control, Darmstadt University of Technology, Landgraf-Georg-Str.4, 64283 Darmstadt, Germany.

Acta Neurochir (2002) [Suppl] 81: 163–165

Information Technology and CPP Management in Neuro Intensive Care

P. H. Mitchell, R. L. Burr, and C. J. Kirkness

Biobehavioral Nursing & Health Systems, University of Washington, Seattle WA, USA

Summary

This study developed and tested the acceptability of a computer interface intended to provide better information about CPP to Neuro Intensive Care nurses. Maintaining adequate CPP is crucial in preventing secondary brain injury, yet current monitoring data displays have poor ergonomics that minimize usable information for clinicians. Information systems developmental methods were used to 1) formulate the model for CPP information display, 2) develop the system with end-users, and 3) install the system in the Neuro Intensive Care Unit. System testing for effects on clinicians and patient outcomes is occurring in a randomized clinical trial. Metaphor graphic and universal graphic displays were tested with 37 staff nurses from three intensive care units using continuous ICP monitoring. Nursing staff preferred an augmented universal data display to the metaphor graphics, endorsing a modified trend area graph with threshold-dependent properties. The preferred model was programmed in Visual Basic and installed on small computers that were randomly allocated as live or blank displays to beds of newly admitted head injury or aneurysmal subarachnoid hemorrhage patients with continuous monitoring. Nursing acceptability of the information interface was achieved through the use of end-user focus groups that resulted in modifying the metaphor graphic approach to a more readily understandable one.

Keywords: Cerebral perfusion pressure; information technology; intensive care.

Introduction

Current clinical management of patients with brain injuries emphasizes maintaining CPP at or above 70 mm Hg, based on the correlation of that threshold with better patient outcomes [2]. CPP can be influenced by nursing care such as positioning, sensory stimuli and suctioning [4], with the potential for multiple daily episodes of diminished perfusion. Minute to minute nursing monitoring and evaluation of CPP responses to both internal stimuli and ongoing care such as positioning or suctioning may reduce the number of these episodes of potential secondary injury and thereby improve overall patient outcome. However, nursing access to meaningful *information* about the patient's minute to minute CPP state is limited, even with current monitoring technology.

Data regarding ICP, ABP and CPP are readily available at the patient's bedside and should be used to guide ongoing nursing evaluation of patient CPP responses to ongoing care. However, current monitoring data displays have poor ergonomics that minimize usable information for clinicians. Biomedical informatics distinguishes data from information in terms of its usefulness in guiding decision-making. *Data* are the ongoing values for the various clinical parameters, such as ABP, ICP, CPP, while *information* is the integration of these values into a clinically relevant picture.

Information requires the interpretation of the meaning of the data, in the context of trends within and among these data, and knowledge of the critical values [1]. The choice and evaluation of a clinical therapeutic involves more than simply tracking data values. Rather, the values in relation to one another and to the tolerable limits must be evaluated. Thus the data available at the bedside have several characteristics that may limit their usefulness to the bedside nurse in integrating them into useful clinical information. First, the data are most commonly displayed by their individual digital values, so that one must mentally subtract a moving ICP value from a similarly moving ABP value to estimate CPP. Further, critical value limits (alarms) are usually set for the individual parameters, not the integrated CPP value. Third, although CPP is readily displayed on the bedside computerized record flowsheet in the units participating in this study, this monitor is usually behind the nurse, is set to display in tabular form, and does not produce audible or visible alarms when critical values are reached. Even if it did, there is a delay between acquisition of the monitoring signal and return of the processed data to the bedside.

Metaphor graphic techniques have been shown to result in faster clinical interpretation of respiratory data than corresponding flow sheet presentation [3]. The metaphor graphic has been described as "custom tailored visual displays designed to look like the real world situation from which the date is collected but not in the literal sense of 'look like'" [3]. They are contrasted with universal graphics (typical trend, bar graphs). Metaphor graphics are dynamic, in that they change with the state of the patient and can be constructed to change in real-time when the analog output of the monitoring system is converted to a machine or computer readable format. For example, respiratory data in artificially ventilated patients was represented by rectangles of different sizes and shadings. Long rectangles represented deeper breathing, while wider rectangles more rapid breathing; deepening color represented more exhaled O_2 and thus less O_2 utilization. Experienced clinicians were able to learn and accurately interpret both the metaphor and spread sheet systems with relatively little error, but there was significantly faster performance in correct interpretation with the graphical system [3]. Thus, we proposed to develop a metaphor graphic system to represent CPP for nurses in the NICU. Both universal graphics and metaphor graphics were tested in order to evaluate staff acceptability.

Materials and Methods

Development and testing of the graphic computer interface to ICP and ABP clinical monitors involved standard approaches to Information System Development (ISD) [5].

Phase One

Model formulation consists of defining and formulating the models for acquisition, representation, processing, display or transmission of biomedical information or knowledge. Metaphor graphic and universal graphic displays of CPP were tested with 37 staff nurses from three intensive care units using ICP monitoring, to formulate the model for CPP information display. Participants in focus groups were shown metaphor and universal graphics representing changing CPP. They were asked which graphic gave them the most information about the patient's state of ICP, ABP and CPP, and what suggestions they had for improving the information.

Phase Two/Three

System development & installation. We then used the preferred graphic model to develop software that created an informational interface between the staff nurse user and the bedside monitoring data. Input processes to the display required sampling continuous analog ICP and ABP pressure signals from Spacelabs and Camino clinical monitors (at 100 samples/sec/channel using a 16 bit A/D converter). Variations related to respiratory and cardiac cycles were smoothed over a five second window. Digital data was provided to a compact pen tablet computer (233 MHZ Pentium, 4.1 GB hard drive, 32 MB SDRAM, 8.4 inch active matrix LCD screen) programmed to calculate CPP dynamically from the ICP and ABP signal. The accuracy and reliability of the programs and system were tested with in-vitro with Spacelabs simulation monitors in the hospital's Clinical Engineering department, and then in-vivo in the neuro intensive care unit. Reproduction of the nominal pressure values of the input clinical monitors was typically within 1 mm Hg.

Results

Nursing staff preferred an augmented universal data display to the metaphor graphics, endorsing a modified trend area graph with threshold-dependent properties. The preferred model was programmed in Visual Basic to the following specifications: rapidly updated dynamic CPP display (worst case 5 second latency) with good temporal resolution, providing strong horizontal line with clinical threshold (70 mm Hg), and a fill area between the x-axis and line graph, with the fill color varying as follows: blue above and red below the threshold. CPP was also displayed digitally, in large font, above the line graph, with 5 second updates. Thus the display provides a visual history of the patient's CPP state as well as the current state, depicted in both graphic and digital form. Figure 1 shows an schematic of the system, with a photo of the graphic interface

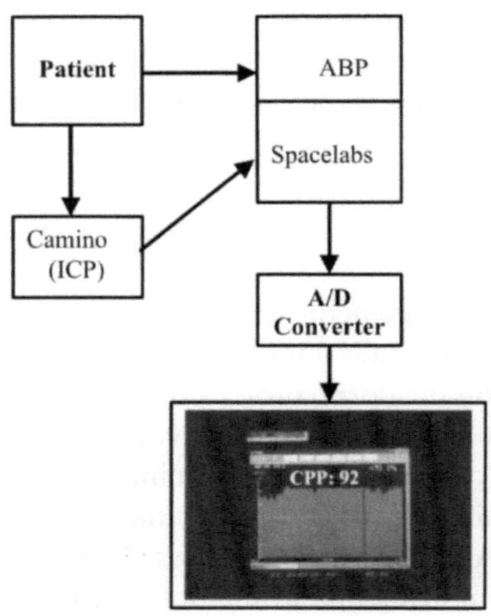

Fig. 1. Computer display of CPP incorporating bedside monitoring signals. ICP and ABP Input from the bedside monitors is processed in the converter and sent to a compact pen tablet computer for display as CPP

in use. Phase Four, system installation and testing, is ongoing in the randomized clinical trial: *Improving Cerebral Perfusion Pressure Management: Information Feedback & Nursing Care*. Patients admitted to the ICUs with acute head injury or aneurysmal subarachnoid hemorrhage and continuous ICP and ABP monitoring are randomly assigned to beds with active or blank CPP displays. Assuming optimal medical and nursing management of the acute condition, we are hypothesizing that patients in beds with active information available regarding CPP will have better maintenance of CPP and measurably improved outcomes at 6 months.

Discussion

Nursing acceptability of the information interface was achieved through the use of end-user focus groups that resulted in modifying the metaphor graphic approach to a more readily understandable one. Medical and nursing acceptability was achieved by meetings with key critical care and service committees, presence at neurosurgery teaching rounds, on-unit briefings and demonstration prior to beginning accrual of patients. System installation and testing of effects on patient care and outcomes are now occurring in the randomized clinical trial.

Acknowledgment

This work was partially funded by the Research Intramural Funding Program, School of Nursing, University of Washington, and a grant from the National Institute of Nursing Research, National Institutes of Health, RO1 NR 04901, to the senior author.

References

1. Blum BI (1986) Clinical information systems: a review. West J Med 45(6): 791–797
2. Brain Trauma Foundation (1996) Guidelines for cerebral perfusion pressure. J Neurotrauma 13(11): 693–697
3. Cole WG, Stewart JG (1994) Human performance evaluation of a metaphor graphic display for respiratory data. Meth Infor Med 33(4): 390–396
4. Mitchell PH (1997) Decreased adaptive capacity. In: Ackerley B, Ladwig G (eds) Nursing diagnosis handbook. Mosby-Yearbook, Inc St Louis, pp 293–297
5. Shneiderman B (1992) Designing the user interface. Strategies for effective human computer interaction. Addison-Wesley, New York

Correspondence: Pamela H. Mitchell, Biobehavioral Nursing and Health Systems, Box 357266, University of Washington, Seattle WA, 98195-7266, USA.

Acta Neurochir (2002) [Suppl] 81: 167–170

Multi-Centre Assessment of the Spiegelberg Compliance Monitor: Interim Results

Y. Yau[1], I. Piper[2], C. Contant[3], G. Citerio[4], K. Kiening[5], P. Enblad[6], P. Nilsson[6], S. Ng[7], J. Wasserberg[8], M. Kiefer[9], W. Poon[7], L. Dunn[2], and I. Whittle[1]

[1] Department of Clinical Neurosciences, University of Edinburgh, UK
[2] Institute of Neurological Sciences, Glasgow, UK
[3] Department of Neurosurgery, Baylor College of Medicine, Houston, Texas
[4] Ospedale San Gerardo, Monza, Italy
[5] Department of Neurosugery, Virchow Hospital, Berlin, Germany
[6] Department of Neurosurgery, University Hospital, Uppsala, Sweden
[7] Department Neurosurgery, Chinese University of Hong Kong, Hong Kong
[8] Department of Neurosurgery, Queen Mary Hospital, Birmingham, UK
[9] Department of Neurosurgery, University Hospital, Homburg, Germany
[10] Department of Neurosurgery, Institute of Neurological Sciences, Glasgow, UK

Summary

Analyses of a multi-centre database of 71 patients at risk of raised ICP showed that in head injured patients (n = 19) and tumour patients (n = 13) clear inverse relationships of ICP vs compliance exist. SAH patients (n = 5) appear to exhibit a biphasic relationship between ICP and compliance, however greater numbers of patients need to be recruited to this group. Patients with hydrocephalus (n = 34) show an initial decrease in compliance while ICP is less than 20 mmHg, thereafter compliance does not show a dependence upon ICP. A power analysis confirmed that sufficient numbers of patients have been recruited in the hydrocephalus group and a ROC analysis determined that a mean compliance value of 0.809 (lower and upper 95% CL = 0.725 & 0.894 resp.) was a critical threshold for raised ICP greater than 10 mmHg. Preliminary time-series analyses of the ICP and compliance data is revealing evidence that the cumulative time compliance is in a low compliance state (< 0.5 ml/mmHg), as a proportion of total monitoring time, increases more rapidly than the cumulative time ICP is greater than 25 mmHg. Before trials testing compliance thresholds can be designed, we need to consider not just the absolute threshold, but the duration of time spent below threshold. A survey may be required to identify a consensus of what is the minimum duration of raised ICP above 25 mmHg needed to instigate treatment.

Keywords: Intracranial pressure; craniospinal compliance; monitoring evaluation.

Introduction

A multi-centre collaborative group (*Brain-IT Group*) has recently been formed and consists of basic scientists and clinicians with a specific interest in the development and assessment of new forms of intensive care monitoring for use in Brain Injured Patients. Each member of the group contributes data to a common database collected according to a standard protocol [1]. A Web-Page has been set up which describes the guidelines and procedures of the group: *http://www.brainit.gla.ac.uk/brainit*. Currently the group is focused on assessing the *Spiegelberg Compliance Monitor*. Raised intracranial pressure (ICP) remains a significant clinical problem in patients with brain trauma, mass lesions and disturbances to cerebrospinal fluid (CSF) dynamics. Measurement of craniospinal compliance offers the potential of earlier identification of processes which lead to raised ICP. In addition to predicting ICP, a measure of compliance in combination with other features of the ICP signal may aid in clinical decisions concerning definitive measures for CSF diversion. A new method for measurement of compliance on a continuous basis has been developed [2] and we report on analyses focused on studying the relationship between compliance and ICP data from 71 patients monitored with the Spiegelberg device.

Methods

The Spiegelberg compliance monitor calculates intracranial compliance ($C = \Delta V/\Delta P$) from a moving average of small ICP perturbations (ΔP) resulting from a sequence of up to 200 pulses of added volume ($\Delta V = 0.1$ ml, total $V = 0.2$ ml) made into a double lumen

Table 1. *Associated Median Compliance (± Median Absolute Deviation) Classed Into 6 ICP Bands (mmHg)*

Group	0–10	10+–>20	20+–>30	30+–>40	40+–>50	50+
HI (n = 19)	0.77 ± .42	0.62 ± .28	0.51 ± .22	0.44 ± .25	0.37 ± .39	0.03 ± 0.03
SAH (n = 5)	0.53 ± .31	0.88 ± .61	0.43 ± .27	0.27 ± .06	0.25 ± .07	0.39 ± .33
Tumour (n = 13)	0.96 ± .37	0.79 ± .36	0.59 ± .24	0.59 ± .21	0.45 ± .21	–
Hydroceph (n = 33)	0.88 ± .39	0.69 ± .30	0.85 ± .30	1.03 ± .32	0.78 ± .07	.92 ± .17

intraventricular balloon catheter. Once a stable average has developed, the device produces a minute by minute measure of intracranial compliance. Neuro-intensive care data collected from 8 centres (Glasgow, Edinburgh, Berlin, Monza, Uppsala, Hong Kong, Homburg, Birmingham) has been recruited to date which include a total of 55000 minutes (38 days) of paired ICP and compliance values. Collected data was grouped by patient type into 4 groups: a) Head Injury (HI) n = 19 patients, b) Hydrocephalus (HYDRO) n = 34 patients, c) Post-Operative tumour (TUMOUR) n = 13 patients, d) Post-Subarachnoid Haemorrhage (SAH) n = 5 patients. Summary statistics were produced for compliance data when grouped into 6 ICP bands and classed by patient type. A receiver-operator characteristic (ROC) analysis was performed to identify critical compliance thresholds for raised ICP. Disease state was defined as ICP > 25 mmHg (>10 mmHg for the hydrocephalus group). The sensitivity and specificity was then calculated for compliance values predicting disease state when compliance was increased from 0.1 to 1.8 ml/mmHg in increments of 0.1. The cross-over point of the sensitivity and 1-specificity curves was used as an estimate of an optimal threshold. To assess the temporal relationship between compliance and ICP, analyses were performed of the proportion of time spent, of total monitoring time, for compliance less than 0.5 ml/mmHg and ICP > 25 mmHg. All analyses were performed with S-Plus 2000.

Results

Table 1 summarises the associated median compliance (± median absolute deviation) classed into 6 ICP bands. Head injured patients (n = 19) and patients after resection of tumours (n = 13) show clear inverse relationships of ICP Vs compliance. Patients with a subarachnoid haemorrhage (n = 5) appear to exhibit a biphasic relationship between ICP and compliance, however greater numbers of patients need to be recruited to this group. Patients with hydrocephalus (n = 34) show an initial decrease in compliance while ICP is less than 20 mmHg, however, above an ICP of 20 mmHg, compliance does not show a dependence upon ICP. Figure 1a shows the relative distribution of ICP between the patient groups. High ICP was predominantly found in the Head Injury, while in the SAH and Tumour groups there was proportionally very little raised ICP within the hydrocephalus group. Figure 1b shows the relative distribution of compliance between the patient groups, which demonstrates all groups showed episodes of lower compliance (≤0.5 ml/mmHg) which can, in the case of the hydrocephalus group occur in the absence of significantly raised ICP above 20 mmHg. This data supports the choice of a 10 mmHg ICP level in the calculation of a critical compliance threshold in this patient population.

Table 2 summarises the results of the ROC analyses expressed as mean and median compliance values (with upper and lower confidence limits). Note that only the hydrocephalus group has recruited sufficient numbers of patients according to an earlier performed power analysis. For the hydrocephalus group it was determined that a mean compliance value of 0.809 (lower and upper confidence limits = 0.725 and 0.894 resp) was a critical threshold for ICP > 10 mmHg.

Figure 2 is a line plot, for a single head injured patient's data with proportion of time spent (of total monitoring time). It shows that compliance was less than 0.5 ml/mmHg and similarly the proportion of time spent with ICP greater than 25 mmHg. Note that the cumulated time compliance is below threshold and rises faster than the cumulative time when ICP is greater than 25 mmHg.

Discussion and Conclusions

In patient groups known to exhibit "tight brains", intracranial compliance, as measured continuously with the Spiegelberg device, shows the expected inverse relationship with ICP. All patient groups show significant periods of lower compliance (< 0.5 ml/mmHg) which, in the case of patients with hydrocephalus, are not necessarily associated with ICP > 20 mmHg. Systematic analyses for identification of compliance thresholds for raised ICP on a patient population basis has now identified a compliance threshold for patients with hydrocephalus which may be used in a subse-

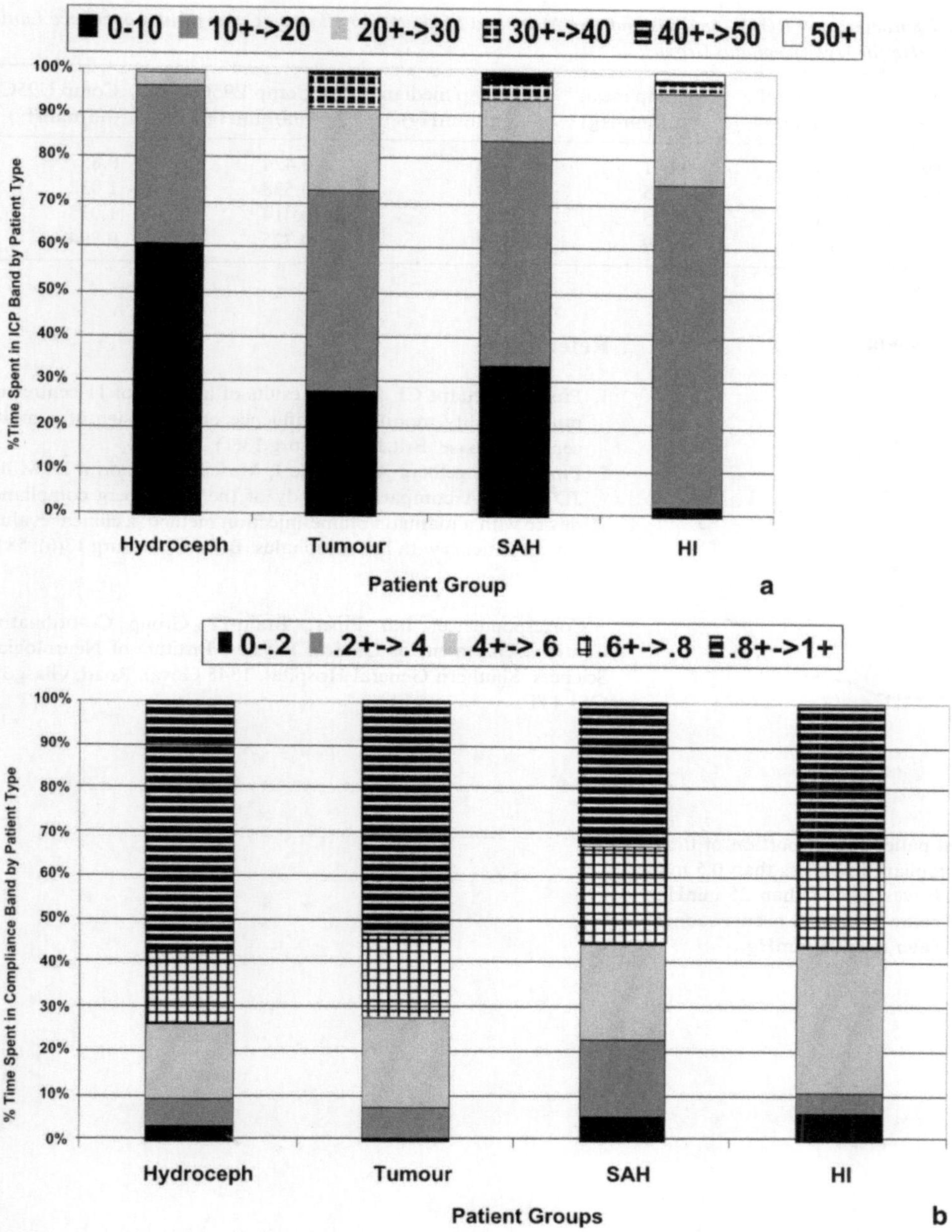

Fig. 1. (a) Bar chart showing the relative distribution of ICP between the patient groups. High ICP was predominantly found in the head injury, SAH and tumour groups whereas proportionally very little raised ICP > 20 mmHg was seen within the hydrocephalus group. (b) Bar chart showing the relative distribution of compliance between the patient groups, which demonstrates all groups showed episodes of lower compliance ($\leq$ 0.5 ml/mmHg) which can, in the case of the hydrocephalus group, occur in the absence of significantly raised ICP above 20 mmHg

quent trial. However, time-series analyses are now revealing that it is not just the absolute compliance value that is critical but that the duration below threshold needs also to be considered. To achieve this and before a trial can be designed, a survey is warranted to identify a consensus of what is the minimum duration of raised ICP above 25 mmHg needed to instigate treatment.

Table 2. *Results of Receiver Operator Characteristic (ROC) Analysis Showing Mean and Median Compliance (Comp) with Confidence Limits for Predicting ICP > 25 mmHg (10 mmHg for Hydrocephalus Group)*

Group	Power analysis (n needed)	N	ICP cutoff (mmHg)	Comp mean (ml/mmHg)	Comp median (ml/mmHg)	Comp L95CL (ml/mmHg)	Comp U95CL (ml/mmHg)
HI	60–70	19	>25	0.641	0.561	0.424	0.857
Tumour	30–40	13	>25	0.785	0.671	0.538	1.032
SAH	30–40	5	>25	0.725	0.632	0.414	1.035
Hydro	30–40	34	>10	0.809	0.800	0.725	0.894

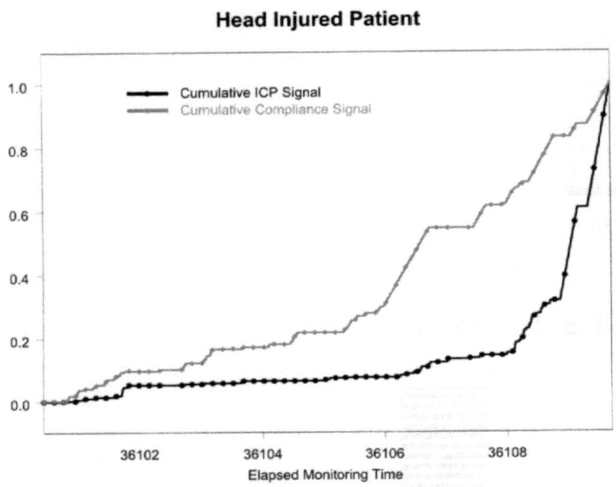

Fig. 2. Plot for a single head injured patient of proportion of time spent (of total monitoring time). Compliance was less than 0.5 ml/mmHg (diamonds) and similarly ICP was greater than 25 mmHg (circles). Note that time compliance below threshold occurs sooner and rises faster than time with ICP greater than 25 mmHg

References

1. Piper I, Contant CF (1999) Results of a survey of 11 centres on multi-modality monitoring: influence on the design of a multi-centre database. Brit J Neurosurg 13(1): 101–118
2. Piper I, Spiegelberg A, Whittle I, Mascia L, Signorini D, Miller JD (1999) A comparative study of the Spiegelberg compliance device with a manual volume-injection method: a clinical evaluation in patients with hydrocephalus. Brit J Neurosurg 13(6): 581–586

Correspondence: Ian Piper, Brain-IT Group Co-ordinating Centre, Department of Clinical Physics, Institute of Neurological Sciences, Southern General Hospital, 1345 Govan Road, Glasgow, G51 4TF.

Acta Neurochir (2002) [Suppl] 81: 171–172

Clinical Experience in the use of the Spiegelberg Automated Compliance Device in the Assessment of Patients with Hydrocephalus

Y. H. Yau[1], I. R. Piper[2], C. F. Contant[3], L. T. Dunn[2], and I. R. Whittle[1]

[1] Department of Clinical Neurosciences, Edinburgh, Scotland, UK
[2] Institute of Neurological Sciences, Glasgow, Scotland, UK
[3] Baylor College of Medicine, Houston, Texas

Summary

Deciding upon shunting in patients with hydrocephalus with possibly related symptomatology, is difficult. The Spiegelberg automated device allows continuous measurements of intracranial compliance. We aimed to evaluate the added information that this new technology can provide, in addition to standard continuous ICP monitoring. Thirty-three patients with hydrocephalus were continuously monitored for ICP and compliance. Patients with abnormal ICP or compliance profiles were selected for shunting. Thirteen patients underwent ventriculo-peritoneal shunting on this basis, with 12 obtaining benefit and one dying as a complication of shunt-related sepsis. The 13 patients undergoing shunting had abnormalities in either intracranial pressure or compliance or both. Only 1 patient had normal ICP, but abnormal compliance and so the true complementary role of continuous compliance measurements cannot be determined. It is proposed that further recruitment be on a larger multi-centre basis. Determination of benefit is required, particularly as a possible time lag of abnormal ICP abnormal compliance over appearing during monitoring can be demonstrated.

Keywords: Intracranial compliance; hydrocephalus, CSF diversion.

Introduction

There remains great difficulty in the management of patients with non-acute hydrocephalus, whether this is associated with a past predisposing cause or entirely idiopathic. Where ventricular enlargement on neuro-imaging is accompanied by disturbance in functions such as gait, cognition and continence; the question of benefit from cerebrospinal fluid (CSF) shunting is raised. Simply inserting a ventriculo-peritoneal shunt carries risks, which if incurred, are met with higher morbidity as patient age and frailty increases. Nevertheless, those patients truly symptomatic as a direct result of their hydrocephalus should be identified, since the balance of benefit from CSF diversion is worthwhile. A number of tests aimed at positively and negatively predicting the outcome from CSF diversion have been utilised by clinicians [1–3]. Amongst these, continuous intracranial pressure (ICP) monitoring, remains one common method in assessing for the need of CSF shunting.

In recent times, the Spiegelberg automated compliance device has improved the practicalities of measuring volume-pressure parameters by providing a means for the continuous measurement of intracranial compliance (ICC), in addition to continuous ICP measurements. We therefore sought to evaluate whether having additional information from continuous ICC measurement would influence the clinical decision to perform CSF diversion during the assessment of patients with Hydrocephalus.

Methods

Patients from two centres, Edinburgh and Glasgow, were studied. Thirty-three patients with cerebral ventriculomegaly on CT/MRI scanning, with symptoms possibly attributable to hydrocephalus were assessed. Overnight ICP monitoring and concurrent automated compliance measurements using an intraventricular air pouch balloon catheter was performed, producing raw data and paper chart recordings. The decision to perform CSF diversion was based upon a broadly defined abnormal ICP profile including a combination of high ICP values, a high proportion of ICP values above 10 mmHg and a significant presence of B waves or other abnormal pressure waves. Low compliance and a large proportion of values below an arbitrary low threshold of 0.5 ml/mmHg were also considered abnormal, requiring CSF diversion. Pre- and post-operative mobility status, including timed 10-metre walk, assessment of standing balance, posture control and function were recorded. Comparative neuropsychometric tests to evaluate areas including orientation, concentration, visuo-spatial perception and frontal lobe function were similarly obtained.

Results

Twenty-two males and 11 females (median age 60 years, range 16 to 86) were assessed. Complications of monitoring included 4 premature catheter dislodgements and one intraventricular haemorrhage. Thirteen underwent CSF shunting, in the form of a ventriculoperitoneal shunt, and all had functional improvement at minimum three months follow-up, except one who died from shunt infection and sepsis. Of the shunted patients, eight had abnormal ICP and compliance, only one patient had a normal ICP profile but low compliance and four had abnormal ICP but normal compliance.

Discussion

Beneficial CSF diversion was achieved in patients with abnormalities in either ICP, ICC or both. Due to the small numbers of patients with normal ICP, but abnormal ICC, the true complementary role of continuous compliance measurements in the assessment of hydrocephalic patients for CSF diversion cannot be determined. It is therefore proposed that further recruitment on a larger multi-centre basis be warranted, with the aim of a randomised trial in evaluating the true benefit of continuous compliance information in this patient group.

The derivation of a poor compliance threshold is based upon a receiver operator characteristic type analysis of the data following the setting of a particular ICP level, above, which is termed abnormal. With the current sample size, taking ICP above 10 mmHg as abnormal, the corresponding compliance threshold has recently been calculated as 0.809 ml/mmHg (95% CI of 0.725–0.894 ml/mmHg). If a compliance of less than 0.809 ml/mmHg simply relates to an ICP of above 10 mmHg, then there appears to be little value in this compliance information. By undertaking a cumulative analysis of the continuous ICP and ICC monitoring data over time, however, a lead time of abnormal compliance over abnormal ICP can be demonstrated (Fig. 1). The clinical implications and value of this remain to be determined.

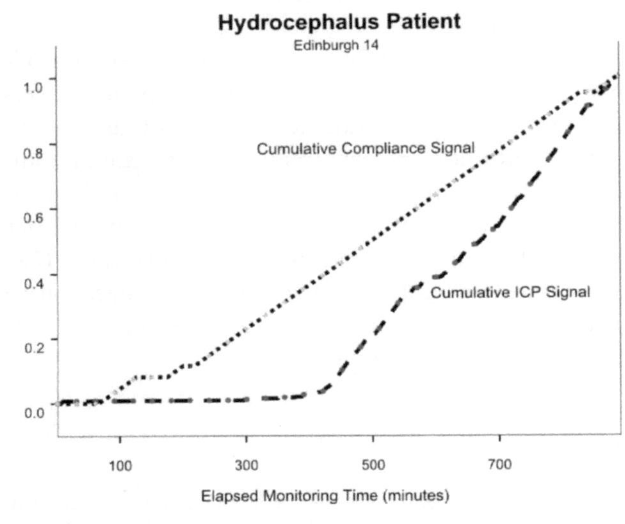

Fig. 1. A cumulative analysis plot of continuous ICP and compliance data during the monitoring period for one Hydrocephalus patient. Each time the ICP is above a set threshold of 10 mmHg, the cumulative ICP signal increments one step. The same occurs with the cumulative compliance signal, each time the compliance falls below the corresponding threshold of 0.8 ml/mmHg. As demonstrated, abnormal compliance leads abnormal ICP throughout

Acknowledgments

This work has been supported by the Scottish Office Department of Health (Grant K/MRS/50/C2662).

References

1. Boon AJ, Tans JT, Delwel EJ, Egeler-Peerdeman SM, Hanlo PW, Wurzer HA, Hermans J (2000) The Dutch normal-pressure hydrocephalus study. How to select patients for shunting? An analysis of four diagnostic criteria. Surg Neurol 53: 201–207
2. Vanneste JA (2000) Diagnosis and management of normal-pressure hydrocephalus. J Neurol 247: 5–14
3. Williams MA, Razumovsky AY, Hanley DF (1998) Comparison of Pcsf monitoring and controlled CSF drainage to diagnose normal pressure hydrocephalus. Acta Neurochir (Wien) [Suppl] 71: 328–330

Correspondence: Y. H. Yau, Department of Clinical Neurosciences, University of Edinburgh, Western General Hospital, Crewe Road, Edinburgh, EH4 2XU, UK.

Acta Neurochir (2002) [Suppl] 81: 173–175

Continuous Cerebral Compliance Monitoring in Severe Head Injury: Its Relationship with Intracranial Pressure and Cerebral Perfusion Pressure

G. Portella, M. Cormio, and G. Citerio

Summary

Cerebral Compliance describes the ability of cranial content to accommodate volume variations. Intracranial vascular compartment is thought to be one of the most important determinants of Compliance. Cerebral perfusion pressure (CPP) has a significant influence upon the calibre of cerebral vessels and consequently, upon blood volume.

This study was designed to investigate the influence of CPP on intracranial volumes balance, described by cerebral compliance, in severe traumatic brain injured patients (TBI).

Nine TBIs were studied. The Spiegelberg ventricular catheter continuously measured ICP and Compliance. Compliance, CPP and ICP were digitally collected for a total of 737 hours of monitoring (44239 total data). Compliance was lower at $CPP < 60$ than at $CPP \geq 60$ (0.51 ± 0.3 versus 0.64 ± 0.3 ml/mmHg).

The ICP level influenced the relation between CPP and Compliance. At $ICP < 20$ (LICP; 80.3% of data) Compliance and CPP were not significantly related. At $ICP \geq 20$ mmHg (HICP; 19.7% of data), Compliance varied with changes in CPP.

When $CPP < 60$ mmHg, Compliance showed a trend to decrease as CPP decreased ($R^2 = 0.85$). At $CPP \geq 60$ mmHg Compliance decreased with CPP ($R^2 = 0.83$). In the range of low CPP vasoparalysis is impending. However, when ICP is pathological, at high CPP our results may express vasodilatation instead of expected vasoconstriction from normal autoregulation.

Keywords: Head injury; compliance; intracranial pressure; cerebral perfusion pressure.

Introduction

Brain compliance expresses the ability of cranial content to accommodate an extra amount of volume. Intracranial vascular compartment is thought to be one of the most important determinants of Compliance and factors influencing this compartment will possibly change Compliance. Variations in cerebral perfusion pressure (CPP) have a significant influence upon cerebral vascular resistances and therefore on cerebral blood volume. The extent and the direction of this influence depend on whether autoregulation, to preserve a constant Cerebral Blood Flow, is still operative or not.

We thought that the new opportunity of continuously monitor cerebral compliance, coupled with other cerebral hemodynamic parameters, could give us some more insight into pathophysiology of intracerebral volumes balance in traumatic brain injury (TBI).

Aim of the study was to investigate the relationships between CPP and Compliance by continuous monitoring of their fluctuations (therapeutically induced and unavoidable) in severe brain injury patients.

Materials and Methods

The measurements were prospectively performed in nine severe head injuries in which a Spiegelberg catheter inserted in a lateral ventricle monitored ICP and Compliance. All patients were sedated, intubated and ventilated to maintain a moderate hyperventilation. Surgical and medical therapy, according to international protocols, were applied with the intent to maintain $ICP < 20$ mmHg and $CPP \geq 60$ mmHg.

The Spiegelberg catheter is a specific ventricular catheter with an air pouch mounted on the tip. The air pouch is automatically filled by 0.2 ml of air every 2.5 sec; the measurement of resulting pressure difference allows the continuous computation of cerebral compliance [3].

One minute average values of ICP, arterial blood pressure (ABP), Compliance and derived CPP and Pressure Volume Index (PVI), were continuously collected at the bedside by a personal computer. The data are summarized as mean $\pm$ standard deviation. For simplicity of analysis, the mean values of Compliance and CPP corresponding at 5 mmHg range of CPP were used to study the relationship between these variables. Linear regression analysis were used for data analysis.

Results

Our study was performed in nine severe head injuries (GCS ≤ 8; 7 male; age 17–76). Lesions were classified by first CT scan as focal in 7 patients and diffuse in the remaining 2 patients. One patient in the group of focal lesion suffered by hemispheric ischemia from traumatic carotid-cavernous fistula. The out-

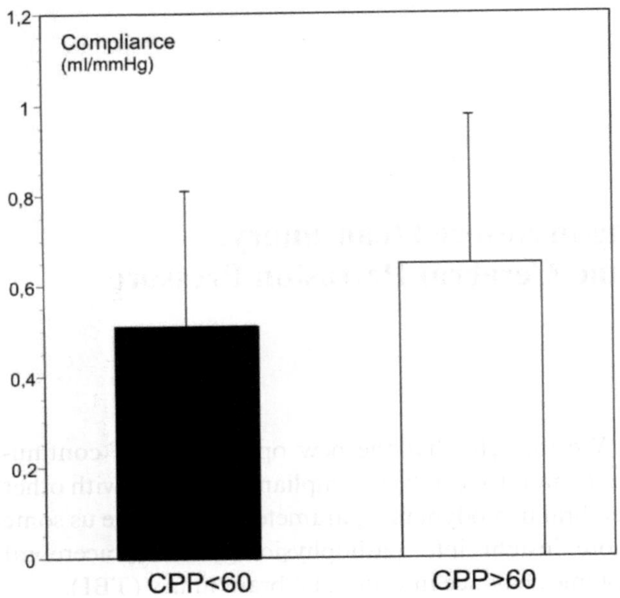

Fig. 1. Compliance was lower at CPP < 60 mmHg

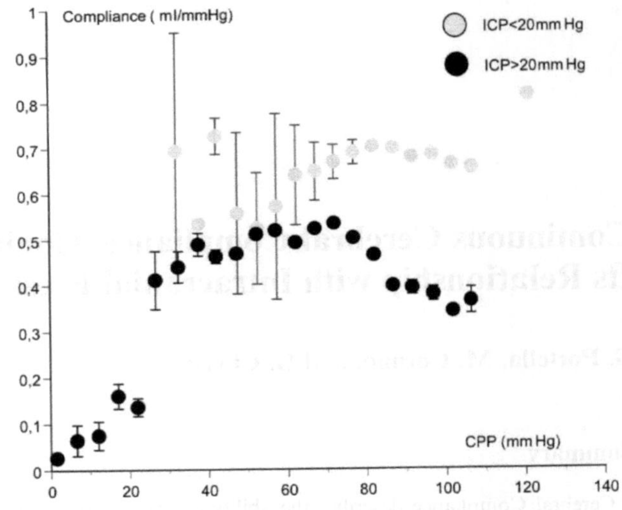

Fig. 2. The relationship between Compliance and CPP is shown. The values are mean $\pm$ SE. The grey symbols represent the values at ICP < 20 mmHg; the black symbol are the values at ICP $\geq$ 20 mmHg

come at the discharge from the ICU was 4 obeying, 3 not obeying and 2 dead from intractable intracranial hypertension.

A total of 44239 digitally recorded data, corresponding to 737 hours of collection, were acceptable for analysis. The average of recorded values were ICP 15.9 $\pm$ 8.9 mmHg, CPP 73.6 $\pm$ 15.1, Compliance 0.62 $\pm$ 0.33 ml/mmHg and PVI 19.6 $\pm$ 11.2 ml. In spite of our efforts to avoid pathologic secondary insults there was an incidence of ICP $\geq$ 20 mmHg of 19.7% of the recorded time and CPP < 60 mmHg in 13% of cases.

Low CPP was caused by a high ICP in 52% of cases and therefore a systemic secondary insult (low ABP) was responsible in the remaining 48% of cases. Cerebral Compliance was lower at CPP < 60 mmHg than at CPP $\geq$ 60 mmHg corresponding to values of 0.51 $\pm$ 0.30 and 0.65 $\pm$ 0.33 ml/mmHg (Fig. 1).

The relationship between CPP and Compliance was different at different level of ICP measured (Fig. 2) At ICP < 20 mmHg Compliance was higher than at ICP $\geq$ 20 mmHg especially at elevated CPP levels. In the normal range of ICP, CPP and Compliance were not related.

Considering pathological values of ICP ($\geq$ 20 mmHg) it was possible to differentiate a complex relationship between CPP and Compliance. At ICP $\geq$ 20 mmHg and CPP < 60 mmHg, Compliance showed a trend to decrease as CPP decreased ($R^2 = 85.8\%$). At ICP $\geq$ 20 mmHg and CPP above 60 mmHg (up to values of 110 mmHg), Compliance decreased at higher CPP levels ($R^2 = 83\%$).

Discussion

Several authors have studied the correlation between CPP and intracranial volume-pressure relationship. From these studies autoregulation has been recognized as the key issue to look at this relation, yet different results have been proposed [1, 2, 5].

We thought that the opportunity to monitor continuously cerebral compliance, coupled with other cerebral hemodynamic parameters, could give some more insight into pathophysiology of intracerebral volume balance related to pressure changes.

In our data setting, the majority of ICP, CPP and compliance values were in a physiological range, probably due to the therapeutic effort to avoid and eventually correct pathological events. Although intracranial and systemic secondary insults couldn't always be avoided: an ICP $\geq$ 20 mmHg and CPP < 60 mmHg were documented in 19.7% and 13% of the recorded time, respectively.

Cerebral Compliance was significantly lower at CPP < 60 mmHg when autoregulatory failure and vessel dilatation are documented to occur [4].

In these conditions, the consequent cerebral vascular engorgement from impending vasoparalysis could be responsible for the lower intracranial volume-buffering capacity.

Looking at the relation between Compliance and CPP, we could discriminate different behaviours depending on whether ICP was higher or lower than 20 mmHg.

Compliance was higher at normal ICP < 20 mmHg than at higher pathological levels, especially at high CPP levels.

When ICP was low, CPP and Compliance were not related suggesting a less impaired cerebral hemodynamic condition and more stable volume balance.

In the range of low CPP and high ICP the trend of Compliance to decrease when CPP decrease seems to support the hypothesis of the impaired autoregulation and impending vasomotor paralysis worsening intracranial volume balance. However, if ICP is pathological, we might suspect a defective autoregulation even at very high CPP, instead of the expected operative autoregulatory response. In these conditions, in fact, we observed a trend of decreasing Compliance when CPP increased, suggesting a pathological passive association between ABP and vessel diameter with subsequent, not counterbalanced, raise of cerebral blood volume.

Our results confirm that low CPP levels are harmful on the intracranial volume balance. However they also suggest that, when ICP is pathological and autoregulation could be impaired, the effort to "over-correct" CPP by increasing MAP doesn't always guarantee intracranial volume equilibrium. It must be underlined that, by these results, no inference is possible regarding the influence of CPP level on metabolic cerebral equilibrium.

References

1. Gray JW, Rosner MJ (1987) Pressure-volume index as a function of cerebral perfusion pressure Part 1: The effect of cerebral perfusion pressure changes and anesthesia. J Neurosurg 67: 369–376
2. Gray JW, Rosner MJ (1987) Pressure-volume index as a function of cerebral perfusion pressure Part 2: The effects of low cerebral perfusion pressure and autoregulation. J Neurosurg 67: 377–380
3. Herman HD (1993) Spigelberg brain-pressure monitor instrumentation, technique, and technology. Neurosurgery 33: 1111–1112
4. Kontos H, Wei E, Navari R, Levasseur J, Rosemblum W, Patterson J (1978) Responses of cerebral arteries and arterioles to acute hypotension and hypertension. Am J Physiol 234(4): H371–H383
5. Muizelaar JP, Marmarou A, Wachi A (1989) ICP and PVI with blood pressure alterations and relation with CBF autoregulation. In: Hoff JT, Betz AL (eds) Intracranial pressure VII. Springer, Berlin Heidelberg New York Tokyo, pp 825–828

Correspondence: G. Citerio M.D., Rianimazione I B, H. Nuovo S. Gerardo, Via Donizetti 106, 20052 Milano, Italy.

Acta Neurochir (2002) [Suppl] 81: 177–180

Intracranial Compliance as a Bed-Side Monitoring Technique in Severely Head-Injured Patients*

K. L. Kiening, W. N. Schoening, W. R. Lanksch, and **A. W. Unterberg**

Department of Neurosurgery, Charité, Virchow Medical Center Humboldt-University at Berlin, Germany

Summary

A recently developed monitoring technology makes an on-line assessment of intracranial compliance (ICC) possible. Aims of our research: 1. Course and values of ICC (critical threshold: <0.5 ml/mmHg) in episodes of pathological intracranial pressure (ICP) (> 20 mmHg) and reduced cerebral oxygenation (brain tissue PO_2 ($PtiO_2$) < 10 mmHg). 2. Mean ICC in different ages. 3. Relationship between ICC and outcome. 4. Evaluation of ICC as routine monitoring parameter by calculation of s.c. time-of-good-data-quality (TGDQ). Computer data assessment of 7 patients with severe closed head-injury was performed providing 830 hours of data. TGDQ resulted from the formula: TGDQ (%) = artifact free time (min) × 100 (%)/total monitoring time (min). Outcome was assessed 6 months posttrauma (Glasgow Outcome Score (GOS). 1. Analysis revealed 43 episodes of pathologically elevated ICP and 39 of critical ICC. In 17 cases overlapping periods were found. In 9 of these ICC preceded ICP. Reduced cerebral oxygenation was neither related with high ICP nor low ICC. 2. ICC was found to be age-related. At a cut-off-point of 20 mmHg in ICP, ICC in children (≤ 16 years) was 0.9, in adults (17–60 years) 0.7 and in elderly (> 60 years) 0.6 ml/mmHg. 3. Adverse outcome was indicated best by high ICP (up to 45% of monitoring time) followed by low ICC (up to 41% of monitoring time). 4. TGDQ in ICC was 72% compared to 95% in ICP and 98% in PtiO2. In predicting adverse outcome, ICP was equal to ICC. The different ICC in each age class points to the need of age-adjusted thresholds. Further refinements of ICC technology are needed to improve ICC data quality and therefore become a useful tool in neuromonitoring.

Keywords: Intracranial compliance; multimodal cerebral monitoring; severe head injury.

Introduction

Since the introduction of continuous intracranial pressure (ICP) measurement [5] into clinical routine, ICP monitoring has become a standard in managing severely head-injured patients in neurointensive care.

Being aware that an increase in ICP is a more or less 'late' sign for intracranial deterioration, it was and is still a goal to identify 'early' monitoring parameters. Measuring intracranial compliance (ICC) and derived terms such as the pressure volume index (PVI), introduced and mathematically quantified by Marmarou [7], offer the potential for such an 'early' detection and should allow prediction of an impending rise of ICP [9, 13]. Several methods of intermittent measurements of intracranial compliance have been described; most of them depending upon manual or semi-manual [3] injection/withdrawal of known fluid volumes into the craniospinal fluid (CSF) compartment resulting in an increase of CSF pressure [7, 6]. In 1990, Piper *et al.* [10] reported a method of automated external volume loading via a closed probe separated from CSF drainage. Meanwhile, this system (Spiegelberg Compliance Monitor) is available for clinical monitoring [11, 12].

We included this new monitoring technology into our multimodal cerebral monitoring system [2] to study 1. intracranial compliance during episodes of raised ICP and reduced cerebral oxygenation (brain tissue PO_2 ($PtiO_2$), 2. a potential age-relation of ICC and 3. impact of ICC on clinical outcome. Furthermore 4. we calculated the s.c. 'time-of-good-data-quality' of ICC, ICP and $PtiO_2$.

Patients and Methods

Patient Characteristics

Permission was granted by the local institutional ethics committee.

During an 18 months period, data assessment of 7 patients with severe closed head injury with a postresuscitation Glasgow Coma Scale (GCS) Score < 9 (all male, age 7 to 75, mean age: 42.3 yrs.

* This work was supported by a grant of the "Kuratorium ZNS".

Table 1. *Patient Characteristics; Percentage of Pathological Monitoring Time of ICP and ICC as well as Outcome*

Patient	Age	Initial GCS	CCT class (Marshall)	% Pathol. ICP	% Pathol. ICC	Outcome (GOS)
1	7	8	II	1.8	1.7	4
2	48	3	evac mass	19.9	12.4	3
3	35	6	III	45.9	36.1	3
4	54	7	evac mass	20.3	2.0	3
5	75	3	IV	15.8	41.4	1
6	29	3	evac mass	24.1	27.9	3
7	57	8	evac mass	43.7	3.4	3

GCS Glasgow Coma Score, *CCT* cranial computed tomography, *evac mass* evacuated mass lesion, *ICP* intracranial pressure, *ICC* intracranial compliance, *GOS* Glasgow Outcome Score.

$\pm$22.6 (SD), median: 48 years) was performed providing 830 hours of data (s. Table 1). Intracranial diagnosis was determined according to Marshalls classification [8].

Patient Management

Patients were sedated, intubated and mechanically ventilated to maintain an arterial $PO_2 > 100$ mmHg. Space occupying lesions greater than 25 cc were surgically evacuated within 2.5–13.25 (median: 5 hrs) hrs post injury. ICP management was done according to the 'guidelines in severe head injury' [1].

Continuous Physiologic Monitoring

All patients were monitored in the neurointensive care unit (NICU) between day 0 and day 10 post trauma (median: 1 to 7). The ICC catheter (Spiegelberg GmbH & Co., Hamburg Germany) measuring ICP and ICC was inserted into the lateral ventricle of the non-lesioned side of brain. With this method, an automated external volume loading is performed via a small balloon, which is integrated close to the tip of the catheter. The balloon is filled with a total volume of 0.2 ml air. The volume is injected during 2.5 seconds, resting for one second, and withdrawn during 2.5 seconds. The difference in ICP between, before and after injection is averaged from 200 cycles of volume loading.

For measuring cerebral white matter $PtiO_2$, a flexible polarographic Clark-type microcatheter [4] was inserted on the same side as the ICC catheter. Additionally, mean arterial blood pressure (MABP), ICP, cerebral perfusion pressure (CPP), arterial oxygen saturation and end-tidal CO_2 were recorded.

A multimodal cerebral monitoring system digitized the analog signals of all parameters with a frequency of 1/min [2].

Off-Line Analyses

Pathological episodes were defined as: ICP > 20 mmHg for >30 min, ICC < 0.5 ml/mmHg for >30 min, PtiO2 < 10 mmHg for >15 min. The critical threshold for ICC was taken from preliminary results of the BrainIT group (s. acknowledgement).

Outcome at six months after injury was determined by the dichotomized Glasgow Outcome Scale (GOS) (favorable: GOS 4–5; unfavorable: GOS 1–3). Information was gathered from the treating physician or the care taker (e.g. relative) by interview.

After clearing the data manually from artifacts, TGDQ was calculated by the formula: TGDQ (%) = artifact free time (min) $\times$ 100 (%)/total monitoring time (min).

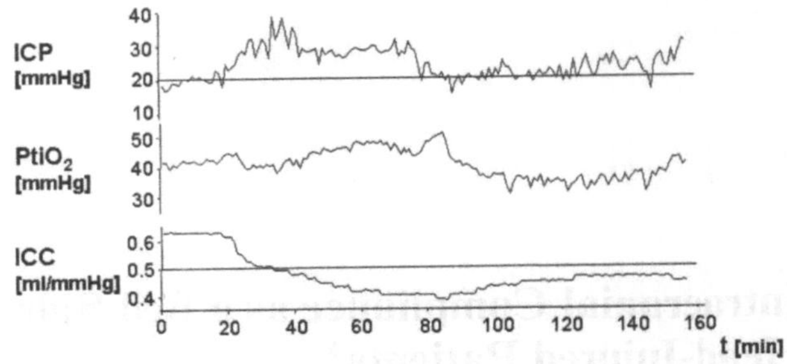

Fig. 1. Episode of pathological ICP. From minute 20–80, ICP increases above 20 mmHg. ICC decreases with a delay of 18 minutes below the critical threshold. $PtiO_2$ is not significantly affected

Statistics

Data are given as either mean or median, as outlined. Data for episode analyses underwent 100 points moving average procedure. Plots of ICP vs. ICC show regression curves of inverse first order polynomial style.

Results

Course and Values of ICC in Episodes of Pathological ICP

The analysis revealed 43 episodes (mean: 143 min; range: 30–540 min) of pathologically elevated ICP and 39 (mean: 221 min; range: 47–450 min) of critical ICC (s. Fig. 1). In 17 cases overlapping periods were found, i.e. ICP and ICC both were pathological. In 9 of these ICC preceded ICP in reaching pathological values. Reduced cerebral oxygenation was not seen in these episodes.

ICC and Age

As shown in Fig. 2 the regression curves (inverse first order, polynomial style) of ICC plotted vs. ICP for the distinct age classes revealed, at a cut-off-point of 20 mmHg, mean ICC values of 0.9 in a 7 year old, 0.7 in a 35 year old and 0.6 ml/mmHg in a 75 year old patient, suggesting an age-relationship of ICC.

ICC and Outcome

One patient showed a favorable outcome, while 5 remained severely disabled and one died. The patient with the favorable outcome had only 2% pathological monitoring time of ICP as well as of ICC. However, in patients with an unfavorable outcome pathological

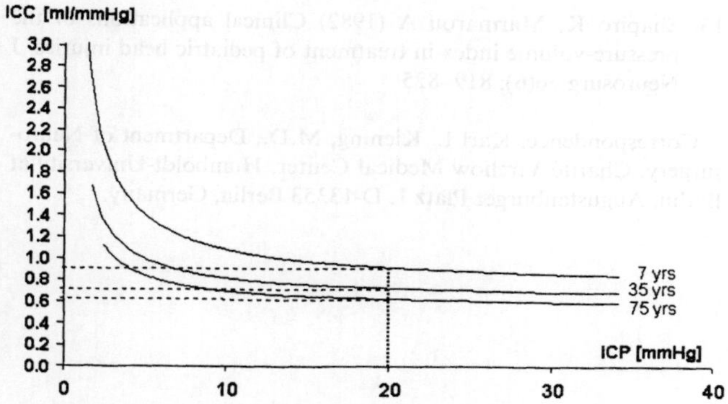

Fig. 2. Regression curves of ICC vs. ICP in three different patients representing the different age classes. At a cut-off-point of 20 mmHg in ICP, mean ICC value is 0.9 in a 7 year old, 0.7 in a 35 year old and 0.6 ml/mmHg in a 75 year old patient

monitoring time was as high as 16–46% regarding ICP (median: 22%) and 2–41% (median: 20%) regarding ICC (s. Table 1).

Time of Good Data Quality (TGDQ)

The total monitoring time was 49827 min (≅ 830 hrs ≅ 34 days). TGDQ in ICC was 72% compared to 95% in ICP and 98% in $PtiO_2$ monitoring.

Discussion

Studies of Piper and Raabe have shown that this new automatic on-line method of intracranial compliance measurement is reliable and correlates well with manual injections methods [11, 12]. But data are still missing concerning its applicability in patients with severe head injury.

ICP and ICC were found to provide about the same percentage of information concerning intracranial hypertension: When ICP was above the critical threshold, ICC was pathological in 40%. The same is true in ICC episodes < 0.5 ml/mmHg, where ICP was elevated above 20 mmHg in 44%. Thus, ICC appears not to overcome ICP in predicting intracranial hypertension. This finding is also underlined by the fact that in overlapping episodes, ICC was the earlier warning parameter in only ~50%.

Our finding of different ICC values in distinct age classes seems to support the theory of an ICC reduction with increasing age. However, this is still an assumption due to the rather small study population. If this preliminary result will be substantiated by further data, defining of age-adjusted ICC thresholds will be necessary.

So far, ICP and ICC are of equal quality in prediction of adverse outcome.

ICC was clearly identified to have a worse TGDQ compared to already established monitoring parameters (ICP, $PtiO_2$). This was due to interference with CSF drainage, occurrence of slit ventricles and problems with Compliance software. A further disadvantage of this technique is that ICC monitoring is not possible following decompressive craniectomy.

We conclude that on-line ICC monitoring may become an additional bed-side monitoring modality in neurointensive care, but system refinements are desperately needed.

Acknowledgments

The patients presented are part of a multicenter databank (BrainIT – study; s. website: www.brainit.gla.ac.uk).

References

1. Guidelines for the treatment of severe head injury (1996). J Neurotrauma 13: 641–734
2. Bardt TF, Unterberg AW, Kiening KL, Schneider GH, Lanksch WR (1998) Multimodal cerebral monitoring in comatose head-injured patients. Acta Neurochir (Wien) 140(4): 357–365
3. Borgesen SE, Gjerris F, Sorensen SC (1978) The resistance of cerebrospinal fluid absorption in humans. A method of evaluation by lumboventricular perfusion, with particular reference to normal pressure hydrocephalus. Acta Neurol Scand 57: 88–96
4. Kiening KL, Unterberg AW, Bardt TF, Schneider GH, Lanksch WR (1996) Monitoring of cerebral oxygenation in patients with severe head injuries: brain tissue PO2 versus jugular vein oxygen saturation. J Neurosurg 85(5): 751–757
5. Lundberg N (1960) Continuous recording and control of ventricular fluid pressure in neurosurgical practice. Acta Psychatr Scand 36 [Suppl] 149: 1–193
6. Marmarou A, Shulman K, LaMorgese J (1975) Compartmental analysis of compliance and outflow resistance of the cerebrospinal fluid system. J Neurosurg 43: 523–534
7. Marmarou A, Shulman K, Rosende RM (1978) A nonlinear analysis of the cerebrospinal fluid system and intracranial pressure dynamics. J Neurosurg 48(3): 332–344
8. Marshall LF, Bowers Marshall S, Klauber MR, van Berkum Clark M (1991) a new classification of head injury based on computerized tomography. J Neurosurg [Suppl] 75: S14–S20
9. Maset AL, Marmarou A, Ward JD, Choi S, Lutz HA, Brooks D, Moulton RJ, DeSalles A, Muizelaar JP, Turner H, Young HF (1987) Pressure-volume index in head injury. J Neurosurg 67(6): 832–840
10. Piper IR, Miller JD, Whittle IR, Lawson A (1990) Automated time-averaged analysis of craniospinal compliance (short pulse response). Acta Neurochir (Wien) [Suppl] 51: 387–390

11. Piper IR, Spiegelberg A, Whittle I, Signorini D, Mascia L (1999) A comparative study of the Spiegelberg compliance device with a manual volume-injection method: a clinical evaluation in patients with hydrocephalus. Br J Neurosurg 13(6): 581–586
12. Raabe A, Czosnyka M, Piper IR, Seifert V (1999) Monitoring of intracranial compliance: correction for a change in body position. Acta Neurochir (Wien) 141(1): 31–36
13. Shapiro K, Marmarou A (1982) Clinical applications of the pressure-volume index in treatment of pediatric head injuries. J Neurosurg 56(6): 819–825

Correspondence: Karl L. Kiening, M.D., Department of Neurosurgery, Charité Virchow Medical Center, Humboldt-University at Berlin, Augustenburger Platz 1, D-13353 Berlin, Germany.

Acta Neurochir (2002) [Suppl] 81: 181–182

An Experimental Evaluation of a new Intraparenchymal Continuous Compliance Probe: Preliminary Studies

Y. H. Yau[1], **I. R. Piper**[3], **R. E. Clutton**[2], and **I. R. Whittle**[1]

[1] Department of Clinical Neurosciences, University of Edinburgh, United Kingdom
[2] Department of Veterinary Clinical Studies, University of Edinburgh, United Kingdom
[3] Department of Clinical Physics, Southern General Hospital, Glasgow, United Kingdom

Summary

The Spiegelberg automated compliance device offers practical benefits over the standard manual injection techniques for assessing volume-pressure status. Currently, however, the system relies on the insertion of an intraventricular catheter. If automated continuous measurement of intraparenchymal compliance could be achieved, then this would be a further practical advance. Automated measurements of compliance using a prototype intraparenchymal probe were assessed in comparison with the current intraventricular probe in a sheep model of diffusely raised ICP. The results show poor correlation between intraventricular compliance (IVC) and intraparenchymal compliance (IPC) at low levels of cerebral perfusion pressure (CPP). The IPC response to decreasing CPP beyond probable levels of blood flow autoregulation suggest that IPC is more dependent on local tissue perfusion factors, rather than overall physical compliance. Further evaluation of compliance in the intraparenchymal compartment versus intraventricular compliance will be needed before adaptation of the automated system for clinical application.

Keywords: Intraventricular compliance; intraparenchymal compliance; continuous monitoring.

Introduction

Information on the volume pressure status of patients with various neuropathological conditions is of value. Methods to derive such information, such as the Pressure Volume Index (PVI) [2] and the Volume Pressure Response (VPR) [3, 4], have been described and utilised for many decades. Their main drawback is the manual bolus injection technique, which is labour-intensive and may incur risks in less experienced hands [5]. The recent availability of the Spiegelberg automated compliance device has brought potential practical advantages with its ability to automatically measure and continuously track intracranial compliance. The current device, however, relies on the insertion of a specialised intraventricular catheter. To further the practical application of the device, modifications to measure compliance in the intraparenchymal compartment should be investigated. Due to the complex nature of brain tissue with both its visco-elastic and incompressible components, it is to be expected that intraparenchymal compliance may differ quantitatively from intraventricular compliance. We therefore aimed to compare continuous measurements from a prototype intraparenchymal compliance probe, with intraventricular compliance using the Spiegelberg automated compliance device.

Methods

The Spiegelberg automated compliance device calculates intracranial compliance ($\Delta V/\Delta P$) from a moving average of small perturbations in the intracranial pressure (ΔP) resulting from a sequence of pulses of added volume (ΔV). The current monitoring system automates these volume additions to an air pouch situated at the tip of a double lumen intraventricular catheter. The resultant ICP perturbations are measured through a fluid-filled inner lumen connected to an external strain gauge pressure transducer. For the prototype intraparenchymal compliance probe, the ICP perturbations were measured via a micro transducer situated at the tip of the probe.

A Spiegelberg intraventricular catheter and a prototype Spiegelberg intraparenchymal probe were placed in 5 anaesthetised and paralysed sheep to allow comparative automated measurements of compliance. Measurements were made throughout a range of ICP (5–50 mmHg) induced by infusions of mock CSF. Continuous mean arterial blood pressure was recorded and cerebral perfusion pressure (CPP) derived. Induced hypercarbia at a constant level of 15–20 mmHg ICP was used to further assess the relationship of IPC to cerebral perfusion.

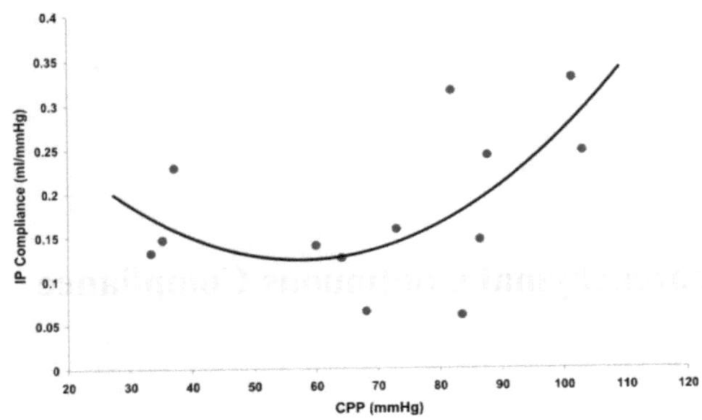

Fig. 1. A plot of intraparenchymal compliance versus cerebral perfusion pressure. This pilot data suggests there may be a biphasic response to the intraparenchymal compliance – CPP relationship. When CPP falls below presumed autoregulatory levels, intraparenchymal compliance may be increasing

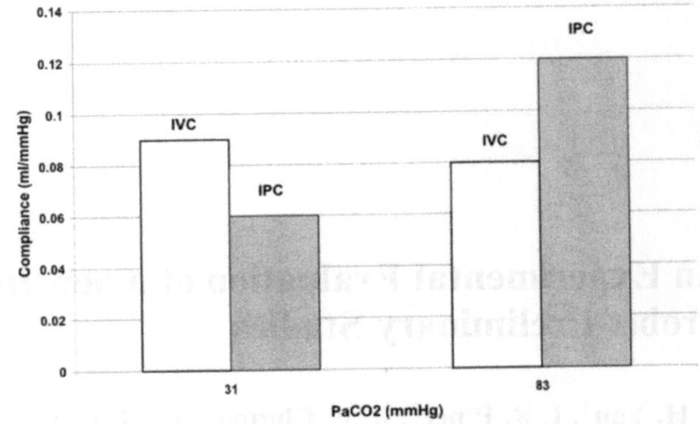

Fig. 2. A plot of change in intraventricular (IVC) and intraparenchymal (IPC) compliance during a change in PaCO2 induced by altering ventilatory parameters. With increased PaCO2, and presumably increased cerebral blood flow, there is relatively little change in IVC. IPC, however, shows a paradoxical rise with increasing PaCO2 and may indicate IPC is more a reflection of the state of local perfusion rather than lumped craniospinal compliance

Results

Thirteen pairs of compliance values were obtained from the intraparenchymal and intraventricular sites. Overall, IPC was higher than IVC at the same level of ICP. Rising ICP and decreasing CPP resulted in the expected decrease in IVC, but there was not a good correlation ($R^2 = 0.654$) between IPC and IVC over the same range of CPP. IPC did, however, appear to be CPP dependent with a suggestion of a biphasic response (Fig. 1). IPC decreased with falling CPP, but further decreases of CPP to below 60–70 mmHg resulted in an increase in IPC. At constant ICP, hypercarbia resulted in a relatively small change in IVC but a rise in IPC to nearly twice its baseline value (Fig. 2).

Discussion

Continuous automated measurements of IPC do not hold a direct correlation with IVC at low CPP. This apparent biphasic response of IPC to increasing ICP and decreasing CPP, beyond the level of cerebral blood flow autoregulation, would support the concept that IPC is dependent upon local tissue cerebral perfusion (similar to what has been described for PVI) [1]. Further studies are required to fully evaluate these physiological and pathophysiological determinants of IPC before accepting a simple adaptation of the current automated compliance device for measuring intraparenchymal compliance.

Acknowledgments

This work has been supported by the Scottish Office Department of Health (Grant K/MRS/50/C2662) and by Spiegelberg (GmbH & Co) KG.

References

1. Gray WJ, Rosner MJ (1987) Pressure-volume index as a function of cerebral perfusion pressure. Part 2: the effects of low cerebral perfusion pressure and autoregulation. J Neurosurg 67: 377–380
2. Marmarou A, Shulman K, LaMorgese J (1975) Compartmental analysis of compliance and outflow resistance of the cerebrospinal fluid system. J Neurosurg 43: 523–534
3. Miller JD, Garibi J (1972) Intracranial volume/pressure relationships during continuous monitoring of ventricular fluid pressure. Intracranial pressure. In: Brock M, *et al* Springer, Berlin Heidelberg New York Tokyo, pp 270–274
4. Miller JD, Garibi J, Pickard JD (eds) (1973) Induced changes of cerebrospinal fluid volume: effects during continuous monitoring of ventricular fluid pressure. Arch Neurol 28: 265–269
5. Piper I (1997) Intracranial pressure and elastance. Head injury: pathophysiology and management of severe closed head injury. In: Reilly P *et al* (eds) Chapman & Hall, Philadelphia

Correspondence: Y. H. Yau, Department of Clinical Neurosciences, University of Edinburgh, Western General Hospital, Crewe Road, Edinburgh, EH4 2XU, UK.

Acta Neurochir (2002) [Suppl] 81: 183–185

An Estimated Compliance Index Derived from Intracranial Pressure Recording

M. L. Daley[1], **M. Pourcyous**[2], **G. Stidham**[3], **S. D. Timmons**[4], and **C. W. Leffler**[5]

[1] Department of Electrical and Computer Engineering, The University of Memphis, Memphis, TN
[2] Departments of Pediatrics, Obstetrics/Gynecology, and Physiology, University of Tennessee Health Science Center, Memphis, TN
[3] Department of Pediatrics, University of Tennessee Health Science Center, Memphis, TN
[4] Department of Neurosurgery, University of Tennessee Health Science Center, Memphis, TN
[5] Departments of Physiology and Pediatrics, University of Tennessee Health Science Center, Memphis, TN

Summary

The purpose of this study is to test the validity of a proposed compliance index, percent change of compliance per mmHg of intracranial pressure (%CC/mmHg), by comparison of values of the index with corresponding experimentally derived values of compliance. The derivation of %CC/mmHg is based on two assumptions: 1) the pressure-volume characteristic of the craniospinal sac can be linearized for small perturbations about an equilibrium; and 2) during a brief interval in which these perturbations occur the pathophysiologic state of the sac does not significantly change.

By rapid infusion of 0.2 ml of mock cerebrospinal fluid (CSF) experimental values of compliance ($n = 44$) were obtained from 10 piglets during monitoring of intracranial pressure (ICP). A strong correlation ($r = 0.89$, $p < .001$, $n = 44$) was obtained between values of %CC/mmHg and corresponding values of experimentally derived compliance (ml/mmHg). The value of the proposed index of compliance, %CC/mmHg, needs to be evaluated in the clinical setting. However, from the view of validation of ICP instrumentation, high values of both mean ICP and mean %CC/mmHg are contradictory and indicative of the occurrence of instrumentation error due to electronic direct current drift.

Keywords: Intracranial pressure; intracranial compliance.

Introduction

Because the direct method for the determination of compliance requires the injection of known value of fluid into the craniospinal sac, it incurs the risk of infection and elevation of ICP [1]. As a result, various methods have been investigated for direct and indirect continuous monitoring of intracranial compliance based on characteristics of the ICP recordings [1–3, 5, 6]. Others have noted that several time-varying factors, including state of vascular tone [1, 2], timing between arterial blood inflow and venous blood outflow, heartrate [3], and timing between arterial blood inflow and movement of CSF to lumbar space [2], influence the shape of the ICP pulse over each cardiac cycle. To avoid these time-varying factors, the proposed index of compliance of this study, percent change of compliance/mmHg, (%CC/mmHg), is based on the assumption that the pathophysiologic state of the system is captured during the brief time interval in which the features of the pulse wave associated with the cardiac cycle are extracted from the pressure recording. The purpose of this study is to test the validity of %CC/mmHg by comparison of values of the index with corresponding experimentally derived values of compliance.

Materials and Methods

Using an approved protocol from the U.T. and U.M. Animal Care and Utilization Committees and procedures similar to those previously described [4], ten α-chloralose anesthetized piglets ranging in weight from 2 to 4 kg were used in this study. Digitized recordings of ICP were obtained with a parenchmally placed Camino transducer, sampled at 250 Hz and artifact screening was accomplished by an updated defined criteria [2].

Analysis Methods: For ICP below 30 mmHg an exponential relationship between pressure and volume is accepted as:

$$P = P_0 \exp(E(V - Veq)). \qquad (1)$$

In the above equation, P_0 represents the value of ICP during normal physiologic conditions, Veq represents an equilibrium value for the craniospinal sac, V represents the volume within the craniospinal sac, and E represents the elastance constant. Assuming a first order series approximation of this function, the maximum and minimum of the fluctuation of ICP associated with the cardiac cycle can be defined as P_2 and P_1 respectively, it can be shown that intracranial compliance ($\Delta V/\Delta P$) can be approximated as:

$$C = P_0(V_2 - V_1)/[(P_2 - P_1)(P_2 + P_1)/2]. \qquad (2)$$

The parameters P_0, V_2, and V_1 are specific to a patient's physiologic state during the recording and are unknown. Generally, the baseline

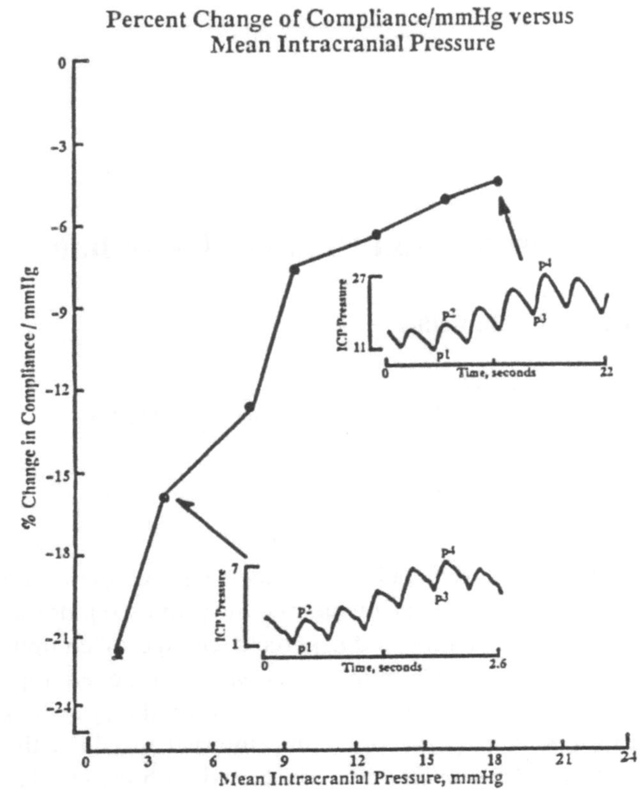

Fig. 1. Percent Change of Compliance/mmHg versus Mean Intracranial Pressure. Group mean and standard error paired values of %CC/mmHg and ICP obtained from ten experiments during induction of severe hypercapnia are plotted. Number of points per plotted mean pair ranges from 4–9. Where error bars not shown, value within symbol of plotted point. Top insert upper right shows example of ICP recording over inhalation phase of mechanical ventilation. Using p2 and p1 to compute compliance C1 and p4 and p3 to compute compliance C2, the computed %CC/mmHg for this recording was −5.1/mmHg at about a mean ICP of 18.4 mmHg. Lower insert shows high-valued ICP recording during normocapnia. Using p1, p2, p3, and p4 as described previously, the computed %CC/mmHg was −15.5 /mmHg at a mean value of 4.8 mmHg. The decreasing negative change of the index with increasing ICP supports the concept that this index is qualitatively related to the derivative of compliance with respect to ICP

of the ICP recording will vary with the frequency of positive pressure ventilation. At the onset of positive pressure inhalation, ICP will rise until the onset of passive pressure expiration (see inserts Fig. 1). Assuming that the parameters P_0 and $(V_2 - V_1)$ do not change during the positive pressure phase of ventilation, it is possible to eliminate the unknown parameters in the expression for compliance by the determination of an index we have termed percent change of compliance/mmHg. Specifically, because percent change of compliance requires division, the unknown parameters P_0, V2, and V1, which are assumed to be constant at the onset and end of the inhalation phase of ventilation, will cancel. Furthermore, to compare the change of compliance from one condition to another, change in compliance was normalized with respect to difference between the mean ICP at onset of inhalation and mean ICP at the end of the inhalation

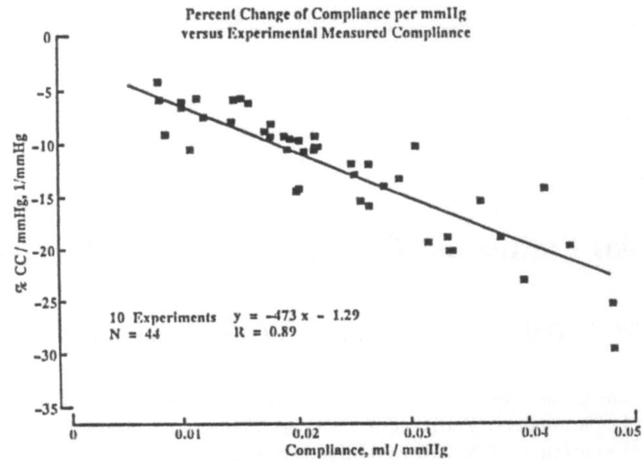

Fig. 2. Percent Change of Compliance per mmHg versus Experimental Measured Compliance. Forty-four measurements of compliance were obtained during the course of 10 laboratory experiments. Correlation between %CC/mmHg and experimental compliance was 0.89 at $p < .001$

phase (see inserts Fig. 1). The %CC/mmHg index is expressed as:

$$\%CC/mmHg = [(C_2 - C_1)/(C_1(P_{final} - P_{initial}))] * 100. \quad (3)$$

By infusing 200 ul of mock cerebrospinal fluid and recording the peak change of pressure, experimental values of compliance were determined.

Results

By varying the partial pressure of carbon dioxide in each laboratory preparation, ICP, cerebral blood volume, and intracranial compliance were manipulated. For the 10 experiments, values of %CC/mmHg were computed from recordings during induction of hypercapnia. Values of %CC/mmHg were grouped according to levels of ICP, and mean paired values were determined (see Fig. 1). To directly evaluate the relationship between %CC/mmHg and compliance, laboratory experiments were completed in which 200 ul of mock cerebrospinal fluid was subdurally infused (see Fig. 2). Both experimental compliance and the corresponding %CC/mmHg were determined and plotted (see Fig. 2). A strong correlation ($r = 0.89$, $p < .001$, $n = 44$) was obtained between values of %CC/mmHg and experimental values of compliance (ml/mmHg).

Discussion

The non-linear inverse relationship between %CC/mmHg and mean ICP is not unexpected (see Fig. 1).

Given an exponential description of the pressure-volume characteristic of the craniospinal sac and a time-invariant elastance constant as expressed in equation (1) above, theoretical compliance is analytically expressed as decreasing exponential function with respect to ICP. However, the proposed index %CC/mmHg is a normalized difference in compliance with respect to a change of pressure and reflects the rate of change of compliance with respect to ICP. Theoretically, the rate of change of compliance with respect to ICP is analytically expressed as a negative decreasing exponential. The experimental relationship between %CC/mmHg and mean ICP qualitatively supports the expected theoretical result. Specifically, when compliance is high, small increases of ICP will produce large decreases in %CC/mmHg, and when compliance is low and the system is tight, large increases of ICP will produce very little change in %CC/mmHg. Because the proposed index reflects the derivative of compliance with respect to intracranial pressure, the strong correlation ($r = 0.89$, $p < .001$) between %CC/mmHg and experimental values of compliance derived by rapid infusion of 200 ul of mock CSF is expected. When compliance is high, %CC/mmHg will also be high, and conversely when compliance is low, the proposed index will also be low.

The derivation of %CC/mmHg requires that heart-rate and other physiologic factors remain relatively constant during the brief inhalation period in which an increase of intrathoracic pressure leads to an increase of cerebral blood volume and correspondingly ICP. Given this constraint, the proposed index has the potential to provide a continuous indication of the state of intracranial compliance. From an instrumentation viewpoint, for example, during long term monitoring the occurrence of high values of %CC/mmHg at high mean ICP values would suggest that an upward d.c. drift in the transducer has occurred. Future studies of the proposed %CC/mmHg should include comparisons to other compliance indices such as the high frequency centroid index [6] and the evaluation of its possible utility in the clinical setting.

References

1. Avezaat CFF, van Eijndhoven JHM, Wyper DJ (1979) Cerebrospinal fluid pulse pressure and intracranial volume-pressure relationships. J Neurol Neurosurg Psychiatry 42: 687–700
2. Czosnyka M, Guazzo E, Whitehouse P, Smielewski Z, Kirkpatrick K, Piechnik S, and Pickard JD (1996) Significance of intracranial pressure waveform analysis after head injury. Acta Neurochir (Wien) 138: 531–542
3. Daley ML, Gallo AE, Mauch W (1986) Analysis of the intracranial pressure pulsation associated with the cardiac cycle. Innovation Et Tech En Biologie Et Medicine 7: 537–544
4. Daley ML and Leffler CW (1998) Correlation coefficient between ICP and arterial pressure: a gauge of cerebral vascular dilation. Acta Neurochir (Wien) [Suppl] 71: 285–288
5. Foltz EL, Blanks JP, Yonemura K (1990) CSF pulsatility in hydrocephalus: Respiratory effect on pulse wave slope as an indicator of intracranial compliance. Neurol Res 12: 67–74
6. Robertson CS, Narayan RK, Contant C, Grossman R, Pahwa R, Caram P, Bray RS, Sherwood AM (1989) Clinical experience with a continuous monitor of intracranial compliance. J Neurosurg 71: 673–680

Correspondence: Michael L. Daley, Ph.D., The University of Memphis, Electrical and Computer Engineering, Campus Box 526574, Memphis, TN 38152.

Acta Neurochir (2002) [Suppl] 81: 187–190

Non-Invasive Assessment of Intracranial Compliance Using a new 2-D "Transit Time" vs "Frequency Centroid" Map

R. P. Penson, R. Allen, and **A. Birch**

Faculty of Technology, Southampton Institute, Southampton, USA

Summary

The objective of this research was to develop a new static two dimensional graphic display indicating changes to intracranial compliance using non invasive ultrasonic Doppler measurements of the Middle Cerebral Artery (MCA) velocity and Arterial Blood Pressure (ABP).

ABP and MCA velocity were measured in a volunteer patient study and the results for hypo-, normo- and hyper-capnia, conditions were recorded. Cross-correlation analysis between ABP and MCA velocity predicted a change in "transit time" between the two parameters and a Fourier Transform analysis of the MCA velocity data predicted a change in "frequency centroid" over the 0 to 10 Hz range indicating change with intracranial compliance.

The results for the hyper-capnia condition were: "Transit Time" – 0 ms, "Frequency Centroid" – 1.9 Hz, for the normo-capnia condition: "Transit Time" – 18 ms, "Frequency Centroid" – 2.5 Hz, for the hypo-capnia condition: "Transit Time" – 38 ms, "Frequency Centroid" – 3.1 Hz.

Plotting the results on a graph with "Frequency Centroid" as the vertical axis and "Transit Time" as the horizontal axis yields a locus possibly indicating a change to intracranial compliance.

Keywords: Intracranial compliance; transit time; frequency centroid; ultrasonic Doppler.

Introduction

The continuous assessment of intracranial dynamics, by means of intracranial pressure (ICP) measurements and/or middle cerebral artery (MCA) blood flow velocity measurements, is important in neurosurgery for patients with intracranial pathology. Changes in these parameters, in the time and frequency domains, can indicate to the clinicians and nursing staff that the intracranial pathology is either worsening, or improving. These indicators can be used to assist the clinical staff in patient management. The work summarised in this paper investigated signal processing techniques for the non invasive assessment of intracranial dynamics, and is supported by work carried out by Penson [1] using a Matlab simulation of a compartmental model of the intracranial haemodynamic system. This non-invasive approach if proved reliable, could lead to not only the improvement to the prediction of trends in the intracranial dynamics, but also a reduction in the risk of infection associated with the current invasive techniques.

A mathematical model based on Karni's lumped parameter equations [4] was developed and simulated, using Simulink software, to enable the relationships between the measurable parameters to be investigated. The primary non-invasive measurement was the MCA velocity determined by standard transcranial Doppler sonography. The secondary non-invasive measurement was arterial blood pressure (ABP) determined by means of a Finapress pressure transducer. The signal processing methods used for analysing the MCA velocity and ABP data was the cross correlation of MCA velocity with ABP and Fourier transform of MCA velocity.

The implementation of a cross correlation computer programme to manipulate the data and the results of the analysis of several sets of data for a range of clinical conditions is discussed. Three sets of data were from an experiment on the author of this paper under normo-, hypo- and hypercapnia conditions. The predictions made by the cross correlation software, embedded into the standard monitoring and display system, at Southampton General Hospital, was very encouraging, indicating that this could well be used to predict changes and trends in intracranial compliance and ICP. The short time Fourier transform (STFT) of the MCA velocity signal, is also discussed to determine if the energy spectrum varied with trauma and pathology. A computer programme was developed to enable short time (4–5 cycles) MCA velocity data to be analysed and the software was embedded into Southampton General hospital's standard data analysis and display software. Analysis of the data for normo-, hypo- and hypercapnia conditions indicated a clear relationship between the frequency centroid in the frequency domain and the intracranial compliance, indicating a relationship with trauma, pathology and ICP.

Finally it is suggested that the "transit time" from the time domain analysis could be combined with the frequency centroid from the STFT analysis by means of a two-dimensional map. This would eliminate the time base from the time domain data presentation, and the time-based moving window from the STFT analysis. In effect the two sets of results could be presented on a two-dimensional static map with "transit time" as the horizontal axis and frequency centroid as the vertical axis.

Methods

In order to obtain a controlled and validated set of results for testing the hypothesis that there will be a changing "transit time" and frequency centroid with changing pathology the author subjected himself to a series of tests at the Medical Physics Department of Southampton General Hospital. The tests involved measuring the ABP using an Ohmeda Plc Finapress finger plethymsograph and the MCA velocity using an EME GmbH TC264 transcranial Doppler ultrasound system, both of which were connected to a 16-channel, Advantec Ltd PCL812 A-D converter, on-line data logger, sampling at every 20 ms and a 486 computer for storing and preprocessing the data.

The first test was carried out under normal conditions of heart rate and breathing ordinary air, which is known as normocapnia conditions. The second test was carried out using a 5% CO_2 in air mixture from a Douglas bag, which induced the condition of hypercapnia, attempting to raise ICP and induce increased intracranial compliance. The third test was carried out during hyperventilation which induced the condition of hypocapnia, attempting to decrease ICP and induce a reduction in intracranial compliance. Each of the tests was recorded for about 20 seconds after a 1 minute stabilisation period to ensure that end-tidal CO_2 remained stable. The data was processed by using high pass filter, cosine window function, cross correlation and Fourier Transform spreadsheet software for normocapnia, hypocapnia and hypercapnia conditions as described above.

Cross correlation of the signal pair was based on the equation given below [2] where f_1 is ABP and f_2 is MCA velocity:

$$r_{xy}(\tau) = \int_{-\infty}^{+\infty} f_1(t) \cdot f_2(t+\tau)\, dt$$

Based on the high pass filtered discrete version of the above equation with a sample time of 20 ms, a table was constructed, in the form of a spreadsheet, to calculate the cross correlation function for each sample period τ, to facilitate "real time" solution by a digital computer. Fourier Transform of the MCA velocity was based on the equation given below [3] where $x(t)$ is the MCA velocity:

$$X(jw) = \int_{-\infty}^{+\infty} x(t) e^{-jwt}\, dt$$

Using the discrete version of the above equation calculations were performed over a 2 second window of raw MCA data in 20 ms steps and over a frequency range of 0 to 15 Hz in steps of 0.15 Hz. In practice a raised cosine window was slid by the time domain data to remove edge effects, a high pass filter applied to remove the offset, the DFT (discrete Fourier transform) calculation performed on each 2 second window of data and the the frequency domain data plotted. This process is known as the sliding window short term Fourier Transform (STFT).

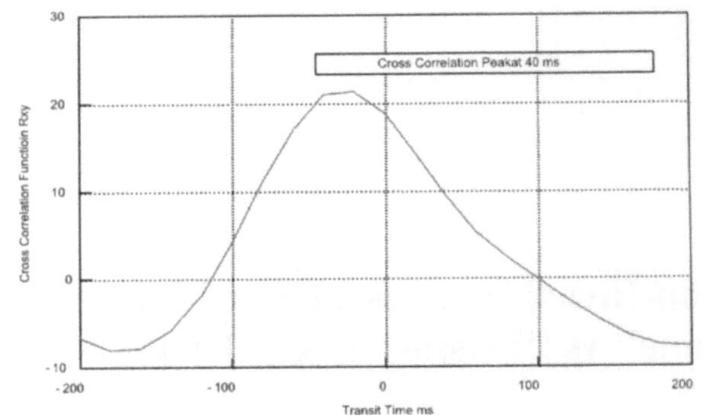

Fig. 1. Results of cross correlation of ABP and MCA velocity during hypocapnia

Results

Figure 1 displays the processed cross correlation data collected from the hypocapnia experiment carried out at Southampton General Hospital as explained above. The vertical axis is a non-scaled measure of the modulus of the cross correlation function and the horizontal scale a measure of time in 100 ms increments. The centre line represents the zero transit time, condition and the actual transit time for a particular set of conditions can be measured horizontally from this line to the peak of the cross correlation coefficient and for this set of data is 40 ms. The cross correlation graphs for normocapnia and hypercapnia display similarly shaped features with peaks at 20 ms and 0 ms respectively. The effect of the CO_2 inhalation appears to modify the intracranial compliance by inducing the autoregulatory system to change the profile of the arterioles, which has the effect of modifying the ICP. The induced changes to the autoregulatory system appear to have a measurable effect on the transit time between the MCA velocity and ABP signals as a function of intracranial compliance and ICP, as predicted by the simulation.

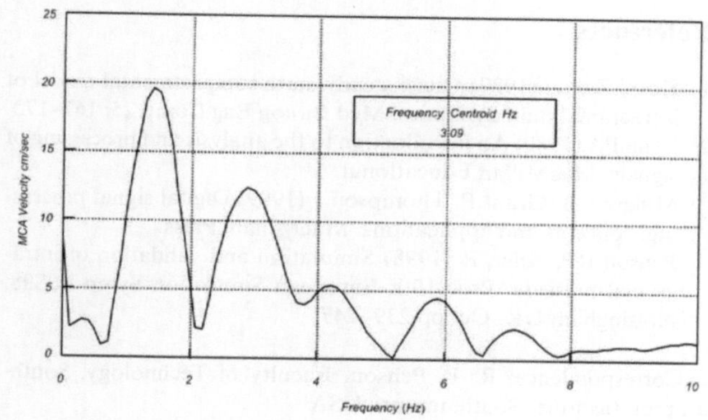

Fig. 2. DFT using STFT analysis of MCA velocity for hypocapnia

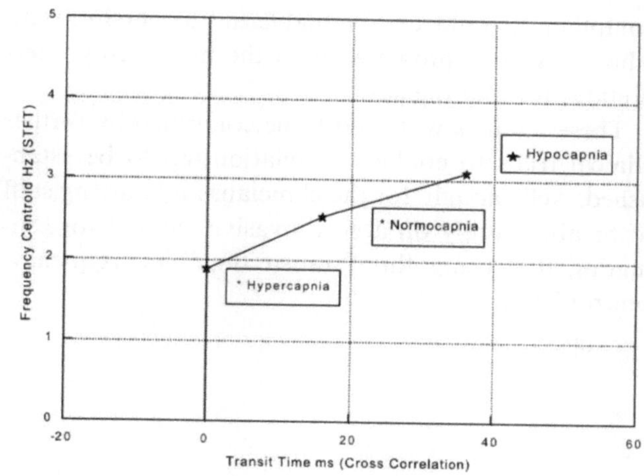

Fig. 3. Two-dimensional map of frequency centroid (STFT) against transit time (cross correlation)

Figure 2 displays the filtered and windowed STFT spectrum of the MCA velocity data for the hypocapnia experiment over the frequency range 0–10 Hz. The spectrum displays a dominant peak at around 1 Hz, corresponding to the heartbeat frequency, two further harmonics at around 2.5 Hz and 3.5 Hz, some high frequency components between 5 and 10 Hz and virtually no harmonic content above 10 Hz. The frequency centroid is calclated to be at 3.09 Hz. The STFT plots for the norm-capnia and hyper-capnia conditions displayed similar overall shapes but with differing amplitudes and frequency centroids. The corresponding frequency centroids were 2.54 Hz and 1.87 Hz respectively.

The results of the frequency domain analysis indicates that the energy distribution in the frequency domain varies with the conditions of hyper-, normo- and hypocapnia, as would be expected, since the MCA velocity profile and the harmonic content also vary, with each of these induced conditions. The implication of this STFT MCA velocity analysis is that intracranial compliance changes can be detected by measuring the change in energy distribution of the frequency spectrum. This change in energy distribution can be most easily achieved by measuring the frequency centroid over the frequency range of 0 to 10 Hz. This frequency centroid variation takes into account the variation of harmonic amplitude and distortion over the frequency range, caused by changing pathology or trauma.

Discussion

As the title of this paper indicates the "transit time" from the time domain analysis could be combined with the frequency centroid from the STFT analysis by means of a two-dimensional map. This would eliminate the time base from the time domain data presentation, and the time-based moving window from the STFT analysis. In effect the two sets of results could be presented on a two-dimensional static map with "transit time" as the horizontal axis and frequency centroid as the vertical axis. The progression of pathology causing changes to intracranial compliance and ICP would be represented by a locus connecting the points, calculated on a moving average basis, representing the combined effect of "transit time" and frequency centroid. Fig. 3 shows this proposed map with the three sets of results from the volunteer patient study plotted. These results represent the change in intracranial compliance from the high value associated with the hypercapnia condition to the low value associated with the hypocapnia condition. From this map changes in intracranial compliance should be easily detectable, and based on the evidence deduced from the limited information obtained, from the volunteer patient study, movement of the locus into the top right hand quadrant would appear to indicate reducing intracranial compliance and possible increases to ICP.

The contour of the locus in Fig. 3, indicates the trend in both the "transit time" and the STFT frequency centroid and movement of this locus into the top right quadrant indicates both a rise in frequency centroid and an increase in "transit time", which appears to be a combined indicator of rising intracranial compliance and ICP. Such a two-dimensional map, with a clear visual indicator of changes to intracranial compliance, could be a valuable aid to nursing staff, who need to be presented with the most easily interpretable form of the data.

These findings will need to be confirmed by further clinical trials to enable the relationship to be established, well enough, for the clinicians and nursing staff to be able to rely on a non invasive method for estimating ICP using this "transit time" vs frequency-centroid map.

References

1. Karni Z *et al* (1987) Quasi-steady-state compartmental model of intracranial fluid dynamics. Med Biolog Eng Comp 25: 167–172
2. Lynn PA (1989) An introduction to the analysis and processing of signals. MacMillan Educational
3. Mulgrew B, Grant P, Thompson J (1999) Digital signal processing: concepts and applications. MacMillam Press
4. Penson RP, Allen R (1998) Simulation and validation of intracranial pressure. Proc 10th European Simulation Symp ESS98, Nottingham UK, Oct pp 239–247

Correspondence: R. P. Penson, Faculty of Technology, Southampton Institute, Southampton, USA

Experimental: Physiology, HI Models, SAH, Ischaemia, Hydrocephalus

Acta Neurochir (2002) [Suppl] 81: 193–195

Approximate Entropy: A Regularity Statistic for Assessment of Intracranial Pressure

A. Beaumont[1] and A. Marmarou[2]

[1] Department of Physiology, Medical College of Virginia, Virginia Commonwealth University, Richmond, VA
[2] Division of Neurosurgery, Medical College of Virginia, Virginia Commonwealth University, Richmond, VA

Summary

Introduction. Waveform analysis of ICP and mABP provideqs important information about cerebrovascular reactivity and intracranial compliance. Traditionally spectral analysis and correlation statistics have been used despite certain limitations. Approximate entropy (ApEn) is an established measure of system regularity; which can change with pathology. This study defines a novel method for application of ApEn to the ICP/mABP waveform, and reports changing ApEn with pathophysiology in the rodent brain.

Methods. Nine Sprague-Dawley rats were anesthetized for mABP, and ICP recording. Rats were exposed to 15 minutes hypotension (45–50 mmHg), followed by resuscitation, equilibration and infusion of a 500 ul subdural hematoma. Raw data, $\text{ApEn}_{\{\text{RAW}\}}$, and wave-period, $\text{ApEn}_{\{\text{PERIOD}\}}$, were assessed for stochastic fluctuations using ApEn ($m = 2$, $r = 0.2$ SD). Results were compared with the established parameters: standard deviation, harmonic transfer function, Pressure Reactivity Index and Correlation Coefficient.

Results. At baseline, $\text{ApEn}_{\{\text{ABP-PERIOD}\}}$ and $\text{ApEn}_{\{\text{ICP-PERIOD}\}}$ were 1.464 ± 0.003, and 0.690 ± 0.020 respectively, suggesting that random heart rate fluctuations are damped during transfer to the ICP waveform. $\text{ApEn}_{\{\text{ICP-PERIOD}\}}$ consistently rose during hypotension (ICP 7 ± 2: $\text{ApEn}_{\{\text{ICP-PERIOD}\}}$ 1.086 ± 0.074, $p < 0.05$) and after SDH infusion (ICP 35 ± 12: $\text{ApEn}_{\{\text{ICP-PERIOD}\}}$ 1.24 ± 0.03, $p < 0.01$). These values were closer to mABP and suggest enhanced transfer of random fluctuations. Significant changes in ApEn were seen in the absence of significant changes in other parameters.

Conclusions. This study defines a system for analyzing the transfer of random fluctuations in mABP waveform to the ICP waveform. ApEn appears to be responsive to changes in intracranial compliance and/or cerebrovascular resistance, therefore more formal studies of the sensitivity and specificity of this novel measure are warranted. These initial findings suggest that ApEn may be a useful adjunct measure of the ICP waveform.

Keywords: Intracranial pressure waves; arterial pressure waves; approximate entropy; intracranial compliance.

Introduction

There is considerable interest in using waveform analysis as a tool to understand the pathophysiology of raised intracranial pressure, and as a clinical tool for monitoring early changes in compliance, or altered autoregulation. Several studies have introduced techniques for this purpose including spectral analysis [1, 4, 6], the Pressure Reactivity Index [2] and the Correlation Coefficient [3].

Approximate Entropy (ApEn) is a measure of system regularity/randomness devised for use in physiological systems [5]. It measures the logarithmic likelihood that runs of patterns that are close for a given number of observations (m), remain close ($\pm$r) on the next incremental comparison. The values m and r are user-defined. Reductions in ApEn imply reduced randomness or increased order – and have been associated with pathology in the cardiovascular, respiratory and endocrine systems.

The relevance of ApEn in ICP dynamics is not known. The aim of this study therefore was to assess whether random fluctuations in the mABP waveform are transmitted to the ICP waveform by calculating ApEn, and to see whether ApEn varies under pathological conditions (hypotension and raised ICP). A secondary aim of the study was to compare ApEn with previously described methods of ICP waveform analysis.

Methods

Adult male Sprague-Dawley rats ($n = 9$) were anesthetized (66% N_20, 33% O_2, 1.5% halothane) and prepared for physiological monitoring including mABP and ICP waveforms (Codman microsensor ICP transducer, 2 mm posterior, 2 mm lateral to bregma). MABP and ICP waveforms were sampled and recorded at 1000 Hz during 60 second windows using a PowerLab system (AD Instruments, GA). Measurements were initially taken at baseline after which mABP was lowered to 45–50 mmHg and sampling repeated. Following resuscitation and equilibration for 30 minutes, 500 μl of au-

Table 1. *Calculated ApEn for the Periodic and Raw Wave Forms*

		Absolute value	ApEn (period)	ApEn (raw)
Baseline				
	mABP	103 ± 6	1.464 ± 0.004	1.028 ± 0.105
	ICP	7 ± 2	0.691 ± 0.212	1.823 ± 0.130
Hypotension				
	mABP	46 ± 3	1.242 ± 0.181	0.820 ± 0.124
	ICP	7 ± 3	1.086 ± 0.074*	0.740 ± 0.012
Post SDH				
	mABP	118 ± 9	1.507 ± 0.065	1.006 ± 0.090
	ICP	35 ± 12	1.242 ± 0.087**	0.682 ± 0.096

mABP Mean arterial blood pressure, *ICP* intracranial pressure, *$p < 0.05$, **$p < 0.01$ cf Baseline.

tologous venous blood was infused into the subdural space, causing ICP to acutely rise. Twenty minutes after this acute rise, whilst ICP remained elevated, a third window of sampling was obtained.

Raw waveform data was processed and passed through an algorithm which automatically identified waveform minima; spurious points were manually removed. The trough-to-trough duration was then calculated for each wave, and a rate-per-trough or waveform period was calculated. Both the raw waveform, and the transformed waveform (periodic profile) were analysed for ApEn according to the methods of Pincus [5], using $m = 2$ and $r = 0.2$ times the standard deviation. Other methods of waveform analysis were then applied for comparison, including standard deviation, harmonic transfer function, Pressure Reactivity Index and Correlation Coefficient.

Results

The calculated ApEn for mACP and ICP are shown in Table 1. Baseline $ApEn_{\{ICP\text{-}PERIOD\}}$ is significantly lower than $ApEn_{\{ABP\text{-}PERIOD\}}$ – suggesting that transmission of random fluctuations in heart rate are transferred to the mABP waveform, but are damped from mABP to the ICP waveform. During hypotension (ICP = 7 ± 2 mmHg) and after SDH (ICP = 35 ± 12 mmHg) $ApEn_{\{ABP\text{-}PERIOD\}}$ remained relatively constant, however $ApEn_{\{ICP\text{-}PERIOD\}}$ significantly increased in both cases suggesting an increase in the transmission of stochastic variation. Similar patterns were not seen in $ApEn_{\{ICP\text{-}RAW\}}$ or $ApEn_{\{ABP\text{-}RAW\}}$.

A comparison between $ApEn_{\{PERIOD\}}$ and other methods of ICP waveform analysis is shown in Table 2. $ApEn_{\{PERIOD\}}$ closely mirrors the changes seen in the harmonic transfer function, and less closely mirrors changes seen in either the Correlation Coefficient or the Pressure Reactivity Index.

Discussion

This study has for the first time applied Approximate Entropy analysis to the periodic function of the ICP/ABP waveform. Changes in $ApEn_{\{ICP\text{-}PERIOD\}}$ during both hypotension and after SDH imply that it may be a useful adjunct technique for the assessment of intracranial pathology, including altered cerebrovascular reactivity and/or intracranial compliance.

Reductions in ApEn have been previously recorded in pathology, and are thought to represent increasing isolation of the system from exogenous physiological signals. The results of this study are opposite to this theory. However since the ICP waveform represents a convolution of the mABP waveform, it is logical that under conditions of reduced intracranial compliance (SDH), or vasodilation (hypotension) there will be a stronger relationship between the two waveforms i.e. greater information transfer. This study demonstrates that this effect also extends to naturally occurring random fluctuations in heart rate which are normally partially damped.

Table 2. *Comparison Beween ApEn and Other Measures of the ICP Waveform Under Different Conditions*

		SD	ApEn	Harmonic transfer	Correlation coefficient	Pressure reactivity index
Baseline						
	mABP	4.63	1.464 ± 0.004			
	ICP	10.75	0.691 ± 0.212	0.00842 ± 0.0010	0.469 ± 0.068	0.180 ± 0.318
Hypotension						
	mABP	5.46	1.242 ± 0.181			
	ICP	7.21	1.086 ± 0.074*	0.0322 ± 0.0091**	0.406 ± 0.079^{NS}	0.377 ± 0.612^{NS}
Post SDH						
	mABP	4.62	1.507 ± 0.065			
	ICP	7.70	1.242 ± 0.037**	0.0451 ± 0.0081***	0.365 ± 0.482^{NS}	0.155 ± 0.514^{NS}

mABP Mean arterial blood pressure, *ICP* intracranial pressure, *$p < 0.05$, **$p < 0.01$, ***$p < 0.001$, *NS* Not Significant *c.f.* Baseline.

Other methods for ICP waveform analysis are better established than ApEn, however ApEn has several advantages which warrant its further investigation. Harmonic transfer function is highly sensitive to noise. Pressure Reactivity Index is a moving Pearson Correlation Coefficient which is related to cerebrovascular reactivity, however its utility depends on underlying slow waves, and a low sampling rate of 0.2 Hz can cause information loss or 'fold-in'. The Correlation Coefficient of Daley *et al.* [3] seems one of the more robust measures, however it is also sensitive to noise. ApEn is inherently insensitive to noise or artefact, to a degree determined by the user-defined value "r", it places no requirement on slow-waves, and does not employ a lossy sampling rate. ApEn may additionally detect changes in wave-transmission before any visual change in waveform, since the periodic function is sensitive to alterations in the rate of wave conduction.

These initial findings are sufficient to establish ApEn as a promising index for assessment of the ICP waveform and intracranial pathology. The precise role, sensitivity and specificity of this measure remain to be defined.

References

1. Chopp M, Portnoy HD (1980) Systems analysis of intracranial pressure. J Neurosurg 53: 516–527
2. Czosnyka M, Smielewski P, Kirkpatrick P *et al* (1998) Continuous monitoring of cerebrovascular pressure-reactivity in head injury. Acta Neurochir (Wien) [Suppl] 71: 74–77
3. Daley ML, Leffler CW (1998) Correlation coefficient between intracranial and arterial pressures: a guage of cerebral vascular dilation. Acta Neurochir (Wien) [Suppl] 71: 285–288
4. Nichols JS, Beel JA, Munro LG (1996) Detection of impaired cerebral autoregulation using spectral analysis of intracranial pressure waves. J Neurotrauma 13: 439–456
5. Pincus SM (1991) Approximate entropy as a measure of system complexity. Proc Natl Acad Sci USA 88: 2297–2301
6. Piper IR, Chan KH, Whittle IR, Miller JD (1993) An experimental study of cerebrovascular resistance, pressure transmission and craniospinal compliance. Neurosurgery 32: 805–816

Correspondence: Prof. Anthony Marmarou, Division of Neurosurgery, P.O. Box, 508, MCV Station, Sanger Hall, Room 8004, 1101 E. Marshall Street, Richmond, Virginia 23298.

Acta Neurochir (2002) [Suppl] 81: 197–199

Simultaneous Measurement of Local Cortical Blood Flow and Tissue Oxygen Saturation by Near Infra-Red Laser Doppler Flowmetry and Remission Spectroscopy in the Pig Brain

B. Walter[1], R. Bauer[1], A. Krug[2], Th. Derfuss[2], F. Traichel[1], and N. Sommer[2]

[1] Friedrich Schiller University, Jena, Germany
[2] LEA Medizintechnik, Giessen, Germany

Summary

In the current study we evaluated the combined use of Near-infrared Laser-Doppler flowmetry (NiLDF) and Remission Spectroscopy (RS) for measurement of regional perfusion and oxygen saturation of the cerebral cortex. An epidural probe for combined measurements of NiLDF and RS was placed above the parietal or frontal cortex of nine anesthetized juvenile pigs. Cerebral perfusion pressure (CPP) was stepwise decreased by intracisternal infusion of artificial CSF at clamped arterial blood pressure (baseline, CPP50, CPP40, CPP30 mmHg, ischemia). Subsequent reperfusion was followed for 3 h. Regional cerebral blood flow (rCBF) was measured with colored microspheres (CMS) and compared with corresponding NiLDF values during CMS injection. Cerebral venous oxygen saturation was measured in blood samples withdrawn from the sagittal sinus and compared with simultaneous recordings of tissue oxygenation during blood withdrawal.

Linear regression analysis resulted in a significant correlation ($p < 0.001$) for changes in regional perfusion during CPP decrease and reperfusion, as measured with CMS and NiLDF ($r = 0.92$, $n = 39$). A significant correlation was also found for tissue oxygen saturation – as measured with RS – and cerebral venous oxygen saturation ($r = 0.85$, $n = 67$). Although the problem of spatial variability remains to be solved, the combined use of NiLDF and RS allows continuous and non-invasive monitoring of changes of key parameters of oxygen metabolism within the cerebral cortex.

Keywords: Cerebral blood flow; tissue oxygenation; Laser-Doppler flowmetry; colored microspheres.

Introduction

The prevention and treatment of secondary insults after traumatic brain injury require an extensive neuromonitoring including measurement of CBF and tissue oxygenation [2]. Laser-Doppler flowmetry (LDF) – alone or combined with other monitoring devices, e.g. ICP, transcranial doppler – has been used to monitor changes of CBF in neurosurgery and neurointensive care [1, 7].

Tissue oxygen spectrometry and LDF have been used to study the relationship between CBF and concentration of reduced hemoglobin during functional activation in the cat cortex [8]. Until now both methods have not been evaluated to measure simultaneously changes of local perfusion and oxygen saturation within a similar tissue volume during CPP changes. Therefore, in the current study we evaluated the combined use of NiLDF and RS for measurement of regional perfusion and oxygen saturation of the cerebral cortex during gradual CPP decrease.

Materials and Methods

Nine female pigs (6–8 weeks old, 17 ± 2 kg) were anesthetized i.v. α-chloralose. All pigs were paralyzed with pancuronium bromide ($0.2\ mg\ kg^{-1}\ h^{-1}$), and were mechanically ventilated. Arterial catheters were inserted through the left and right saphenous artery (PU, 1.4 mm o.d.) for blood pressure monitoring and withdrawal of arterial blood samples. A catheter was inserted into the left atrium for injection of colored microspheres (CMS) and a cuff was placed around the trunk of the pulmonary artery for arterial blood pressure control. Trepanations were made for insertion of a sagittal sinus catheter (2.5 Ch, PU; advanced to the confluens sinuum) and placement of an epidural multiple glass fiber probe above the left frontal or parietal cortex. The probe was connected with a 4-channel NiLDF Monitor and a remission spectrometer (Optoflow®, AbTisSpek®, LEA Medizintechnik, Giessen, Germany). For ICP measurement a fiberoptic catheter (Camino) was placed within the left parietal cortex. All probes were fixed with skull screws and dental acrylic.

Experimental protocol: After recovery from surgery and measurement of baseline values the MABP was clamped at about 80 mmHg and CPP was stepwise decreased to 50, 40 and 30 mmHg, and zero

Table 1. *Summary of Physiological Parameters (Mean ± SD)*

	Baseline	CPP 50	CPP 40	CPP 30	Reperfusion
Sao_2 [%]	93 ± 1	91 ± 4	91 ± 3	89 ± 5	91 ± 6
Hb_a [mmol/l]	6.0 ± 1.1	6.4 ± 1.1	6.4 ± 1.3	6.5 ± 1.2*	6.0 ± 1.0
pH_a	7.42 ± 0.05	7.39 ± 0.08	7.40 ± 0.10	7.37 ± 0.06	7.43 ± 0.06
Pao_2 [mmHg]	118 ± 14	102 ± 17	105 ± 24	91 ± 28	105 ± 35
$Paco_2$ [mmHg]	40 ± 3	38 ± 3	40 ± 3	38 ± 5	37 ± 4
CPP [mmHg]	104 ± 15	51 ± 2*	41 ± 4*	32 ± 3*	94 ± 13
MABP [mmHg]	108 ± 15	86 ± 9*	83 ± 14*	77 ± 6*	97 ± 12
ICP [mmHg]	3 ± 3	35 ± 9*	42 ± 14*	46 ± 5*	3 ± 5
CBF [$mL\ min^{-1}\ 100\ g^{-1}$]	57 ± 18	43 ± 12*	27 ± 9*	17 ± 8*	51 ± 25
regional CBF [$mL\ min^{-1}\ 100\ g^{-1}$]	59 ± 14	44 ± 14*	27 ± 10*	15 ± 8*	51 ± 23

The pressure data represent the electrical mean during CMS injection and reference blood withdrawal during each experimental stage (baseline, CPP50, CPP40, CPP30, Reperfusion). The reperfusion value was measured 120 min after ischemia.
* $p < 0.05$: CPP50, CPP40, and CPP30 versus baseline; *Sao_2* arterial oxygen saturation, *CPP* cerebral perfusion pressure; *ICP* intracranial pressure; *MAPB* mean arterial blood pressure.

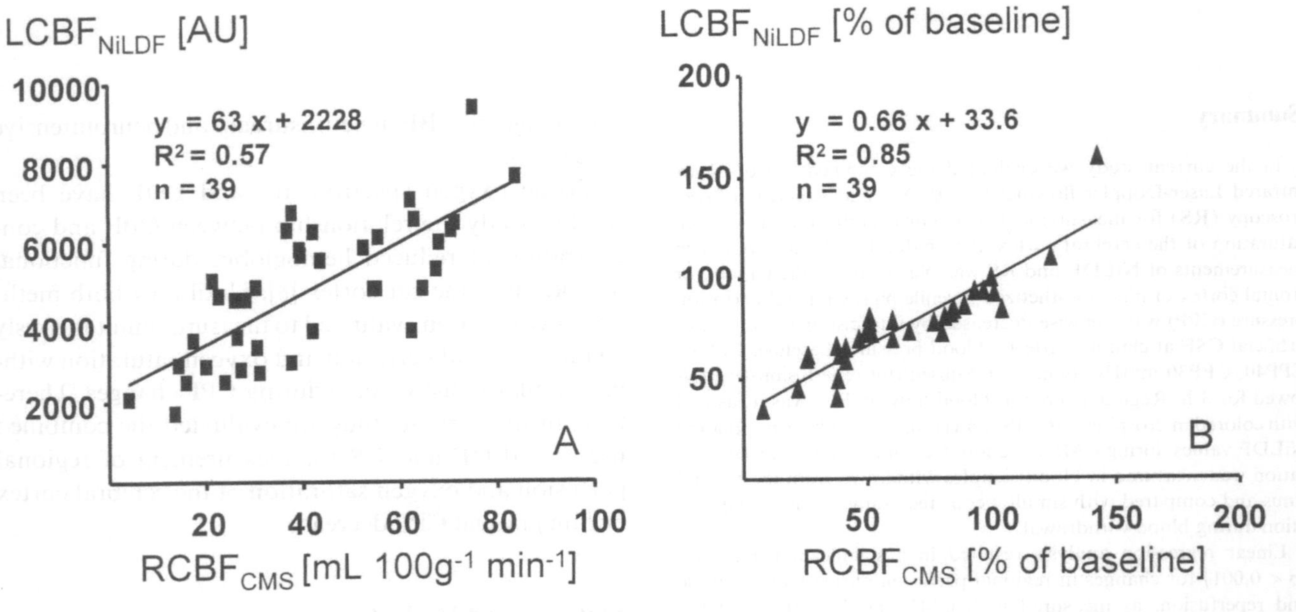

Fig. 1. (A) Correlation of regional CBF ($RCBF_{CMS}$) as measured with colored microspheres and local CBF ($LCBF_{NiLDF}$) as measured with NiLDF ($r = 0.75$; $p < 0.001$). (B) Correlation of normalized CBFs (baseline = 100%) for both measurement methods ($r = 0.92$, $p < 0.001$). The solid line represents the linear regression model

(ischemia) (15 min each stage) by intracisternal infusion of artificial CSF. Subsequently, reperfusion was followed for 180 minutes. For measurement of regional CBF (rCBF) CMS ($2–3 \times 10^6$) were injected at baseline and CPP50, CPP40, CPP30 and at 120 min of reperfusion. After injection of CMS arterial and sagittal sinus blood samples for measurement of oxygen saturation, blood hemoglobin and blood gases were drawn. At the end of the experiment the animals were sacrificed and the brain tissue samples were processed for CMS counting and calculation of rCBF as described elsewhere [9].

Changes of physiological parameters between experimental stages were compared using the one way repeated measures ANOVA. Dunn's method was used for pairwise multiple comparison of single stages with baseline values. The correlation of CBF measurements and oxygen saturation measurements was tested by linear regression analysis and calculation of the Spearman correlation coefficient and the coefficient of determination.

Results

Physiologic variables of all animals are summarized in Table 1. Figure 1 summarizes all CBF measurements obtained with CMS and NiLDF. The correlation coefficient of CBF_{CMS} and CBF_{NiLDF} measurements was best with a fiber separation (illuminating – detecting fiber) of 4 mm (Fig. 1a; $r = 0.75$). Moreover,

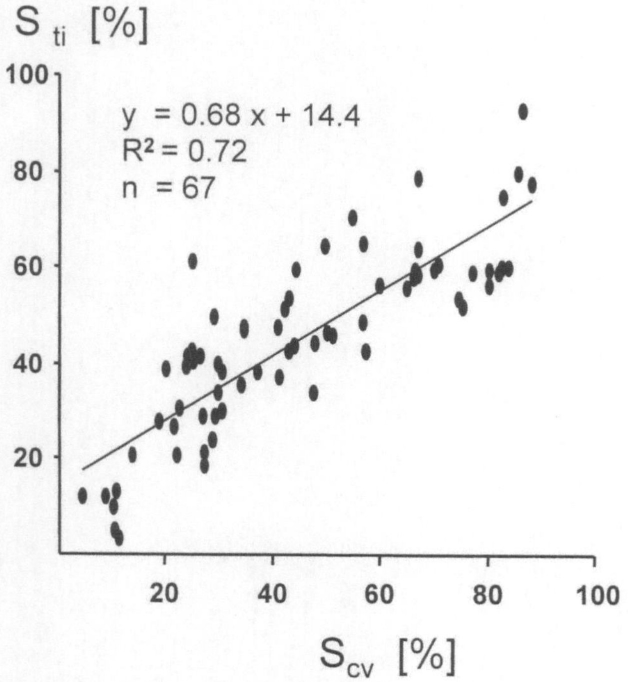

Fig. 2. Correlation of mixed cerebral venous blood oxygen saturation (S_{CV}) – measured in the confluens sinuum, and local tissue hemoglobin oxygen saturation (S_{ti}) measured by remission spectroscopy in the frontal or parietal cortex ($r = 0.85$, $p < 0.001$)

when regional CBF_{CMS} and local CBF_{NiLDF} values were normalized (baseline = 100%), the correlation coefficient increased to $r = 0.92$ (Fig. 1b). As shown in Fig. 2 there was also a satisfactory correlation of local tissue oxygen saturation as measured with RS – and oxygen saturation of mixed cerebral venous blood.

Discussion

In the current study the use of NiLDF and RS was evaluated for continuous measurement of regional CBF and tissue oxygenation. The correlation coefficient which was obtained in our study is comparable with values reported from other investigators [3, 5]. Although the Optoflow®-system allows a considerable larger fiber separation when compared with other LDF monitors, measurement of absolute blood flow values seems not possible. This may be due to the spatial variability of blood flow measurements using single fibers [8, 9]. Moreover, local tissue oxygenation was significantly correlated with cerebral venous oxygen saturation.

In summary, we have shown that the combined use of NiLDF and RS allows continuous optical monitoring of key parameters of oxygen metabolism within the cerebral cortex under clinically relevant conditions. The combined use of both methods may be an adjunct to more global or intermittent measurements of CBF and cerebral oxygen metabolism.

Acknowledgments

The authors express sincere gratitude to R. M. Zimmer and L. Wunder for their technical assistance. Supported by BMBF 01ZZ9622

References

1. Bolognese P, Miller JI, Heger IM, Milhorat TH (1993) Laser-Doppler flowmetry in neurosurgery. J Neurosurg Anesthesiol 5: 151–158
2. Dearden NM (1998) Mechanisms and prevention of secondary brain damage during intensive care. Clin Neuropathol 17: 221–228
3. Eyre JA, Essex TJ, Flecknell PA, Bartholomew PH, Sinclair JI (1988) A comparison of measurements of cerebral blood flow in the rabbit using laser Doppler spectroscopy and radionuclide labelled microspheres. Clin Phys Physiol Meas 9: 65–74
4. Kempski O, Heimann A, Strecker U (1995) On the number of measurements necessary to assess regional cerebral blood flow by local laser Doppler recordings: a simulation study with data from 45 rabbits. Int J Microcirc Clin Exp 15: 37–42
5. Kirkeby OJ, Rise IR, Nordsletten L, Skjeldal S, Hall C, Risoe C (1995) Cerebral blood flow measured with intracerebral laser-Dopplerflow probes and radioactive microspheres. J Appl Physiol 79: 1479–1486
6. Kirkeby OJ, Rise IR, Risoe C (1997) Local variations in the cerebral microcirculatory response to hypercapnia and haemorrhage. Acta Neurochir (Wien) 139: 981–986
7. Kirkpatrick PJ, Smielewski P, Czosnyka M, Pickard JD (1994) Continuous monitoring of cortical perfusion by laser Doppler flowmetry in ventilated patients with head injury. J Neurol Neurosurg Psychiatry 57: 1382–1388
8. Malonek D, Dirnagl U, Lindauer U, Yamada K, Kanno I, Grinvald A (1997) Vascular imprints of neuronal activity: relationships between the dynamics of cortical blood flow, oxygenation, and volume changes following sensory stimulation. Proc Natl Acad Sci U S A 94: 14826–14831
9. Walter B, Bauer R, Gaser E, Zwiener U (1997) Validation of the multiple colored microsphere technique for regional blood flow measurements in newborn piglets. Basic Res Cardiol 92: 191–200

Correspondence: Bernd Walter, Institute of Pathophysiology, Friedrich Schiller University, 07740 Jena, Germany.

Acta Neurochir (2002) [Suppl] 81: 201–204

Cerebral Veno-Arterial pCO2 Difference as an Estimator of Uncompensated Cerebral Hypoperfusion

S. Rossi, A. Colombo, S. Magnoni, E. Roncati Zanier, V. Conte, and N. Stocchetti

Department of Anesthesia and Intensive Care, Ospedale Maggiore Policlinico IRCCS, Milano, Italy

Summary

The aim of the present study was to assess the veno-arterial difference in pCO2 (ΔpCO2) as an indicator of ischemia compared to the arteriovenous O2 difference (AVDO2).

Staircase cerebral blood flow (CBF) reductions were obtained in seven domestic pigs by inducing intracranial hypertension: CBF 100%, 50–60% of baseline, 20–30% of baseline. ICP, MAP, CPP and CBF (Laser-Doppler method) were continuously recorded. The superior sagittal sinus was punctured to determine AVDO2 and ΔpCO2. AVDO2 was 5.9 (± 1.78, range 3.3–7.4), 7.01 (± 1.31, range 5–8.9) and 8.17 (± 1.51, range 6.0–11.3) ml/100 ml in the three CBF steps ($p = 0.001$). CBF impairment was accompanied by the following increases in ΔpCO2: from 10 (± 4, range 4–15) mmHg to 14.5 (± 4.11, range 10–27) mmHg, and to 31.2 (± 9.0, range 17–39) mmHg ($p < 0.001$).

When CBF declines AVDO2 increases, indicating greater extraction of O2 to satisfy the aerobic metabolism. However, this mechanism can no longer compensate once a critical CBF threshold is reached. ΔpCO2 rises slowly during moderate CBF reduction because of defective washout; the rise is impressive during marked CBF impairment when anaerobic metabolism takes place with proton buffering in CO2 and H2O. Therefore, when the brain's ability to compensate for low blood flow is exceeded, CO2 production outweighs O2 extraction.

Keywords: Ischemia; hypoperfusion; veno-arterial difference in pCO_2.

Introduction

The development of ischemia is a common pathway of cerebral damage [3, 5].

When cerebral blood flow (CBF) declines, the arteriovenous oxygen difference (AVDO2) increases, indicating greater O2 extraction to satisfy aerobic metabolism. However, if CBF falls below a critical threshold, this decrease cannot be compensated by a further increase in O2 extraction. It follows that, when the shift from aerobic to anaerobic metabolism takes place, AVDO2 is not a good indicator of metabolic derangement. In experimental models and in the clinical setting, in cases of sepsis, hypovolemic shock and cardiocirculatory arrest, an increase in the veno-arterial difference of pCO2 has been designated a reliable indicator of hypoperfusion and subsequent ischemia, but data on the veno-arterial difference of pCO2 during moderate and severe hypoperfusion in the brain are lacking [2, 6, 9, 10]. This study addressed the question whether arteriovenous pCO2 gradients are good indicators of compensated or uncompensated cerebral hypoperfusion.

Methods

The experiments were conducted in accordance with the guidelines for animal research published by the European Union and acknowledged by Italian Law no 116/92.

ICP was measured by a parenchymal fiberoptic device (Camino Lab). Cerebral perfusion pressure (CPP) was calculated as the difference between mean arterial pressure (MAP) and ICP. CBF estimation was obtained continuously by laser Doppler flowmetry (Peri-flux, Perimed) and was calculated as the change in signal as percentage of baseline. A burr hole through the sagittal suture gave access to the superior sagittal sinus and was punctured for monitoring venous blood gases and venous hemoglobin oxygen saturation (SsO2).

Arterial pressure was monitored through a catheter inserted into a deep branch of the external carotid artery. Intermittent samples were drawn simultaneously from the superior sagittal sinus and from the artery, and processed for blood gases, pH, hemoglobin and oxyhemoglobin concentrations by a gas-analyzer (ABL 30 Radiometer) and a CO-oximeter (OSM 2 Radiometer). AVDO2 was calculated as follows:

$$Hb^{*}1.34^{*}(SaO2\% - SsO2\%) + 0.003(paO2 - psO2).$$

The difference between the superior sagittal sinus paCO2 (pvCO2) and arterial pCO2 (paCO2) was calculated and called ΔpCO2. The model was developed to reduce CBF in three stable steps: baseline (CBF 100%), CBF 50–60% of baseline, 20–30% of baseline. CBF was reduced by inducing intracranial hypertension by infusing saline

Table 1. *Mean Arterial Blood Pressure (MAP), Intracranial Pressure (ICP), Hemoglobin (Hb), Arterial Blood Gases and Internal Temperature During the Three Stages of the Experiment*

	MAP (mmHg)	ICP (mmHg)	Hb (g/dl)	PaO2 (mmHg)	PaCO2 (mmHg)	pH	T °C
CBF 100%	107.8 (±13.8)	8 (±3.1)	9.0 (±1.25)	120 (±19.9)	38 (±2.58)	7.40 (±0.064)	37.8 (±0.30)
CBF 50–60% of Baseline	91.42 (±12.7)	38.5 (±6.5)	8.3 (±1.43)	121 (±24.5)	37.1 (±3.07)	7.41 (±0.054)	37.5 (±0.45)
CBF 20–30% of Baseline	75.28 (±14.6)	45 (±10)	7.9 (±1.13)	113 (±26.9)	37.7 (±1.97)	7.40 (±0.044)	37.9 (0.29)
Repeated-Measures Analysis	P < 0.05	P < 0.001	NS	NS	NS	NS	NS

(warmed to 38 °C), into the left lateral ventricle through a catheter connected with an infusion pump. During each step arterial and venous blood was sampled twice, when the end-point was reached and at the end of the phase. The Cushing response elicited by the ICP increase was inhibited by the infusion of $\alpha - \beta$ blockers (repeated bolus of labetalol 0.5–1 mg/kg). Data were summarized as mean ± standard deviation. Intracranial and extracranial parameters at different CBF values were compared using repeated-measures analysis of variance. A $p \leq 0.05$ was considered as statistically significant.

Results

ICP, MAP and CPP changes, and blood gases during the phases of the experiment are presented in Table 1. AVDO2 increased significantly during the three stages; however, the change from moderate to severe CBF impairment was less pronounced than from intact to moderately impaired CBF (Fig. 1, upper panel). The $\Delta pCO2$ increased significantly from 10 (±4) mmHg at baseline, to 14.5 (±4.11) mmHg, and to 31.2 (±9.0) mmHg in the two reduction steps ($p < 0.01$) (Fig. 1, lower panel). The relationships between each value of AVDO2, $\Delta pCO2$, and CBF are depicted in Fig. 2. The best fitting for AVDO2 and $\Delta pCO2$ was obtained by an exponential curve ($y = ae^{bx}$). For AVDO2 $r^2 = 0.32$, $a = 8.38$ and $b = -0.01$. For $\Delta pCO2$ $r^2 = 0.64$, $a = 36.82$ and $b = -0.06$.

Discussion

Ischemia takes place when a decrease in tissue perfusion exceeds the tissue's ability to increase oxygen extraction from the blood. It consists of inadequate oxygen delivery, inadequate removal of waste products, decrease in high energy phosphates and decrease in production of ATP, shift of metabolism from aerobic to anaerobic with production of lactate and a drop in intracellular pH. Although ischemia is a complex

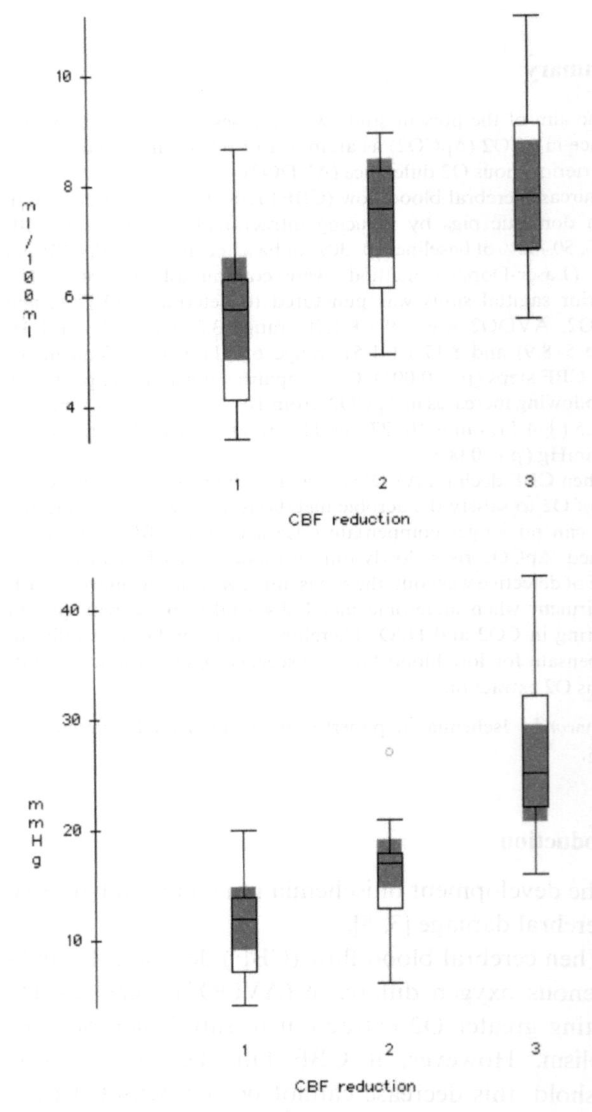

Fig. 1. Boxplots showing AVDO2 and ΔpCO2 during the three-step CBF reduction. *1* intact CBF, *2* moderate CBF reduction, *3* severe CBF impairment

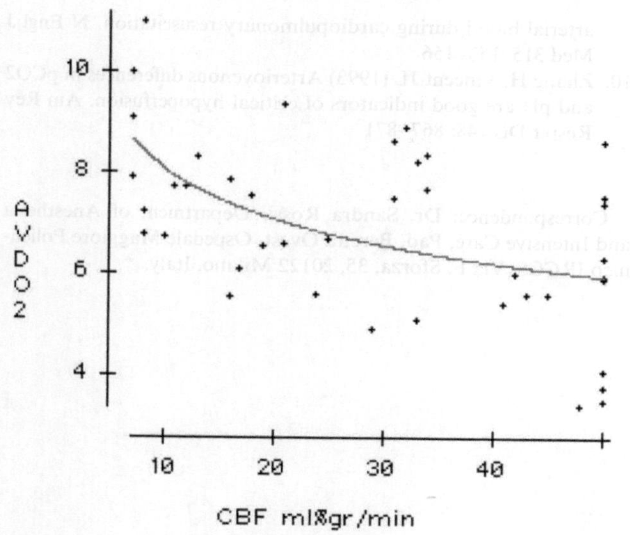

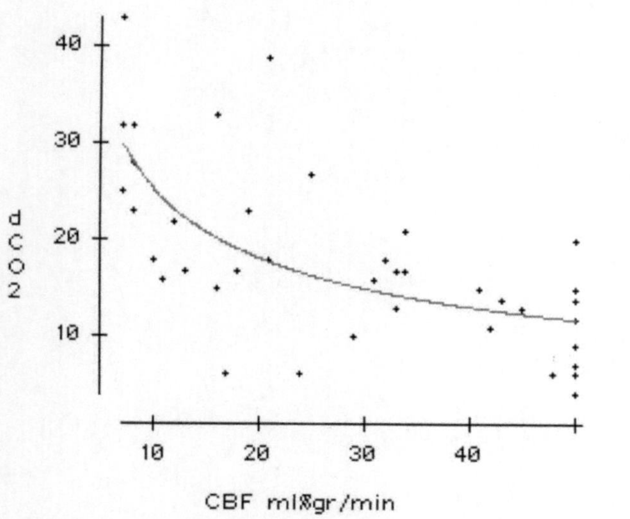

Fig. 2. Scatterplots showing the relation between estimated CBF and AVDO2 and ΔpCO2. CBF was calculated assuming intact CBF as 50 ml/100 g/min

process, inadequate oxygen delivery with respect to the tissue's metabolic demand can be considered the decisive link in the chain, oxygen being the terminal electron acceptor for oxidative phosphorylation. For this reason AVDO2 has been widely used as an estimator of the adequacy of oxygen delivery to meet metabolic demand.

Our animal model, which has been described elsewhere [8], is useful for studying the relationship between CBF and metabolism during moderate CBF impairment and during severe hypoperfusion, the latter reasonably consistent with the phase of shift from aerobic to anaerobic metabolism [1]. The AVDO2 and ΔpCO2 values confirm this. When CBF declines AVDO2 increases, indicating greater extraction of O2 to satisfy the aerobic metabolism. However, once a certain CBF threshold is reached, this mechanism can no longer compensate. This was suggested by Robertson *et al.*, in 100 severely head injured patients. In that study most patients with an extremely low CBF (less than 20 ml/100 g/min) had normal or low AVDO2 values [7]. ΔpCO2 rises slowly during moderate CBF reduction, but the rise is impressive during the last CBF reduction step. This biphasic behavior is probably due to the two main mechanisms responsible for venous hypercarbia: the decreased removal of CO2 during hypoperfusion and the shift from aerobiosis to anaerobiosis. During ischemia hydrogen ions are generated as a by-product of lactic acid and from the hydrolysis of ATP and ADP. These hydrogen ions are buffered by bicarbonate from which CO2 is generated. The first mechanism is responsible for the rise in CO2 during the mild CBF reduction, and the second accounts for the majority of the anaerobically produced CO2.

In conclusion: the rise in ΔpCO2 is a useful indicator of cerebral hypoperfusion and is quantitatively related to the severity of the perfusion failure. ΔpCO2 rises slowly during moderate CBF reduction because of defective washout; it rises steeply during marked CBF impairment when the metabolism becomes anaerobic. Therefore, when the brain's ability to compensate for low blood flow is exceeded, CO2 production outweighs O2 extraction.

References

1. Astrup J (1982) Energy-requiring cell functions in the ischemic brain. J Neurosurg 56: 482–493
2. Bakker J, Vincent JL, Gris P, Leon M, Coffernils M, Kahn RJ (1992) Veno-arterial carbon dioxide gradient in human septic shock. Chest 101: 509–515
3. Bouma GJ, Muizelaar JP, Choi SC, Newlon PG, Young HF (1991) Cerebral circulation and metabolism after severe traumatic brain injury: the elusive role of ischemia. J Neurosurg 75: 685–693
4. Gattinoni L, Lissoni A (1998) Pathophysiology and diagnosis of acid-base disturbances in patients with critical illness. Critical care nephrology. In: Ronco, Bellomo (eds), Kluwer Academic Publishers, pp 297–311
5. Graham DI, Adams JH, Doyle D (1978) Ischaemic brain damage in fatal non-missile head injury. J Neurol Sci 39: 213–234
6. Johnson BA, Weil MH (1991) Redefining ischemia due to circulatory failure as dual defects of oxygen deficits and carbon dioxide excesses. Crit Care Med 19: 1432–1438

7. Robertson CS, Narayan RK, Gokaslan ZL, Pahwa R, Grossman RG, Caram P, Allen E (1989) Cerebral arteriovenous oxygen difference as an estimate of cerebral blood flow in comatose patients. J Neurosurg 70: 222–230
8. Rossi S, Stocchetti N, Longhi L *et al* (2000) Brain oxygen tension, oxygen supply and oxygen consumption during arterial hyperoxia in a model of progressive cerebral ischemia. J Neurotrauma (in press)
9. Weil MH, Rackow EC, Trevino R, Grundler W, Falk JL, Griffel MI (1986) Difference in acid-base state between venous and arterial blood during cardiopulmonary resuscitation. N Engl J Med 315: 153–156
10. Zhang H, Vincent JL (1993) Arteriovenous differences in pCO2 and pH are good indicators of critical hypoperfusion. Am Rev Respir Dis 148: 867–871

Correspondence: Dr. Sandra Rossi, Department of Anesthesia and Intensive Care, Pad. Beretta Ovest, Ospedale Maggiore Policlinico IRCCS, Via F. Sforza, 35, 20122 Milano, Italy.

Acta Neurochir (2002) [Suppl] 81: 205–207

Glial and Neuronal Serum Markers after Controlled Cortical Impact Injury in the Rat

C. Woertgen[1], R. D. Rothoerl[1], M. Wiesmann[2], U. Missler[2], and A. Brawanski[1]

[1] Department of Neurosurgery, University of Regensburg, Germany
[2] Department of Neuroradiology, University of Lübeck, Germany

Summary

The aim of this study was to investigate the time course and the correlation of glial fibrillary acidic protein (GFAP), protein S-100B, and neuron specific enolase (NSE) serum levels to the severity of traumatic brain injury in rats. Male Wistar rats (n = 65 S-100B, NSE group and n = 55 GFAP group) underwent a severe cortical impact injury (100PSI, 2 mm deformation). Blood samples were drawn directly after trauma, 1 h, 6 h, 12 h, 24 h, and 48 h post trauma as well as in sham operated animals directly after craniotomy, after 6 h and 48 h. Serum levels at different severities were estimated in 20 rats (45PSI, 75PSI, 2 mm deformation). We found a time-dependent release of NSE and GFAP into serum after trauma. The highest NSE values were detected six hours after trauma (31.5 µg/l, mean, $p < 0.0001$), the highest GFAP levels were measured one hour after trauma (0.079 µg/l, mean, $p < 0.0014$). Additionally we found a close relationship between NSE serum levels and the severity of traumatic brain injury (45PSI = 12.7 µg/l, 75PSI = 16.17 µg/l, 100PSI = 28.45 µg/l, $p < 0.05$). S-100B serum levels showed an increase (0.92 µg/l, $p < 0.005$) but no time-dependant release. S-100B and GFAP showed no relationship to trauma severity. Serum levels of GFAP, S-100B and NSE are significantly elevated in the early phase after experimental traumatic brain injury. In this experimental model of cortical impact injury only NSE, but not GFAP and S-100B serum levels are time-dependantly correlated with the severity of cortical impact.

Keywords: Traumatic brain injury; glial serum markers; neuronal serum markers.

Introduction

Serum markers like Neuron Specific Enolase (NSE), S-100B are known to give useful additional information for outcome prediction after severe head injury [4, 5]. Experimental investigations concerning this issue are sparse. Missler *et al.* recently introduced for the first time, an dissociation-enhanced lanthanide immunoassay (DELFIA) to quantify glial fibrillary acidic protein (GFAP) serum concentrations, and this protein seems to be a further potential serum marker of central nervous system damage [3]. The aim of this study was to investigate the time course and the correlation of GFAP, protein S-100B, and NSE serum levels to the severity of traumatic brain injury in rats.

Methods

The experimental protocol was approved by the local animal protocol review committee. A detailed description of the experimental methods is given elswhere [6]. Male Wistar rats (n = 65 S-100B, NSE group and n = 55 GFAP group) underwent a severe cortical impact injury (Dixon *et al.* 1991 and 1997, 100PSI, 2 mm deformation). Blood samples were drawn directly after trauma, 1 h, 6 h, 12 h, 24 h, and 48 h post trauma as well as in sham operated animals directly after craniotomy, after 6 h and 48 h. Serum levels at different severities were estimated in 20 rats (45PSI, 75PSI, 2 mm deformation). Serum samples were analyzed on NSE and S-100B concentrations with a commercial available light immuno assay (LIA-mat® NSE Prolifigen® and LIA-mat® Sangtec® 100, Byk-Sangtec Diagnostica GmbH & Co.KG, Dietzenbach, Germany). To quantify glial fibrillary acidic protein (GFAP) serum concentrations a dissociation-enhanced lanthanide immunoassay (DELFIA) was used [3].

The statistical workup: Continuous variables compared across groups were examined using analysis of variance followed by analysis for statistical significance using the Fisher's Protected Least Significant Difference post hoc test. The significance level was $P < 0.05$.

Results

Time Course of NSE Serum Level after Trauma

Directly after trauma the NSE serum level had increased to 10.6 µg/l (control 8.82 µg/l, mean), 1 hour later we found 28.45 µg/l, 6 hours after trauma 31.5 µg/l NSE (mean, $p < 0.0001$ from control). After

12 and 24 hours the concentration decreased to 23.47 μg/l and 22.1 μg/l (mean). After 2 days the NSE concentration dropped to 17.56 μg/l (mean). The NSE levels of the control and direct group differed significantly from the 1,6,12 and 24 hour groups. In the 45 PSI group the NSE serum level was 12.7 μg/l (mean), in the middle group 16.17 μg/l (mean) and in the high group 28.45 μg/l NSE (mean, $p < 0.05$ from each other and control).

Time Course of GFAP Serum Level after Trauma

Directly after trauma the GFAP serum level was 0.019 μg/l (mean). One hour later the GFAP serum level was significantly elevated to 0.079 μg/l (control 0.013 μg/l, mean, $p < 0.05$ from control, direct, 12, 24, 48 hours group) The following groups showed steadily decreasing serum levels. But up to 24 hours after trauma the GFAP serum levels were still significantly elevated compared to the control group (6 hour group 0.038 μg/l, 12 hour group 0.028 μg/l, 24 hours group 0.024 μg/l and 48 hours group 0.019 μg/l, mean). One hour after trauma induction with a low level, we found a GFAP serum level of 0.062 μg/l (mean), in the medium group the GFAP serum level was 0.12 μg/l (mean $p < 0.05$ from low group). After a severe trauma the GFAP serum level was 0.079 μg/l (mean, $p < 0.05$ from control, n.s. from low and medium group).

Time Course of S-100B Serum Level after Trauma

Directly and one hour after traumatic brain injury the mean S-100B concentration was 0.92 μg/l and 0.93 μg/l respectively (control 0.38 μg/l). After six hours we found 0.85 μg/l S-100B, after twelve hours 0.88 μg/l and after 24 hours 0.84 μg/l (all $p < 0.05$ from control). Two days after trauma the mean S-100B value was at 1.03 μg/l (n.s. from control). The mean serum levels at different severities were 1.05 μg/l at 45 PSI, 1.01 μg/l at 75 PSI, and 0.93 μg/l at 100 PSI ($p < 0.05$ from control, n.s. from each other).

Discussion

In different clinical studies the protein S-100B showed a good correlation to outcome especially in the early stage after traumatic brain injury [4, 7]. Thus it seems that the S-100B protein is able to reflect the severity of central nervous system trauma in the clinical setting. The results in our experimental study confirm the clinical findings of a rapid release of GFAP into serum after traumatic brain injury [3]. The GFAP serum concentration one hour after trauma was the highest during 48 hours after trauma. However, when looking at different severities of trauma, the GFAP and S-100B serum levels showed no unequivocal sevierity dependent release after a cortical impact injury. An elevation of the protein S-100B could be observed up to 24 hours after trauma. Concerning the NSE serum levels a time dependent release into the serum after a cortical impact injury could be demonstrated. In addition we found a close relationship between NSE serum levels and severity of trauma. Li *et al.* found that 4 to 6 hours after trauma almost all neurons had lost theire NSE immunoreactivity [2]. In accordance to these findings we found the highest NSE serum levels six hours after trauma reflecting neuronal cell death. Furthermore after controlled cortical impact injury we saw no severity dependent release of S-100B and GFAP into the serum, indicating that the Cci device is not able to induce a severity dependent trauma of glial tissue as demonstrated by Fox [1]. There are no comparable data regarding serum concentrations of GFAP after experimental nervous sytem damage published in the literature. In different clinical studies the NSE serum level did not correlate to clinical assessment and outcome after traumatic brain injury. According to the literature and our experimental results it can be concluded that the NSE serum level seems to reflect only the direct neuronal damage after traumatic brain injury in a time dependent manner. However clinical outcome after traumatic brain injury is dependent on glial and neuronal damage. This fact could explain the clinical failure of the NSE serum level to be of prognostic value.

In summary we were able to quantify GFAP, NSE and S-100B serum levels in rats after controlled cortical impact injury. We found a time dependent release of GFAP and NSE into the serum with an early peak after trauma. However different trauma severities were not reflected by glia marker like GFAP and S-100B serum levels in this experimental setting. In contrast NSE serum levels were able to reflect trauma severity after cortical impact injury.

References

1. Fox GB, Fan L, LeVasseur RA, Faden AI (1998) Sustained Sensory/Motor and cognitive deficits with neuronal apoptosis

following controlled cortical impact brain injury in the mouse. J Neurotrauma 15: 599–614
2. Li R, Fujitani N, Jia JT, Kimuta H (1998) Immunihistochemical indicators of early brain injury: An experimental study using the fluid-percussion model in cats. Rhe Am J Forensic Med Pathol 19: 129–136
3. Missler U, Wiesmann M, Wittmann G, Magerkurth O, Hagenström H (1999) Measurements of glial fibrillary acidic protein in human blood: analytical method and preliminary clinical results. Clin Chem 45: 138–141
4. Raabe A, Grolms C, Sorge O, Zimmermann M, Seifert V (1999) Serum S-100B protein in severe head injury. Neurosurgery 45: 477–483
5. Ross SA, Cunningham RT, Johnston CF, Rowlands BJ (1996) Neuron-specific enolase as an aid to outcome prediction in head injury. Brit J Neurosurgery 10(5): 471–476
6. Rothoerl RD, Brawanski A, Woertgen C (2000) S-100B protein serum levels after controlled cortical impact injury in the rat. Acta Neurochir (Wien) 142: 199–203
7. Woertgen C, Rothoerl RD, Metz C, Brawanski A (1999) Comparison of clinical, radiological and serum marker as progostic factors after severe head injury. J Trauma 47: 1126–1130

Correspondence: Chris Woertgen M.D., Department of Neurosurgery, University of Regensburg, Franz-Josef-Strauss Allee 11, 93042 Regensburg, Germany.

Acta Neurochir (2002) [Suppl] 81: 209–212

Long-Time in-Vivo Metabolic Monitoring Following Experimental Brain Contusion Using Proton Magnetic Resonance Spectroscopy

M. U. Schuhmann[1], **D. Stiller**[3], **M. Skardelly**[1], **S. Thomas**[2], **M. Samii**[1,2], and **T. Brinker**[2]

[1] Department of Neurosurgery, Medical School Hannover, Germany
[2] Department of Neurosurgery, Nordstadt Hospital Hannover, Germany
[3] Special Lab Non-Invasive Brain Imaging, Leibniz Institute of Neurobiology Magdeburg, Germany

Summary

In a Sham-controlled study we applied proton magnetic resonance spectroscopy (^{1}H-MRS) at 4.7 T to a model of experimental traumatic brain contusion. The time course of cerebral metabolite changes was monitored in serial investigation in 14 Sprague Dawley rats up to 4 weeks after trauma. 6 animals served as controls. ^{1}H-MRS spectra were acquired from a voxel covering the hippocampus/basal ganglia ipsi and contralateral to the lesion. Metabolites ratios of the injured hemisphere were compared to those ipsilateral in Sham animals and to those of the contralateral side in the trauma animals. NAA/Cr ratio and Glu/Cr ratio, possible markers of neuronal loss, persistently decreased after trauma to a minimum of −40% and −20% versus controls, respectively. One week after trauma Cho/Cr ratio was strongly increased by 73%. This might indicate a high inflammatory activity at that time. Lac/Cr ratio showed long-lasting and continuing increases up to 2000% versus controls as a sign of permanently shifted posttraumatic energy metabolism. ^{1}H-MRS proved to be a useful non-invasive method for in-vivo monitoring of posttraumatic metabolism also in models of brain contusion. In single cases however, accompanying haemorrhage can potentially prevent useful data acquisition.

Keywords: Proton magnetic resonance spectroscopy; neuronal loss; traumatic brain injury.

Introduction

Volume selective proton magnetic resonance spectroscopy (^{1}H-MRS) is a non-invasive method for in-vivo monitoring of brain metabolites in a defined anatomical area. It permits to monitor metabolite kinetics over time as well as comparative studies between different brain regions. In a pilot study we evaluated the use of ^{1}H-MRS following experimental traumatic brain contusion [7] since previously the method was only applied to diffuse brain injury or fluid percussion injury. In the present Sham-controlled study we clarified the time course of metabolite changes following unilateral cortical contusion injury. ^{1}H-MRS spectra were acquired from a voxel covering the hippocampus/basal ganglia ipsi and contralateral to the lesion. Metabolites ratios of the injured hemisphere were compared to those ipsilateral in Sham animals and to those of the contralateral side in trauma animals.

Materials and Methods

20 male Sprague Dawley rats (250–350 g) were investigated at 1 h, 4 h, 24 h, 7 d and 28 d after injury. 14 rats received trauma, 6 served as controls. Anaesthesia was induced with 5% Isoflurane in N_2O/O_2 (2:1) and maintained at 1.5–2%. Animals were intubated and ventilated for surgical procedures or breathed spontaneously during MR investigations. The left parietal bone was exposed via a midline incision. Using a high-speed drill a left-sided 7 mm craniotomy was centred 3 mm posterior and 4 mm lateral to bregma. Animals received a Controlled Cortical Impact Injury (*CCII*) with a device similar to the development of Lighthall [5]. Impact velocity was determined with a laser-optic system (optoNCDT, Mikro Epsilon Messtechnik, Ortenburg, Germany). A 5 mm round impactor tip was accelerated to 4.02 ± 0.28 m/s with a vertical deformation depth of 2.5 mm.

MRI technique: All animals underwent serial investigations using a Bruker Biospec 47/20 scanner at 4.7 T running Paravision® software (Bruker GmbH, Ettlingen, Germany). For homogeneous excitation a 72 mm birdcage resonator and for detection an anatomically shaped 3-cm surface coil were used. Coronal T_2-weighted RARE_8 sequences (TR 3100 ms, TE 79.4 ms, slice thickness 1.5 mm, FOV 3.2 cm, matrix 256^2) were generated for anatomically precise placement of the spectroscopy voxel. For volume selective spectroscopy a PRESS-sequence (TR 2500 ms, TE 20 ms, 128 accumulations) was used. Voxel position (size 3 mm^3) was chosen right below the contusion covering the hippocampus and basal ganglia. The corresponding contralateral position and the ipsilateral spot in Sham-operated animals were taken as reference. MRS echoes were baseline corrected and exponentially filtered (LB 2 Hz), followed by zero filling before fast Fourier transformation. Metabolite spectra were phase corrected manually (0th and 1st order). Peak areas and intensities were determined by Lorentzian deconvolution algorithm

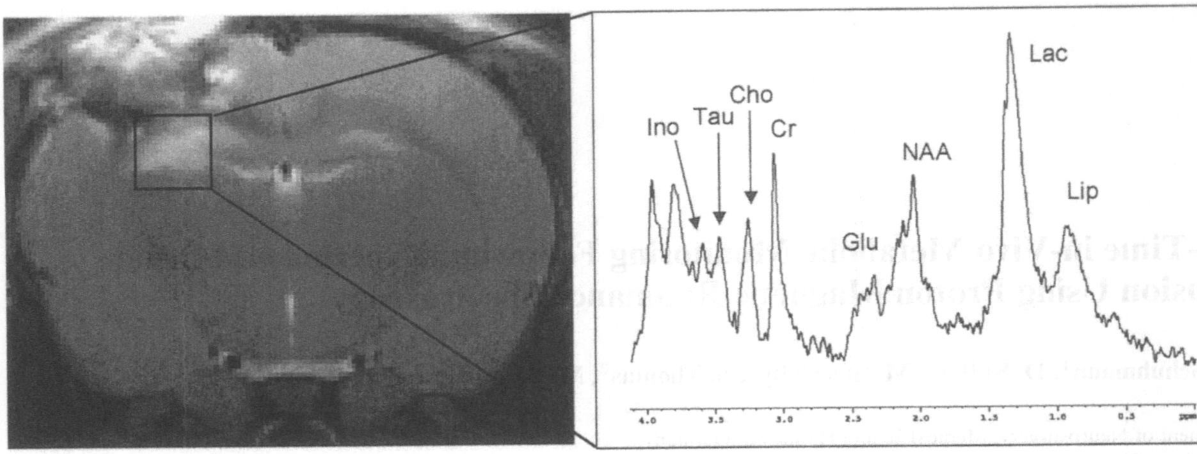

Fig. 1. Left shows voxel position ipsilateral to contusion in high-resolution MRI. Right displays the resulting MR spectrum. Peaks of chemical shift of several metabolites are marked: *Ino* Inositol, *Tau* Taurine, *Cho* Choline, *Cr* Creatine, *Glu* Glutamate, *NAA* N-acetyl aspartate, *Lac* Lactate, *Lip* Membrane Lipids

(Bruker XWIN-NMR software package) for inositol (Ino), choline (Cho), creatine + phosphocreatine (Cr), glutamate (Glu), N-acetyl aspartate (NAA), lactate (Lac), and Taurine (Tau). A semiquantitative analysis was performed taking the Cr peak as reference point and calculating ratios for the remaining metabolites. Differences were accepted in case of $p < 0.05$ in non-parametric tests.

Results

Figure 2 demonstrates changes of metabolites of the injured side versus the contralateral side and versus Sham. NAA/Cr ratio decreases on the injured side immediately after trauma, to a minimum of −40% versus Sham at 24 h. Lower levels on the injured side remained until 4 weeks after trauma. All changes were significant versus both controls. The Glu/Cr ratio showed a very similar behaviour with a decrease on the injured side of −15 to −20% at 4 h after trauma. Glu/Cr ratio remained low during the further course. All changes after 4 h were significant. The choline containing compounds Cho and Ino qualitatively showed almost identical behaviour. Cho/Cr ratio is displayed. A tendency to rise on the trauma side is evident, with significant increases at 4 h (+27%) and 1 week (+73%). At 4 weeks ratios had returned to the level of the contralateral side. Lac/Cr ratio increased on the injured side continuously up to 4 weeks by 400–2000%. Lactate was detected in 3 of 21 spectra of Sham controls (14%), however in 25 of 47 (53%) spectra of the contralateral side. The Tau/Cr ratio was increased versus Sham at 4 h and thereafter (29–59%), however differences versus the contralateral side were significant at 1 and 4 weeks only.

Discussion

In the region of interest (hippocampus/basal ganglia), which is the zone just below the contused parietal cortex, we observed significant metabolite changes compared to the contralateral side or to Sham operated animals. The persisting decrease of N-acetyl aspartate and Glutamate immediately or 4 h after trauma might indicate persistent neuronal cell loss. Both metabolites are considered as markers of neuronal integrity. NAA is unequivocally specific to neurons and a decrease of NAA in MRS has been shown to be equivalent to neuronal loss [2]. In humans after TBI a decrease of NAA correlated positively to adverse outcome and neuropsychologic dysfunction [1, 6]. The observation of lower NAA levels at 4 h and 24 h, when oedema is more prominent, compared to 7 d and 4 weeks might be due to an alteration of NAA relaxation times by the oedema. This could potentially contribute to an error in estimation of neuronal loss of ~2.5% per 10% change of relaxation time [2]. Choline and Inositol have been reported elevated following days to weeks after human trauma [6] either as a sign of membrane breakdown/synthesis or inflammation. In rats the inflammatory activity is known to reach a maximum on day 4–6 after experimental brain contusion and to persist for months [3, 4]. The strong increase of Cho/Cr at 1 week might therefore be an indicator of increased inflammatory reactions. The long-lasting and increasing lactate accumulation on the injured side as well as the increased rate of lactate detection on the contralateral side indicates a persis-

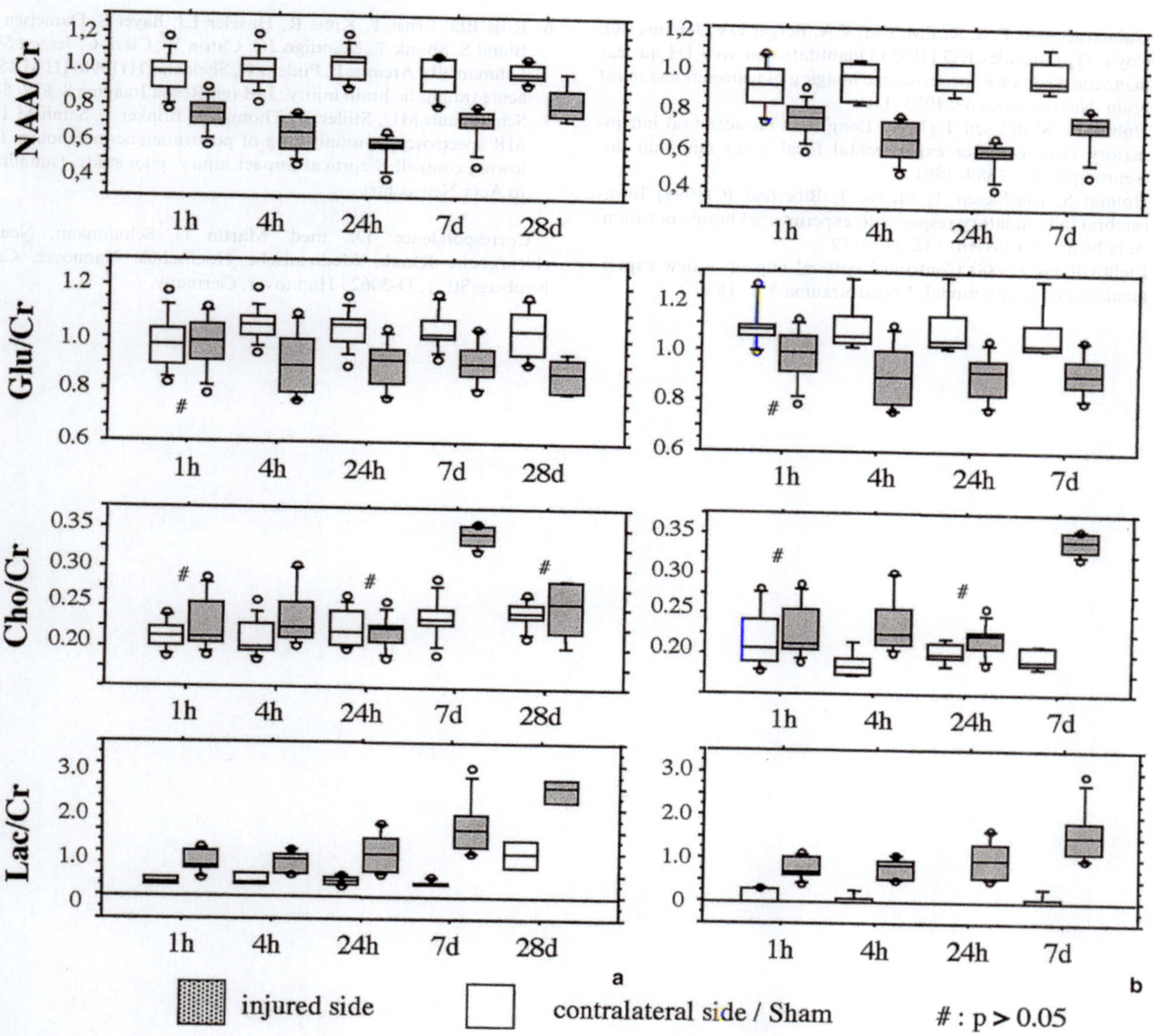

Fig. 2. Time course of metabolite ratios of the injured side in comparison to ratios of the contralateral side (a) or Sham controls (b). *Ino* Inositol, *Tau* Taurine, *Cho* Choline, *Cr* Creatine, *Glu* Glutamate, *NAA* N-acetyl aspartate, *Lac* Lactate

tent posttraumatic shift of energy metabolism towards anaerobic glycolysis. At a post-acute time > 24 h when hypoperfusion and ischemia in this model should have resolved there is still high lactate suggesting e.g. persistent hyperglycolysis.

In summary, we successfully applied ^{1}H-MRS in a Sham controlled setting to a contusional trauma model. In individual cases however, the disturbed magnetic field homogeneity caused by an intracontusional haemorrhage can potentially prevent acquisition of useful spectra. To increase the clinical usefulness of the method, future research has to link the observed metabolite changes to known posttraumatic mechanisms. Furthermore the exact quantification of metabolites instead of semiquantitative ratios versus creatine, which might not be as stable in this model as generally supposed, will improve results.

References

1. Friedman SD, Brooks WM, Jung RE, Chiulli SJ, Sloan JH, Montoya BT, Hart BL, Yeo RA (1999) Quantitative proton MRS predicts outcome after traumatic brain injury. Neurology 52: 1384–1391

2. Guimaraes AR, P. S, R. PM, Carr CA, Berger UV, Jenkins BG, Coyle JT, Gonzáles RG (1995) Quantitative in vivo 1H nuclear magnetic resonance spectroscopic imaging of neuronal loss in rat brain. Neuroscience 69: 1095–1101
3. Holmin S, Mathiesen T (1999) Long-term intracerebral inflammatory response after experimental focal brain injury in rat. Neuroreport 10: 1889–1891
4. Holmin S, Mathiesen T, Shetye J, Biberfeld P (1995) Intracerebral inflammatory response to experimental brain contusion. Acta Neurochir (Wien) 132: 110–119
5. Lighthall JW (1988) Controlled cortical impact: a new experimental brain injury model. J Neurotrauma 5: 1–15
6. Ross BD, Ernst T, Kreis R, Haseler LJ, Bayer S, Danielsen E, Bluml S, Shonk T, Mandigo JC, Caton W, Clark C, Jensen SW, Lehman NL, Arcinue E, Pudenz R, Shelden CH (1998) 1H MRS in acute traumatic brain injury. J Magn Reson Imaging 8: 829–840
7. Schuhmann MU, Stiller D, Thomas S, Brinker T, Samii M 1H-MR spectroscopic monitoring of posttraumatic metabolism following controlled cortical impact injury: pilot study. (submitted to Acta Neurochir)

Correspondence: Dr. med. Martin U. Schuhmann, Neurochirurgische Klinik, Medizinische Hochschule Hannover, Carl-Neuberg-Str. 1, D-30625 Hannover, Germany.

Acta Neurochir (2002) [Suppl] 81: 213–215

Determination of Contusion and Oedema Volume by MRI Corresponds to Changes of Brain Water Content Following Controlled Cortical Impact Injury

M. U. Schuhmann[1], **D. Stiller**[3], **M. Skardelly**[1], **M. Mokktarzadeh**[1], **S. Thomas**[2], **T. Brinker**[2], and **M. Samii**[1,2]

[1] Department of Neurosurgery, Medical School Hannover, Germany
[2] Department of Neurosurgery, Nordstadt Hospital Hannover, Germany
[3] Special Lab Non-Invasive Brain Imaging, Leibniz Institute of Neurobiology Magdeburg, Germany

Summary

The time-course of brain contusion/oedema development as visualised by high-resolution MRI was compared to brain water content following experimental brain contusion. 36 Sprague-Dawley rats underwent Controlled Cortical Impact Injury (*CCII*), 24 served as controls. In 16 animals serial T_2 weighted MRI investigations at 1 h, 4 h, 24 h and 7 d after *CCII* were performed, in 44 rats hemispheric brain water content was determined at the same time points by wet dry weight method. MRI lesion volume (mm^3) and brain water content of injured hemisphere (%) showed for absolute and relative values a strictly parallel course. Significant posttraumatic increases had a maximum at 24 hours. Values on day 7 were below those of 1st h in both methods. The simple non-invasive MRI method quantifies contusion and surrounding penumbra according to elevated tissue water signal. The invasive wet dry weight method quantifies changes of hemispheric brain water content that are likely to take place in contusion core and surrounding penumbra. Therefore, from a theoretical aspect both methods seem comparable. Following experimental brain contusion, the simple MRI method might be an equally sufficient way to describe post-traumatic or post-therapeutic changes of lesion size and brain oedema.

Keywords: Magnetic resonance imaging; brain oedema; brain water content; brain injury.

Introduction

Magnetic resonance imaging (MRI) has become available for use in experimental traumatic brain injury with the advance of high-field scanners having a sufficient resolution to precisely visualise posttraumatic anatomical changes in rats. Structural damage as well as changes in tissue water can be sufficiently detected by a rather simple T_2 weighted sequences with shorter scanning times, compared to time consuming diffusion weighted imaging. Furthermore the non-invasive methods allows these measurements as an addition to other investigations in the same animals without the need for a separate control group. Determination of brain water content (%BW) either by wet dry weight method or by gravimetry is the gold standard for assessment of posttraumatic hemispheric or local oedema development. We compared the time courses of brain contusion/penumbra volume development, as measured by T2 weighted MRI, to changes in hemispheric %BW for the first week following experimental brain contusion.

Materials and Methods

60 Sprague Dawley rats (250–350 g) were investigated at 1 h, 4 h, 24 h, and 1 week after injury. 36 rats received trauma, 24 served as controls. Anaesthesia was induced with 5% Isoflurane in N_2O/O_2 (2:1) and maintained with 1.5–2%. Animals were intubated and ventilated for surgical procedures or breathed spontaneously during MR investigations. With the head mounted in a stereotactic frame the left parietal bone was exposed via a midline incision. Using a high-speed drill a left-sided 7 mm craniotomy was centred 3 mm posterior and 4 mm lateral to bregma. Animals received a Controlled Cortical Impact Injury (*CCII*) with a device similar to the development of Lighthall [4]. Impact velocity was determined with a laser-optic system (optoNCDT, Mikro Epsilon Messtechnik, Ortenburg, Germany). A 5 mm round impactor tip was accelerated to 4.18 ± 0.32 m/s with a vertical deformation depth of 2.5 mm. 44 animals were sacrificed at assigned time points, brains quickly removed and meticulously separated in the midline. Hemispheres were dried at 110 °C for 48 h. %BW was determined as difference between wet and dry weight. %BW of injured left hemisphere was compared to the contralateral right side and to controls. Relative changes vs. values at 1 h were calculated. MRI technique: 16 animals underwent serial investigations using a Bruker Biospec 47/20 scanner at 4.7 T running Paravision® software (Bruker GmbH, Ettlingen, Germany). For homogeneous excitation a 72 mm birdcage resonator and for detection an anatomically shaped 3-cm surface coil were used. Coronal T2-weighted RARE_8 sequences (TR 3100 ms, TE

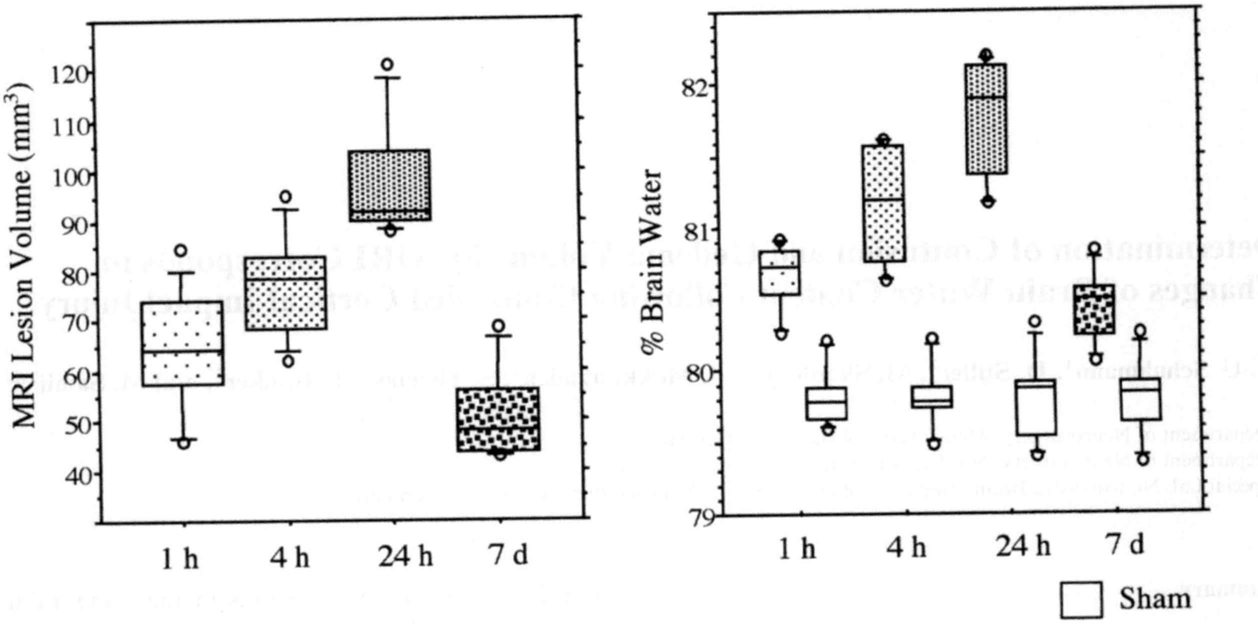

Fig. 1. Left shows the time course of the contusional lesion volume following CCII as assessed by T_2 weighted high-resolution MRI. Left shows the corresponding time course of brain water content (%BW) of the injured hemisphere vs. the contralateral side following same trauma. Results of Sham animals, lacking any difference to the contralateral side, are not displayed

79.4 ms, slice thickness 1.5 mm, FOV 3.2 cm, matrix 256^2) were generated. Volumes of contusion/surrounding oedema zone and of hemisphere were determined by planimetry. Absolute and relative (vs. hemisphere) changes of lesion volume and relative changes vs. values at 1 h were calculated. Differences were accepted in case of $p < 0.05$ in non-parametric Mann Whitney U test.

Results

Lesion (contusion/oedema) volumes as defined on MRI images increased from 64.3 ± 12.5 mm^3 at 1 h to 97.5 ± 11.9 mm^3 at 24 h and decreased to 50.8 ± 9.4 mm^3 at 7 d. Relative lesion volumes (vs. hemisphere) changed from $14.1 \pm 2.4\%$ to $21.6 \pm 2.2\%$ and returned to $13.8 \pm 2.6\%$. Changes at 4 h, 24 h and 7 d relative to 1 h were $27.3 \pm 29.6\%$, $61.2 \pm 23.3\%$, and $-12.8 \pm 20.4\%$, respectively. All changes were significantly different. Scans of Sham operated animals showed no changes.

%BW of injured hemisphere increased significantly vs. contralateral side or Sham to $80.7 \pm 0.25\%$, $81.2 \pm 0.46\%$, $81.8 \pm 0.44\%$, and $80.4 \pm 0.26\%$ at 1 h, 4 h, 24 h and 7 d, respectively. %BW of contralateral side ($79.7 \pm 0.33\%$) or Sham ($79.8 \pm 0.52\%$) remained unchanged. Changes of the injured hemisphere at 4 h, 24 h and 7 d relative to 1 h were $0.54 \pm 0.64\%$, $1.6 \pm 0.55\%$, and $-0.32 \pm 0.34\%$, respectively.

Discussion

Determination of %BW either of the whole hemisphere or of single brain slices is a widely established method to quantify brain oedema. In the same model, however with slightly different parameters of trauma application, others determined a %BW at 24 hours for the injured hemisphere and contralateral side of $82.8 \pm 0.1\%/79.9 \pm 0.2\%$ [5], and $82.5 \pm 0.5\%/81.3 \pm 0.1\%$ [3], respectively. Another group, using a more severe trauma level, showed L-R differences in %BW of $1.69 \pm 0.18\%$ at 2 h, of $3.00 \pm 0.08\%$ at 24 h, and of $0.94 \pm 0.21\%$ at 7 d, respectively [1]. We measured slightly lower L-R differences of $1.35 \pm 0.5\%$ at 4 h, of $2.02 \pm 0.34\%$ at 24 h, and of $0.64 \pm 0.36\%$ at 7 d, respectively, however, the time course pattern was identical. Although absolute values might differ it is evident that in the *CCII* model a reliable oedema development is present. Most changes of %BW will occur in the contusion core, where necrotic tissue and a disrupted blood brain barrier exist and in the surrounding oedematous penumbra zone, where the cascades of posttraumatic secondary and progressive brain damage take place. Exactly these two compartments of the contusional lesion are visualised by T_2 weighted MRI, which displays areas of increased water signal versus

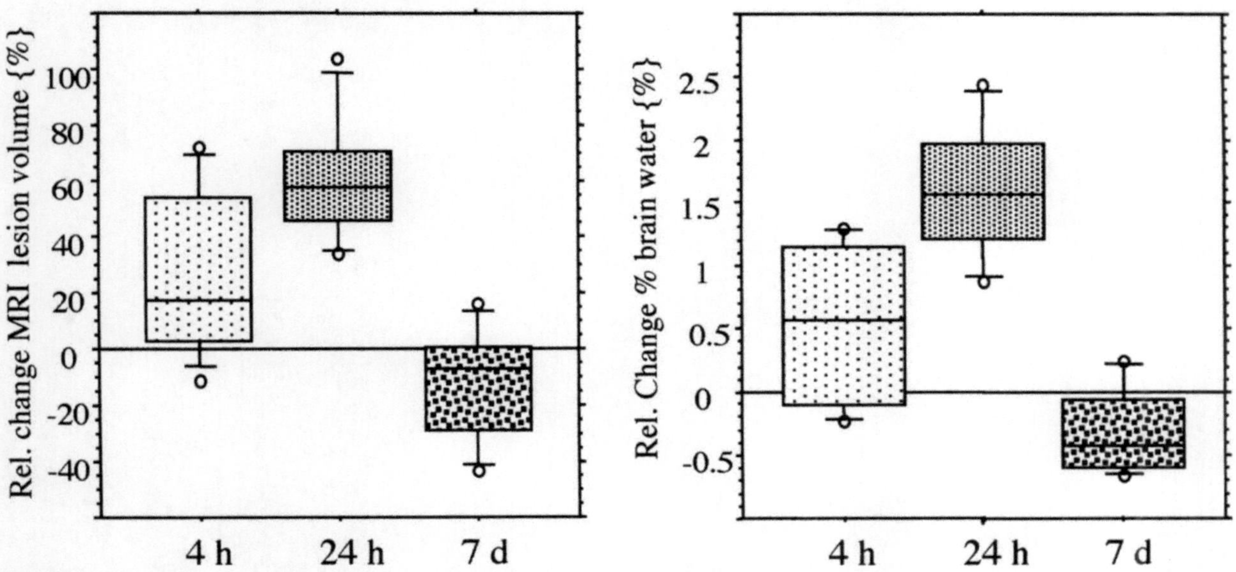

Fig. 2. Comparison of relative changes versus values at 1 h post CCII. (Left) MRI lesion volume; (Right) brain water content

normal tissue. A good differentiation between the surrounding oedema and the contusion core was only possible if the latter had undergone haemorrhagic transformation, however this was not a consistent finding. Consequently the total lesion volume determined at 24 h by MRI in our study (97.5 ± 11.9 mm^3) was above histological determinations of contusion volume at 24 h alone (50–77 mm^3) found by others [2, 3, 5]. Kochanek *at al.* demonstrated a similar relation between smaller histological contusion volume (31.6 ± 10.3 mm^3) and larger MRI delineated lesion volume (47.1 ± 14.3 mm^3) at 7 d after *CCII* [1].

In conclusion, very similar time courses of lesion volume in T_2 weighted MRI and brain water content suggests a strong correlation between these two parameters. Additionally the non-invasiveness of MRI facilitates intra-individual follow-up studies as addition to other in-vivo investigations. We suggest that this method might be equally useful as determination of %BW if brain oedema has to be quantified after experimental brain contusion.

References

1. Kochanek PM, Marion DW, Zhang W, Schiding JK, White M, Palmer AM, Clark RS, O'Malley ME, Styren SD, Ho C, Dekosky ST (1995) Severe controlled cortical impact in rats: assessment of cerebral edema, blood flow, and contusion volume. J Neurotrauma 12: 1015–1025
2. Kroppenstedt SN, Kern M, Thomale UW, Schneider GH, Lanksch WR, Unterberg AW (1999) Effect of cerebral perfusion pressure on contusion volume following impact injury. J Neurosurg 90: 520–526
3. Kroppenstedt SN, Schneider GH, Thomale UW, Unterberg AW (1998) Neuroprotective properties of aptiganel HCL (Cerestat®) following controlled cortical impact injury. Act Neurochir (Wien) [Suppl] 71: 114–116
4. Lighthall JW (1988) Controlled cortical impact: a new experimental brain injury model. J Neurotrauma 5: 1–15
5. Stroop R, Thomale UW, Pauser S, Bernarding J, Vollmann W, Wolf KJ, Lanksch WR, Unterberg AW (1998) Magnetic resonance imaging studies with cluster algorithm for characterization of brain edema after controlled cortical impact injury (CCII). Acta Neurochir (Wien) [Suppl] 71: 303–305

Correspondence: Dr. med. Martin U. Schuhmann, Neurochirurgische Klinik, Medizinische Hochschule Hannover, Carl-Neuberg-Str. 1, D-30625 Hannover, Germany.

Acta Neurochir (2002) [Suppl] 81: 217–219

Secondary Insults Worsen Blood Brain Barrier Dysfunction Assessed by MRI in Cerebral Contusion

A. Beaumont[1], **A. Marmarou**[1], **P. Fatouros**[2], and **F. Corwin**[2]

[1] Division of Neurosurgery, Medical College of Virginia, Richmond, VA, USA
[2] Division of Radiation Physics, Medical College of Virginia, Richmond, VA, USA

Summary

Object. Understanding the cause of post-traumatic intracranial hypertension requires information about the pathophysiology of edema formation. Secondary insults are known to exacerbate edema formation following experimental contusion, however the influence of these insults on blood brain barrier (BBB) integrity is not known. This study non-invasively assesses the influence of hypoxia and hypotension on BBB permeability following experimental cortical contusion.

Methods. Sprague-Dawley rats (350–380 g) were divided into three groups. Group A: (n = 3) Sham, Group B (n = 8) focal injury (controlled cortical impact 6.0 m/sec, 3 mm depth), Group C (n = 8), focal injury with secondary insult. Cortical BBB integrity was assessed four hours post-trauma using an i.v. bolus of 0.2 mmol/kg Gd-DTPA with serial T1 MR images, over 30 minutes. Absolute tissue concentrations of Gd were measured empirically using known references. The time course of accumulation was analyzed with respect to BBB permeability.

Results. BBB permeability was greatest in the site of contusion, and Gd accumulation was greatly enhanced by secondary insult ($p < 0.01$). Regions of lowest ADC and maximal swelling correlated with regions of maximal BBB permeability ($p < 0.05$).

Conclusions. Secondary insults enhance BBB dysfunction in contusion. Positive relationships between low ADC, tissue swelling and BBB dysfunction suggest synergy between underlying cytotoxic swelling and BBB permeability in contusion. These data also suggest that restoration of BBB integrity after injury may be an energy dependent process. These findings have important implications for the pathophysiology of ICP elevations following cerebral contusion.

Keywords: Traumatic brain injury; blood brain barrier; contusion; secondary insult.

Introduction

Understanding the cause of post-traumatic intracranial hypertension requires information about the pathophysiology of edema formation. Measurements of Apparent Diffusion Coefficients of water (ADCw) in recent studies have shown that cerebral edema in traumatic brain injury (TBI) is principally cellular. Secondary insults are known to exacerbate cellular edema and neuronal injury following TBI including contusion [1, 2]. The influence of secondary insults on blood brain barrier (BBB) integrity is not known, although one study on diffuse injury suggests that hypoxia and hypotension prolong BBB opening after injury [3]. The aim of this study therefore was to non-invasively assess the influence of hypoxia and hypotension on BBB permeability following experimental cortical contusion.

Methods

In outline, adult-male Sprague-Dawley rats (350–380 g) were exposed to either cortical contusion alone, or in combination with hypoxia and hypotension. Four hours after injury, animals were placed in a 2.35 T magnet, and infused with an iv bolus of 0.2 mmol/kg gadolinium-DTPA (Gd-DTPA), while obtaining rapid, seria, T1 images. Changes in signal intensity were used to calculate gadolinium concentration in tissue from known standards. The time course of gadolinium accumulation was then examined, and conclusions made about barrier permeability.

Rats were anesthetised (O_2/N_2O/halothane) and divided into 3 groups. Group 1 (n = 3) Sham injury; Group 2 (n = 6) cortical contusion (6 m/sec, 2 mm depth), and Group 3 (n = 5); cortical contusion with a 30 minute secondary insult of hypoxia and hypotension (mABP = 30–40 mmHg, FiO2 = 12%). Contusion injury was performed as described previously and secondary insults were induced by a reduction of inspired O_2 for 30 mins following injury, after which anesthetic parameters were returned to normal.

BBB permeability was assessed 4 hours following injury using contrast enhanced MRI in a 2.35 T, 40 cm bore magnet (Biospec, Bruker Instruments, Billerica, MA) equipped with a 12 cm inner diameter actively shielded gradient insert. RF excitation and reception was performed using a 4.5 cm helmet coil. Initial measures of ADCw and tissue water content were made using methods described previously [1]. Serial T1 images were then obtained from a 3 mm thick slice, 7.5 mm posteriorly. Imaging parameters used were

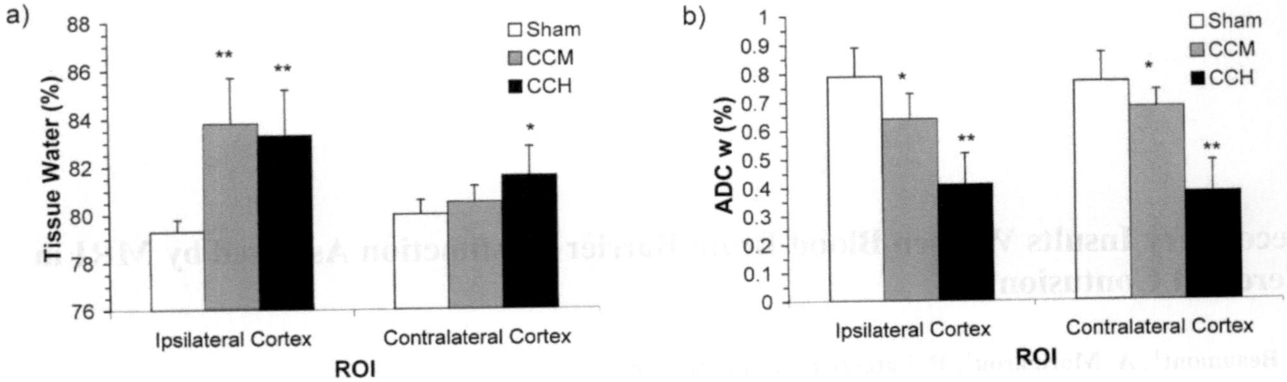

Fig. 1. Tissue water (a) and ADCw values (b) in sham, contusion and contusion with secondary insult groups, 4 hours post injury. (*Sham* sham injury, *CCM* cortical contusion, *CCH* contusion with secondary insult, * $p < 0.05$, ** $p < 0.01$)

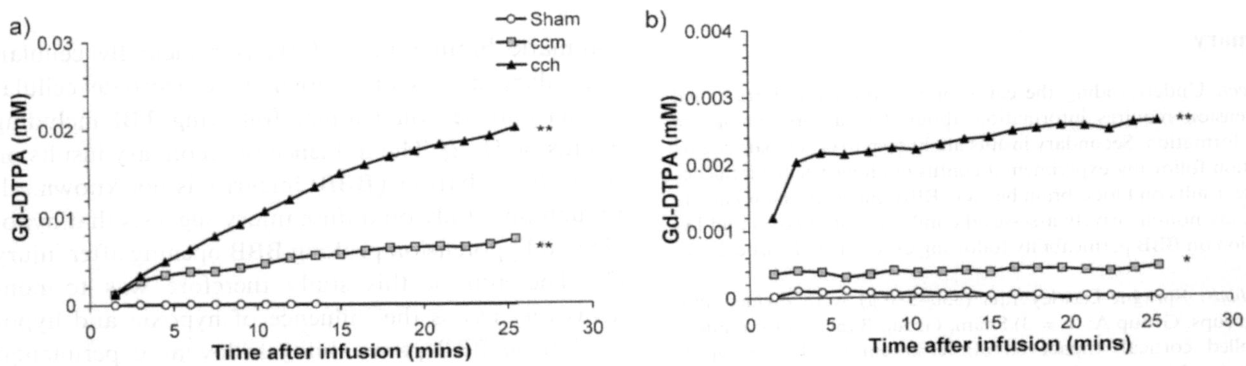

Fig. 2. Profiles of Gd-DTPA uptake into brain for a) Ipsilateral and b) Contralateral cortex, with bolus contrast infusion 4 hours post-injury. Gd-uptake is clearly correlated with injury severity, and the different profiles of uptake suggest the influence of injury dependent variables (*Sham* sham injury, *CCM* cortical contusion, *CCH* contusion with secondary insult, * $p < 0.05$, ** $p < 0.01$)

TR = 100 msec, TE = 14 msec, FOV 4 cm^2, with a 64 × 64 matrix. Five baseline images were acquired to establish non-contrast signal intensity. An i.v. bolus of Gd-DTPA was then given (0.2 mmol/kg), whilst imaging. Signal intensity changes were measured and converted to tissue concentrations of gadolinium using a standard curve based on varying concentrations of Gd-DTPA in 2% agarose gels (0–2 mM). Tissue concentration of gadolinium was used as a marker of BBB permeability, which was compared with ADCw and tissue water content changes. Statistical analysis included Student-t, Kruskal-Wallis and Wilcoxon Signed Rank Test.

Results

Tissue water content and ADCw for ipsilateral and contralateral cortex are summarized in Fig. 1. Edema formation was accompanied by a marked reduction in ADCw. Secondary insults greatly increased tissue water content and lowered ADCw in areas adjacent to the site of impact ($p < 0.01$). Concentration changes of Gd-DTPA are shown for all groups in Fig. 2. In Sham animals, there was a small increase in signal intensity consistent with Gd in the plasma fraction of the ROI. Several different profiles of Gd accumulation were seen after injury and therefore gadolinium uptake is influenced by injury-dependant variables. In all anatomical regions the extent of Gd accumulation was proportional to severity of injury; maximal accumulation was seen in the second insult group ($p < 0.01$). Statistical analysis of tissue water, ADCw and peak Gd concentration shows that tissue with maximal swelling and lowest ADCw values also has the greatest accumulation of gadolinium. ($p = 0.018$ for ADC vs Gd, and $p = 0.028$ for Water vs Gd).

Discussion

This study has demonstrated for the first time that secondary insults worsen the severity and extent of

BBB damage in cerebral contusion. Areas of maximal BBB disruption are associated with areas of maximal tissue swelling and reduced ADCw (cellular swelling). The fact that hypoxia and hypotension influence the status of the BBB up to four hours after injury suggests that secondary insults are either directly injurious to the barrier, or a component of BBB repair after injury may be energy dependent.

Based on ADCw values, swelling in this model is markedly cellular. The finding of a strong relationship between tissue water accumulation, low ADC and marked barrier opening seems contrary to the theory of vasogenic swelling. These data are however consistent with previous reports [4] which have suggested that BBB disruption following injury exacerbates underlying cytotoxic edema by providing a low resistance pathway for the movement of water and cations.

References

1. Barzo P, Marmarou A, Fatouros P, Hayasaki K, Corwin F (1997) Contribution of vasogenic and cellular edema to traumatic brain swelling measured by diffusion weighted imaging. J Neurosurgery 87: 900–907
2. Portella G, Beaumont A, Corwin F, Fatouros P, Marmarou, A. Characterising edema associated with cortical contusion and secondary insult using magnetic resonance spectroscopy. Acta Neurochir (Wien) [Suppl] (in press)
3. Barzo P, Marmarou A, Fatouros P, Corwin F, Dunbar J (1996) Magnetic resonance imaging-monitored blood-brain barrier changes in experimental traumatic brain injury. J Neurosurg 85: 1113–1121
4. Beaumont A, Marmarou A, Hayasaki K *et al* The permissive nature of blood brain barrier opening in edema formation following traumatic brain injury. Acta Neurochir (Wien) [Suppl] (in press)

Correspondence: Prof. Anthony Marmarou, Division of Neurosurgery, P.O. Box, 508, MCV Station, Sanger Hall, Room 8004, 1101 E. Marshall Street, Richmond, Virginia 23298.

Acta Neurochir (2002) [Suppl] 81: 221–223

Neuronal Activity Determined by Quantitative EEG and Cortical Microdialysis is Increased Following Controlled Cortical Impact Injury in Rats

O. W. Sakowitz, A. W. Unterberg, and **J. F. Stover**

Charité – Department of Neurosurgery, Berlin, Germany

Summary

Following brain injury increased glutamate release is linked to sustained neuronal activation resulting in excitotoxic tissue damage. Isoflurane anesthesia has been shown to decrease electroencephalographic (EEG) activity and extracellular (e.c.) glutamate, possibly attenuating excitotoxic tissue damage. However, based on clinical experience EEG activity can fluctuate despite stable isoflurane concentrations. Therefore, the aims of this study were to investigate the impact of neuronal activity assessed by quantitative EEG on e.c. glutamate during isoflurane anesthesia following controlled cortical impact injury (CCII).

In 10 rats balanced anesthesia using isoflurane was induced at 4 hours after CCII. Under steady-state conditions maintaining isoflurane at 1.8 vol%, EEG was recorded for 3 hours. During this period, e.c. glutamate was sampled in the pericontusional cortex by microdialysis.

Despite maintaining isoflurane at 1.8 vol%, neuronal activity expressed as low frequency EEG power showed marked fluctuations. Spontaneous increases in neuronal activity coincided with elevated e.c. glutamate levels and vice versa. Overall, EEG power correlated significantly with pathologically elevated e.c. glutamate levels ($n = 58$; $R^2 = 0.54$; $p < 0.05$).

Despite unchanged isoflurane concentrations fluctuations in neuronal activity were reflected by altered EEG power and e.c. glutamate concentrations. Therefore, neuronal activity needs to be considered for the interpretation of e.c. glutamate levels.

Keywords: Anesthesia; glutamate; excitotoxicity; isoflurane.

Introduction

The excitatory amino acid transmitter glutamate is known for its pivotal role to increase neuronal activity under physiological conditions and induce cell damage under pathological conditions by activating postsynaptic glutamate receptors [5]. Following traumatic brain injury, glutamate is elevated within the extracellular space and CSF under experimental and clinical conditions [4, 7, 8]. Based on these findings, reduction in glutamate is considered beneficial in terms of attenuating postsynaptic neuronal activity. In reverse, any increase in glutamate can be detrimental and therefore should be avoided.

As outlined by Patel *et al.* [6] anesthetic depth is an essential key factor known to influence e.c. glutamate levels. The volatile anesthetic isoflurane has been shown to reduce e.c. glutamate concentrations dose-dependently [6]. However, clinical experience reveals that neuronal activity determined by electroencephalographic recordings (EEG) fluctuates during steady-state conditions where administration of anesthetic agents is kept constant. Therefore, spontaneous changes in neuronal activity could result in equivalent alterations in e.c. glutamate.

To investigate this hypothesis, changes in neuronal activity and e.c. glutamate concentrations were measured by quantitative EEG and microdialysis during 3 hours of balanced anesthesia using isoflurane following focal traumatic brain injury in rats.

Materials and Methods

Controlled Cortical Impact Injury (CCII)

CCII was induced by accelerating a pneumatic impactor (diameter 5 mm; penetration depth 1 mm, velocity 7 ms^{-1}) in 10 male Sprague Dawley rats (300–350 g). This resulted in a significant left temporoparietal contusion and brain edema as recently published [7].

Balanced Anesthesia

Spontaneously breathing rats were anesthetized with isoflurane in a mixture of N_2O and O_2 (2:1). At the chosen isoflurane concentration maintained at 1.8 vol%, arterial blood gases remained within physiological limits (table 1) waiving the need for intubation. To mimic the clinical situation, balanced anesthesia (isoflurane combined with N_2O and O_2) was induced at 4 hours after trauma and maintained for 3 hours. This corresponds to the time-frame of initial hospitalization and surgical treatment following traumatic brain injury.

Table 1. *Arterial Blood Gases, Blood Glucose, and Mean Arterial Blood Pressure (MABP) Remained Stable During the Entire Study Period*

Parameters	60 minutes	120 minutes	180 minutes
pH	7.391 ± 0.02	7.411 ± 0.02	7.409 ± 0.01
$paCO_2$ [mmHg]	45.6 ± 3.2	41.3 ± 1.3	43.3 ± 1.7
paO_2 [mmHg]	190 ± 5	181 ± 11	182 ± 10
base excess	1.73 ± 0.5	1.45 ± 0.8	2.28 ± 0.48
hemoglobin [g/l]	15.4 ± 0.2	14.9 ± 0.2	14.4 ± 0.2
blood glucose [mg/dl]	185 ± 22	151 ± 12	158 ± 16
MABP [mmHg]	89 ± 2	88 ± 3	89 ± 3

Physiological Parameters

During anesthesia mean arterial blood pressure (MABP) and arterial blood gases were determined (Table 1). Rectal temperature was maintained between 37 and 38 °C.

Electroencephalographic Recordings (EEG)

Neuronal activity was assessed by attaching two Ag/AgCl electrodes to the free skull bone (right parietal and left frontal region) and one to the tail as zero reference. EEG signals were amplified and digitized using a custom-build system. To avoid electrical interference a 50 Hz notch filter was applied. Wide-band filtered data was sampled at 32 Hz and recorded on a PC-computer system. Off-line signal analysis in terms of quantitative EEG was performed using an automated artifact rejection algorithm on 1-minute epochs. Spectral power was calculated from artifact-free epochs using a Hanning-window prior to the Fast Fourier Transformation. Only the most dominant coefficients (1–3 Hz, delta power) were assessed and expressed in μV^2.

Microdialysis and Determination of e.c. Glutamate

Microdialysis catheters (CMA 12/membrane length 2 mm) were inserted in the cortex of 10 traumatized and 3 non-traumatized rats at a depth of 2 mm. Identical placement was achieved in all rats using the coordinates of the stereotaxic frame (−8 mm from bregma and −3 mm from the saggital suture). In traumatized rats, the microdialysis catheter was placed within the pericontusional cortex. Catheters were perfused with artificial cerebrospinal fluid at 2 μl/min and samples were collected in 30 minute intervals. Glutamate was then analyzed enzymatically using the bed-side analyzer CMA 600 and corrected for recovery determined before and after each experiment.

Statistical Analysis

Results are presented as mean ± SEM. Parameters were compared for significant differences using one-way analysis of variances (ANOVA) and Student's *t*-test, where appropriate. Differences were rated significant at $p < 0.05$.

Results

Physiological Parameters

During balanced anesthesia with isoflurane, arterial blood gases, and MABP remained within physiological limits (Table 1).

Table 2. *During Balanced Anesthesia with Isoflurane Maintained at 1.8 vol% Neuronal Activity and e.c. Glutamate Determined by Quantitative EEG and Microdialysis were Significantly Increased Over Time (*$p < 0.05$ ANOVA)*

	30 min	60 min	90 min	120 min	150 min	180 min
EEG power [μV^2]	15 ± 2	17 ± 4	21 ± 3*	26 ± 4*	34 ± 5*	34 ± 5*
e.c. glutamate [μM]	19 ± 3	17 ± 3	18 ± 4	20 ± 5	23 ± 5	29 ± 6*

Neuronal Activity

During three hours of anesthesia maintaining isoflurane at 1.8 vol% neuronal activity expressed as EEG power was significantly increased over time (Table 2). While EEG power remained stable within the first hour, EEG power increased steadily during the following 2 hours, reaching highest values by 150 and 180 minutes (Table 2).

E.c. Glutamate Concentrations

Compared to non-traumatized rats, e.c. glutamate was significantly increased at 4 hours after CCII (19 ± 3 vs. 0.8 ± 0.1 μM; $p < 0.05$). During the first 2 hours of balanced anesthesia with isoflurane e.c. glutamate remained stable. By 3 hours, however, glutamate was significantly increased (Table 2).

Neuronal Activity and e.c. Glutamate

A representative example depicting spontaneous fluctuations in both neuronal activity and e.c. glutamate levels is shown in Fig. 1. Increased EEG power coincided with elevated e.c. glutamate while attenuated EEG power was reflected by decreased e.c. glutamate. Pooling EEG power and glutamate allowed to statistically investigate a mutual dependency between neuronal activity and e.c. glutamate concentrations. EEG power correlated significantly with e.c. glutamate concentrations ($r = 0.544$; $n = 58$; $p < 0.01$).

Discussion

During steady-state conditions of balanced isoflurane anesthesia, neuronal activity and e.c. glutamate levels were significantly increased over time, possibly reflecting glutamate-mediated neuronal activation and sustained neuronal release of glutamate.

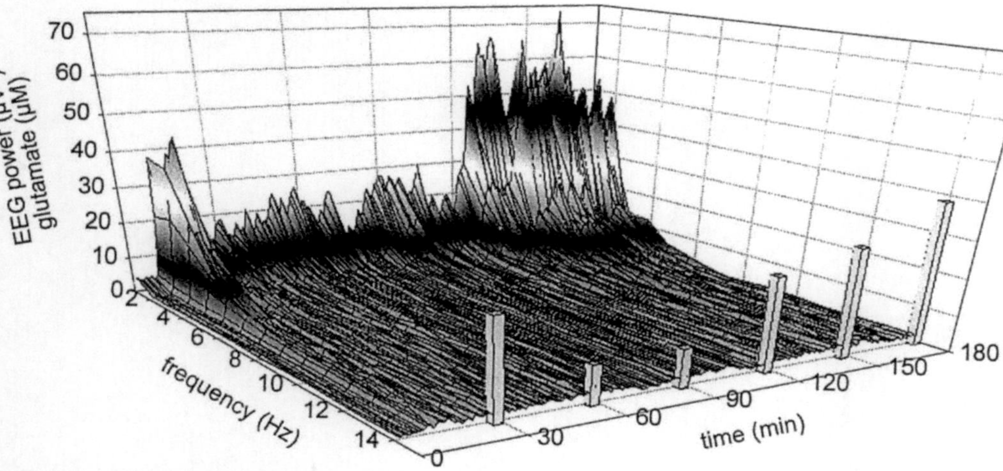

Fig. 1. This example of a single experiment depicts the relationship between EEG power (µV^2) and e.c. glutamate concentrations (µM). Increased neuronal activity coincided with elevated e.c. glutamate and vice versa. Note that the changes in EEG power occur predominantly within the lower frequency bands

Within cortical structures glutamate is the predominant excitatory transmitter known to induce cortical neuronal activity by activating postsynaptic glutamate receptors [5]. An increase in neuronal activity elevates e.c. glutamate levels as seen e.g., during different depth of anesthesia [6] and seizure activity [4].

Isoflurane anesthesia has been shown to attenuate neuronal activity and e.c. glutamate concentrations, most likely by reducing presynaptic glutamate release [1] and interfering with postsynaptic glutamate receptor binding [2, 3]. As reported by Patel *et al.* [6] this effect is dose-dependent as increasing isoflurane results in a burst-suppression pattern and decreased e.c. glutamate concentrations. Our present findings are in line with these observations. Under pathological conditions as encountered following traumatic brain injury any additional increase in e.c. glutamate is thought to aggravate underlying tissue damage [5] and should therefore be avoided. Based on the present results it appears useful to adjust isoflurane concentration according to underlying neuronal activity with the aim of decreasing e.c. levels of the excitotoxic transmitter glutamate.

At present the exact reasons for the observed fluctuations in neuronal activity and e.c. glutamate concentrations in face of unchanged isoflurane concentration cannot be explained. It remains to be clarified if a similar pattern also occurs in non-traumatized rats or if these changes are related to trauma-induced disturbance of cerebral homeostasis.

Based on the present findings anesthetic depth influences neuronal activity and e.c. glutamate concentrations following focal traumatic brain injury and therefore needs to be considered for the interpretation of e.c. glutamate.

References

1. Liachenko S, Tang P, Somogyi GT, Xu Y (1999) Concentration-dependent isoflurane effects on depolarization-evoked glutamate and GABA outflows from mouse brain slices. Br J Pharmacol 127: 131–138
2. MacIver B, Mikulec AA, Amagasu SM, Monroe VA (1996) Volatile anesthetics depress glutamate transmission via presynaptic actions. Anesthesiology 85: 823–834
3. Martin DC, Plagenhoef M, Abraham J, Dennison RL, Aronstam RS (1995) Volatile anesthetics and glutamate activation of N-Methyl-D-Aspartate receptors. Biochem Pharmacol 49: 809–817
4. Nilsson P, Ronne-Engström E, Flink R, Ungerstedt U, Carlson H, Hillered L (1994) Epileptic seizure activity in the acute phase following cortical impact trauma in rat. Brain Res 637: 227–232
5. Obrenovitch TP, Urenjak J (1997) Altered glutamatergic transmission in neurological disorders: from high extracellular glutamate to excessive synaptic efficacy. Prog Neurobiol 51: 39–87
6. Patel PM, Drummond JC, Cole DJ, Goskowicz RL (1995) Isoflurane reduces ischemia-induced glutamate release in rats subjected to forebrain ischemia. Anesthesiology 82: 996–1003
7. Stover JF, Schöning B, Beyer TF, Woiciechowsky C, Unterberg AW (2000) Temporal profile of cerebrospinal fluid glutamate, interleukin-6, and tumor necrosis factor-α in relation to brain edema and contusion following controlled cortical impact injury in rats. Neurosci Lett 288: 25–28
8. Stover JF, Pleines UE, Morganti-Kossmann MC *et al* (1999) Thiopental attenuates energetic impairment but fails to normalize cerebrospinal fluid glutamate in brain-injured patients. Crit Care Med 27: 1351–1357

Correspondence: John F. Stover, M.D., Charité – Department of Neurosurgery, Augustenburger Platz 01, 13353 Berlin, Germany.

Acta Neurochir (2002) [Suppl] 81: 225–227

Norepinephrine is Superior to Dopamine in Increasing Cortical Perfusion Following Controlled Cortical Impact Injury in Rats

S.-N. Kroppenstedt, O. W. Sakowitz, U.-W. Thomale, A. W. Unterberg, and J. F. Stover

Department of Neurosurgery, Charité, Virchow Medical Center, Humboldt-University Berlin, Germany

Summary

Following traumatic brain injury catecholamines are routinely applied to increase cerebral perfusion. To date, it remains controversial if infusion of catecholamines is associated with diminished cerebral perfusion due to catecholamine-mediated vasoconstriction. The aims of the present study were to investigate the effects of norepinephrine and dopamine on cortical perfusion and brain edema following controlled cortical impact injury (CCII) in rats.

Four hours after CCII, rats (n = 22) received either norepinephrine or dopamine with the aim of increasing MABP to 120 mm Hg for 90 minutes. Control rats were given NaCl. Cortical perfusion was measured before, during, and after catecholamine infusion using Laser Doppler flowmetry. Brain swelling was determined directly after the study period (8 hrs after CCII).

Following CCII cortical perfusion was reduced by 40% compared to pre-trauma values in all rats. Parallel to the increases in MABP, cortical perfusion was significantly elevated under norepinephrine and dopamine, respectively ($p < 0.05$). Despite similar MABP values this increase was mostly sustained under norepinephrine. In control rats cortical perfusion remained diminished. Brain swelling was similar in all groups.

Both norepinephrine and dopamine significantly increased cortical perfusion following CCII. Norepinephrine, however, was superior to dopamine in CBF. Based on increased CBF and unchanged brain swelling catecholamine-mediated vasoconstriction does not seem to occur under the present study design.

Keywords: Brain edema; catecholamines; cerebral blood flow; traumatic brain injury.

Introduction

In recent years the necessity to maintain a significant cerebral perfusion pressure has been high-lighted. Therefore, following traumatic brain injury catecholamines are commonly applied to increase cerebral perfusion. However, due to their potential vasoconstrictory effect on intracerebral vessels [1, 8, 7] it remains controversial if catecholamines might impair local CBF, despite adequate CPP elevation, and therefore increase tissue damage.

The aims of this study were to investigate the acute effects of norepinephrine and dopamine on cerebral blood flow (CBF) and brain edema following controlled cortical impact injury in rats.

Material and Methods

Animal Preparation and Experimental Brain Injury

In the present study, 22 male Sprague-Dawley rats (300–350 g) were anesthetized with 1–1,5 vol% isoflurane in a 2:1 mixture of N_2O/O_2 breathing spontaneously via a mask. For blood pressure monitoring a catheter was placed in the right femoral artery. A craniotomy was performed over the left hemisphere. A standard controlled cortical impact (CCI) was applied to the left hemisphere (impact depth: 1 mm, impact velocity: 7 m/s) keeping the dura intact. After impact injury, the scalp incision was closed, anesthesia was stopped and animals were returned to their cages. For later measurements of CBF and venous infusion, animals were again anesthetized and catheters were placed in the right femoral vein and artery.

Measurement of CBF

Local cortical blood flow (lCBF) was measured using a laser flow blood perfusion monitor (DRT4, Moor Instruments, England) with the needle probe attached to a micromanipulator. Over the traumatized hemisphere, lCBF data were collected from 46 different locations by moving a 0.8 mm LD needle probe in 0.2 mm steps over the brain surface (scanning) with a total distance of 9 mm. The median of 46 lCBF measurements from each animal is termed regional CBF (rCBF). RCBF is expressed in % changes to pre-trauma values.

Experimental Groups and Study Protocol

Baseline CBF was measured over the left hemispheres in all rats before trauma. At 4 hours following cortical contusion, CBF was measured again. Thereafter, rats received either physiological saline (n = 10), 1–2 μg/kg/min norepinephrine (n = 5) or 40–50 μg/kg/min dopamine (n = 7) with the aim of increasing mean arterial blood pressure to 120 mmHg for 90 minutes. RCBF was measured repeatedly during the infusion period, i.e. at 30, 60 and 90 minutes after beginning the infusion. Thirty minutes after stopping the infusions a final rCBF measurement was performed. During the entire study period arterial blood pressure was continuously monitored. Arterial blood gases were determined after each rCBF measurement. At 8 hours brains were removed to determine hemispheric swelling and water content, as described previously [5].

The experimental protocol was approved by the committee for animal research in Berlin, Germany.

Statistical Analysis

Data are expressed as mean ± SEM for all groups. Changes over time were evaluated for statistical significance by using a one way repeated measures analysis of variance. Comparison of data between groups was performed using a one way analysis of variance for multiple comparison (SigmaStat®, Jandel Scientific). Differences were considered significant at $p < 0.05$.

Results

Arterial blood gas analysis (pH, pCO_2, pO_2) revealed no significant differences between the different groups at any investigated time point. All variables were within normal limits.

Cerebral Blood Flow

At 4 hours after trauma, CBF was significantly reduced in all rats compared to pre-trauma levels (controls: 58 ± 5%; norepinephrine: 64 ± 9%; dopamine: 62 ± 7%; $p < 0.05$; Fig. 1). MABP did not differ significantly between the groups (controls: 90 ± 2 mmHg; norepinephrine: 91 ± 2 mmHg; dopamine: 89 ± 2 mmHg, $p > 0.05$). During the 90 minute

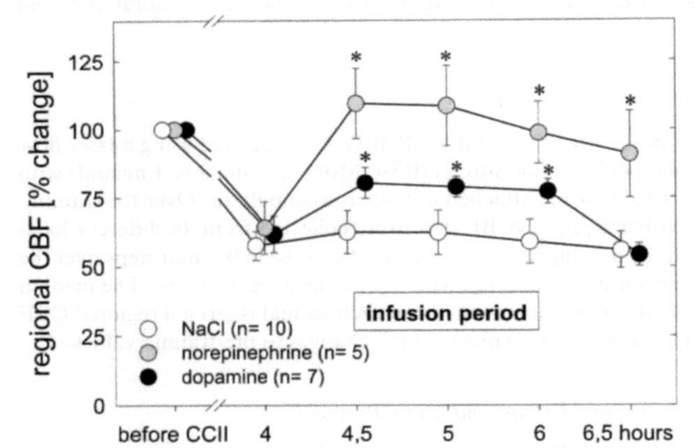

Fig. 1. Time course of regional CBF (*controls*: white circles; *norepinephrine*: grey circles; *dopamine*: black circles) assessed by laser Doppler scanning of the traumatized hemisphere. Data are shown as scatter plots (mean ± SEM; rCBF is expressed in % changes to pre-trauma values). Infusion of norepinephrine and dopamine significantly increased posttraumatic rCBF (*: $p < 0.05$ vs rCBF 4 hours after trauma). RCBF increase was higher under norepinephrine

infusion period with physiological saline MABP and rCBF remained unchanged [controls: 89 ± 2 mmHg and 61 ± 4% (mean)]. In the norepinephrine and dopamine group, MABP was significantly increased to 120 mmHg during the entire infusion period [norepinephrine: 120 ± 2 mmHg; dopamine: 119 ± 2 mmHg (mean)]. Parallel to this increase in MABP, rCBF was significantly increased [norepinephrine: 106 ± 7%; dopamine: 79 ± 3%; (mean), Fig. 1]. The CBF increase was more sustained under norepinephrine. After stopping the infusion, MABP (93 ± 3 mmHg) and rCBF dropped significantly to pre-infusion values in the dopamine group. In the norepinephrine group, however, rCBF remained elevated, MABP being 97 ± 3 mmHg.

Hemispheric Swelling and Water Content

There was no significant difference ($p > 0.05$) in posttraumatic hemispheric swelling between rats receiving physiological saline, norepinephrine or dopamine (Table 1). Nevertheless, there was a trend towards higher swelling in catecholamine-treated animals. Posttraumatic water content in the non-traumatized and traumatized hemisphere did not differ significantly between the groups ($p > 0.05$, Table 1).

Discussion

Changes in CBF

Under the present study design, elevation of MABP by infusing norepinephrine and dopamine increased posttraumatic rCBF. However, despite similar MABP pressure values this increase was mostly sustained under norepinephrine. These differences in rCBF increase suggest further CPP-independent

Table 1. *Posttraumatic Hemispheric Swelling and Water Content Determined at 8 Hours Following Controlled Cortical Impact. Neither Hemispheric Swelling nor Water Content in Traumatized Hemispheres Differed Significantly Between the Groups ($p > 0.05$)*

	Swelling [%]	Hemispheric water content [%]	
		Non-traumatized	Traumatized
Saline (n = 11)	5.9 ± 0.9	79.1 ± 0.08	79.9 ± 0.09
Norepinephrine (n = 5)	7.7 ± 0.8	79.2 ± 0.13	80.1 ± 0.11
Dopamine (n = 6)	8.0 ± 1.5	79.2 ± 0.13	80.2 ± 0.22

mechanisms, as e.g. catecholamine-mediated activation of neurons. In the early phase following CCI the blood brain barrier is damaged as determined by extravasation of Evans Blue [2].

Thus, norepinephrine could have entered brain tissue, and thereby stimulated neurons. This, in turn, could result in an additional increase in rCBF. Investigations comparing cortical activity using electroencephalographic recordings during posttraumatic infusion of norepinephrine and dopamine are forthcoming.

Changes in Brain Edema Formation

Improved posttraumatic CBF at an increased MABP level did not significantly affect brain edema formation. In contrast, there was a trend towards increased edema formation. In previous investigations increases in MABP to 120 mmHg by infusing phenylephrine for 15 minutes and 3 hours or dopamine for 3 hours did not influence posttraumatic brain edema formation and did not reduce contusion volume, or improve neurological outcome [3, 4, 6]. The current treatment failed to reveal neuroprotective properties. This could be related to flow-independent changes following traumatic brain injury as, e.g., release and accumulation of cytotoxic mediator compounds, such as free radicals or glutamate.

In summary, both, norepinephrine and dopamine significantly increase rCBF following CCI. However, norepinephrine is superior to dopamine in elevating rCBF. Brain edema remained unchanged. Thus, under the present study design no signs of catecholamine-mediated vasoconstriction were found. To mimick the clinical situation the effect of prolonged infusion of catecholamines needs to be investigated.

References

1. Altura BM, Gebrewold A, Lassoff S (1980) Biphasic responsiveness of rat pial arterioles to dopamine: direct observations on the microcirculation. Br J Pharmacol 69: 543–544
2. Baskaya MK, Rao AM, Dogan A, Donaldson D, Dempsey RJ (1997) The biphasic opening of the blood-brain barrier in the cortex and hippocampus after traumatic brain injury in rats. Neurosci Lett 226: 33–36
3. Cherian L, Chacko G, Goodman JC, Robertson CS (1999) Cerebral hemodynamic effects of phenylephrine and L-arginine after cortical impact injury. Crit Care Med 27: 2512–2517
4. Kroppenstedt SN, Kern M, Thomale UW, Schneider GH, Lanksch WR, Unterberg AW (1999) Effect of cerebral perfusion pressure on contusion volume following impact injury. J Neurosurg 90: 520–526
5. Kroppenstedt SN, Stroop R, Kern M, Thomale UW, Schneider GH, Unterberg AW (1999) Lubeluzole following traumatic brain injury in the rat. J Neurotrauma 16: 629–637
6. Talmor D, Roytblat L, Artru AA, Yuri O, Koyfman L, Katchko L, Shapira Y (1998) Phenylephrine-induced hypertension does not improve outcome after closed head trauma in rats. Anesth Analg 87: 574–578
7. von Essen C, Kistler JP, Lees RS, Zervas NT (1981) Cerebral blood flow and intracranial pressure in the dog during intravenous infusion of nitroglycerin alone and in combination with dopamine. Stroke 12: 331–338
8. von Essen C, Zervas NT, Brown DR, Koltun WA, Pickren KS (1980) Local cerebral blood flow in the dog during intravenous infusion of dopamine. Surg Neurol 13: 181–188

Correspondence: John F. Stover, M.D., Department of Neurosurgery, Charité – Virchow Medical Center, Humboldt-University Berlin, Augustenburger Platz 1, 13353 Berlin, Germany.

Acta Neurochir (2002) [Suppl] 81: 229–231

Cortical Hypoperfusion Precedes Hyperperfusion Following Controlled Cortical Impact Injury

U.-W. Thomale[1], K. Schaser[2], S.-N. Kroppenstedt[1], A. W. Unterberg[1], and J. F. Stover[1]

[1] Department of Neurosurgery, Charité, Virchow Medical Center, Humboldt-University of Berlin, Germany
[2] Department of Trauma Surgery, Charité, Virchow Medical Center, Humboldt-University of Berlin, Germany

Summary

Impaired cerebral perfusion contributes to tissue damage following traumatic brain injury. In this longitudinal study persistence of reduced cortical perfusion employing laser doppler flowmetry was investigated following controlled cortical impact injury (CCII).

Before, 30 minutes, 6, 24, and 48 hours after CCII, perfusion in pericontusional cortex was determined by moving a laser doppler probe in 50 × 0.2 mm steps over the traumatized hemisphere in 5 rats. Arterial blood gases and mean arterial blood pressure were monitored.

Mean arterial blood pressure and arterial blood gases remained stable during the entire experiments. At 30 minutes and 6 hours following CCII, cortical perfusion was significantly diminished by 24% and 43% ($p < 0.05$), respectively compared to pre-trauma levels. At 24 and 48 hours after CCII, pericontusional blood flow was significantly increased by 64% and 123%.

Cortical hypoperfusion found within the early phase following trauma is reversible and precedes a long lasting phase of hyperperfusion. Changes in tissue mediators (endothelin, acidosis, NO) could account for these findings.

Keywords: Traumatic brain injury; cerebral blood flow; laser doppler flowmetry.

Introduction

Diminished cerebral perfusion following traumatic brain injury is accepted to contribute to secondary tissue damage. In the early phase following traumatic brain injury a decrease in regional cerebral blood flow (rCBF) was shown within the traumatized cortex. rCBF determined by autoradiography was significantly decreased at 30 minutes and 4 hours following CCII, reaching ischemic values (< 20 ml/100 g/min) within the contusion [3]. At 2 and 24 hours after CCII, Kochanek *et al.* determined a decrease in rCBF by 78% and 67% within the injured parietal cortex using autoradiographic studies [6]. Furthermore, perfusion magnetic resonance imaging measurements revealed a reduced rCBF by 48% in injured cortex at 24 hours following CCII compared to the contralateral cortex [4]. Changes in regional cerebral perfusion following traumatic brain injury might be important for adapted therapeutical strategies to prevent secondary insults to pericontusional brain tissue. The aim of this study was to investigate the temporal profile of rCBF in the pericontusional cortex following a focal contusion in rats using laser doppler flowmetry.

Material and Methods

A total of 5 male Sprague Dawley rats (250–350 g) were anesthetized with isoflurane (1.5–2%) in a mixture of N_2O and O_2 (2:1). The right femoral artery was catheterized allowing to monitor mean arterial blood presure (MABP) and determine arterial blood gases (ABG). A left temporo-parietal trephination from lamdba to bregma and temporally to the zygomatic arch was performed. The Controlled Cortical Impact Injury model was used to apply a moderate left temporo-parietal focal contusion as described previously [9] using the following settings: impact velocity 7.4 m/s, penetration depth 0.5 mm, impact diameter 5 mm and contact time 300 ms. For rCBF measurements Laser Doppler Flowmetry (LDF, Moor Instruments Ltd., England) was performed. For this, a Laser Doppler probe was stereotactically placed over the cortex and moved in 0.2 mm steps over a total distance of 10 mm along the pericontusional cortical region from frontal to occipital cortex. rCBF was assessed as Laser Doppler Units. For each time point two measurements were performed and all data were collected to calculate the corresponding mean value. The study protocol was designed to determine the temporal profile of cortical perfusion during the early posttraumatic phase up to 48 hours after CCII. For this, rCBF was measured before trauma, 30 minutes, 6, 24 and 48 hours after trauma. Statistical analysis was performed by ANOVA and Student's-*t*-test using the software Sigma Stat 3.0 (Jandel Scientific, Erkrath, Germany). All results are given as means with standard error of mean. Differences were rated significant at a probability less than 0.05.

Table 1. *Arterial Blood Gases and Blood Glucose Values were Determined Before, 30 Minutes, 6, 24, and 48 Hours after CCII. All Variables Remained Within Physiological Limits*

	Before	30 Minutes	6 Hours	24 Hours	48 Hours
pH	7.42 ± 0.02	7.39 ± 0.001	7.41 ± 0.001	7.44 ± 0.02	7.40 ± 0.02
$paCO_2$	40.3 ± 1.2	42.6 ± 1.2	41.0 ± 2.1	41.4 ± 3.7	43.6 ± 2.4
paO_2	200.5 ± 12.0	190.0 ± 11.0	195.0 ± 20.4	219.7 ± 7.9	190.5 ± 4.3
Glucose	124.2 ± 10.9	110.2 ± 4.6	107.8 ± 4.1	121.2 ± 9.9	142.0 ± 9.8

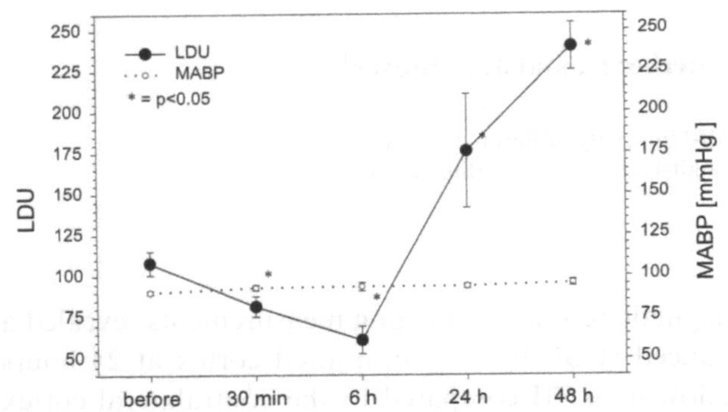

Fig. 1. Time course of MABP (dotted line) and LDU (solid line) following CCII. MABP remained stable during the entire experiments. LDU was significantly decreased in the early phase (30 minutes, 6 hours) after CCII (*$p < 0.05$). At 24 and 48 hours after CCII, LDU was significantly increased, reflecting hyperperfusion (*$p < 0.05$)

Results

Physiological parameters remained within the normal range at all time points. Values of ABG and blood glucose are given in Table 1. MABP remained stable during the entire study period with values ranging from 90 to 96 mmHg. The time course of MABP (dotted line) and Laser Doppler units (LDU, solid line) during the entire experiments are depicted in Fig. 1. Before trauma a mean value of 108 ± 7 LDU was determined. At 30 minutes following trauma there was a significant reduction to 81 ± 6 LDU, correspondence to a decrease by 24% ($p < 0.05$). A further reduction of rCBF was observed at 6 hours after CCII by 43% (61 ± 8 LDU; $p < 0.05$). At later time points after CCII the hypoperfusion was followed by a long lasting period of hyperperfusion. At 24 hours after contusion rCBF was significantly increased by 64% compared to baseline values (176 ± 35 LDU; $p < 0.05$). By 48 hours following CCII hyperperfusion reached highest values, as cortical perfusion was increased by 123% compared to baseline values (240 ± 15 LDU; $p < 0.05$).

Discussion

In the early phase after trauma a reversible and significant reduction in cortical perfusion was determined in the pericontusional cortex. This hypoperfusion precedes a long lasting phase of hyperperfusion seen in the late phase at 24 and 48 hours following CCII.

Hypoperfusion

Hypoperfusion seen in the early phase is most likely caused by different mechanisms. The direct biomechanical injury of brain tissue and smaller vessels can cause reductions in rCBF due to immediate cerebrovascular injury. Furthermore, histological investigations of the focal lesion after CCII showed thrombotic occlusions in pial vessels [8], possibly explaining the decrease in regional blood flow in the pericontusional cortex as seen in the present study. In addition, leukocyte sticking and plugging has been described in the early phase after focal contusion in rabbits [5], possibly accounting for the reductions in rCBF due to aggregation of white blood cells. In addition, vasospasm resulting in rCBF is related to the influence of subarachnoid blood on the vessel wall. Furthermore, trauma-related imbalance between vasodilating and vasoconstricting mediators is discussed to contribute to reduced rCBF in the early phase after traumatic brain injury. Among others, reduced nitric oxide (NO) [1] and increased endothelin [2] are associated with decreased cerebral perfusion.

Changes in systemic parameters, as e.g., hyperventilation and decreased MABP do not account for the observed posttraumatic cortical hypoperfusion as these variables remained within normal limits.

Hyperperfusion

By 24 and 48 hours after CCII hyperperfusion was encountered within pericontusional structures. Systemic factors as altered arterial blood gases (pH, $paCO_2$) or changes in systemic blood pressure do not account for the observed increase in rCBF. Investigations of CSF of the same animals could exclude infectious meningitis as a cause for the observed hyperperfusion. Rats did not develop fever, which rules out underlying infection. Therefore, the observed increase in rCBF is most likely related to local alterations associated with traumatic tissue lesion. Mediators like nitric oxide or bradykinin [10] are known vasodilators, resulting in elevated rCBF. Local changes of tissue pH (acidosis) have been described following traumatic brain injury [7] and might explain increases in regional perfusion. Furthermore, local inflammatory response and penetration of neutrophils within the lesion may also release mediators as e.g., cytokines [9], possibly contributing to increased cortical perfusion. It is still unclear if the late phase of hyperperfusion is reactive to the acute hypoperfusion following CCII. In addition, it remains to be investigated if the observed hyperperfusion aggravates or prevents further cell damage. Reasons for the altered rCBF and possible implications for temporally adapted therapeutical strategies need to be elucidated.

References

1. Alagarsamy S, DeWitt DS, Johnson KM (1998) Effects of moderate, central fluid percussion traumatic brain injury on nitric oxide synthase activity in rats. J Neurotrauma 15: 627–633
2. Armstead WM (1999) Role of endothelin-1 in age-dependent cerebrovascular hypotensive responses after brain injury. Am J Physiol 277: H1884–1894
3. Bryan RM, Jr, Cherian L, Robertson C (1995) Regional cerebral blood flow after controlled cortical impact injury in rats. Anesth Analg 80: 687–695
4. Forbes ML, Hendrich KS, Kochanek PM, Williams DS, Schiding JK, Wisniewski SR, Kelsey SF, DeKosky ST, Graham SH, Marion DW, Ho C (1997) Assessment of cerebral blood flow and CO_2 reactivity after controlled cortical impact by perfusion magnetic resonance imaging using arterial spin-labeling in rats. J Cereb Blood Flow Metab 17: 865–874
5. Hartl R, Medary MB, Ruge M, Arfors KE, Ghajar J (1997) Early white blood cell dynamics after traumatic brain injury: effects on the cerebral microcirculation. J Cereb Blood Flow Metab 17: 1210–1212
6. Kochanek PM, Marion DW, Zhang W (1995) Severe Controlled Cortical Impact in Rats: Assessment of cerebral edema, blood flow, and contusion volume. J Neurotrauma 12: 1015–1025
7. Krishnappa IK, Contant CF, Robertson CS (1999) Regional changes in cerebral extracellular glucose and lactate concentrations following severe cortical impact injury and secondary ischemia in rats. J Neurotrauma 16: 213–224
8. Maeda TYK, Kawamata T, Aoyama N, Mori T (1997) Hemodynamic depression and microthrombosis in the peripheral areas of cortical contusion in the rat: role of platelet activating factor. Acta Neurochir (Wien) [Suppl] 70: 102–105
9. Stover JF, Schöning B, Beyer TF, Woiciechowsky C, Unterberg AW (2000) Temporal profile of cerebrospinal fluid glutamate, interleukin-6, and tumor necrosis factor-α in relation to brain edema and contusion following Controlled Cortical Impact Injury in rats. Neurosci Lett 288: 25–28
10. Unterberg A, Wahl M, Baethmann A (1984) Effects of bradykinin on permeabilty and diameter of pial vessels in vivo. J Cereb Blood Flow Metab 4: 574–585

Correspondence: John F. Stover, M.D., Department of Neurosurgery, Charité, Virchow Medical Center, Humboldt-University of Berlin, Augustenburger Platz 1, 13353 Berlin, Germany.

Acta Neurochir (2002) [Suppl] 81: 233–235

Effects of Brain Hypothermia on Brain Edema Formation after Intracerebral Hemorrhage in Rats

N. Kawai, T. Nakamura, and **S. Nagao**

Department of Neurological Surgery, Kagawa Medical University, Kagawa, Japan

Summary

Patients with intracerebral hemorrhage (ICH) may deteriorate progressively after the initial ictus because of the brain edema around the hematoma. Recently, thrombin has become known to play an important role in the brain edema formation after ICH. In this study, we examined the effect of brain hypothermia on brain edema formation after hematoma and thrombin injection into the brain in rats and clarified the mechanism of hypothermia on brain damage. Anesthetized Sprague-Dawley rats received an injection of 100 microL of autologous blood or 10 units of bovine thrombin into the basal ganglia. Animals were divided into the normothermic and hypothermic groups, which were housed in a room at 25 °C and in a cold room at 5 °C respectively, for 24 hours. Brain water content was significantly reduced with hypothermia in the cortex (80.8 vs. 79.7% $p < 0.05$) after hematoma induction. After thrombin injection, brain water content was also significantly reduced with hypothermia in the basal ganglia (84.5 vs. 82.2%; $p < 0.01$), accompanied by a significant reduction in blood-brain barrier (BBB) permeability to Evan's blue (29.4 vs. 11.6 ng/g tissue; $p < 0.05$) and in accumulation of polymorphonuclear leukocytes (3.03 vs. 0.27 U of myeloperoxidase/g tissue; $p < 0.01$). This study indicates that brain hypothermia significantly reduces brain edema formation after hematoma and thrombin injection into the brain in rats. Inhibition of thrombin-induced BBB breakdown and inflammatory response with hypothermia appear to contribute to brain protection in this model.

Keywords: Brain edema; hypothermia; intracerebral hemorrhage; thrombin.

Introduction

Patients with intracerebral hemorrhage (ICH) may deteriorate progressively after the initial ictus because of the accumulation of edema fluid around the hematoma. Mass-related effects on cerebral blood flow (CBF) have been proposed to explain ischemic brain injury due to hematoma. Experimentally, however, mild and transient ischemia seen immediately after ICH could not account for large changes in brain edema formation. Recently, a toxic effect of the clot itself has been implicated in the pathogenesis of brain ischemia that follows ICH. Among neurotoxic substances from the clot, thrombin was demonstrated to be involved in the development of brain edema formation following ICH [3, 4]. Thrombin induces blood-brain barrier (BBB) disruption and death of parenchymal cells without significant CBF alteration [5]. There is also evidence that thrombin has an effect regarding inflammation including chemotaxis of polymorphonuclear (PMN) leukocytes.

In the present study, we have examined the effect of brain hypothermia on hematoma-induced and thrombin-induced brain edema formation. Effects of hypothermia on BBB permeability and accumulation of PMN leukocytes were also determined to clarify the protective mechanism of hypothermia on thrombin-induced brain damage.

Materials and Methods

Adult male Sprague-Dawley rats were used in this study. The rats were anesthetized with intraperitoneal sodium pentobarbital (65 mg/kg).

Experimental Model

The rat was positioned in a stereotactic frame and a blunt 26-gauge needle was inserted into the left basal ganglia under stereotactic guidance (coordinates: 0.2 mm anterior, 6 mm ventral and 3 mm lateral to the bregma). A 100 µl of autologous blood or solution containing 10 U of bovine thrombin was infused into the brain. After surgery, animals were divided into normothermic and hypothermic groups, housed in a room maintained at 25 °C and in a cold room maintained at 5 °C respectively, for 24 hours.

Experimental Protocols

This study was performed in three parts in both normothermic and hypothermic rats. The first part evaluated the effect of temperature on hematoma-induced and thrombin-induced brain edema formation. In the second and third part, BBB permeability to Evan's blue dye and accumulation of PMN leukocytes were examined to clarify the protective mechanism of hypothermia on thrombin-induced brain edema formation.

Part 1. Brain Water Content. Brain water content was determined using drying-weighing method in the normothermic (n = 7) and hypothermic (n = 6) rats after hematoma induction into the basal ganglia. Effect of brain temperature on thrombin-induced brain edema formation was also determined in the normothermic (n = 10) and hypothermic (n = 10) rats.

Part 2. Blood-Brain Barrier Permeability to Evan's Blue. The integrity of the blood-brain barrier was investigated using Evan's blue dye extravasation in the normothermic (n = 6) and hypothermic (n = 6) rats after the thrombin injection. Evan's blue (2% in saline, 2 ml/kg) was injected intravenously and allowed to circulate for 30 minutes. Dye was extracted and its fluorescence was determined with a luminescence spectrophotometer (excitation at 620 nm and emission at 680 nm).

Part 3. Myeloperoxidase Activity. Myeloperoxidase (MPO) activity, an indicator of tissue PMN leukocytes accumulation [6] was determined in the normothermic (n = 6) and hypothermic (n = 6) rats after the thrombin injection. The procedure described by Bradley *et al.* [1] was used for quantification of MPO activity.

Results

There were no significant differences in the values of physiological parameters between the normothermic and hypothermic groups. The brain temperature in rats housed in a cold room maintained at 5 °C reduced temporarily to approximately 31 °C and recovered to 35 °C which lasted during the experiment.

Brain hypothermia significantly reduced the hematoma-induced brain edema formation compared to the normothermic group in the ipsilateral cortex (80.8 ± 0.4 vs. 79.7 ± 0.1%; $p < 0.05$). An increase in thrombin-induced brain edema formation was also significantly suppressed with brain hypothermia in the ipsilateral basal ganglia (84.3 ± 0.2 vs. 82.4 ± 0.1%; $p < 0.01$) (Fig. 1).

Blood-brain barrier was significantly protected from the breakdown with brain hypothermia compared to normothermic treatment in the ipsilateral cortex (24.3 ± 4.5 vs. 9.2 ± 2.5 ng/g tissue; $p < 0.05$) and basal ganglia (29.4 ± 5.3 vs. 11.6 ± 3.0 ng/g tissue; $p < 0.05$) after the thrombin injection (Fig. 2a).

Hypothermic treatment significantly inhibited the accumulation of PMN leukocytes (MPO activity) into the brain tissue compared to normothermic treatment in the ipsilateral cortex (0.56 ± 0.15 vs. 0.11 ± 0.04 U/g tissue; $p < 0.05$) and basal ganglia (3.03 ± 0.79 vs. 0.27 ± 0.16 U/g tissue; $p < 0.01$) after the thrombin injection (Fig. 2b).

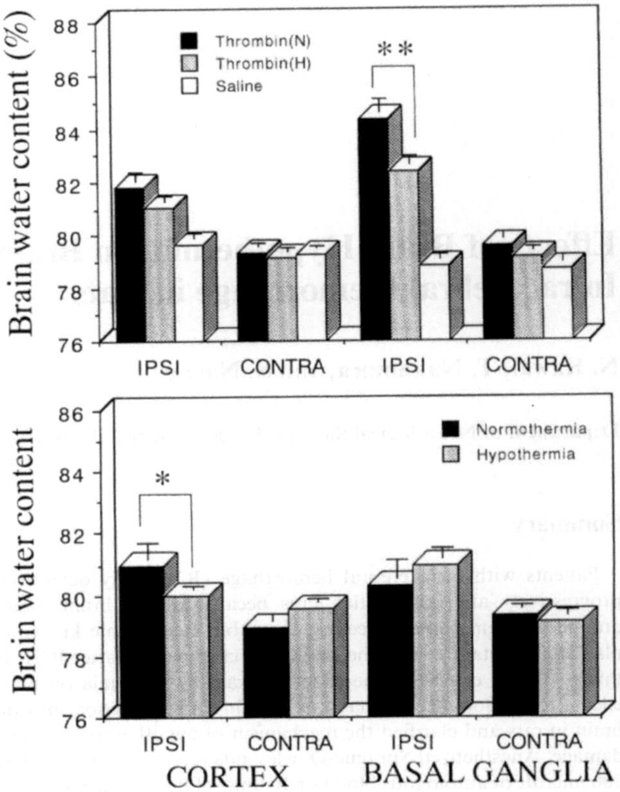

Fig. 1. Bar graphs comparing the brain water content in the normothermic, hypothermia animals after thrombin – (top) and hematoma – (bottom) injected animals. Measurements were made with drying-weighing method after 24 hours of thrombin and hematoma injection into the basal ganglia. Brain slices were divided into the ipsilateral (IPSI) and contralateral (CONTRA) hemispheres, and the cortex was separated from the basal ganglia bilaterally. Values are mean ± SEM. Hypothermia significantly reduced the thrombin-induced brain edema formation in the ipsilateral basal ganglia (** $p < 0.01$) and hematoma induced brain edema formation in the ipsilateral cortex (* $p < 0.05$) compared to the normothermic treatment

Discussion

There is no experimental evidence that the degree or duration of hypoperfusion around the intracerebral hematoma is sufficient to produce ischemic brain damage. Attention has recently focused on the direct role of the biochemical substances in clot in generating cerebral edema. Studies indicate that thrombin is directly involved in the pathogenesis of cerebral edema, and direct cell toxicity and later BBB disruption by thrombin are triggering mechanisms for the edema formation that follows ICH [3, 4, 5]. Studies also indicate that thrombin has effects related to inflammation including chemotaxis of leukocytes. The adhesion of leukocytes to the endothelium is the requisite first step

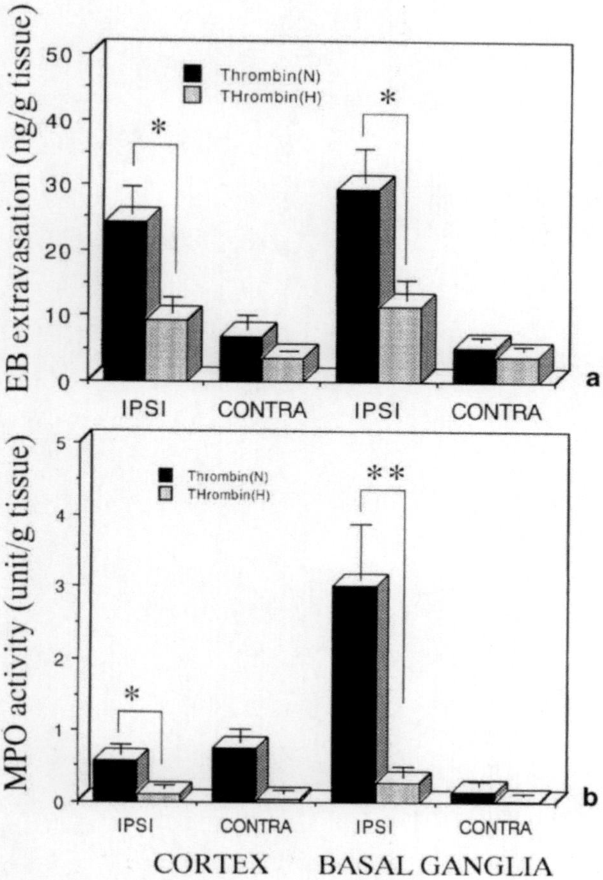

Fig. 2. Bar graphs comparing the BBB permeability to Evan's blue (EB) (a) and myeloperoxidase (MPO) activity (b) in the ipsilateral and contralateral cortices and basal ganglia after 24 hours of thrombin injection into the basal ganglia. Values are mean ± SEM. Hypothermic treatment significantly reduced the BBB permeability to EB in the ipsilateral cortex (*$p < 0.05$) and basal ganglia (*$p < 0.05$) compared to the normothermic group. Hypothermia also significantly inhibited the accumulation of PMN leukocytes in the ipsilateral cortex (*$p < 0.05$) and basal ganglia (**$p < 0.01$) compared to the normothermic group

to acute inflammation. The migration of leukocytes into the injured tissue, together with red blood cells and plasma proteins, may cause capillary plugging and a reduction of microvascular blood flow. Also, a variety of leukocyte derived compounds, including oxygen free radicals are capable of increasing vascular permeability and promoting cell death directly.

Brain hypothermia protects the BBB from damage [2] and, therefore, may exert a protective effect by reducing the passage of potentially harmful bloodborne substances across the endothelial barrier and subsequent vasogenic brain edema. In our experiment, brain hypothermia dramatically reduced brain edema in the basal ganglia at 24 hours after thrombin injection. BBB disruption to EB was suppressed by hypothermic treatment in a similar fashion, suggesting that hypothermia-induced decrease in brain edema was mainly mediated by the protection of BBB integrity. Emerging evidence also suggests that hypothermia attenuates the cell-mediated inflammatory response to cerebral injury [7]. The direct relationship between brain edema and reduced PMN leukocytes accumulation observed in our study suggests that the neuroprotective effects of hypothermia was mediated, in part, by effects on the acute inflammatory response.

References

1. Bradley PP, Priebat DA, Christensen RD *et al* (1982) Measurement of cutaneous inflammation: estimation of neutrophil content with an enzyme marker. J Invest Dermatol 78: 206–209
2. Dietrich WD, Busto R, Halley M *et al* (1990) The importance of brain temperature in alterations of the blood-brain barrier following cerebral ischemia. J Neuropathol Exp Neurol 49: 486–497
3. Lee KR, Betz AL, Keep RF *et al* (1995) Intracerebral infusion of thrombin as a cause of brain edema. J Neurosurg 83: 1045–1050
4. Lee KR, Colon GP, Betz AL *et al* (1996) Edema from intracerebral hemorrhage: the role of thrombin. J Neurosurg 84: 91–96
5. Lee KR, Kawai N, Kim S *et al* (1997) Mechanisms of edema formation after intracerebral hemorrhage: effects of thrombin on cerebral blood flow, blood-brain barrier permeability, and cell survival in a rat model. J Neurosurg: 272–278
6. Matsuo Y, Onodera H, Shiga Y *et al* (1994) Correlation between myeloperoxidase-quantified neutrophil accumulation and ischemic brain injury in the rat: effects of neutrophil depletion. Stroke 25: 1469–1475
7. Toyoda T, Suzuki S, Kassell NF *et al* (1996) Intraischemic hypothermia attenuates neutrophil infiltration in the rat neocortex after focal ischemia-reperfusion injury. Neurosurgery 39: 1200–12005

Correspondence: Nobuyuki Kawai, M.D., Department of Neurological Surgery, Kagawa Medical University, 1750-1 Ikenobe, Miki-cho, Kita-gun, Kagawa 761-0793, Japan.

Acta Neurochir (2002) [Suppl] 81: 237–239

Appropriate Cerebral Perfusion Pressure During Rewarming after Therapeutic Hypothermia

A. Aoki[1], K. Mori[1], M. Maeda[1], M. Miyazaki[2], and H. Iwase[2]

[1] Department of Neurosurgery, Juntendo University, Izunagaoka Hospital, Japan
[2] Casualty Center, Juntendo University, Izunagaoka Hospital, Japan

Summary

This study evaluated the cerebral ischemic parameters during the rewarming period after therapeutic hypothermia to determine the critical cerebral perfusion pressure (CPP) threshold to avoid ischemic deterioration. Cat experimental head injury was induced by inflation of an epidural rubber balloon to maintain intracranial pressure at 30 mmHg under hypothermia. During the rewarming period, CPP was maintained at ≥120 mmHg, 90 mmHg, and 60 mmHg by controlling the blood pressure. CBF, $CMRO_2$, $AVDO_2$, and cerebral venous oxygen saturation ($ScvO_2$) were measured. Brain extracellular glutamate concentrations were also measured by a dialysis electrode. Histological preparations of all brains were examined under an electron microscope. The cerebral metabolic parameters in animals with CPP of more than 90 mmHg returned to the base values after rewarming. However, $ScvO_2$ was significantly lower (27 ± 6%) and $AVDO_2$ was significantly higher (9.4 ± 1.8 ml/100 g/min) after rewarming in the animals with CPP = 60 mmHg, which indicated misery perfusion. Animals with CPP = 60 mmHg also showed increased extracellular glutamate concentration and histological ischemic damage (mitochondrial swelling). CPP of 60 mmHg during the rewarming period is associated with irreversible ischemia, which indicates continuation of cerebral vasoconstriction. Therefore, a CPP of greater than 90 mmHg is required to avoid cerebral ischemia.

Keywords: Hypothermia; cerebral perfusion pressure; rewarming.

Introduction

Mild hypothermia has a protective effect during the treatment of cerebral ischemia and head injury because small differences in brain temperature can determine the extent of ischemic brain injury [2]. However, hypothermia is associated with various disadvantages including acidosis, coagulopathy, arrhythmia, and electrolyte imbalance. Ischemic deterioration after therapeutic hypothermia is one of the most notable clinical complications related to hypothermia. Hypothermia may cause cerebral vasoconstriction and misery perfusion in the brain if the cerebral perfusion pressure (CPP) is not high enough, but this risk of relative ischemia can be avoided by vasopressor administration [3]. The present study investigated various parameters of cerebral ischemia during the rewarming period to determine the critical CPP threshold to avoid ischemic deterioration using an experimental head injury model.

Materials and Methods

Twenty-eight cats were anesthetized by continuous infusion of ketamine (10 mg/kg/hr) and pancuronium bromide (1 mg/kg/hr). A tracheostomy was performed for mechanical ventilation to maintain the arterial carbon dioxide tension at 35–45 mmHg. The basic blood gas management was α-stat management but acidosis and hypopotassemia caused by hypothermia were promptly corrected. Cerebral blood flow (CBF) was measured by a hydrogen clearance method using a platinum electrode in the thalamus. Intracranial pressure (ICP) was monitored by a fiberoptic transducer inserted into the occipital lobe. The superior sagittal sinus was cannulated with a catheter to obtain samples of cerebral venous blood to calculate $AVDO_2$, cerebral venous oxygen saturation ($ScvO_2$), $CMRO_2$, and CBF equivalent ($CBF/CMRO_2$). Deep brain temperature was monitored by a needle probe in the occipital lobe. A rubber balloon in the epidural space was inflated to increase and maintain ICP at 30 mmHg throughout the experiment. The deep brain temperature was decreased from 37 °C to 29 °C by surface cooling with a water-circulating blanket and maintained at 29 °C for three hours and then the animals were rewarmed gradually to 37 °C and maintained at 37 °C for three hours. The animals were divided into three groups according to the CPP maintained during the rewarming period by controlling the blood pressure with administration of trimethaphan camsylate (CPP ≥ 120 mmHg, N = 10; CPP = 90 mmHg, N = 7; CPP = 60 mmHg, N = 6). The parameters of cerebral metabolism were measured at each brain temperature. Five cats were also anesthetized and cooled and then rewarmed at these CPP levels and extracellular glutamate concentration was monitored by a dialysis electrode placed in the frontal cortex. Histological preparations of all animal brains were examined under an electron microscope.

Results

Parameters of Cerebral Metabolism During Rewarming

CBF decreased with hypothermia and recovered to the base values after rewarming in the CPP ≥ 120 mmHg group (36.2 ± 18.9 ml/100 g/min) and the CPP = 90 mmHg group (31.0 ± 15.0 ml/100 g/min), but CBF recovery was significantly reduced in the CPP = 60 mmHg group (17.3 ± 9.1 ml/100 g/min, $P < 0.05$). CBF/$CMRO_2$ ratio decreased with hypothermia but recovered to the base value after rewarming in the CPP ≥ 120 mmHg group (20.0 ± 4.0 ml blood/ml O_2) and the CPP = 90 mmHg group (17.4 ± 4.0 ml blood/ml O_2), but the recovery of CBF/$CMRO_2$ was significantly reduced in the CPP = 60 mmHg group (11.0 ± 2.0 ml blood/ml O_2, $P < 0.05$). The poor recovery of CBF equivalent was caused by the poor recovery of CBF during rewarming in the animals with CPP = 60 mmHg.

Figure 1 shows the change in $ScvO_2$ at various brain temperatures. $ScvO_2$ decreased with hypothermia but recovered to the base values after rewarming in the CPP ≥ 120 mmHg group (55 ± 7%) and the CPP = 90 mmHg group (46 ± 11%), but the recovery of $ScvO_2$ in the CPP = 60 mmHg group was significantly worse (27 ± 6%, $P < 0.05$). Figure 2 shows the change in $AVDO_2$ at various brain temperatures. $AVDO_2$ increased with hypothermia but recovered to the base values after rewarming in the CPP ≥ 120 mmHg group (6.4 ± 1.3 ml/100 g/min) and the CPP = 90 mmHg group (6.3 ± 1.9 ml/100 g/min), but the recovery of $AVDO_2$ in the CPP = 60 mmHg group was significantly worse (9.4 ± 1.8 ml/100 g/min, $P < 0.05$). The low $ScvO_2$ and high $AVDO_2$ in the CPP = 60 mmHg group during the rewarming period indicated that relative ischemia (misery perfusion) occurred.

Brain Extracellular Glutamate Concentration During Rewarming

The extracellular glutamate concentration was reduced during hypothermia but recovered after rewarming. Some animals with CPP = 60 mmHg showed remarkable increases of extracellular glutamate concentrations during the rewarming period.

Electron Microscopic Examination

The mitochondria of the cortex neurons remained normal in the CPP ≥ 120 mmHg and 90 mmHg groups, whereas mitochondria in the CPP = 60 mmHg group showed remarkable swelling, and intra-cytoplasmic vacuoles and slight fragmentation of endoplasmic reticulum were also recognized.

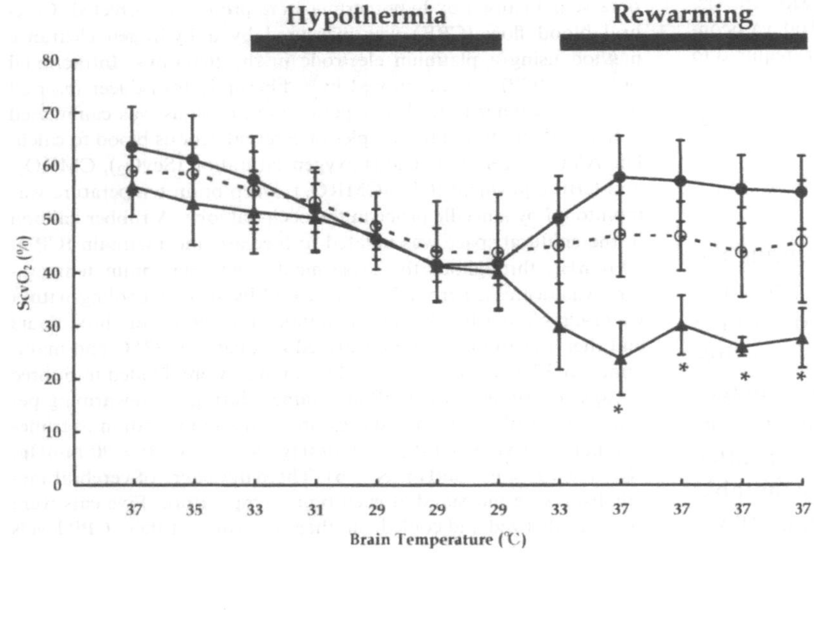

Fig. 1. Change in cerebral venous oxygen saturation ($ScvO_2$) in animals with cerebral perfusion pressure maintained at ≥120 mmHg (●), 90 mmHg (○), or 60 mmHg (▲) during rewarming. Asterisk: $P < 0.05$

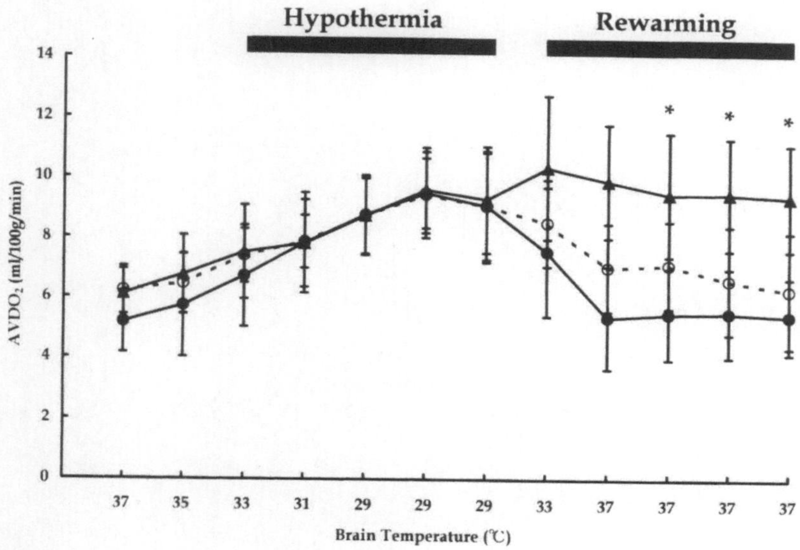

Fig. 2. Change in arteriovenous oxygen difference ($AVDO_2$) in animals with cerebral perfusion pressure maintained at ≥120 mmHg (●), 90 mmHg (○), or 60 mmHg (▲) during rewarming. Asterisk: $P < 0.05$

Discussion

The present study showed that $ScvO_2$ and $AVDO_2$ were never restored to the baseline levels but remained significantly lower and higher, respectively, after rewarming in the CPP = 60 mmHg group. These results indicate that secondary ischemic damage occurred during rewarming period if the CPP was not sufficiently high. Such metabolic misery perfusion was associated with increased extracellular glutamate concentration and histological signs of subcellular ischemic damage. We speculate that cerebral vasoconstriction caused by hypothermia in the rewarming period and secondary ischemic damage cannot be avoided if the CPP is not high enough. Ischemic neuronal damage is one of the most important determinants of neurological outcome after severe head injury. Recently, protocols intended to maintain CPP at over 70 mmHg have significantly improved the outcome in patients with severe head injury [4]. The present study showed that a CPP higher than 90 mmHg is required to avoid the potential risk of relative ischemia during the rewarming period. Maintenance of a high CPP during the rewarming period is one of the most important factors to achieve a successful outcome after hypothermic therapy for severe head injury.

The present study used α-stat gas management, but this relatively hyperventilated state might cause vasoconstriction. pH-stat management has been recommended for therapeutic hypothermia because cerebral oxygen delivery is better in pH-stat management [1]. However, pH-stat management causes hypercarbia and loss of cerebral autoregulation [5]. Further investigation is needed to evaluate the combined effects of optimal CPP and other related factors such as rate of rewarming and blood gas management.

Acknowledgments

This work was supported in part by a grant awarded to Prof. M. Maeda (No. 09671449) from the Japan Ministry of Education, Science and Culture.

References

1. Bauer R, Fritz H, Walter B, Schlonski O, Jochum T, Hoyer D, Zwiener U, Reinhart K (2000) Effect of mild hypothermia on cerebral oxygen uptake during gradual cerebral perfusion pressure decrease in piglets. Crit Care Med 28: 1128–1135
2. Busto R, Dietrich WD, Globus MY, Valdes I, Scheinberg P, Ginsberg MD (1987) Small differences in intraischemic brain temperature critically determine the extent of ischemic neuronal injury. J Cereb Blood Flow Metab 7: 729–738
3. Mori K, Maeda M, Miyazaki M, Iwase H (1999) Misery perfusion caused by cerebral hypothermia improved by vasopressor administration. Neurol Res 21: 585–592
4. Rosner MJ, Rosner SD, Hohnson AH (1995) Cerebral perfusion pressure: Management protocol and clinical results. J Neurosurg 83: 949–962
5. Verhaegen MJJ, Todd MM, Hindman BJ, Warner DS (1993) Cerebral autoregulation during moderate hypothermia in rats. Stroke 24: 407–414

Correspondence: Aya Aoki, M.D., Department of Neurosurgery, Juntendo University, Izunagaoka Hospital, 1129 Nagaoka, Izunagaoka-cho, Tagata-gun, Shizuoka, 410-2295, Japan.

Acta Neurochir (2002) [Suppl] 81: 241–242

Diffuse Brain Injury Complicated by Acute Subdural Hematoma and Secondary Insults in the Rodents: The Effect of Surgical Evacuation

S. Sawauchi, A. Beaumont, S. Signoretti, Y. Tomita, J. Dunbar, and A. Marmarou

Division of Neurosurgery, Medical College of Virginia, Richmond, Virginia, USA

Summary

Head Trauma associated with acute sudural hematoma (SDH) and complicated by secondary insult is a grave clinical combination with complex pathophysiology. The aim of this study was to develop a clinically relevant injury model, which can be used to study the interaction between injury mechanisms. We present a novel model of SDH combined with diffuse brain injury (DBI) and a hypoxic secondary insult, and investigate the effects of surgical evacuation.

Adult Sprague-Dawley rats were given a 300 µl SDH and 20 minute-hypoxia following Impact Acceleration DBI. Hematoma was evacuated at one hour post-injury. Physiological parameters were measured for 5 hours, together with assessment of brain water content.

Secondary insult after traumatic SDH was associated with significant brain swelling and stimulated refractory rise in ICP. In traumatic SDH complicated by secondary insult, brain swelling is exacerbated by surgical evacuation.

Keywords: Acute subdural hematoma; diffuse brain injury; intracranial pressure; surgical treatment.

Introduction

Post-traumatic acute subdural hematoma (SDH) is commonly associated with brain swelling showing a rapidly devastating course [1]. The role and effects of surgical intervention in the treatment of this severe condition are not fully understood, specially when referring to post-surgical refractory in intracranial pressure (ICP). In this study, we present a novel experimental SDH model combined with diffuse brain injury coupled with secondary insult, and investigate the effects of surgical evacuation of the hematoma.

Materials and Methods

Adult Sprague-Dawley rats (n = 23) were randomly divided into three experimental groups; 1) SDH+Trauma group (n = 4), 2) Hypoxia with non-evacuation group (n = 11): SDH + Trauma + Hypoxia, 3) Hypoxia with evacuation group (n = 8): SDH + Trauma+Hypoxia+Evacuation.

Animals were anesthetized, intubated and mechanically ventilated for the entire experimental period. Trauma was induced by the impact acceleration head injury model (weight 450 gm and height 2 m) [2]. Immediately after trauma, the hematoma was induced by infusing 300 µl non-heparinized autologous venous blood into the subdural space through a 23 gauge blunt-tipped needle. Hypoxia was induced by reducing the level of inspired O_2 (13%) for 20 minutes concurrent with production of the hematoma. One hour after induction of the SDH, the hematoma was evacuated through the craniotomy. After the evacuation, the bone flap was replaced and sealed tightly. Five hours after the induction of SDH, the rat was sacrificed by halothane overdose.

We analysed the profiles of the physiological parameters including mean arterial blood pressure (ABP), ICP and cerebral blood flow (CBF) of the contralateral hemisphere. At the end of the experiment, we measured brain water content using the wet weight and dry weight method.

Result

Physiological Assessment: SDH + Trauma

ICP reached a peak value during the hematoma induction and remained stable, although elevated compared with baseline. ABP did not show significant changes. CBF exhibited a transient reduction during the injection of the hematoma, followed by a gradual increase to baseline levels.

Physiological Assessment: Hypoxia with Non-Evacuation

The animals undergone to the hypoxic insult were retrospectively divided into two types based on intracranial hemodynamic parameters. In Type 1 animals, ICP after the resuscitation remained stable, followed by a delayed gradual increase with cerebral perfusion pressure (CPP) remaining above 60 mmHg. CBF exhibited a transient reduction during the hypoxic period, showing a gradual recovery to the level of baseline level. In Type 2 animals, the resuscitation caused a rapid increase of ICP above 100 mmHg, followed by a decline to 50 mmHg with CPP remaining below 10 mmHg for the remainder of the protocol. CBF recovered only temporarily after resuscitation, and showed marked reduction below 1%.

Physiological Parameters: Hypoxia with Evacuation

In Type 1 group, evacuation reduced ICP, which remained stable for the remainder of the protocol. In these animals surgery resolved CBF to hyperemic values. In Type 2 group, evacuation acutely reduced ICP. However, this reduction was only transient and followed by a steadily increase. CBF recovered following evacuation, but then gradually decreased to ischemic levels.

Brain Water Content

The water content of the hematoma hemisphere in Hypoxia with non-evacuation/Type 1 and Type 2 was significantly higher compared to the SDH+Trauma group, not exposed to hypoxia. In Hypoxia with evacuation/Type 1 group, removal of the hematoma had a beneficial effect revealing significant decrease of the water content. On the contrary, in Hypoxia with evacuation/Type 2 group, both hemispheres showed significantly higher water content than non-evacuation group. Surgical evacuation in Type 2 worsened the brain edema formation.

Discussion

Swelling of the hemisphere is the most threatening lesion associated with acute SDH being responsible of the highest mortality rate and most importantly of the highest incidence of refractory rise of ICP [1]. To date, there are no univocal explanations of the pathogenesis of post-traumatic, post-operative brain swelling. To reproduce this clinical scenario, we generated an experimental model in which ICP increases progressively after the evacuation of an acute SDH.

Interestingly, the combination of severe DBI with a SDH of 300 μl, followed by 20 minutes of hypoxic insult showed two major categories of pathophysiological behavior. In Type 1 animals, evacuation of the hematoma was helpful to maintain the adequate CBF and CPP, and limited brain edema formation. Contrarily, in Type 2 animals, surgical procedure, although performed early was not beneficial: it failed to restore normal CBF, allowing only a transient recovery and simply delayed the rise of ICP, compared to the non-evacuated group. In terms of brain edema, surgical intervention on Type 2 was even detrimental, resulting in increased water content. Surgical evacuation in these conditions only allowed ischemic-reperfusion damages, leading to brain edema and refractory intracranial hypertension.

In conclusion, Secondary insults after traumatic SDH are associated with significant brain swelling and can stimulate a refractory rise in ICP. In traumatic SDH complicated by secondary insult, surgical evacuation delays ICP rise but worsens brain edema.

References

1. Lobato RD, Sarabia R, Cordobes F *et al* (1988) Posttraumatic cerebral hemispheric swelling. J Neurosurg 68: 417–423
2. Marmarou A, Foda MAA, van den Brink W *et al* (1994) A new model of diffuse brain injury in rats. Part I: Pathophysiology and biomechanics. J Neurosurg 80: 291–300

Correspondence: Anthony Marmarou, Ph.D., Division of Neurosurgery, Medical College of Virginia, P.O. Box 950508, Richmond, Virginia 23298-0508, USA.

Acta Neurochir (2002) [Suppl] 81: 243–244

Diffuse Brain Injury Complicated by Acute Subdural Hematoma in the Rodents: The Effect of Early or Delayed Surgical Evacuation

S. Sawauchi, A. Beaumont, S. Signoretti, Y. Tomita, C. Marmarou, and A. Marmarou

Division of Neurosurgery, Medical College of Virginia, Richmond, Virginia, USA

Summary

Of all the possible clinical factors affecting the outcome of patients suffering acute subdural hematomas (SDH), timing of surgical evacuation is certainly the most debated. The purpose of this study was to develop an experimental model able to reproduce the clinical behavior of post-traumatic SDH as observed in head injured patients. We present a novel model of SDH combined with diffuse brain injury (DBI), and investigate the effects of early and delayed surgical evacuation.

Following Impact Acceleration DBI, adult Sprague-Dawley rats were given a 400 μl SDH. Hematoma was then evacuated at one (rapid evacuation) or four hours (delayed evacuation) post-injury. Physiological parameters were measured for 5 hours, followed by the assessment of brain water content.

In this experimental model, there is strong evidence that trauma acts synergistically with SDH enhancing brain edema formation and increasing ICP. In absence of secondary insult, rapid evacuation of traumatic SDH limits exposure to high ICP, reduces brain edema and is beneficial.

Keywords: Acute subdural hematoma; diffuse brain injury; intracranial pressure; surgical treatment.

Introduction

The definitive treatment for acute subdural hematoma (SDH) is the surgical removal. However, the timing of evacuation is still debated, and the consequent pathophysiological effects are not fully understood. In this study, we present a novel experimental model of SDH and investigate the influence of rapid and delayed surgical evacuation following SDH alone and SDH combined with diffuse traumatic brain injury.

Materials and Methods

Adult Sprague-Dawley rats (n = 28) were randomly divided into two main experimental groups such as SDH Alone (n = 14) and SDH+Trauma (n = 14). Furthermore, both groups were subdivided into three groups such as non-evacuation, rapid evacuation and delayed evacuation.

Animals were anesthetized, intubated and mechanically ventilated for the entire experimental period of 5 hours. In the SDH Alone group, the hematoma was induced by infusing 400 μl venous blood into the subdural space. In the SDH + Trauma group, the Impact Acceleration injury model (weight 450 gm and height 1 m) was used to induce diffuse traumatic brain injury [3]. Immediately after trauma, 400 μl blood was infused. In rapid evacuation group, surgery was performed one hour post-injury. In delayed evacuation group, surgery was performed four hours post-injury. Hematoma was evacuated through a parietal craniotomy. After the evacuation, the bone flap was replaced and sealed tightly.

The profiles of the physiological parameters including mean arterial blood pressure (ABP), intracranial pressure (ICP), cerebral blood flow (CBF) of the contralateral hemisphere were analysed. At the end of the experiment, we also measured the brain water content using the wet/dry weight method.

Result

Physiological Assessment: SDH Alone

In non-evacuation group, rise in ICP during the hematoma induction was immediate, reaching a maximum value of 57 mmHg, followed by a gradual decrease to 17 mmHg. ABP did not show any significant changes. CBF exhibited a transient reduction during the hematoma induction, followed by a gradual increase up to 148% of the baseline. Although for a longer period of time ICP remained higher in the delayed evacuation group compared to the rapid evacuation group, the CBF profile in the two groups was the same. Similarly, there were no significant differences in ICP temporal course and ABP. Most importantly, ICP did not rise above 20 mmHg.

Physiological Assessment: SDH + Trauma

In non-evacuation group, increased in ICP equalled a maximum value of 77 mmHg during the hematoma induction, followed by a gradual decrease to 25 mmHg. Blood pressure did not show any significant changes. CBF exhibited a transient reduction during the hematoma induction, followed by a gradual increase up to 114% of the baseline. Both rapid and delayed evacuation reduced ICP to stable value of 11 mmHg and 9 mmHg, respectively. However, in rapid evacuation, mean ICP value from the end of hematoma induction to the end of experiment was significantly lower than delayed evacuation.

Brain Water Content

In the SDH Alone group, there were no significant differences in brain edema formation among the non-evacuated, rapid and delayed evacuated groups. In rapidly evacuated SDH+Trauma group, water content on the subdural side was significantly lower than in the delayed evacuated group.

Discussion

In the clinical setting, several interacting factors determine the need to evacuate an acute SDH, mainly the neurological status, volume of the hematoma, and ICP values. Seelig *et al.* [5] and Haselberger *et al.* [1] had reported that the time interval from injury to surgical evacuation is the most critical factors in determining outcome. However, this principle was challenged in 1991, by Wilberger *et al.* [7]. These investigators concluded that ICP control is more critical to outcome than the absolute timing of the hematoma removal. Moreover, other studies have observed a lack of benefit for early operative intervention [2, 4]. Servadei *et al.* [6] reported that when ICP is persistently higher than 25 mmHg, patient needs prompt surgical removal, before brain stem compression occurs. According to this report, the purpose of the evacuation is to avoid further brain injury secondary to ICP increase, therefore a surgical evacuation will be beneficial only if ICP is higher than the threshold value of 25 mmHg.

Our data indicates that in SDH Alone, where the average ICP was always below 20 mmHg, neither rapid nor delayed evacuation affected brain edema formation. However, when trauma was added to this SDH model, the average ICP values were higher than 20 mmHg and the prompt evacuation of the hematoma significantly reduced brain edema, achieving better ICP control, compared to the delayed evacuation.

We conclude that in this experimental model, additional trauma acts synergistically with SDH enhancing brain edema formation and increasing ICP. In traumatic SDH without secondary insult, early surgical evacuation limits exposure to high ICP, reduces brain edema and is beneficial.

References

1. Haselsberger K, Pucher R, Auer LM (1988) Prognosis after acute subdural or epidural haemorrhage. Acta Neurochir (Wien) 90: 111–116
2. Kotwica Z, Brzezinski J (1993) Acute subdural hematoma in adults: An Analysis of outcome. Acta Neurochir (Wien) 121: 95–99
3. Marmarou A, Foda MAA, van den Brink W *et al* (1994) A new model of diffuse brain injury in rats. Part I: Pathophysiology and biomechanics. J Neurosurg 80: 291–300
4. Massaro F, Lanotte M, Faccani G *et al* (1996) One hundred and twenty-seven cases of acute subdural haematoma operated on: Correlation between CT scan finding and outcome. Acta Neurochir (Wien) 138: 185–191
5. Seelig MJ, Becker DP, Miller JD *et al* (1981) Traumatic acute subdural hematoma. Major mortality reduction in comatose patients treated within four hours. N Engl J Med 304: 1511–1518
6. Servadei F, Nanni A, Nasi MT *et al* (1995) Evolving brain lesions in the first 12 hours after head injury: Analysis of 37 comatose patients. Neurosurgery 37: 899–907
7. Wilberger JE, Harris M, Diamond DL (1991) Acute subdural hematoma: morbidity, mortality, and operating timing. J Neurosurg 74: 212–218

Correspondence: Anthony Marmarou, Ph.D., Division of Neurosurgery, Medical College of Virginia, P.O. Box 950508, Richmond, Virginia 23298-0508, USA.

Acta Neurochir (2002) [Suppl] 81: 245–247

Traumatic Subarachnoidal Hemorrhage in the Developing Rat

S. Thomas[1], F. Tabibnia[1], B. Herrmann[1], M. U. Schuhmann[2], T. Brinker[1], and M. Samii[1]

[1] Department of Neurosurgery, Nordstadt Hospital, Hannover, Germany
[2] Medical School, Hannover, Germany

Summary

The aim of the present study was to utilize an experimental traumatic subarachnoidal hemorraghe model in the developing rat.

Diffuse brain injury was produced in intubated and ventilated 21 to 25 days old Sprague-Dawley rats (N = 10) using a modification (1 m/100 g) of the Marmarou-model. Before induction of the injury heparin was administered i.v. and antagonised after injury by protamine. Mean arterial blood pressure and intracranial pressure was measured continuously. Histopathological investigations were performed. The results were compared to readings in adult animals (N = 12) subjected to a 1.5 m/500 g injury.

In the developing rat ICP increased immediately following injury from 11.4 ± 2.1 mm Hg to 55.9 ± 20.3 mm Hg. It remained elevated till the end of the experiment 1 h after injury. MABP increased from 79.8 ± 8.7 mm Hg to 100.2 ± 21.7 mm Hg immediately following injury, returning to 61.3 ± 28.7 mm Hg at the end of the experiment resulting in a marked decrease of CPP. The mortality rate was 60%. All brains showed a severe subarachnoidal hemorrhage in the basal cisterns.

The increase of ICP following injury is attributable to the bleeding similar as in adult animals. The high mortality is due to the marked decrease of CPP. Rat pups are more vulnerable to t-SAH compared to adult rats.

Keywords: Traumatic subarachnoidal hemorrhage; rat pup; ICP; blood pressure.

Introduction

Traumatic brain injury is a major cause of morbidity and mortality in children [1]. A subgroup of patients with severe traumatic brain injury suffered a traumatic subarachnoidal hemorrhage (t-SAH) occurring with an incidence of 23% to 39% [2, 3].

In previous studies in our laboratory an experimental t-SAH-model was established in adult rats and ICP-and MABP-pattern were determined [7].

The aim of the present study was to utilize the t-SAH-model for the first time in the developing rat and to determine changes of ICP, MABP, CPP, and histology. The results obtained in developing animals were compared to findings in adult animals. According to the "Kennard principle" there is a better performance and milder deficits after brain injury if sustained early in life [4]. Therefore, the rat pups were expected to do better following t-SAH compared to adult rats.

Material and Methods

21–25 days old Sprague-Dawley rats (N = 10; 46–54 g) were intubated and ventilated with a gas mixture of 1.0–2.0% isoflurane, 70% N_2O and 30% O_2. Polyethylene catheters (PE-10) were placed into the femoral artery and continuous blood pressure recordings were obtained until one hour after injury. Measurements of ICP were performed using a catheter (PE-10) placed subdurally through a lateral-frontal burr hole into the anterior fossa.

The injury device first described by Marmarou *et al.* was used to produce a diffuse trauma [5, 7]. Following a midline scalp incision the skin and periosteum were reflected and a stainless steel disc was mounted on the skull using cyanoacrylate. A brass weight (100 g) fell free onto the helmet guided by a 1 m Plexiglas tube. The animal was placed in prone position on a foam (20 × 20 × 50 cm; spring constant 30/50) held within a wooden frame. The lower end of the tube was placed directly above the helmet. Immediately following the initial impact the box was slid horizontally to prevent a second impact. Five minutes before trauma heparin (10 I.E./g) was injected i.a.. Five minutes following trauma the equivalent dose of protamine (10 I.E./g) was administered and anesthesia reinstated.

All brains were processed for hematoxylin-eosin staining using 20 μm coronal sections. Surviving animals were perfused transcardially one day after injury and the brains were removed and postfixed in 4%-formalin. Sections were studied under light-microscopy for cell loss and hemorrhages.

The results were compared to readings in adult animals (N = 12) subjected to a 1.5 m/500 g injury.

All measurements were stored and analyzed using commercially available software (Dasy Lab V.3, Datalog, Mönchengladbach, Germany). Statistical analysis was performed using Wilcoxon signed rank test for paired data. Data are presented as mean ± SD.

Results

A t-SAH was achieved in all injured animals as determined by histological evaluation. However, the extension of blood extravasation was quite heterogeneous.

The mortality rate for developing animals was 60% (6/10). Death occurred usually within one hour after injury. The animals did not start breathing following termination of mechanical ventilation. In the adult animals the mortality rate was 41.6% (5/12).

In the developing rats ICP increased immediately following injury from 11.4 ± 2.1 mm Hg to 55.9 ± 20.3 mm Hg ($p < 0.05$). It remained elevated till the end of the experiment, one hour after injury (46.25 ± 30.9 mm Hg). In the adult rats the initial increase of ICP from 8.6 ± 3.7 mm Hg to 40.9 ± 36.5 mm Hg ($p < 0.05$) was similar as in the rat pups. However, in the adult rats ICP returned to base-line levels (7 ± 5.1 mm Hg) within one hour following injury.

In the rat pups MABP increased slightly from 79.8 ± 8.7 mm Hg to 100.2 ± 21.7 mm Hg (n.s.) immediately following injury returning to lower levels (59.4 ± 11.1 mm Hg) within 3 minutes. It remained diminished till the end of the experiment (61.3 ± 28.7 mm Hg). The adult rats exhibited an increase of MABP immediately after injury from 148.8 ± 15.9 to 175.8 ± 52.6 mm Hg (n.s.) returning to lower levels 77.9 ± 37.7 mm Hg within 15 min and 85.4 ± 42.9 mm Hg one hour after injury.

The elevation of ICP and decrease of MABP resulted in a marked reduction of CPP. In the developing animals CPP was about 15 mm Hg lasting from 3 min till 60 min after trauma. In the adult animals the lowest CPP value was 62.8 mm Hg at 15 min following trauma.

Gross pathological examination of the t-SAH animals did not reveal any skull fractures. Following removal of the brain extended subarachnoidal hemorrhage was observed within the basal cisterns and in the whole subarachnoidal space. Histological investigation confirmed the gross pathological inspection and showed in addition diffuse neuronal cell loss in all cortical areas, the hippocampus, and brainstem. In addition minor perivascular bleedings were detected in the brainstem.

Discussion

The present study is the first description of the t-SAH-model in the developing rat. A modification of the weight-drop-model can be applied to produce a reproducible t-SAH in the developing rat with a significant increase of ICP, moderate decrease of MABP, and significant reduction of CPP.

The marked increase of ICP is due to the actual bleeding caused by the rupture of subarachnoidal vessels and similar as in adult animals. The slight increase of MABP in both developing and adult animals immediately following injury is in contrast to our previous findings [7]. However, the injury is quite heterogeneous indicated by the large standard deviation values.

The mortality rate of 41.6% for the adult animals is in the range of mortalities reported in clinical studies

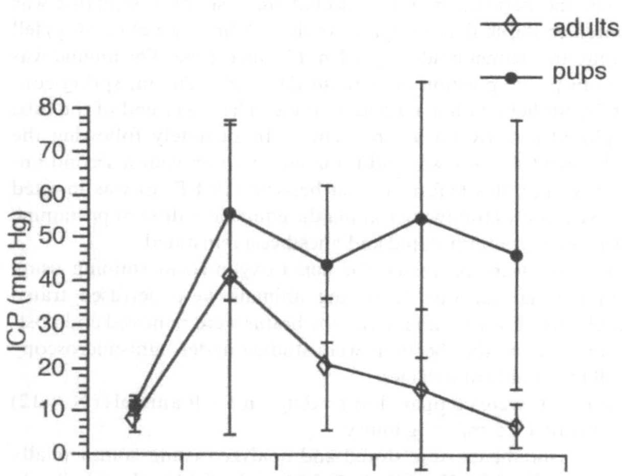

Fig. 1. Intracranial pressure (mean ± SD) before and after injury

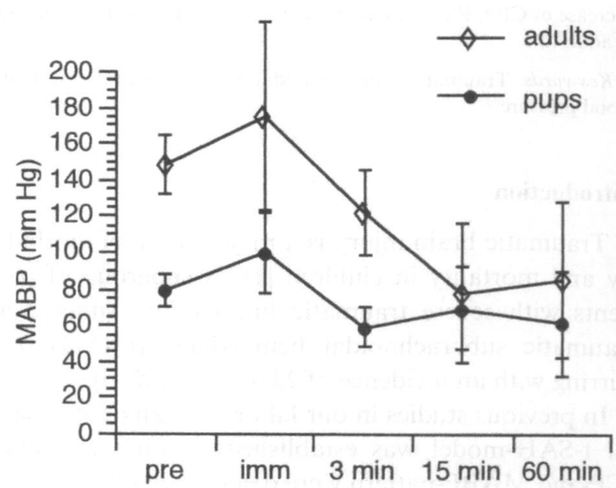

Fig. 2. Mean arterial blood pressure (mean ± SD) before and after injury

and very close to the 42% in the HIT II study. In contrast to findings in adult animals where only a moderate reduction of CPP was observed, the rat pups exhibited a significant reduction of CPP, far below the threshold of ischemia. Therefore, the higher mortality in the developing animals may be attributable to the significant decrease of CPP.

In conclusion, the present model offers a simple possibility to perform experimental studies on t-SAH in developing and adult rats. The results of the study indicate that 21 to 25 days old rat pups are more sensitive to t-SAH compared to adult ones. The "Kennard principle", indicating a better outcome if brain injury is sustained early in life, has to be rejected in developing rats with t-SAH.

References

1. Aldrich EF, Eisenberg HM, Saydjari C, Luerssen TG, Foulkes MA, Jane JA, Marshall LF, Young H (1992) Diffuse brain swelling in severely head-injured children. A report from the NIH Traumatic Coma Data Bank. J Neurosurg 76: 450–454
2. Eisenberg HM, Gary HE, Aldrich EF *et al* (1990) Initial CT findings in 753 patients with severe head injury. A report from the NIH Traumatic Coma Data Bank. J Neurosurg 73: 688–698
3. Kakarieka A (1997) Traumatic subarachnoidal haemorrhage. Springer, Berlin Heidelberg New York Tokyo
4. Kennard MA (1936) Age and other factors in motor recovery from precentral lesions in monkeys. Am J Physiol 115–138
5. Marmarou A, Foda MAA, Van den Brink W, Campbell J, Kita H, Demetriadou K (1994) A new model of diffuse brain injury in rats. Part I: pathophysiology and biomechanics. J Neurosurg 80: 291–300
6. Thomas S, Tabibnia F, Schuhmann MU, Hans VHJ, Brinker T, Samii M (1998) Traumatic brain injury in the developing rat pup: studies of ICP, PVI and neurological response. Acta Neurochir (Wien) [Suppl] 71: 135–137
7. Thomas S, Tabibnia F, Herrmann B, Schuhmann MU, Brinker T, Samii M (1999) Traumatic subarachnoidal hemorrhage: Introduction of a new experimental model in the rat. J Neurotrauma 16: 959

Correspondence: Sebastian Thomas, M.D., Neurochirurgische Klinik, Nordstadt Hospital, Haltenhoffstrasse 41, 30167 Hannover, Germany.

Acta Neurochir (2002) [Suppl] 81: 249–251

Experimental Intracerebral Hemorrhage: Effect of Lysed Erythrocytes on Brain Edema and Blood-Brain Barrier Permeability

R. R. Bhasin[1], G. Xi[1], Y. Hua[1], R. F. Keep[1,2], and J. T. Hoff[1]

[1] Department of Surgery (Neurosurgery), University of Michigan, Ann Arbor, Michigan
[2] Department of Physiology, University of Michigan, Ann Arbor, Michigan

Summary

Understanding the mechanism of edema formation following intracerebral hemorrhage (ICH) is important for developing treatment protocols for this condition. This study examines the role of red blood cell (RBC) lysis and hemoglobin in edema formation following ICH. Significant brain edema developed after 24 hours in rats infused with lysed RBCs and this was associated with a 3-fold increase blood brain barrier (BBB) permeability to α-aminoisobutyric acid. We have previously shown that intracerebral injection of packed RBCs does not cause edema formation at one day but does at three days. In this study, we found that packed RBCs did not cause significant BBB disruption at one day but produced a 4-fold increase in BBB permeability at three days. These studies show that following ICH the leakage of substances inside the RBC, facilitated by cellular lysis, results in delayed edema. This was confirmed by both experimentally induced lysis and naturally occurring in-vivo lysis.

Keywords: Intracerebral hemorrhage; blood brain barrier; hemoglobin; erythrocyte lysis.

Introduction

Intracerebral hemorrhages are ruptures of the vasculature within the brain. Many patients deteriorate quickly following ICH due to perihematomal edema development leading to elevations in intracranial pressure that can cause herniation, brain stem compression, and mass effect with secondary ischemia. However, the pathological mechanisms behind edema development are not well understood.

Animal studies have shown that specific blood products have the capability to induce brain swelling. Thrombin can induce a significant brain edema within 24 hours of injection into the brain, as well as disrupt the BBB [3]. It has been shown that red blood lysis is an key event in the natural progression of ICH to perihematomal swelling [6].

Current understanding of parenchymal edema development allows for mechanisms of water entry into brain tissue: either cytotoxic or vasogenic. Direct cell cytotoxicity could account for swelling, as well as BBB disruption. We hypothesized from the earlier thrombin studies that RBC lysis may also induce BBB disruption. In addition, we hypothesized that hemoglobin should also open the BBB, but to a lesser degree, given that it produced less edema than lysed RBCs. Lastly, we investigated whether intact RBCs following natural lysis would also produce the same results as the experimentally lysed RBCs.

Materials and Methods

The protocols in this study were approved by the University of Michigan Committee on the Use and Care of Animals. Male Sprague-Dawley rats, weighing between 350–450 grams, were used in experiments. Animals were anesthetized with pentobarbital (40 mg/kg IP). The right femoral artery was catheterized for blood pressure monitoring and blood sampling for ICH induction and blood gases. The rats were positioned in a stereotactic frame and a cranial burr hole (1.0 mm) was drilled on the skull (0.2 mm anterior, 5.5 mm ventral, 4.0 mm lateral to bregma). Either no infusion, saline, packed RBCs, or lysed RBCs were microinfused into the right caudate nucleus at a rate of 10 μl/min through a 26-gauge needle [6]. Rats were sacrificed and 4 mm sections of tissue around the hematoma (ipsilateral), as well as the opposite side (contralateral), were cut for analysis. To prepare packed RBCs, blood (0.5 ml) was centrifuged at 14,000 G for 2 min. Plasma and buffy coat were discarded. To prepare lysed RBCs, packed cells were frozen in liquid nitrogen for 5 minutes and then allowed to thaw in room temperature water. Rat hemoglobin (Sigma) was prepared in saline at a concentration of 300 mg/ml. Because native hemoglobin is readily oxidized in air the infusate was predominately met-hemoglobin. *Brain Water Content Groups:* Animals received either saline (20 μl, n = 4), hemoglobin (20 μl, n = 5), or lysed RBCs (20 μl, n = 5). Following 24 hours, brain water (wet-dry weight method) and sodium contents were measured [6]. *BBB Groups:* Animals either received a needle stab (n = 5), packed RBCs (50 µl, n = 11), lysed RBCs (20 µl, n = 5), or hemoglobin (20 µl, n = 5). BBB permeability was assessed by measuring the permeability surface area (PS) product of [^{3}H]-α-aminoisobutyric acid (AIB) [3]. Measurements were made at 24 hours, except for five packed RBC animals which were measured at 72 hours. Data were analysed by one-factor ANOVA or Student's t-test. Values are presented as means ± S.D. Significance is denoted by probability value less than 0.05.

Results

Cerebral Water Content (24 hours): There were no significant differences in blood pH, glucose, hematocrit, pO_2, pCO_2, or blood pressure among any of the groups. Perihematomal tissue water contents were 84.7 ± 0.2, 81.3 ± 1.1 79.1 ± 0.3% for the lysed RBC, hemoglobin and saline groups, respectively (Figure 1) while tissue sodium contents were 659 ± 102, 481 ± 105 and 229 ± 19 mEq/kg dry weight for the same three groups. Edema and sodium content were higher in the lysed RBC group than the other two groups ($p < 0.05$ for both), while the hemoglobin group was significantly higher than the saline group ($p < 0.05$). There were no significant differences between groups in contralateral tissues or cerebellum.

Blood-Brain Barrier (24 hours): Infusion of lysed RBCs resulted in a marked increase ($p < 0.05$ for all) in AIS PS product to 7.93 ± 0.84 µl/g/min in the perihematomal basal ganglia compared to 2.96 ± 0.54, 3.29 ± 1.68 and 2.63 ± 0.50 µl/g/min in the packed RBC, hemoglobin and sham groups (Fig. 2). Hemoglobin did not produce significant increases in permeability probably because our preparation consisted predominately of met-hemoglobin, while lysed RBCs contains oxy-hemoglobin.

In vivo lysis (72 hours): In contrast to the 24 hour results, intracerebral injection of packed red blood cells produced marked BBB disruption after 72 hours (AIB PS product 5.07 ± 3.12 and 1.35 ± 0.49 µl/g/min in the ipsi- and contralateral hemispheres, respectively; $p < 0.05$). This degree of disruption is similar to that found with lysed RBCs at 24 hours.

Discussion

These results indicate that factors within RBCs have the capability to induce BBB disruption, as well as produce significant parenchymal edema. The key event in both processes is lysis of intact RBCs, either experimentally or naturally induced, with the release of intracellular contents into the surrounding tissue. Although our results show that hemoglobin can account for a significant percentage of the changes in that occur in ICH, it is likely the hemoglobin exerts its prolonged effects through its breakdown products.

The brain expresses the enzyme hemeoxygenase which is critical in the breakdown of the hemoglobin molecule to its constituent parts. Once exposed to the enzyme following RBC lysis, hemoglobin is broken down into bilirubin, carbon monoxide and ferrous iron. Each of these substances has the potential for neuronal toxicity. Free radicals are generated in an

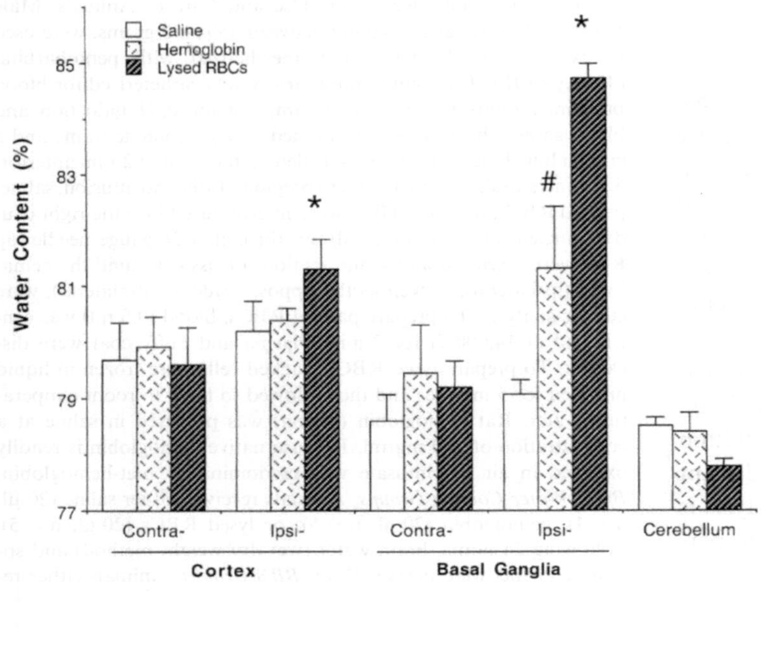

Fig. 1. Brain tissue water content 24 hours after infusion of saline, hemoglobin or lysed RBCs. Values are means ± S.D., n = 4–5. * = $p < 0.05$ vs. hemoglobin and saline. # = $p < 0.05$ vs. saline

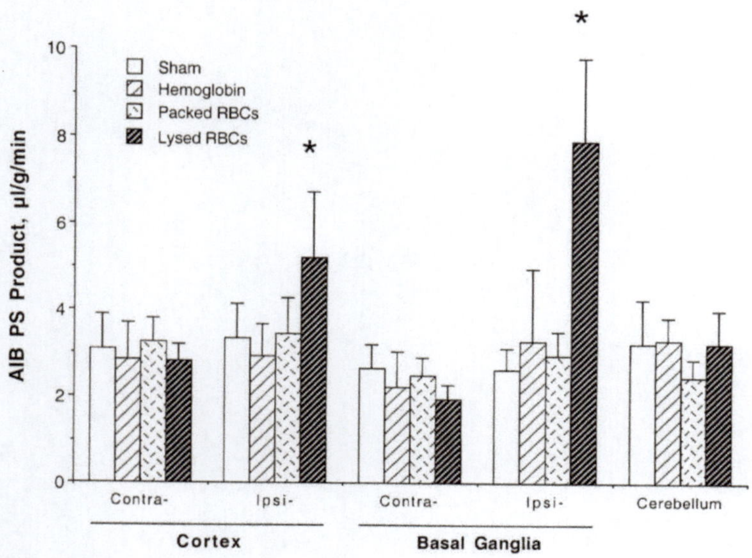

Fig. 2. Effect of hemoglobin, packed RBC, or lysed RBC infusion or a sham operation on AIB PS product 24 hours later. Values are means ± S.D., n = 5–6. * = $p < 0.05$ vs. all groups

ICH blood clot both from the ferrous iron contained within heme as well as the auto-oxidation of oxyhemoglobin in which a spontaneous reduction-oxidation reaction to met-hemoglobin forms the superoxide free radical [1]. Free radicals target the lipid membranes of cells causing alterations in membrane fluidity and integrity, eventually leading to leakage of ions across cellular membranes. They can also oxidize amino acids leading to inactivation of enzymes, receptors, or structural proteins [2]. Bilirubin also has the potential for neuronal excitoxicity [4], although low levels of bilirubin can be neuroprotective through a free radical scavenger mechanism.

Possible mechanisms of perihematomal edema development involve either vasogenic changes from damage to the endothelium of penetrating blood vessels of the BBB or by direct cytotoxic damage to neuronal cells or local astrocytes that are involved in maintaining extracellular homeostasis. It has been shown that oxyhemoglobin can induce apoptosis in cultured endothelial cells, possibly through free radial damage to the endothelial vessel wall tissue [1]. The temporal pattern of edema formation after infusion of lysed on packed eryrthrocytes (this study and [6]) is similar to the pattern of BBB disruption. A second mechanism for edema development is direct neuronal cytotoxicity caused by hemoglobin. Neuronal toxicity results in leakage of fluid, ions, and proteins into cells creating an increased osmotic pressure for fluid retention. Exposure of cultured rat spinal cord cells to hemoglobin produces a concentration-dependant cell toxicity as measured by lactate dehydrogenase release [5].

Following ICH, a cascade of events triggered by cellular lysis appears to be critical for edema development. These involve significant changes at the BBB that contribute to the increased cerebral water content and, potentially, morbidity.

Acknowledgment

This study was supported by grants NS-17760, NS-34709 and NS-39866 from the National Institutes of Health.

References

1. Ogihara K, Zubkov A, Bernake D, Lewis A, Parent A, Zhang J (1999) Oxyhemoglobin induced apoptosis in cultured endothelial cells. J Neurosurg 91: 459–465
2. Facchinetti F, Dawson V, Dawson T (1998) Free radicals as mediators of neuronal injury. Cell Mol Neurobiol 18: 667–683
3. Lee KR, Kawai N, Kim S, Sagher O, Hoff JT (1997) Mechanisms of edema formation after intracerebral hemorrhage: effects of thrombin on cerebral blood flow, blood-brain barrier permeability, and cell survival in a rat model. J Neurosurg 86: 272–278
4. McDonald J, Shapiro S, Silverstein F, Johnston M (1998) Role of glutamate receptor mediated excitotoxicity in bilirubin-induced brain injury in the Gunn rat model. Exp Neurol 1150: 21–29
5. Regan R, Guo Y (1998) Toxic effects of hemoglobin on spinal cord neurons in culture. J Neurotrauma 15: 645–653
6. Xi G, Keep R, Hoff JT (1998) Erythrocytes and delayed brain edema formation following intracerebral hemorrhage in rats. J Neurosurg 89: 991–996

Correspondence: Guohua Xi, M.D., R5550 Kresge I, University of Michigan, Ann Arbor, Michigan 48109-0532.

Acta Neurochir (2002) [Suppl] 81: 253–256

Brain Edema after Intracerebral Hemorrhage: The Effects of Systemic Complement Depletion

G. Xi[1], Y. Hua[1], R. F. Keep[1,2], J. G. Younger[3], and J. T. Hoff[1]

[1] Department of Surgery (Neurosurgery), University of Michigan, Ann Arbor, Michigan
[2] Department of Physiology, University of Michigan, Ann Arbor, Michigan
[3] Department of Emergency Medicine, University of Michigan, Ann Arbor, Michigan

Summary

The complement cascade is activated after experimental intracerebral hemorrhage (ICH) and may play an important role in edema formation. This study investigated the effects of systemic complement depletion on brain edema formation following ICH. Thirty-six pentobarbital-anesthetized Sprague-Dawley rats were used. Treatment animals were complement-depleted with cobra venom factor (CVF) while controls received an equal volume of saline injection (i.p.). In both treatment and control rats, autologous blood (100-μL) was infused stereotactically into the right basal ganglia. Rats were sacrificed one and three days later for brain water and ion content measurements and immunohistochemical studies. Immunohistochemistry was used to detect complement C3d, C5a, and C9. Western blot analysis was applied for C9 semiquantitation. Perihematomal brain edema was reduced by systemic complement depletion at one and three days. The water content of the cerebellum (a tissue distant from the hematoma site) was unaffected by complement depletion. Immunocytochemistry found complement depletion significantly reduced perihematomal C9 deposition, C3d production, and C5a positive cell accumulation. In conclusion, complement depletion by CVF attenuates brain edema in ICH perhaps by inhibiting the inflammatory response and membrane attack complex (MAC) formation.

Keywords: Cerebral hemorrhage; brain edema; complement; membrane attack complex (MAC).

Introduction

In a recent study, we found that the complement cascade is activated after ICH and that N-acetylheparin, an inhibitor of complement activation, reduces ICH-related brain edema [1]. The complement system is an important self-defense immune system. However, it causes tissue injury if it is activated inappropriately. Complement activation and complement-mediated brain injury have been found in variety of central nervous system diseases [4]. Cobra venom factor (CVF) is a nontoxic glycoprotein that is purified from cobra venom and can cause systemic complement depletion. Systemic depletion of complement by CVF attenuates experimental cerebral vasospasm after subarachnoid hemorrhage, reduces ischemic brain damage in cerebral ischemia and reduces the recruitment of inflammatory cells in experimental allergic encephalomyelitis.

The purpose of the present study was to investigate whether systemic complement depletion by CVF attenuates complement system activation within the brain and brain edema formation following ICH. We chose to measure brain water content, the complement cascade activation indicator C3d, anaphylatoxin C5a, and a key complement component for MAC formation C9 in the rat ICH model with and without CVF treatment.

Materials and Methods

The protocols for these animal studies were approved by the University of Michigan Committee on the Use and Care of Animals. Thirty-six male Sprague-Dawley rats (weighing 300–400 g) were used. For all surgical procedures, rats were anesthetized with pentobarbital (40 mg/kg, i.p.) and aseptic precautions were utilized. The ICH model involved catheterization of the right femoral artery for continuous blood pressure and blood gas monitoring and blood sampling. Body temperature was maintained at 37.5 °C. Autologous blood (100 μL) was then infused into the right caudate nucleus through a 26-gauge needle [5].

This study was divided into five parts. Each part consisted of a control group and a CVF-treated group. All rats received intracerebral 100-μL autologous blood infusion and were killed at different time points for different purposes. In the first and second parts, rats ($n = 5$ per group) were killed 24 hours or 72 hours later for brain water and ion contents. In the third and fourth parts, four groups of two to three animals each were investigated. They were killed 24 hours or 72 hours later for complement C3d, C5a, and C9 immunohistochemistry. In the fifth part, brains were removed for

C9 Western blot analysis. Brain edema was quantified by wet/dry weight and ion contents were measured by flame photometry [5]. Ion content was expressed in milliequivalents per kilogram of dehydrated brain tissue (mEq/kg dry wt). Our methods for immunohistochemistry and Western blot have been described previously [6]. The primary antibodies were rabbit anti-human C3d polyclonal antibody (DAKO), goat anti-rat C5a polyclonal antibody (gift from Dr. P. A. Ward, University of Michigan), rabbit anti-rat C9 polyclonal antibody (gift from Dr. P. Morgan, University of Wales). CVF-treated animals were given intraperitoneal injections of 25 units of CVF in 36, 24, and 12 hours prior to induction of an ICH. To confirm complement depletion in CVF treated animals, total serum hemolytic activity was measured prior to injury using the CH_{50} technique. All data in this study are presented as mean ± standard deviation. Data were analyzed with Student's t test. Significance levels were measured at $p < 0.05$.

Results

In all animals treated with the CVF protocol, total serum hemolytic activity was undetectable ($CH_{50} <$ 20). Complement C3 titers were in each case $\leq 1:160$ (with $>1:640$ being normal in our laboratory). Complement depletion by CVF reduced brain edema in the ipsilateral basal ganglia (78.8 ± 0.6% vs. 81.5 ± 0.8% in control, $p < 0.01$; Fig. 1) one day following ICH. The reduction of water content was associated with a reduction in sodium ion accumulation (243 ± 24 vs. 369 ± 59 mEq/kg dry wt in control, $p < 0.001$) and a reduction in potassium ion loss (373 ± 19 vs. 317 ± 24 mEq/kg dry wt in control, $p < 0.05$). Complement-depleted rats also had less edema (81.5 ± 1.5 vs. 83.6 ± 0.9% in control, $p < 0.05$; Fig. 1) in the ipsilateral basal ganglia three days after ICH. Cerebellar water content was unaffected by CVF treatment (78.2 ± 0.3 vs. 78.0 ± 0.1% in control, $p > 0.05$). C3d immunoreactivity was detected around the hematoma and in the clot three days after ICH in non-CVF treated rats. However, there were only a few C3d immunoreactive particles found in the clot in complement-depleted animals. Perihematomal complement C5a positive cells were also detected after ICH in non-CVF treated rats, with most of the C5a positive cells appearing to be neutrophils. In contrast, it was difficult to find C5a positive cells around the hematoma in CVF-treated rats. Although Western blot analysis for complement C9 showed no difference between CVF-treated and control group 24 hours post-ICH, significant complement C9 deposition was found on the neurons around the hematoma in non-CVF treated animals, but not in those treated with CVF (Fig. 2).

Discussion

The present study shows that systemic complement depletion by CVF reduces edema formation one and

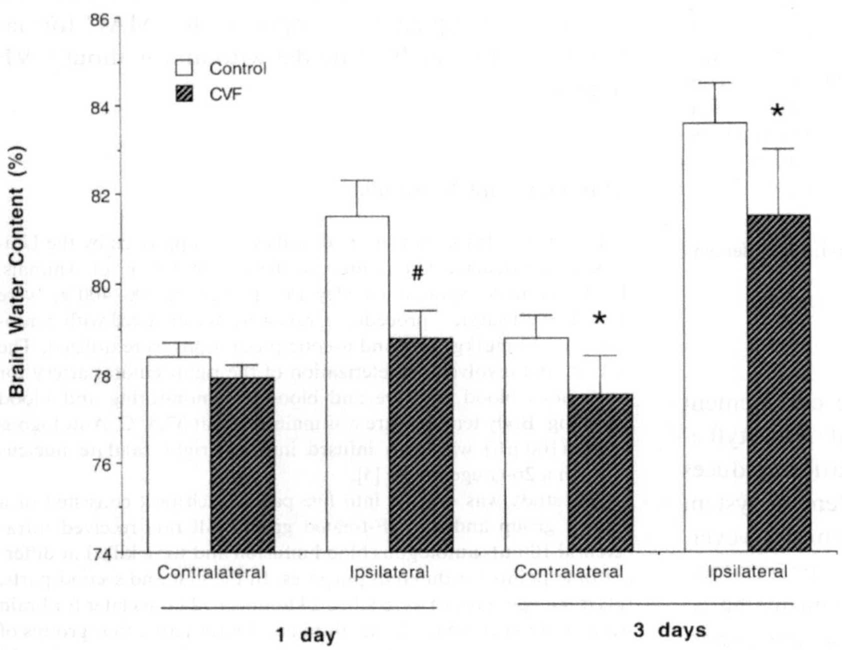

Fig. 1. Water content of the ipsi- and contralateral basal ganglia 24 and 72 hours after ICH. Control = control group and CVF = CVF-treated group. Values are expressed as mean ± SD; n = 5–6. *$p < 0.05$, #$p < 0.01$ vs. control group

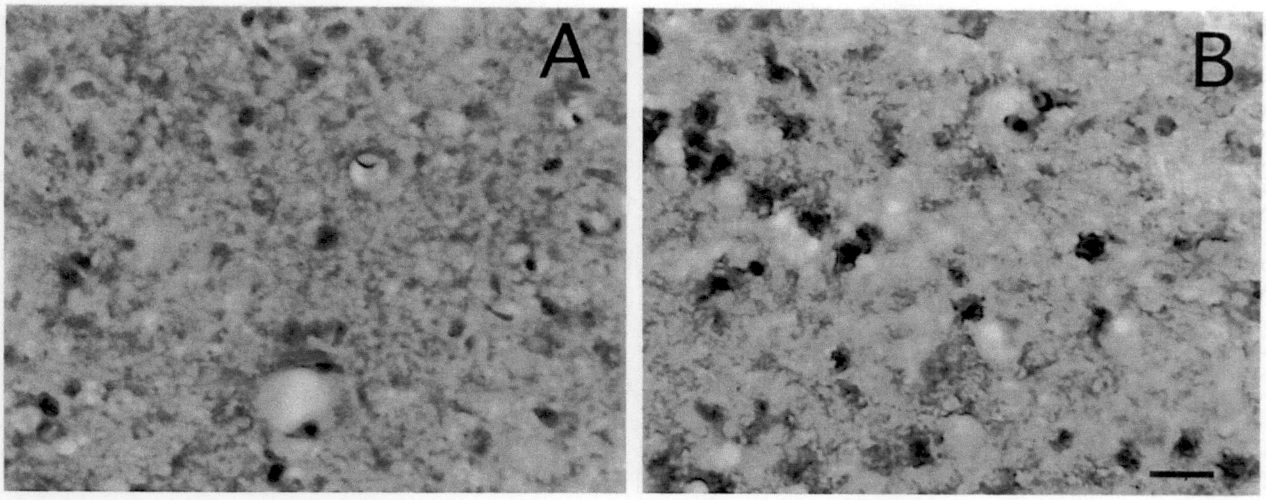

Fig. 2. Complement C9 immunoreactivity around the hematoma in CVF-treated (A) and control rats (B) 3 days following ICH. Scale bar = 20 μm

three days after ICH. The reduction of brain edema in CVF-treated rats is associated with less C3d production, fewer C5a positive cells and a marked decrease of C9 deposition on cell membranes around the hematoma. All these data suggest that complement activation after ICH is involved in brain edema formation and inhibiting complement activation may provide a novel treatment for brain edema following ICH.

After ICH, the complement cascade is activated locally in or around the hematoma in our rat model [1]. C3d is a segment of complement C3 and an indicator of complement activation. The absence of C3d around the hematoma in CVF-treated rats confirms that the complement system is depleted, not only in the blood (C3 titers) but also in the brain.

Complement depletion reduced edema formation at both 24 and 72 hours after ICH. These two time points were chosen because there are multiple causes for edema formation following ICH [5]. For example, the clotting cascade has a major role in early edema formation [2] while erythrocyte lysis plays a role later [5]. That complement depletion affects edema formation at both time points suggests that complement cascade activation triggers multiple mechanisms.

Complement-mediated brain injury is probably related to an inflammatory response. After activation of the complement cascade, anaphylatoxins C3a and C5a are generated. C3a and C5a cause blood-brain barrier leakage by degranulating mast cells and leukocytes. C5a is also a potent chemoattractant for leukocytes and contributes to inflammatory cell injury [3]. The present results show that the numbers C5a positive cells are dramatically reduced in CVF-treated animals.

MAC formation after complement activation may exacerbate ICH-induced brain injury. The MAC is a macromolecular complex that consists of C5b to C9, which forms a transmembrane pore and eventually causes cell lysis. That complement depletion reduces brain edema after ICH may, at least in part, be through a reduction in MAC formation. In ICH, MAC may contribute to brain edema formation by inducing erythrocyte lysis and hemoglobin release. Hemoglobin is neurotoxic and can induce brain edema [5]. MAC may also directly insert into neurons, astrocytes and endothelial cells causing neuronal injury and blood-brain barrier disruption. The reduction of C9 deposition in CVF-treated animals indicates that complement depletion by CVF does not deplete C9, but abolishes MAC formation in our ICH model.

In summary, we have shown that complement depletion by CVF reduces brain edema following ICH. The reduction of brain edema may be associated with inhibition of inflammatory response and inhibition of MAC-mediated erythrocyte lysis and brain injury.

Acknowledgment

This study was supported by grants NS-17760, NS-34709 and NS-39866 from the National Institutes of Health.

References

1. Hua Y, Xi G, Keep RF, Hoff JT (2000) Complement activation in the brain after experimental intracerebral hemorrhage. J Neurosurg 92: 1016–1022
2. Lee KR, Colon GP, Betz AL, Keep RF, Kim S, Hoff JT (1996) Edema from intracerebral hemorrhage: the role of thrombin. J Neurosurg 84: 91–96
3. Lucchesi BR (1993) Complement activation, neutrophils, and oxygen radicals in reperfusion injury. Stroke 24: I41–I47
4. Morgan BP, Gasque P, Singhrao S, Piddlesden SJ (1997) The role of complement in disorders of the nervous system. Immunopharmacology 38: 43–50
5. Xi G, Keep RF, Hoff JT (1998) Erythrocytes and delayed brain edema formation following intracerebral hemorrhage in rats. J Neurosurg 89: 991–996
6. Xi G, Keep RF, Hua Y, Xiang JM, Hoff JT (1999) Attenuation of thrombin-induced brain edema by cerebral thrombin preconditioning. Stroke 30: 1247–1255

Correspondence: Guohua Xi, M.D., R5550 Kresge I, University of Michigan, Ann Arbor, Michigan 48109-0532.

Acta Neurochir (2002) [Suppl] 81: 257–263

Metabolic Alterations in Cerebrospinal Fluid from Double Hemorrhage Model of Dogs

W. Yin, R. Tibbs, K. Aoki, A. Badr, and J. Zhang

Department of Neurosurgery, University of Mississippi Medical Center, Jackson, MS

Summary

Objective. Even though cerebral vasospasm after subarachnoid hemorrhage (SAH) causes cerebral ischemia or infarction, the metabolic alterations in cerebrospinal fluids (CSF) after SAH have not been studied. This study was undertaken to measure the levels of glucose, lactate, pyruvate and glutamate in CSF from double hemorrhage dog models.

Method. Thirty-two mongrel dogs of either sex, weighing 15–30 kg, underwent double hemorrhage by percutaneous needle puncture of the cisterna magna and injection of autologous blood on day 0 and day 2. The dogs were then sacrificed on day 3, 5 and 7, after collecting CSF. In another study, the dogs were treated with mitogen-activated protein kinase (MAPK) inhibitors PD98059 and U0126, and caspase-2 and caspase-3 inhibitors from day 3 to day 6 after initial blood injection. CSF was collected on day 7 before dogs were sacrificed. The concentration of glucose, lactate, pyruvate and glutamate in CSF was measured by photometrical method.

Result. Compared with CSF collected on day 0, glucose was decreased on days 5–7, lactate was increased on days 2–7, pyruvate was increased on days 2–7, and glutamate was increased on days 3–7 ($P < 0.05$). In the groups treated with MAPK or caspase inhibitors, most of the metabolic alterations remained unchanged as compared with CSF from untreated dogs. Clinically, caspase inhibitors-2 and -3, and MAPK inhibitor U0126 all failed to prevent vasospasm. MAPK inhibitor PD98059 partially prevented vasospasm.

Conclusion. Our data demonstrated a metabolic alteration of glucose, glutamate, lactate and pyruvate in CSF during cerebral vasospasm. This metabolic change is consistent with the time course of cerebral vasospasm. This study suggests that brain energy metabolites and excitative amino acids are altered during cerebral vasospasm.

Keywords: Glucose; lactate; pyruvate; glutamate; CSF; vasospasm.

Introduction

Subarachnoid hemorrhage (SAH) is characterized by high mortality, increased intracranial pressure, decreased cerebral blood flow, and deceased cerebral perfusion pressure [2]. A consequence of SAH-induced vasospasm, cerebral infarction, produces an unrecoverable ischemic tissue core surrounded by a potentially amenable penumbra. Abnormalities of oxidative and energy metabolism appear to be involved in multiple pathological alterations during vasospasm. However, a possible metabolic alteration in vasospasm has not been studied.

Extracellular glutamate contribute to excitotoxicity and neuronal death. Extracellular glutamate concentrations can be taken as a marker of the severity of ischemic neuronal injury. Lactate was normally considered to be a product of anaerobic glycolysis and therefore a good marker for neuropathological event [14]. Lactic acidosis also disturbs ionic homeostasis and might have its own adverse effects on the development of secondary brain damage. Furthermore, after release, glutamate uptake induces astrocytic glycolysis, leading to lactate production that then becomes the preferred energy substrate for neurons, undergoing excitotoxic or transmitter-induced ionic stress [14]. In animal model of cerebral ischemia, extracellular glucose was decreased, glutamate and lactate increased following ischemic insult [14, 16].

This study is undertaken to investigate possible changes of lactate, pyruvate, glucose and glutamate in cerebrospinal fluid (CSF) after experimental SAH.

Materials and Methods

Experimental SAH Model

Thirty-two adult mongrel dogs of either sex, weighing 18–24 kg, were used for the dog double hemorrhage model. The dogs were anesthetized with thiopental (10 mg/kg) and mechanically ventilated during the experiments. The body temperature was kept at 37 °C with a heating blanket, and mean arterial blood pressure and blood gases were monitored through a catheter inserted into the femoral artery and maintained within normal range. Experimental subarachnoid hemorrhage was induced according to the method of Varsos *et al.* [17]. Cerebral angiography was performed on Exposcop 7000 (Ziehm International Medical Systems, Riverside, CA). One of the vertebral arteries was catheterized with a 4F catheter via the femoral artery, and the baseline vertebrobasilar angiogram was obtained. The cisterna magna was punctured transcutaneously, and 0.4 ml/kg of CSF was withdrawn. An equivalent amount of arterial blood was withdrawn from the femoral artery and immediately and slowly injected into the cisterna magna. The dogs were then tilted 20 degrees, head down, in a prone position, for 10 minutes to permit pooling of the blood around the basilar artery. The first injection was considered to be day 0 SAH. On day 2, the same blood injection procedure was repeated without angiography.

The dogs were divided randomly into three groups:

(1) The first group of dogs was used for a time course study. Dogs were sacrificed on day 3 ($n = 4$), 5 ($n = 4$) or 7 ($n = 4$) after double hemorrhage. Angiograph was taken and CSF was collected before sacrifice.

(2) The second group of dogs was treated with vehicle (DMSO, $n = 4$), and MAPK inhibitors PD98059 ($n = 4$), and U0126 ($n = 4$). MAPK inhibitors PD98059, U0126, and DMSO were injected intracisternally on day 3 and continued daily through day 6. Angiograph was repeated on day 7, and CSF was collected before sacrifice.

(3) The third group of dogs was treated with caspase-2 ($n = 4$) and caspase-3 ($n = 4$) inhibitors. The inhibitors were injected intracisternally on day 3 and continued daily through day 6. Angiograph was repeated on day 7, and CSF was collected before sacrifice.

For the drug treatment, 1 ml of CSF was withdrawn through the suboccipital puncture. MAPK inhibitors PD98059, U0126, and caspase-2 and caspase-3 inhibitors or DMSO (about 40 μl) were diluted with 1 ml of CSF and then injected back into the cisterna magna. The doses of antagonists were calculated individually for each dog to reach similar drug levels in the dogs' CSF. The calculations took into account the relative size of the CSF space to obtain a final concentration in CSF of 10 μM, assuming that canine CSF volume is 2.0 ml/kg. Dogs were sacrificed by an overdose of pentobarbital (120 mg/kg).

This protocol was evaluated and approved by the University of Mississippi Medical Center Animal and Ethics Review Committee.

Measurements of Arterial Diameter

The arterial diameter was measured in a double-blinded fashion from zoomed angiograms. In order to eliminate differences in the enlarged angiograms, a penny was placed on the dog's chin during the angiography run. The coin was used as a standard, and all values of the arterial diameter were relatively adjusted to the size of the coin. Two researchers independently measured the arterial diameter on the magnified angiograms at the distal, central, and proximal portions of the basilar artery. The mean of these three measurements was taken for the arterial diameter. The mean of the measurements of both researchers was taken as the final diameter.

Measurement of Glucose, Lactate, Pyruvate, and Glutamate

The CSF was placed in a CMA 600 microdialysis analyzer (CMA/Microdialysis AB, Sweden). All reagents were obtained from CMA/Microdialysis AB. By completely automated enzymatic reaction techniques, concentrations of glucose, lactate, pyruvate and glutamate were obtained and displayed on a computer screen. The assays consisted of standard enzymatic phosphorylation and/or oxidation reaction steps and spectrophotometric detection.

Chemicals and Inhibitors

PD98059 (BIOMOL Research Laboratories, Inc, Plymouth Meeting, PA) and U0126 (Promega, Madison, WI) were commercially obtained. Caspase-2 Inhibitor I (Z-VDVAD-FMK) and Caspase-3 Inhibitor II (Z-DEVD-FMK) were purchased from CALBIOCHEM (San Diego, CA). All drugs were diluted in dimethyl sulfoxide (DMSO) to 10 mM.

Data Analysis

Data are expressed as the mean ± the standard error of the mean. Statistical differences between angiographic values in the control and other groups were compared using a one-way analysis of variance (ANOVA) and then the Tukey-Kramer multiple comparison procedure (95% lower and upper confidence interval) if a significant variance was found. A value of $P < 0.05$ was considered statistically significant.

Result

Time Course of Cerebral Vasospasm

The caliber of the basilar artery was calculated as the ratio of the mean basilar artery diameter on day 7, as a percentage of that on day 0. The residual diameter of the basilar arteries was 80.8 ± 13.4% ($P > 0.05$), 67.3 ± 6.4% ($P < 0.05$, ANOVA) and 53.4 ± 5.5% ($P < 0.005$, ANOVA) on day 3, 5, and 7, respectively.

Effects of p44/42 MAPK Inhibitors on Angiographic Vasospasm

The MAPK kinase inhibitor treatment groups were compared with the vehicle group because MAPK kinase inhibitors were diluted with DMSO. The residual diameter of the basilar arteries in the vehicle (DMSO) treatment group on day 7 was 52.7 ± 3.4%, similar to the diameter of dogs from SAH without treatment groups, indicating intrathecal injection of DMSO did not alter the vessel diameter. The residual diameter of the basilar arteries in the PD98059 and U0126 groups on day 7 was 79.0 ± 11.8% and 63.1 ± 8.6%, respectively. These results showed that PD98059 significantly attenuated the vasoconstriction ($P < 0.05$, ANOVA), compared with SAH or DMSO-treated groups. U0126 failed to significantly reduce vasospasm.

Effect of Caspase Inhibitors on Angiographic Vasospasm

The effect of caspase-2 and -3 inhibitors were compared with vehicle groups because the caspase inhib-

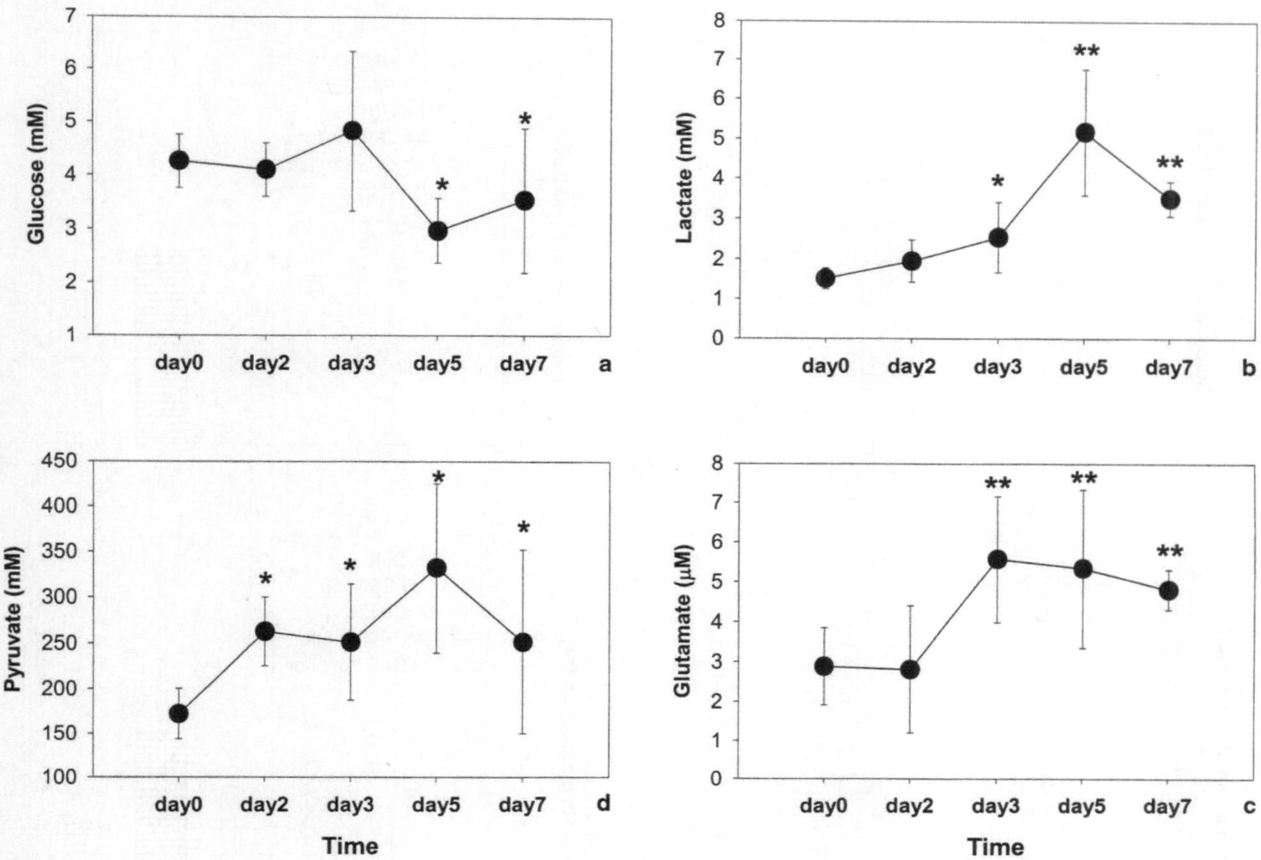

Fig. 1. Time course of metabolic alterations. A dynamic change of glucose (a), lactate (b), pyruvate (c), and glutamate (d) in CSF was shown. Compared with CSF collected on day 0, glucose was decreased on day 5 and day 7. Lactate was increased on day 2–7. Pyruvate was increased on day 2–7. Glutamate was increased on day 3–7. * and ** indicate $P < 0.05$, < 0.01 (vs. CSF from day 0, ANOVA), respectively

itors were diluted with DMSO. The residual diameter of the basilar arteries in the caspase-2 and caspase-3 inhibitors groups on day 7 was $56.2 \pm 2.7.8\%$ and $64.1 \pm 5.5\%$, respectively. These results showed that caspase-2 and -3 inhibitors failed to significantly reduce ($P > 0.05$, ANOVA) vasospasm.

Metabolic Alteration in CSF

Comparing with CSF collected on day 0 (4.26 ± 0.5 mM), glucose was decreased ($P < 0.05$, ANOVA) on day 5 (2.97 ± 0.6 mM) and day 7 (3.53 ± 1.35 mM), respectively (Fig. 1). Lactate was increased ($p < 0.01$, ANOVA) compared with CSF collected on day 0 (1.51 ± 0.26 mM) on day 2 (1.95 ± 0.53 mM), day 3 (2.54 ± 0.87 mM), day 5 (5.18 ± 1.59 mM) and day 7 (3.5 ± 0.43 mM), respectively (Fig. 2). Pyruvate was increased ($P < 0.05$, ANOVA) compared with CSF collected on day 0 (172.2 ± 28.1 mM) on day 2 (262.7 ± 37.5 mM), day 3 (250.95 ± 63.4 mM), day 5 (332.15 ± 92.9 mM) and day 7 (251.07 ± 101 mM), respectively. Glutamate was increased ($p < 0.01$, ANOVA) compared with CSF collected on day 0 (2.88 ± 0.97 μM) on day 3 (5.57 ± 1.59 μM), day 5 (5.34 ± 2.0 μM) and day 7 (4.8 ± 0.5 μM), respectively (Figure 1).

Effect of MAPK and Caspase Inhibitors on Metabolic Alteration

Most of the metabolic alterations remained unchanged after treatment of dogs with MAPK or caspase inhibitors as compared with CSF from day 7-SAH dogs (Fig. 2). The increase of lactate in CSF from day 7-SAH dogs was reduced ($P < 0.05$, ANOVA) by U0126 treatment (from 3.5 ± 0.43 reduced to 2.13 ± 0.23 mM). The increase of glutamate in the CSF from day 7-SAH dogs was decreased ($P < 0.05$, ANOVA) by caspase inhibitor 3 (from 4.8 ± 0.5 to 3.58 ± 0.3 μM).

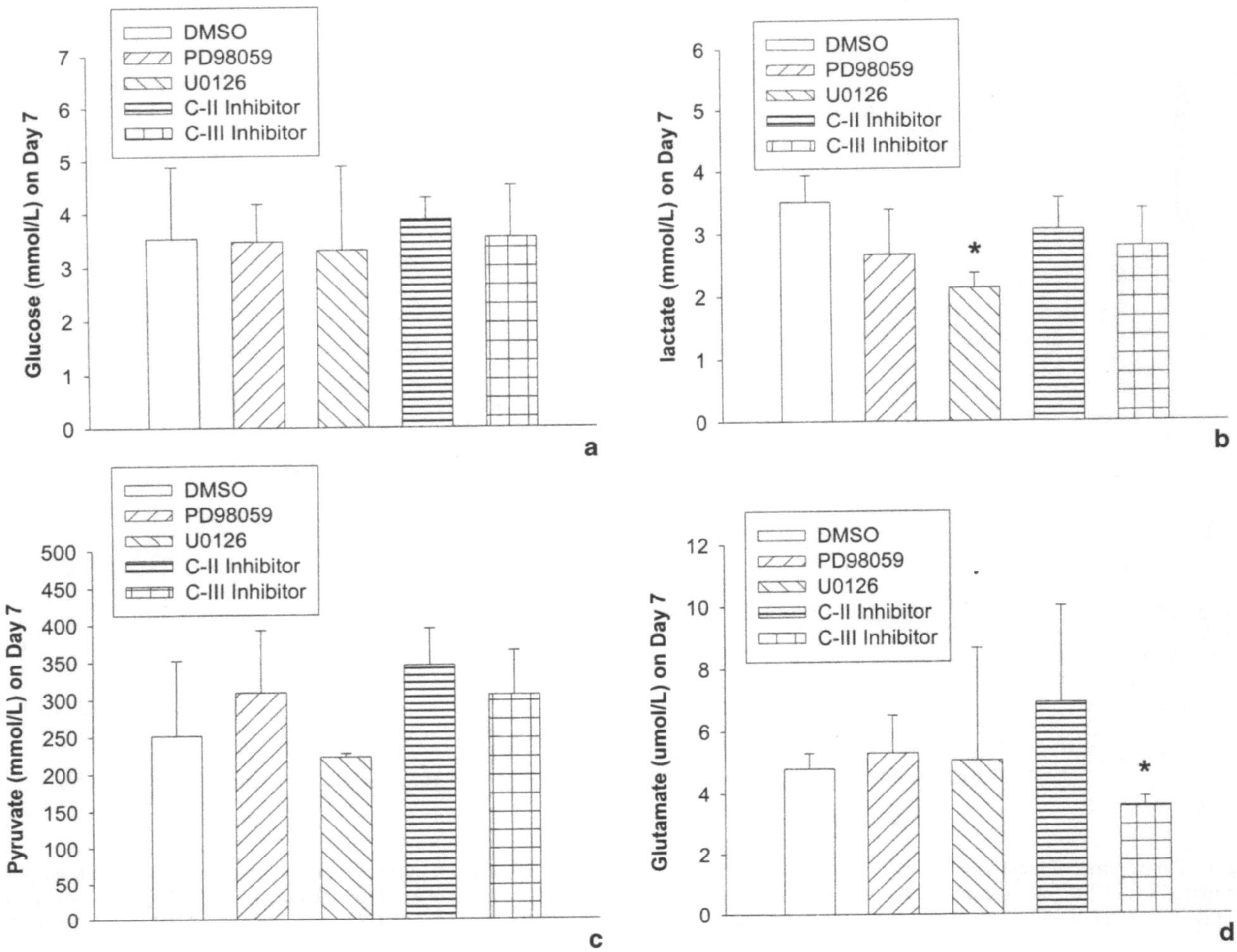

Fig. 2. Metabolic changes after treatment. The effect of PD98059 and U0126, caspase-2, and caspase-3 inhibitors on glucose (a), lactate (b), pyruvate (c), and glutamate (d) in CSF collected on day 7 from dogs after double hemorrhage. Most of the metabolic alterations remain unchanged as compared with CSF collected from untreated dogs. The level of lactate was reduced ($P < 0.05$, ANOVA) by U0126 treatment. The level of glutamate was decreased ($P < 0.05$, ANOVA) by caspase inhibitor 3. * indicates $P < 0.05$ (vs. CSF on day 7 of untreated dogs, ANOVA). c2 inhibitor = caspase-2 inhibitor; c3 inhibitor = caspase-3 inhibitor

Discussion

The following results were obtained in this study. (a) Compared with CSF collected on day 0, lactate, pyruvate, and glutamate was increased but glucose decreased during cerebral vasospasm. The alteration of those chemicals is consistent with the time course of vasospasm. (b) With the except of MAPK inhibitor PD98059, all other drugs (U0126, caspase-2 and caspase-3 inhibitors) failed to reverse vasospasm. However, regardless of the clinical effect of those inhibitors, most of the metabolic alterations remain unchanged as compared with CSF from untreated dogs.

Metabolic Products of Cerebral Ischemia

Glucose is the main energy source of the brain. Cerebral blood flow reduction or impairment of glucose transporters, may have influenced the extracellular glucose content and that normal uptake and metabolic processes were extremely disturbed next to severely contused brain tissue [16]. Another possible reason for glucose decreases may be due to glutamate-induced increased energy demand.

Glutamate is highly concentrated in the cerebral cortex and is the most abundant amino acid neurotransmitter in the mammalian brain. As such, it is important in a variety of normal neural functions. Excess stimulation by glutamate, however, can be toxic to neurons. Previous study showed that vasoconstriction was associated with decreased cerebral blood flow, ischemic glutamate release and premature mortality after experimental SAH [8]. The origin of the elevated glutamate concentrations in CSF remains unknown, even though the following factors may be possibly involved. (a) CSF reflects a high extracellular fluid glutamate concentration; (b) glutamate may influx from plasma through the broken blood-brain barrier; (c) glutamate could originate from the cytosol of dead cells [15]. Under normal condition, glutamate is found in the extracellular space within the central nervous system, ranging from 1 to 3 μM. Beyond this level, glutamate might be toxic to cells. In cultured neurons, as low as 2–5 μM of glutamate has been found to be toxic, whereas in neuron-glial co-cultures up to 100 μM glutamate may be needed for toxicity. It was showed that toxicity of glutamate depended on the energetic state of the nervous tissue and a low level of glucose or oxygen might potentiate the toxicity.

Lactic acid has widely been accepted as an indicator of anaerobic metabolism caused by ischemia and it is also massively released at non-ischemic blood flow levels during ischemia [14]. The lumbar CSF concentrations of lactate and pyruvate are considered to reflect those in the brain [1]. Lactate and pyruvate will both increase as a consequence of increased glycolysis [14]. Some studies demonstrated that SAH is associated with generalized brain edema, causing a reduction of global cerebral blood flow, loss of autoregulatory mechanism, vasospasms and thrombosis. This leads to cerebral ischemia and consequently to glycolysis by means of anaerobic metabolism [9]. Because lactate penetrates the blood-brain barrier at a very low rate, measurement of CSF lactate is a useful index of cerebral metabolism. The increase in brain lactate would be expected to worsen cellular acidosis and thereby worsen cellular injury [4].

An elevation of the CSF level of pyruvate during SAH probably indicated an acceleration of pyruvate production from glucogenic amino acids with an inhibition of flux through pyruvate dehydrogenease. Therefore the shunting to pyruvate exceeds the capacity to enter the Krebs citric acid cycle in the central nervous system after SAH, that may accelerate glycolysis while decelerate gluconeogenesis, decrease the expenditure of energy in central nervous system metabolism so that it will increase neural excitability [10].

Metabolic Changes During Cerebral Vasospasm

Cerebral arteries respond to SAH with a biphasic contraction that begins minutes after the bleed and a delayed vasospasm occurs more than 3–5 days later. Although a great deal is known about the mechanisms and management of delayed vasospasm, less is known about the metabolic alterations. Examination of CSF neurochemistry has been used to study possible neurotransmitter changes in patients and animals in cerebral ischemia. Previous studies showed that important chemical substances involved in the development of cerebral ischemia can be retrieved from the CSF, for example, energy-related substances such as lactate, pyruvate, glucose, and excitatory amino acids such as glutamate. Changes of them may serve as biochemical markers of impending ischemia [11]. We have demonstrated in this study a dynamic change of glucose, lactate, pyruvate and glutamate in CSF from SAH dogs and this change reflected an ischemic state of brain metabolism during cerebral vasospasm.

Metabolic changes in CSF did not occur immediately or two days after blood injection. Most of the metabolic changes occurred on day 3 and lasted up to day 7. This change is consistent with the time course of cerebral vasospasm and reflected the ischemic changes during cerebral vasospasm. An increased level of CSF lactate and pyruvate may reflect the metabolic derangement of the mitochondia, or the decreased regional cerebral blood flow. The generation of these metabolic products might be highly related to a decreased cerebral blood flow and an energy perturbation during ischemia [2]. Furthermore, a decrease of glucose and an increase of glutamate in CSF may aggravate cerebral ischemia caused by cerebral vasospasm. Persson *et al.* [11] reported an increased lactate and excitatory amino acids in the extracellular fluid in the frontal cortical tissue early after SAH, and this change might contribute to the pathology of frontal lobe. It is likely that a persistent lactic acidosis and increase of glutamate may directly damage or enhance the vulnerability of the tissue to secondary ischemia [11].

Metabolic Changes after Treatment. Numerous publications have reported endothelial and smooth muscle cell damage in animal models or in the patients suffering cerebral vasospasm, however, the mechanism and the pattern of cell death remains unclear [18]. The gradual onset and nonocclusive stenosis of cerebral arteries in vasospasm produces wide areas of marginal reduction in cerebral blood flow. This phenomenon is similar to the penumbra occurring after vascular occlusion [18]. It is more likely that this "mild stimulation" in vasospasm induces apoptosis rather than necrosis in endothelial cells. We have reported previously that oxyhemoglobin produces apoptosis in cultured endothelial cells [19], and in a patient died of cerebral vasoapsm [22]. Apoptosis in the endothelial layer and the detachment of endothleial cells expose internal lamina and collagen. The exposed internal lamina and collagen might trigger platelet activation and even thrombus formation. In the absence of endothelial barrier, neurotransmitters, toxins, and other vasoactive agents in the blood stream might activate receptors in smooth muscle and trigger contraction.

We have also demonstrated that mitogen-activated protein kinase (MAPK) is involved in cerebral vasospasm. Hemolysate and endothelin-1, causative agents for vasospasm, produced contraction and enhanced MAPK immunoprecipitation in rabbit basilar artery [20, 21]. A similar observation of MAPK involvement in cerebral vasospasm was reported in a dog double hemorrhage model [23]. MAPK activity was increased after the blood injection, and the activity peaked on day 2 and remained elevated for up to 7 days in canine basilar arteries.

Those studies offered rational of using MAPK and caspase inhibitors as a new treatment for cerebral vasospasm. In this study, MAPK and caspase inhibitors were administered intracisternally from day 3 through day 6 after double blood injections on days 0 and 2. The chosen approach was more clinically oriented to simulate the treatment of patients with vasospasm rather than beginning the treatment immediately after or prior to SAH. This study used a relatively lower concentration of MAPK and caspase inhibitors due to the uncertainty of their cytotoxicity. With the except of PD98059 is partially effective, none of the other inhibitors prevented or reversed vasospasm. Consistently, most of the metabolic alterations remain unchanged after treatment compared with CSF from day 7-SAH dogs. Even though the level of lactate was reduced by a MAPK inhibitor U0126 ($P < 0.05$), and the level of glutamate was reduced by caspase-3 inhibitor, the other metabolic products remained unaltered.

In conclusion, brain energy metabolites and excitative amino acids are altered during cerebral vasospasm. The metabolic changes in CSF are consistent with the time course of cerebral vasospasm. A decrease of glucose and an increase of glutamate, lactate, pyruvate in CSF reflected a state of cerebral ischemia and may aggravate cerebral ischemia caused by cerebral vasospasm.

Acknowledgments

This work was partially supported by a grant-in-aid to J.Z. from the American Heart Association.

References

1. Alessandri B, Doppenberg E, Bullock R (1999) Glucose and lactate metabolism after severe human head injury: influence of excitatory neurotransmitters and injury type. Acta Neurochir (Wien) 75: 21–24
2. Alessandri B, Doppenberg E, Zauner A (1999) Evidence for time-dependent glutamate-mediated glycolysis in head-injured patients: a microdialysis study. Acta Neurochir (Wien) 75: 25–28
3. Bennani NR, Jeandel C, Lefebvre E (1998) Abnormal substrate levels that depend upon mitochondrial function in cerebrospinal fluid from Alzheimer patients. Gerontology 44: 300–304
4. Dietrich HH, Dacey RG (2000) Molecular keys to the problems of cerebral vasospasm. Neurosurgery 46: 517–530
5. Fujikawa H, Tani E, Yamaura I (1999) Activation of protein kinases in canine basilar artery in vasospasm. J Cereb Blood Flow Metab 19: 44–52
6. Leblasnc MH, Qian XB, Cai ZW (1997) The effect of glucose during ishcemia on brain ATP, lacttate and glutamate in piglets. Biol Neunate 72: 243–254
7. Leib SL, Boscacci R, Gratzl O (1999) Predictive value of CSF lactate level versus CSF/Blood glucose ratio for the diagnosis of bacterial meningitis following neurosurgery. Clin Infec Dis 29: 69–77
8. Matsuishi T, Sakai T, Naito E (1996) Elevated cerebrospinal fluid lactate/pyruvate ratio in Machado-Joseph disease. Acta Neurol Scan 93: 72–75
9. Mayberg MR (1998) Cerebral vasospasm. Neurosurg Clin North Am 9: 615–627
10. Miyazaki M, Hashinoto T, Yoneda Y (1998) Adrenocorticotropic hormone therapy for infantile spasms alters pyruvate metabolism in the central nervous system. Brain Develop 20: 312–318
11. Nilsson OG, Brandt L, Ungerstedt U (1999) Bedside detection of brain ischemia using intracerebral microdialysis: subarachnoid hemorrhage and delayed ischemic deterioration. Neurosurgery 45: 1176–1181
12. Ogihara K, Zubkov AY, Bernanke DH (1999) Oxyhemoglobin-induced apoptosis in cultured endothelial cells. J Neurosurg 91: 459–465
13. Persson L, Valtysson J, Enblad P (1996) Neurochemical monitoring using intracerebral microdialysis in patients with subarachnoid hemorrhage. J Neurosurg 84: 606–616
14. Podell M, Hadjiconstantinou M (1997) Cerebraospinal fluid r-aminobutyric acid and glutamate values in dogs with epilepsy. Am J Vet Res 58: 451–459
15. Sehba FA, Ding WH, Chereshnev I (1999) Effects of s-Nitrosoglutathione on acute vasoconstriction and glutamate release after subarachnoid hemorrhage. Stroke 30: 1955–1961
16. Shiogai T, Nara I, Saruta K (1999) Continuous monitoring of cerebrospinal fluid acid-base balance and oxygen metabolism in patients with severe head injury: pathophysiology and treat-

ments for cerebral acidosis and ischemia. Acta Neurochir (Wien) 75: 49–55
17. Spranger M, Schhwab S, Kremppien S (1996) Excess glutamate levels in the cerebrospinal fluid predict clinical outcome of bacterial meningitis. Arch Neurol 53: 992–1011
18. Stover JF, Pleines UE, Morganti-kossmann MC (1997) Neurotransmitters in cerebrospinal fluid reflect pathological activity. Eur J Clin Invest 27: 1038–1046
19. Varsos VG, Liszczak TM, Han DH (1983) Delayed cerebral vasospasm is not reversible by aminophylline, nifedipine, or papaverine in a two hemorrhage canine model. J Neurosurg 58: 11–17
20. Yamamoto T, Rossi S, Stiefel M (1999) CSF and ECF glutamate concentrations in head injured patients. Acta Neurochir (Wien) 75: 17–19
21. Zubkov AY, Ogihara K, Tumu P (1999) Mitogen-activated protein kinase mediation of hemolysate-induced contracton in rabbit basilar artery. J Neurosurg 90: 1091–1097
22. Zubkov AY, Ogihara K, Bernanke DH (2000) Apoptosis of endothelial cells in vessels affected by cerebral vasospasm. Surg Neurol 53: 260–266
23. Zubkov AY, Rollins KS, Parent AD (2000) Mechanism of endothelin-1-induced contraction in rabbit basilar artery. Stroke 31: 526–533

Correspondence: John H. Zhang, M.D., Ph.D., Department of Neurosurgery, University of Mississippi Medical Center, 2500 North State Street, Jackson, MS, 39216-4505.

Acta Neurochir (2002) [Suppl] 81: 265–268

Effect of Ischemic Preconditioning on Edema Formation and Cerebrovascular Injury Following Focal Cerebral Ischemia

T. Masada[1], **Y. Hua**[1], **G. Xi**[1], **S. R. Ennis**[1], and **R. F. Keep**[1,2]

[1] Department of Surgery (Neurosurgery), University of Michigan, Ann Arbor, Michigan, USA
[2] Department of Physiology, University of Michigan, Ann Arbor, Michigan, USA

Summary

Many studies have shown that a brief period of ischemia can protect against a subsequent severe ischemic event and this has been termed ischemic preconditioning (IPC). Most studies have been focused on neuroprotection, with only a little attention on cerebrovascular effects. This study examines the effect of IPC, induced by 15 minutes of middle cerebral artery occlusion (MCAO) in the rat, on brain edema formation and cerebrovascular injury induced by a permanent MCAO induced three days later. Brain edema formation was significantly reduced in IPC treated rats compared to non-IPC treated rats. IPC-treated rats also had reduced blood-brain barrier disruption and reduced cerebrovascular expression of heat shock protein 70, a marker of cell stress. These results indicate that IPC reduces cerebrovascular injury from subsequent permanent focal cerebral ischemia. Understanding the mechanisms involved may provide new therapeutic strategies for stroke.

Keywords: Focal cerebral ischemial; blood-brain barrier; heat shock protein 70.

Introduction

Ischemic preconditioning (IPC), or ischemic tolerance, describes a phenomenon whereby a brief period of ischemia can protect against a subsequent prolonged ischemic event. First shown in brain with models of global ischemia [5], it has also been shown to occur in models of focal ischemia [2]. Most studies have been focused on neuroprotection following IPC. Little attention was paid to vascular effects although cerebral edema is important in determining morbidity and mortality following cerebral ischemia [1] and cerebral hemorrhage (i.e. endothelial cell dysfunction) is a major limitation on the use of tissue plasminogen activator treatment for cerebral ischemia [7]. This study, therefore, was designed to examine the effect of IPC on edema formation and cerebrovascular injury following middle cerebral artery occlusion (MCAO) in the rat. Cerebrovascular injury was assessed by measurement of blood-brain barrier (BBB) permeability to [^{3}H]inulin and by examining heat shock protein 70 (HSP70) immunoreactivity in the vasculature. HSP70 is a marker of cell stress, including endothelial cell stress [6], as well as being a potential protective agent.

Materials and Methods

The protocols in this study were approved by the University of Michigan Committee on the Use and Care of Animals. Male Sprague-Dawley rats, with final weights between 275–350 g, were used in these experiments. Animals were anesthetized with pentobarbital (40 mg/kg ip.) and either underwent IPC, 15 min of transient MCAO, using the thread method of Zea Longa [8] or a sham occlusion. They were then allowed to recover. After 3 days, both sets of rats underwent permanent thread MCAO, again using the method of Zea Longa. They were then used for measurement of either infarct volume (24 hours after the permanent occlusion), brain edema (at 24 hours), BBB permeability (at 6 hours) or the number of HSP70 immunoreactive blood vessels (at 0–24 hours after permanent occlusion).

Infarct Volume

Twenty-four hours after permanent MCA occlusion, seven IPC-treated and eight non-IPC treated rats were decapitated and the brains rapidly removed. The brains were sliced at 2 mm intervals prior to staining with 2,3,5-triphenyltetrazolium (TTC) for determination of infarct volume.

Brain Edema

Twenty-four hours after permanent MCAO, eight IPC-treated and nine non-IPC treated rats were decapitated and the brains rapidly removed. The cerebral cortices ipsi- and contralateral to the MCA occlusion were divided into core, intermediate and outer zones depending on their relation to the MCA as described in Dickinson and Betz [3]. Water content of these samples was determined by the wet weight-dry weight method, and sodium content by flame photometry.

Blood-Brain Barrier Permeability

Six hours after permanent MCAO, seven IPC-treated and six non-IPC treated rats were used to measure the BBB [^{3}H]inulin permeability. An influx rate constant (K_i) was measured using a method similar to that described in Dickinson and Betz [3], using a 30 min circulation time for [^{3}H]inulin and a 2 min circulation time for [^{14}C]inulin, which was used to correct for vascular volume. Brain sampling was as for edema measurements.

Immunohistochemistry

IPC and non-IPC treated rats were sacrificed after different durations (0, 3, 6 and 24 hours) of permanent ischemia for HSP70 immunohistochemistry. The brains underwent transcardiac fixation prior to sectioning (50 μm) on a vibratome. A 1:500 dilution of the primary antibody (mouse anti-rat HSP70, StressGen) and a 1:800 dilution of the second antibody (biotinylated goat anti-mouse IgG, Chemicon) were used.

Statistics

Data are presented as means ± S.E. Data were analyzed by Student's t-test and statistical significance was accepted at $p < 0.05$.

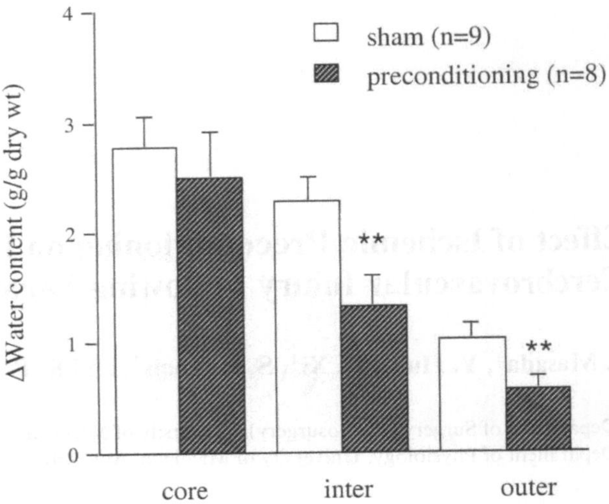

Fig. 1. The difference in water content between ipsi-and contralateral tissue samples 24 hours after permanent MCAO. Core, intermediate and outer zones were sampled from rats that had undergone ischemic preconditioning or a sham operation three days prior to permanent MCAO. Values are means ± S.E., n = 8–9. ** indicates a significant difference between the sham and preconditioning groups at the $p < 0.01$ level

Results

There were no significant differences in blood pH, glucose, pO_2, pCO_2, or hematocrit between the IPC and non-IPC treated animals. Rats that underwent IPC had significantly smaller infarcts after 24 hours of permanent MCAO than non-IPC treated animals (253 ± 42 vs, 431 ± 31 mm [3]; $p < 0.01$). They also had significantly less edema formation in the intermediate and outer zones, although edema formation in the core zone was not significantly different (Fig. 1). Contralateral brain water content was unaffected by IPC. The reduced edema formation in the intermediate and outer zones in IPC-treated rats was matched by a reduction in the accumulation of sodium during ischemia. Thus, in the intermediate zone, the difference in sodium content between ipsi- and contralateral hemispheres was 487 ± 47 mEq/kg dry weight in non-IPC treated rats but only 288 ± 63 mEq/kg in IPC treated rats ($p < 0.05$). Similarly, in the outer zone, the differences were 193 ± 34 mEq/kg dry weight in non-IPC treated rats but only 109 ± 27 mEq/kg in IPC treated rats ($p < 0.05$).

To examine whether the reduction in edema formation with IPC was associated with reduced cerebrovascular injury, the K_i for [^{3}H]inulin uptake into brain was measured. In non-IPC treated rats, six hours of permanent MCAO resulted in a 3-fold increase in K_i in the ipsilateral core compared to the contralateral hemisphere (Fig. 2a) and smaller increases in the intermediate and outer zones (data not shown). In rats that underwent IPC, this increase in permeability in the core was markedly attenuated (Fig. 2a), as was the increase in the intermediate and outer zones (data not shown). This attenuated BBB disruption was associated with a reduction in the number of HSP70 immunoreactive blood vessels found following permanent MCAO (Fig. 2b). Such vessels were found in the cortex three, six and twenty-four hours after the onset of MCAO in non-IPC treated rats. At each of those time points, IPC treated rats had significantly fewer HSP70 immunoreactive blood vessels.

Discussion

This study demonstrates that IPC markedly reduces the brain edema formation and the cerebrovascular injury that follows a subsequent period of permanent focal cerebral ischemia. A reduction in cerebrovascular injury with IPC was demonstrated by both a marked attenuation in BBB disruption and a reduced number of blood vessels expressing the stress protein HSP70 with IPC.

Edema formation following cerebral ischemia is commonly thought to have cytotoxic and vasogenic components [1]. The reduction in BBB disruption (as assessed by the [^{3}H]inulin) indicates that there may be

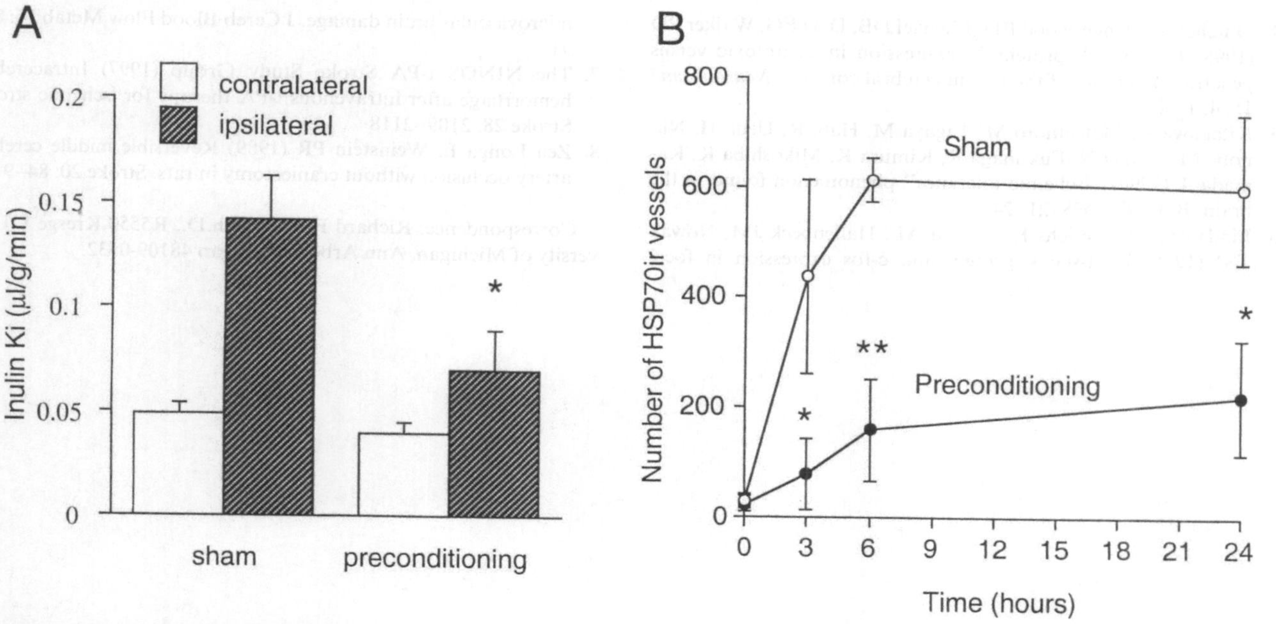

Fig. 2. Comparison of cerebrovascular injury in rats undergoing ischemic preconditioning or a sham operation three days prior to permanent MCAO. (A) The influx rate constant (K_i) for [^{3}H]inulin in ipsi- and contralateral core samples six hours after permanent MCAO. Values are means ± S.E., n = 6–7, * indicates $p < 0.05$ vs. sham. (B) The number of heat shock protein 70 immunoreactive blood vessels at different times after permanent MCAO. Values are means ± S.E. of counts from a coronal section (2.2 mm anterior from Bregma), n = 3–4, * indicates $p < 0.05$ vs. sham, ** indicates $p < 0.01$ vs. sham

a reduction in the vasogenic component. However, IPC also reduced infarct volume, suggesting that there may also be a reduction in cytotoxic edema formation.

That there is a reduction in both infarct size and cerebrovascular injury with IPC raises questions as to whether there is a link between these two phenomena. Is the reduction in cerebrovascular injury due to less parenchymal cell injury? Two observations suggest that this is not the case. 1) Parenchymal cell injury induced by excitotoxic amino acids does not appear to induce vascular HSP70 (e.g. [4]) suggesting that ischemia-induced vascular HSP70 may be a direct effect of ischemia on the vasculature. 2) The effect of IPC on infarct volume is primarily penumbral [2] whereas in the current study there was a marked effect on BBB permeability in the core of the MCA territory. Conversely, is the reduction in parenchymal cell injury due to less cerebrovascular injury? The neuroprotective effect of IPC does not appear to be related to an increase in cerebral blood flow [2], but it is possible that reducing BBB disruption may prevent the entry of potentially harmful compounds from blood to brain. It appears, however, most likely that IPC has independent protective effects on the vasculature and on parenchymal cells. It should be noted that many of the mechanisms that have been proposed to be involved in IPC, such as an upregulation in free radical scavengers and inhibitors of inflammation, are likely to have effects on multiple cell types.

In conclusion, this study has demonstrated that IPC reduces cerebral edema formation and cerebrovascular injury during subsequent permanent focal cerebral ischemia. Understanding the mechanisms involved may provide new therapeutic windows for stroke.

Acknowledgment

This study was supported by grants NS-34709 and NS-39866 from the National Institutes of Health.

References

1. Betz AL (1996) Alterations in cerebral endothelial cell function in ischemia. Advances in neurology. In: Siesjo BK, Wieloch T (eds) Lippincott-Raven, Philadelphia, pp 301–313
2. Chen J, Graham SH, Zhu RL, Simon RP (1996) Stress proteins and tolerance to focal cerebral ischemia. J Cereb Blood Flow Metab 16: 566–577
3. Dickinson LD, Betz AL (1992) Attenuated development of ischemic edema in vasopressin-deficient rats. J Cereb Blood Flow Metab 12: 681–690

4. Dutcher SA, Underwood BD, Michael DB, Diaz FG, Walker PD (1998) Heat shock protein 72 expression in excitotoxic versus penetrating injuries of the rodent cerebral cortex. *J Neurotrauma* 15: 421–432
5. Kitagawa K, Matsumoto M, Tagaya M, Hata R, Ueda H, Niinobe M, Handa N, Fukunaga R, Kimura K, Mikoshiba K, Kamada T (1990) "Ischemic tolerance" phenomenon found in the brain. Brain Res 528: 21–24
6. Lindsberg PJ, Frerichs KU, Siren AL, Hallenbeck JM, Nowak TSJ (1996) Heat-shock protein and c-fos expression in focal microvascular brain damage. J Cereb Blood Flow Metab 16: 82–91
7. The NINDS t-PA Stroke Study Group (1997) Intracerebral hemorrhage after intravenous t-PA therapy for ischemic stroke. Stroke 28: 2109–2118
8. Zea Longa E, Weinstein PR (1989) Reversible middle cerebral artery occlusion without craniectomy in rats. Stroke 20: 84–91

Correspondence: Richard F. Keep, Ph.D., R5550 Kresge I, University of Michigan, Ann Arbor, Michigan 48109-0532.

Acta Neurochir (2002) [Suppl] 81: 269–270

ICP Monitoring Following Bilateral Carotid Occlusion in GFAP-Null Mice

H. Nawashiro[1], S. Huang[1], M. Brenner[2], K. Shima[1], and J.-M. Hallenbeck[3]

[1] Department of Neurosurgery, National Defense Medical College, Saitama, Japan
[2] Department of Neurobiology and Department of Physical Medicine & Rehabilitation University of Alabama at Birmingham
[3] Stroke Branch, NINDS, NIH Bethesda, USA

Summary

To investigate the possible role of glial fibrillary acidic protein (GFAP) in cerebral ischemia, we have monitored the intracranial pressure (ICP) and local cerebral blood flow (lCBF) following bilateral carotid artery occlusion (BCAO) in GFAP-null mice and their wild type littermates. GFAP-null mice (B6,129-G*fap*^{tmlMes}) were obtained from Jackson Laboratories. The ICP and lCBF was continuously monitored during 15 minutes BCAO and reperfusion. The variation of the circle of Willis was also investigated in both GFAP-null and wild type mice. The breakdown of blood brain barrier (BBB) was assessed by immunohistochemical staining against mouse immunogloblins (IgG). A significantly more profound and immediate decrease in lCBF after BCAO was observed in GFAP-null mice ($p < 0.04$, ANOVA). GFAP-null mice also showed a significant increase (% change) in ICP after reperfusion ($p < 0.05$, ANOVA). There were no gross differences in the circle of Willis between GFAP-null and wild type mice. No abnormal IgG immunoreactivity was observed in the forebrain of both animals. These results indicate a high susceptibility to cerebral ischemia in GFAP-null mice and suggest an important role for astrocytes and GFAP in the progress of ischemic brain damage and increased ICP after cerebral ischemia with reperfusion.

Keywords: Glial fibrillary acidic protein; mice; cerebral ischemia; intracranial pressure.

Introduction

Astrocytes perform a variety of neuroprotective function in the adult brain. Glial fibrillary acidic protein (GFAP) is an astrocyte specific intermediate filament component. To investigate the possible roles of GFAP in cerebral ischemia, we have monitored the intracranial pressure (ICP) and local cerebral blood flow (lCBF) following bilateral carotid artery occlusion (BCAO) in GFAP-null mice and their wild type littermates. The breakdown of blood brain barrier (BBB) was also assessed by immunohistochemical staining against mouse immunoglobulins (IgG).

Materials and Methods

GFAP-Null Mice

GFAP-null mice (B6,129-G*fap*^{tmlMes})[6] were obtained from Jackson Laboratories (Bar Harbor, Maine, USA). Mice of mixed B6,129 genetic background heterozygous for the GFAP-null allele were crossed to generate the homozygous GFAP-null mice and wild type littermates used for these experiments [3]. Mature mice weighing 19.0 to 24.3 g from several different litters were included in the study.

Bilateral Transient Carotid Artery Occlusion

Animals were anesthetized with 2% halothane for induction and 1.0% halothane for maintenance in 30% O2 and 70% N2O through a face mask. The right femoral artery was catheterized with a PE-10 polyethylene tube for continuous monitoring of arterial blood pressure. A 10 mm cervical ventral midline skin incision was made. The bilateral common carotid arteries were exposed and isolated. A micro aneurysmal clip, 85 gr pressure (Roboz Surgical Instrument, Rockville, MD, USA) was applied to the common carotid artery for 15 minutes. Reperfusion of the carotid artery was visually confirmed with the operating microscope. Body and temporal muscle temperature were monitored and maintained at 36.5 °C to 37.5 °C during and after occlusion for 15 minutes.

Measurement of Intracranial Pressure and Local Cerebral Blood Flow

The ICP, lCBF and mean arterial blood pressure was continuously monitored during 15 minutes bilateral carotid occlusion and reperfusion. ICP was measured using a Codman ICP micro-sensor that was placed over the right frontal cortex (2 mm lateral to the midline and 1 mm anterior to the bregma). lCBF was measured by laser-Doppler flowmetry (LFN-50; Biomedical Science, Kanazawa, Japan) placed over the contralateral frontal cortex.

Comparison of Cerebrovascular Anatomy

To investigate the difference in cerebrovascular anatomy, the circle of Willis was visualized using carbon black in GFAP-null mice ($n = 6$) and wild-type littermates ($n = 7$). After receiving deep anesthesia, animals were given an intracardiac injection of carbon black and then killed.

Assessment of the Breakdown of BBB by Immunohistochemical Staining for Mouse Immunoglobulins

Twenty-four hours after the insult, the mice were injected with a lethal dose of thiopental (150 mg per kilogram of body mass, i.p.) and fixed transcardially by perfusion with 4% paraformaldehyde in 150 mM NaCl and 50 mM sodium phosphate (pH 7.4) (PBS). The adequacy of perfusion was confirmed by the absence of intravascular blood on light microscopy. Paraffin-embedded 3-μm-thick tissue sections were used for conventional histology and immonohistochemistry. After removal of paraffin with xylene, endogenous peroxidase activity was blocked by incubation in 3% hydrogen peroxide for 10 min at room temperature, and nonspecific antibody binding was blocked by incubation with normal rabbit serum for 20 minutes at room temperature. The sections were then incubated for 1 h with a polyclonal rabbit antibody to mouse IgG. The sections were washed with PBS, treated with biotinylated gout anti-rabbit immunoglobulin for 10 min, washed with PBS again, incubated with peroxidase-labeled streptavidin for 5 min, and finally incubated with 3,3′-diaminobenzidine solution.

Ethics

Procedures involving animals were approved by the National Defense Medical College Animal Care and Use Committee and were consistent with the Japanese Experimental Animal Research Association standards as defined in the Guidelines for Animal Experiments (1987).

Results

A significantly more profound and immediate decrease in lCBF after BCO was observed in GFAP-null mice ($n = 6$) ($p < 0.04$, ANOVA followed by Bonerroi/Dunn test). GFAP-null mice also showed a significant increase (% change) in ICP after reperfusion ($p < 0.05$, ANOVA followed by Bonerroi/Dunn test). There were no gross differences in the circle of Willis between GFAP-null ($n = 6$) and wild type mice ($n = 7$). No breakdown of the BBB to endogenous IgG was detected in the forebrains of both animals.

Discussion

In the previous study, we have found that GFAP-null mice were more sensitive to middle cerebral artery occlusion (MCAO) with transient carotid artery occlusion than were wild-type littermates [4]. The result suggested that astrocytes normally provided a protective function after ischemia, and that this function was compromised in GFAP-null mice. An alternative explanation was that the absence of GFAP results in malfunctioning of the central nervous system causing greater sensitivity to ischemia. There were multiple candidate functions attributed to astrocytes that could affect neuronal survival after ischemia, including regulation of extracellular glutamate and potassium, contributing to the BBB, and control of brain volume. The breakdown of the BBB does not seem to be a possible mechanism of increased susceptibility to cerebral ischemia in GFAP-null mice because we observed no exaggerated breakdown of BBB after reperfusion in this animal model of cerebral ischemia. Rapid swelling of perivascular astrocytes was one potential mechanism for the greater drop in lCBF in the GFAP-null mice during BCAO. Normal matured astrocytes have been shown to undergo swelling within 30 minutes of MCAO [2], and the absence of GFAP may increase the susceptibility of these cells to cytotoxic edema [1]. Further study will be needed to clarify the morphological evidence of cellular swelling or the quantitative measurement of the extracellular space after cerebral ischemia in GFAP-null mice and wild type littermates.

Conclusion

These results indicate a high susceptibility to cerebral ischemia in GFAP-null mice and suggest an important role for astrocytes and GFAP in the progress of ischemic brain damage and increased ICP after cerebral ischemia with reperfusion.

References

1. Ding M, Eliasson C, Betsholtz C, Hamberger A, Pekny M (1998) Altered taurine release following hypotonic stress in astrocytes from mice deficient for GFAP and vimentin. Brain Res Mol Brain Res 12: 77–91
2. Garcia JH, Liu KF, Yoshida Y, Chen S, Lian J (1994) Brain microvessels: factors altering their patency after the occlusion of a middle cerebral artery (Wistar Rat) Am J Pathol 145: 728–740
3. McCall MA, Gregg RG, Behringer RR, Brenner M, Delaney CL, Galbreath EJ, Zhang CL, Pearce RA, Chiu SY, Messing A (1996) Targeted deletion in astrocyte intermediate filament (Gfap) alters neuronal physiology. Proc Natl Acad Sci USA 93: 6361–6366
4. Nawashiro H, Brenner M, Fukui S, Shima K, Hallenbeck JM (2000) High susceptibility to cerebral ischemia in GFAP-null mice. J Cereb Blood Flow Metab (in press)

Correspondence: Hiroshi Nawashiro, M.D., D.M.Sc., Department of Neurosurgery, National Defense Medical College, 3-2 Namiki, Tokorozawa, 359-8513 Saitama, Japan.

Acta Neurochir (2002) [Suppl] 81: 271–273

Spinal Cerebrospinal Fluid Pathways and their Significance for the Compensation of Kaolin-Hydrocephalus

W. Luedemann[1], **D. Kondziella**[1], **K. Tienken**[2], **P. Klinge**[1], **T. Brinker**[1], and **D. Berens von Rautenfeld**[2]

[1] Department of Neurosurgery, Medical School Hannover, Hannover, Germany
[2] Department of Anatomy, Medical School Hannover, Hannover, Germany

Summary

Aim. To study the mechanisms of CSF-outflow in hydrocephalus we used radiological and histological methods to examine pathways of CSF absorbtion.

Two, four and six weeks after occlusion of the cisterna magna by kaolin solution, CSF-dynamics were determined. Direct magnification radiography was used to visualize the outflow of X-ray contrast. Ten rats in each group were sacrificed for histological analysis following ventricular perfusion with marker proteins.

ICP was increased to 15 ± 1 mmHg (mean ± SD) compared to control animals (7 ± 2 mmHg) in the four week group. Six weeks following kaolin injection no increase in ICP (6 ± 1 mmHg) could be demonstrated. Outflow resistance was markedly raised in all animals (1074 ± 315 mmHg min^{-1} ml^{-1}) displaying highest values (2160 ± 960) in the four week group as compared to control animals (504 ± 71). Cisternography demonstrated blocked cranial absorption and CSF-outflow along lumbosacral nerve roots.

Histological examination showed syrinx formation in the cervical and thoracic spinal cord. Marker proteins left the subarachnoid space along thoracic and lumbo-sacral spinal rootlets.

The radiological and histological findings and the normalisation of ICP after six weeks at doubled CSF-outflow resistance indicated a recruitment of spinal perineural CSF outflow pathways for the compensation of the disturbed cranial CSF-absorption.

Keywords: Hydrocephalus; CSF-absorption; syringomyelia.

Introduction

The absorption of cerebrospinal fluid (CSF) takes place in the arachnoid granulations into the venous sinus [7, 8], but also into the lymphatics [5] along the cranial nerves [3, 4], resp. along spinal nerves and major intracranial vessels [9].

Recent studies underline the quantitative importance of lymphatic CSF-absorption in comparison with the blood vascular load. In sheep more than 50% of an intracranial injected markerprotein was found in lymphatic vessels [1].

To investigate the significance of these alternative CSF-pathways for the compensation of hydrocephalus, we used the kaolin-induced hydrocephalus in the rat. Special attention was paid to the spinal CSF-pathways.

Material and Methods

Hydrocephalus was induced under general anesthesia in 30 rats by injection of 0.1 ml saturated kaolin solution through the atlanto-occipital membrane using microsurgical technique. Two, four and six weeks after occlusion of the cisterna magna CSF-outflow dynamics (i.e. ICP, pressure dependent outflow resistance curve [2]) were determined using a ventricular perfusion with continuous ICP-monitoring. Direct magnification radiography (Feinfocus, Garbsen, Germany) was used to visualize the outflow of X-ray contrast after ventricular infusion.

Ten rats in each group were sacrificed for histological and ultrastructural analysis following ventricular infusion under controlled ICP elevation up to 25 mmHg with the low molecular ferritin (cathionized ferritin, 2.5 mg in a total infusion volume of 0.5 ml) and the high molecular marker protein horseradish peroxidase (HRP, 2.3 mg in a total infusion volume of 0.5 ml).

Results

Intracranial pressure (ICP) is increased up to 15 ± 1 mmHg (mean ± SE) compared to control animals (7 ± 2 mmHg) in the four week group. Two weeks after induction the ICP was 9 ± 1 mmHg. Six weeks following kaolin injection no increase in ICP (6 ± 1 mmHg) could be demonstrated anymore. Outflow resistance was markedly raised in all animals (1074 ± 315 mmHg min^{-1} ml^{-1}) displaying highest

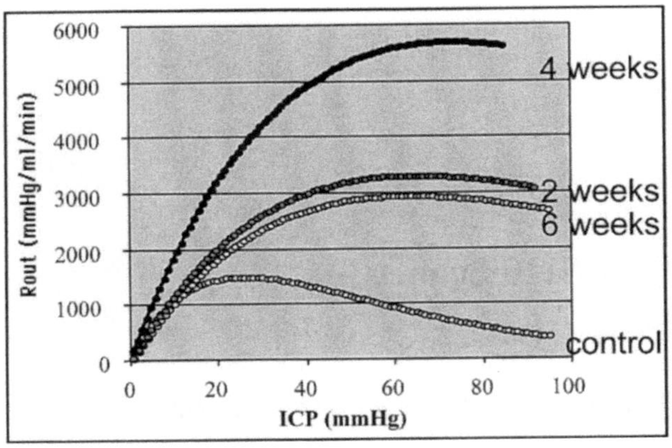

Fig. 1. Pressure/Resistance plots, demonstrating the increasing and decreasing impairment of CSF-absorption in the time-course of kaolin hydrocephalus

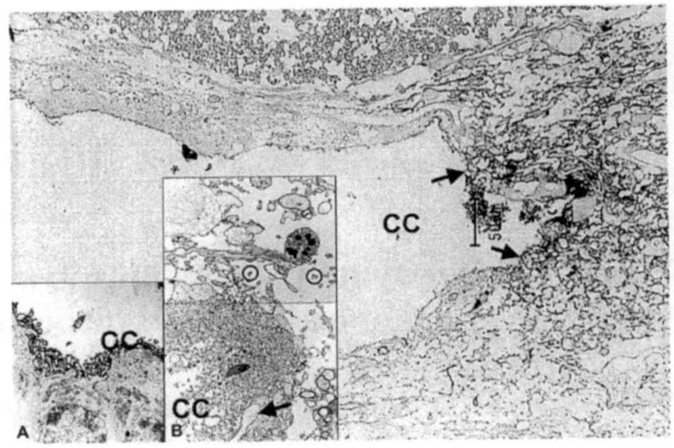

Fig. 2. Microscopic view of the central canal (*CC*) of the thoracic spinal cord. The picture shows the rupture of the central canal lining with ferritin (circles) passing between the ependymal layers (arrows), ×100. Inset A: Transmission electron microscopic view of normal ependymal layer with apical ferritin particles ×8000. Inset B: Transmission electron microscopic view of ruptured ependymal layer (arrows) with ferritin particles (circles) passing through ×15000

values (2160 ± 960) in the four week group as compared to control animals (504 ± 71). The pressure dependent outflow resistance curves (Fig. 1.) confirmed the initial increased values and the decrease in the six week group.

Cisternography demonstrated the blocked cranial absorption and contrasting syrinx formation of the cervical and thoracic spinal cord. The central canal was enlarged and communicated with the enlarged ventricles. The spinal subarachnoid space was contrasted in the thoracic and lumbosacral region.

Histological examination showed syrinx formation predominantely in the cervical spinal cord. The enlarged central canal was partly ruptured and marker proteins were found penetrating the spinal cord (Fig. 2.). In these areas ferritin particles were detectable in the spinal cord, predominantly in the dorsal column. Ferritin particles were also found around the spinal nerves.

Discussion

The results presented show that spinal CSF-absorption plays an important role under pathological conditions. It has a surprising capacity to compensate for CSF circulation disturbances. Previous studies have shown the dilation of the central canal [6], but were not able to detect tracer proteins. In this study it was achieved to demonstrate the spinal CSF-outflow pathway through the central canal to the spinal subarachnoid space and into the spinal funnels. The spinal CSF-absorption is suggested to be mainly into the lymphatics [10].

It is unknown, whether spinal CSF-absorption is important under physiological conditions or even in humans. With the upright gait and the changing hydrostatic pressures man could have different characteristics of the spinal absorption areas. The significance of spinal CSF absorption might be the explanation for hydrocephalic conditions in spinal pathologies.

References

1. Boulton M, Flessner M, Armstrong D, Hay J, Johnston M (1997) Lymphatic drainage of the CNS: effects of lymphatic diversion/ligation on CSF protein transport to plasma. Am J Physiol 272: R1613–1619
2. Brinker T, Beck H, Klinge P, Oi S, Samii M (1998) Sinusoidal Intrathecal Infusion for Assessment of CSF Dynamics in Kaolin-Induced Hydrocephalus. Acta Neurochir (Wien) 140: 1069–1075
3. Brinker T, Ludemann W, von Rautenfeld DB, Brassel F, Becker H, Samii M (1997) Breakdown of the meningeal barrier surrounding the intraorbital optic nerve after experimental subarachnoid hemorrhage. Am J Ophthalmol 124: 373–380
4. Brinker T, Luedemann W, von Rautenfeld D, Samii M (1997) Dynamic properties of lymphatic pathways for the absorption of cerebrospinal fluid. Acta Neuropathol 94: 493–498
5. Foldi M, Csillik B, Zoltan OT (1968) Lymphatic drainage of the brain. Experientia 24: 1283–1287
6. Hochwald GM, Nakamura S, Camins MB (1981) The rat in experimental obstructive hydrocephalus. Z Kinderchir 34: 403–410

7. Key E, MG. R (1875) (eds) Studien in der Anatomie des Nervensystems und des Bindegewebes. Samson&Wallin, Stockholm
8. Tripathi R (1973) Ultrastructure of the arachnoid mater in relation to outflow of cerebrospinal fluid. Lancet ii: 8–11
9. Weller RO, Kida S, Zhang ET (1992) Pathways of fluid drainage from the brain – morphological aspects and immunological significance in rat and man. Brain Pathol 2: 277–284
10. Zenker W, Bankoul S, Braun JS (1994) Morphological indications for considerable diffuse reabsorption of cerebrospinal fluid in spinal meninges particularly in the areas of meningeal funnels. An electronmicroscopical study including tracing experiments in rats. Anat Embryol (Berl) 189: 243–258

Correspondence: Wolf Luedemann, M.D., Departement of Neurosurgery, Medical School Hannover, OE 7240, Carl Neubergstr.1, D-30625 Hannover, Germany.

Acta Neurochir (2002) [Suppl] 81: 275–277

Temporal and Regional Profile of Neuronal and Glial Cellular Injury after Induction of Kaolin Hydrocephalus

P. Klinge[1], A. Mühlendyck[1], S. Lee[1], W. Lüdemann[1], S. Groos[2], M. Samii[1], and T. Brinker[1]

[1] Department of Neurosurgery, Medical School and Nordstadt Hospital, Hannover, Germany
[2] Institute of Functional Anatomy, Medical School Hannover, Germany

Summary

Aim. To study regional and temporal pattern of glial and neuronal reaction to induction of kaolin hydrocephalus in adult rats.

Emzyme- and immunohistochemistry was performed in 20 adult rats with kaolin-hydrocephalus after 2, 4, 6 and 8 weeks to glial glutamatergic transmission activity (GLDH) and neuronal nitrous oxide synthetic activity (nNOS). Also, glial fibrillary acidic protein (GFAP), 68 kd neurofilament protein (NF68) and synaptophysin (SYN38) and basic fibroblastic growth-factor (bFGF) were stained. Results were quantified by imaging analysis (SCION IMAGE©) and expressed as relative immunopositive area.

After 2 weeks, nNos-activity increased in cortical and hippocampal neurones (CA1 and CA3) and GLDH-activity also showed increases, most significant in periventricular white matter (25.7 ± 3.8 vs. 15.5 ± 4.9; $p < 0.001$) and hippocampus ($p < 0.01$). After 4 or 6 weeks, global cortical GLDH-activity showed further marked increases (25.7 ± 3.9 vs. 11.3 ± 1.5; $p < 0.05$), while sustained structural changes have occurred: GFAP decreased in periventricular (3.3 ± 0.5 vs. 6.3 ± 1.2; $p < 0.01$), hippocampal and cortical astrocytes (0.9 ± 0.34 vs. $5.0 \pm 0.7\%$; $p < 0.01$), whereas NF68 in cortical efferent neurones increased ($6.5 \pm 1.5\%$ vs. 4.7 ± 0.1; $p < 0.01$) followed by a decrease in cortical and hippocampal (CA1) SYN 38 ($p < 0.05$).

Acute glial and neuronal reactions were almost functional and in chronic stages sustained structural changes predominated. Since neuronal reactions were pronounced in selective vulnerable areas glial reaction was not restricted to periventricular astrocytes.

Keywords: Kaoline hydrocephalus; selective vulnerability; immunostaining; astrocytes.

Introduction

"Periventricular gliosis" is generally regarded as pathognomonic to the astrocytic response after induction of experimental hydrocephalus [2]. Although, morphologically well described, there are still controversies about its pathophysiological mechanisms and whether there is any relevance to neuronal function and neurological impairment in hydrocephalus disease [2]. Therefore we performed enzyme- and immunocyto-chemical studies on regional and temporal relationship of the glial and neuronal response to induction of kaolin hydrocephalus.

Material and Methods

Twenty (5 controls) adult rats (Sprague-Dawley 280–320 g) were investigated 2 (acute), 4 (subacute), 6 and 8 (chronic) weeks after injection of 0.01 ml kaolin (4.5 I.E.) into the cisterna magna. For histological processing the animals were anaesthetised with Isoflurane® and euthanasised with 35 I.E. Ketamine ®, brains were removed in toto, cut into three sections (bregma level: −3.3 mm and −5.5 mm) and fresh-frozen in isopentane ® chilled nitrous (−70 °C). After embedding in a cryomatrix, specimens were stored at −80 °C. Kryosections (5 μm) were mounted on Poly-L-Lysine®-coated slides and stored at −21 °C after drying for 3–4 hours at room temperature. Immunostaining was performed using peroxidase-anti-peroxidase techniques. The following antibodies for investigation of functional and structural cellular reactions were used:

- anti-Glial Fibrillary Acidic Protein (GFAP; polyclonal 1:200)
- anti-Neurofilament 68 (68 kd-subunit) (NF 68; monoclonal 1:1000)
- anti-Synaptophysin 38 (SYN38; monoclonal 1:20)
- anti-Neuronal Nitrous-oxide-synthase (nNOS; polyclonal 1:400)
- anti-Basic Fibroblastic-growth-factor (bFGF; monoclonal 1:200)

For enzyme histochemical studies of astrocytic glutamat dehydrogenase-activity (GLDH) kryosections were immediately processed [3]. Histological sections were viewed with the aid of a photomicroscope (×40 or ×20 objective) and digitally captured. A public-domain image-analysis program (Scion-Image©) was used to quantify staining results. The immunoreactive area was expressed as relative area of positive staining per optical field (black pixels) or as the degree of blackening (density) regarding GLDH-staining. Statistics were performed by Anova post-hoc testing (Fisher's PLSD).

Results

In the acute phase (2 weeks) increased nNos-activity in cortical and hippocampal neurones (CA1 and CA3) was observed (Fig. 1.). Parallel, enzymatic activity of

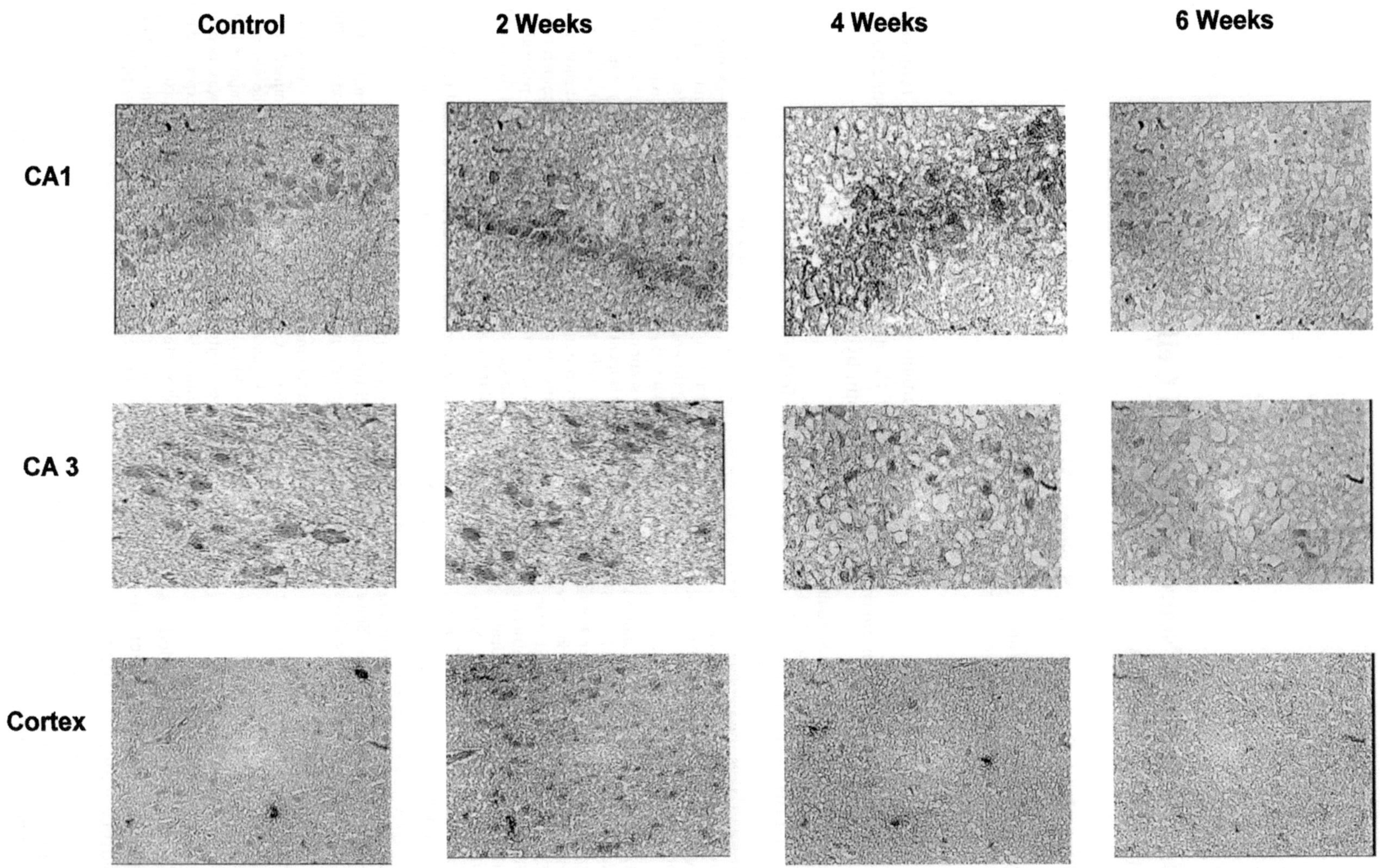

Fig. 1. Time course of nitrous oxide synthase (nNOS) in the stratum pyramidale of the CA1- and CA3-section and superficial cortex: in the acute period neuronal enzymatic activity was increased in vulnerable areas (CA1 > CA3) and disappeared in the subacute and chronic stages (×40 objective magnification)

GLDH in astrocytes showed increases, however, most significant in periventricular white matter (25.7 ± 3.8 vs. 15.5 ± 4.9 8 (controls); $p < 0.001$) and hippocampus (30.7 ± 7.4 vs. 15.3 ± 4.2 (controls); $p < 0.01$). In CA1, also immunoreactivity to NF 68 (4.5 ± 0.2 vs. 6.5 ± 0.13 (control); $p < 0.01$) and SYN 38 (0.03 ± 0.01 vs. 0.1 ± 0.05 (control); $p < 0.05$) was reduced. While neuronal enzymatic activity (nNos) decreased in subacute stages (4 weeks), further global increases in enzymatic activity of astrocytes (GLDH) was observed, specifically in the cortex (25.7 ± 3.9 (6 weeks) vs. 11.3 ± 1.5 (control); $p < 0.05$). This was paralleled by sustained structural changes in cortical neurones: Immunoreactivity against NF 68 increased in pyramidal neurones, specifically in the frontal and parietal cortex (6.5 ± 1.5 (4 and 6 w) vs. 4.7 ± 0.1 (control); $p < 0.01$). Also, bFGF-activity in cortical areas (3.9 ± 0.5 (6 w) vs. 2.3 ± 0.3 (4 w); $p < 0.05$) was found which was followed by a dramatic decrease of synaptophysin in CA1 and superficial cortex after 8 weeks (0.7 ± 0.2 vs. 2.0 ± 1.2 (control); $p < 0.05$); (Fig. 2). In late stages (6 and 8 weeks), also structural changes in astrocytes were predominating with overall significant reductions in GFAP-staining in peri-ventricular (3.3 ± 0.5 (4 w) vs. 6.3 ± 1.2 (control); $p < 0.01$), hippo-campal (2.9 ± 0.4 (4 w) vs. 5.7 ± 0.9 (control)%; $p < 0.05$) and cortical astrocytes (0.9 ± 0.34 (6 w) vs. 5.0 ± 0.7 (control); $p < 0.01$); figure 2.

Discussion

Most relevant result of the present study was that temporal changes in astrocytes were rather global and not restricted to periventricular regions, while neuronal reaction in vulnerable areas was more pronounced. Specifically in chronic stages, when severe structural damage in neuronal cell-types occurred (NF68, bFGF, SYN 38), global "activation" of astrocytes (GLDH and GFAP) was initiated.

The observed increases in cortical neurofilament in subacute stages indicating sustained (but reversible) axonal degradation [5] is in concordance with clinical observation that found elevated NF-concentrations in patients with chronic hydrocephalus [4]. It is suggested, however, that the observed temporal profile in astrocytic response reflects a "biphasic" nature and that late glial changes were rather secondary to sustained neuronal injury since it is known that astrocytic activation might occur in the vicinity of synaptic damage [1].

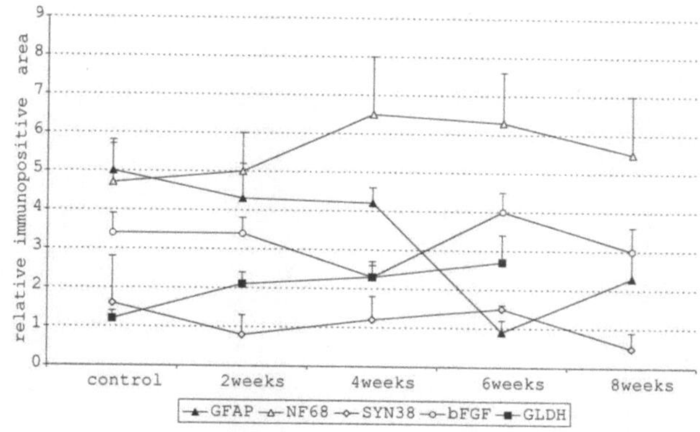

Fig. 2. Qualitative temporal changes of cortical enzyme- and immuno-staining results (black pixels) to astrocytic GLDH-activity, intermediate filaments (GFAP and NF68), presynaptic vesicles (SYN 38) and bFGF; for significant changes see results (mean values ± 1SD)

References

1. Aldskogius H, Svensson M (1999) Glial response to synaptic damage and plasticity. J Neurosci Res 58: 33–41
2. Del Bigio MR, Bruni JE (1988) Periventricular pathology in hydrocephalus rabbits before and after shunting. Acta Neuropathol 77: 186–195
3. Kugler P, Weeger T, Horvath E (1995) Glutamat dehydrogenase in astrocytes of the rat dentate gyrus following lesions of the enthorninal cortex. Neuroscience 64: 173–182
4. Tullberg M, Rosengren L, Blomsterwall RPT (1998) CSF neurofilament and glial fibrillary acidic protein in normal pressure hydrocephalus. Neurology 50: 1122–1127
5. Yaghmai A, Povlishock JT (1992) Traumatically induced reactive change as visualized through the use of monoclonal antibodies targeted to neurofilament subunits. J Neuropathol Exp Neurol 51: 158–176

Correspondence: Thomas Brinker, M.D., Ph.D., Department of Neurosurgery, Nordstadthospital Hannover, Haltenhoffstraße 41, 30167 Hannover, Germany.

Brain Biochemical Monitoring and Imaging

Acta Neurochir (2002) [Suppl] 81: 281–283

Mechanisms of the Mass Effect of Cerebral Contusion: ICP Monitoring and Diffusion MRI Study

T. Kawamata, Y. Katayama, T. Mori, N. Aoyama, and **T. Tsubokawa**

Department of Neurological Surgery, Nihon University School of Medicine, Tokyo, Japan

Summary

Objective. Cerebral contusion is sometimes associated with a non-hemorrhagic mass effect which progresses rapidly within 12–48 hours post-trauma. In order to determine the mechanisms underlying such a mass effect, we analyzed data obtained from ICP monitoring and diffusion MRI in a total of 38 patients with cerebral contusion.

Methods. Diffusion imaging and ADC mapping were performed employing 1.5 T echo planar MRI. ADC values were expressed as a ratio relative to the values of intact brain areas.

Results. In 6 patients, ICP became uncontrollable medically and surgical resection of the contused brain tissue was eventually performed. Within 24 hours post-trauma, diffusion images revealed a low intensity core and a high intensity rim in the contusion. The ADC ratio increased in the central area (1.13 ± 0.21) and decreased in the peripheral area (0.67 ± 0.14). A crescent-shaped zone of very high ADC ratio (1.45 ± 0.14) was observed at the border between these two areas during the period of 24–48 hours.

Conclusions. It appears that the capacitance of edema fluid accumulation is elevated by cellular disintegration in the central area, whereas the resistance to edema fluid propagation is elevated by cellular swelling in the peripheral area. We suggest that such events facilitate extracellular edema fluid accumulation within contused brain tissue and contribute, together with cellular swelling itself, to the non-hemorrhagic mass effect of cerebral contusion.

Keywords: Cerebral contusion, brain edema, diffusion MRI, brain tissue osmolality.

Introduction

Severe cerebral contusion is sometimes associated with early massive edema within 12–48 hours post-trauma. This often results in progressive intracranial pressure (ICP) elevation and clinical deterioration [4]. The previous studies have provided data which are consistent with the idea that the early contusion edema, in contrast to delayed peri-contusion edema [2, 7], does not display the characteristics of vasogenic edema, and is, at least partially, cytotoxic in nature [1, 3]. We previously proposed another mechanism for the early contusion edema; viz. that an elevated osmolality within the area of contusion necrosis, a direct consequence of mechanical impact (contusion necrosis proper [8]), plays an important role in edema formation in cerebral contusion [6]. The cellular elements in this area, both neuronal as well as glial, uniformly undergo shrinkage, and then disintegration, homogenation and cyst formation. In the present study, we attempted to characterize the evolution of this area during the period of early contusion edema based on ICP monitoring, diffusion images and ADC mapping in patients with cerebral contusion in a total of 38 patients with cerebral contusion.

Materials and Methods

A total of 29 patients with cerebral contusion were investigated in diffusion MRI study. These patients were selected on the basis of the following criteria: GCS ≥ 9, no hypoxic episodes, no massive ICP increase, no massive intracerebral hematoma, no severe multiple injury and no severe systemic complications, to avoid severe secondary pathogenesis for edema formation in the contusion. Following conventional T1- and T2-weighted imaging, diffusion images were obtained and ADC mapping was computed from various b factor diffusion images. With reference to the T1- and T2-weighted, and diffusion images, several regions of interest (ROI) for ADC were defined in the central area and the peripheral area of cerebral contusion. When contusion hemorrhage was observed on the T1- and T2-weighted images, the area of hemorrhage was carefully excluded from the ROI. The ADC ratio (= ADC in contusion/ADC in normal brain) was calculated by dividing the ADC values in the ROI by a reference ADC value which was obtained from normal brain tissue. In another group of patients with severe cerebral contusion, most of whom demonstrated progressive neurological deterioration, ICP was monitored with an intraventricular catheter.

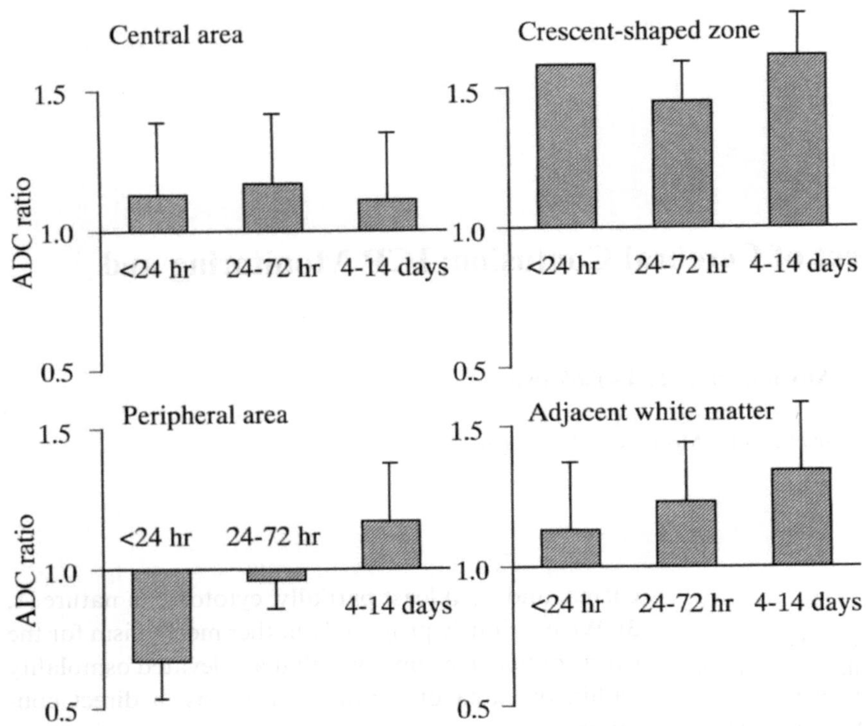

Fig. 1. The ADC ratio in the central area of contusion (upper left), in the crescent-shaped zone (upper right), in the peripheral area of contusion (lower left), and in the adjacent white matter (lower right). The ADC ratio increased in the central area and decreased in the peripheral area within 24 hours post-trauma. The crescent-shaped zone showed very high ADC ratio. Interstitial edema developed into the adjacent white matter at more than 24 hours post-trauma

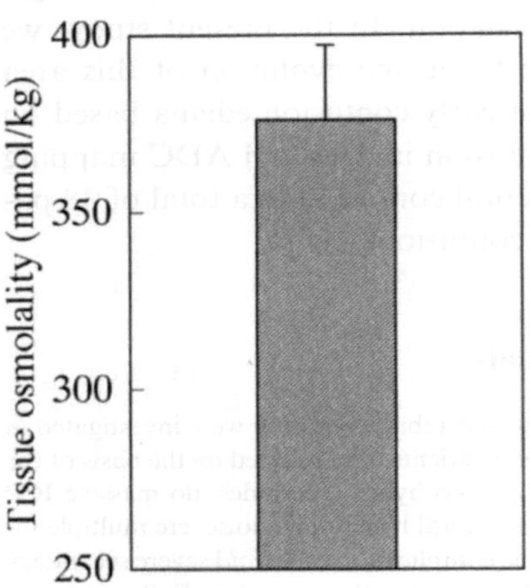

Fig. 2. Tissue osmolality in the contused brain increased to 376 ± 21 mmol/kg, which was approximately 70 mmol/kg higher than that in the normal brain. Such a marked increase in osmolality may cause edema fluid accumulation in the contusion

Results

An increase in ICP was always observed in parallel with the neurological deterioration. In 6 patients, ICP became uncontrollable medically within 36 hours post-trauma and surgical resection of the contused brain tissue was eventually performed. In some surgical cases, tissue osmolality in the contusion brain was measured using a vapor pressure osmometer. The tissue osmolality increased into 376 ± 21 mmol/kg, which was approximately 70 mmol/kg higher than that in the normal brain. Within 24 hours post-trauma, diffusion images revealed a low intensity core in the central area and a high intensity rim in the peripheral area of contusion. The ADC ratio increased in the central area (1.13 ± 0.21) and decreased in the peripheral area (0.67 ± 0.14). These findings suggest the occurrence of cellular disintegration and tissue homogenization in the central area and cellular swelling in the peripheral area. A crescent-shaped zone of very high ADC ratio (1.45 ± 0.14) was observed at the border between these two areas after 24 hours post-trauma in patients who demonstrated a large low intensity core on diffusion images. This appears to represent edema fluid accumulation within the region of tissue homogenization. Interstitial edema (a high ADC ratio) extending along white matter fibers developed around the peripheral area of contusion at more than 24 hours post-trauma (1.23 ± 0.21).

Discussion

An early histopathological investigation reported by Lindenberg *et al.* [8] demonstrated the presence of two components in cerebral contusion; one comprises the area of contusion necrosis proper and the other is the surrounding area in which microthrombosis and cellular swelling are observed. These two components are clearly separated by a line of demarcation. The central area of cerebral contusion which demonstrates high ADC values appears to correspond to the area of contusion necrosis proper, since cellular disintegration and homogenization in this area would result in an expansion of the extracellular space [5]. The peripheral area of cerebral contusion in which the ADC values decrease, appears to correspond to the surrounding area, since cellular swelling which is predominant in this area would result in a shrinkage of the extracellular space.

It appears that expansion of the extracellular space in the central area increases the capacitance for edema fluid accumulation [5]. In contrast, the shrinkage of the extracellular space in the peripheral area increases the resistance for edema fluid propagation or resolution. Since the ADC values of the crescent-shaped zone at the border between the central and peripheral areas is very high, this zone may represent edema fluid accumulated within the area of contusion necrosis proper.

The result of osmolality measurement clearly demonstrated that a marked increase in tissue osmolality occurs in the core of contusion (contusion mecrosis proper) [6]. It is uncertain whether or not such a marked increase in osmolality is osmotically active and causes edema fluid accumulation. We hypothesize that the barrier formed by swollen cells in the peripheral area may prevent edema fluid propagation and also helps to create an osmotic potential within the central area. Since blood flow is greatly decreased but is not completely interrupted in contused brain tissue, water is continuously supplied from the blood into the central area. We suggest that a combination of these events facilitates edema fluid accumulation in the central area and contributes to the mass effect of early contusion edema. The therapeutic effect of surgical resection (contusion necrotomy) is not only due to simple internal decompression, but also due to removal of the origin of edema formation itself.

In conclusion, the present findings imply that multiple mechanisms exist in early contusion edema. Diffusion images and ADC mapping offer powerful tools for investigating spatially as well as temporally heterogeneous mechanisms of contusion edema.

Reference

1. Barzó P, Marmarou A, Fatouros P *et al* (1996) Magnetic resonance imaging-monitored acute blood-brain barrier changes in experimental traumatic brain injury. J Neurosurg 85: 1113–1121
2. Bullock R, Statham J, Patterson D, Wyper D, Hadley D, Teasdale E (1990) The time course of vasogenic oedema after focal human head injury: evidence from SPECT mapping of blood brain barrier defects. Acta Neurochir (Wien) 51: 286–288
3. Ito J, Marmarou A, Barzó P *et al* (1996) Characterization of edema by diffusion-weighted imaging in experimental traumatic brain injury. J Neurosurg 84: 97–103
4. Katayama Y, Tsubokawa T, Miyazaki S, Kawamata T, Yoshino A (1990) Oedema fluid formation within contused brain tissue as a cause of medically uncontrollable elevation of intracranial pressure in head trauma patients. Acta Neurochir (Wien) 51: 308–310
5. Katayama Y, Tsubokawa T, Kinoshita K, Himi K (1992) Intraparenchymal fluid-blood levels in traumatic intracerebral hematomas. Neuroradiol 34: 381–383
6. Katayama Y, Mori T, Maeda T *et al* (1999) Pathogenesis of the mass effect of cerebral contusions: rapid increase in osmolality within the contusion necrosis. Acta Neurochir (Wien) (in press)
7. Kushi H, Katayama Y, Shibuya T, Tsubokawa T, Kuroha T (1994) Gd-DTPA enhanced magnetic resonance imaging of cerebral contusions. Acta Neurochir (Wien) 60: 472–474
8. Lindenberg R, Freytag E (1957) Morphology of cortical contusion. Arch Path 63: 23–42

Correspondence: Ttsuro Kawamata, M.D., Ph.D., Department of Neurological Surgery, Nihon University School of Medicine, 30-1 Oyaguchi Kamimachi, Itabashi-ku, Tokyo 173-8610, Japan.

Acta Neurochir (2002) [Suppl] 81: 285–287

Incidence of Intracranial Hypertension Related to Jugular Bulb Oxygen Saturation Disturbances in Severe Traumatic Brain Injury Patients

P. Schoon, L. Benito Mori, G. Orlandi, C. Larralde, and **M. Radrizzani**

"Prof. Dr. Luis Güemes" General Hospital, Haedo, Buenos Aires, Argentina

Summary

Objective. To analyze the Intracranial Hypertension (IH) development related to jugular bulb oxygen saturation (SjO_2) disturbances in severe traumatic brain injury patients (sTBI).

Materials and Methods. One hundred and thirty-five sTBI patients were reviewed. Those without IH at admission ($n = 116$) were included. All patients underwent ICP and SjO_2 continuous monitoring. Two groups were distinguished according to the SjO_2 values during the first 24 hours. Group A: those with abnormal SjO_2 (SjO_2 more than 75% or less than 55%) and Group B: those with normal SjO_2 (55–75%). Differences in IH development and outcome between groups were analyzed. Causes of abnormally low SjO_2 were identified.

Results. IH developed in 56,9% of patients, between 12 and 48 hours from admission. Group A had a significantly higher incidence of IH than Group B ($p < 0.001$) and it also had a worse outcome than Group B (GOS 1–2) ($p < 0.005$). Patients from Group A had a risk of IH 4.5 fold higher than Group B. Considering only patients who developed IH, an abnormal SjO_2 value increased 2.3 fold the risk of death compared to those without SjO_2 disturbances. Main causes of SjO_2 desaturation were hyperventilation (40.7%), hypovolemia (28.4%) and anemia (21%).

Conclusions. Early detection of disturbances in oxygen supply-demand relationship and prevention or resolution of the secondary insults which produce these disturbances, might lead to a reduction in the incidence of intracranial hypertension.

Keywords: Jugular venous oxygen saturation; intracranial hypertension; cerebral monitoring; head injury.

Introduction

Intracranial Hypertension (IH) is a common feature in patients with severe traumatic brain injury (sTBI) and it was widely observed that a persistent raise in intracranial pressure is related to poor outcome [6]. Besides the presence of intracranial collections, it has been described that raised intracranial pressure (ICP) might be a consequence of the pathophysiological mechanisms that occur early after head injury such as disturbed autoregulation, increase in cerebral blood volume and cerebral blood flow, brain swelling or cerebral ischemia, among others. In vulnerable brain, the presence of secondary injuries may spread the neuronal damage. Some of such disturbances might be detected by the assessment of the Cerebral Blood Flow (CBF)/Cerebral Metabolic rate of O_2 ($CMRO_2$) relationship. Monitoring of jugular bulb oxygen saturation (SjO_2) allows a global assessment of this relationship [12] and might be useful, not only to monitor the results and assurance of some therapeutic procedures against IH, but to warn about the occurrence of some secondary insults that might lead to IH as well.

The purpose of this study was to evaluate the relationship between the development of IH and previous SjO_2 disturbances, and to identify causes of jugular desaturations, in a series of sTBI patients.

Material and Methods

One hundred and thirty-five consecutive patients with closed sTBI (GCS after resuscitation ≤ 8) were reviewed. Only patients without IH at admission (116 patients) were included in the study. Time from trauma to admission was less than six hours in 62% of patients and less than eight hours in all of them. The age was between 16 and 67 (mean 30.9 years), 75 males and 41 females, mean GCS was 6.48.

All patients underwent SjO_2 and ICP monitoring. SjO_2 was monitored with a 4,5 Fr. fiberoptic catheter inserted percutaneously in the internal jugular vein homolateral to the most severe injury or in the right side if diffuse damage was present. ICP was monitored with ventricular or parenchymal fiberoptic catheters. All patients underwent continuous monitoring of mean arterial pressure, arterial oxygen saturation and end tidal CO_2 ($ETCO_2$). Routine proceedings included head elevation at 30 degrees in neutral plane, mechanical ventilation with proper sedation and relaxation to maintain an $ETCO_2$ between 35 and 40 mmHg, analgesia and fenitoin. All patients were managed with a pathophysiological approach that emphasized early evacuation of extra-axial collections and prevention of secondary injury. Therapeutic goals included an ICP < 20 mmHg, a Cerebral Perfusion Pressure (CPP) ≥ 70 mmHg and SjO_2 values

Table 1. *Intracranial Hypertension Incidence and Outcome Between Groups*

Group	SjO_2	Patients (%)	IH incidence	GOS 1–2
A	<55%	52 (44,8%)	76,9% } a	73% } b
	>75%	28 (24,2%)	71,4%	64%
B	55%–75%	36 (31%)	16,6%	22%
Total		166 (100%)	56,9%	53,4%

SjO_2 Jugular oxygen saturation; IH intracranial hypertension; *GOS* Glasgow Outcome Scale; $^a p < 0.001$; $^b p < 0.005$.

between 55% and 75%. Whenever SjO_2 was out of normal values during more than 10 minutes, catheter position was tested and jugular blood samples were taken to confirm oxygen saturation by a laboratory oximeter.

Two groups of patients were distinguished according to the SjO_2 values during the first 24 hours from admission or until IH developed: those patients with "abnormal" SjO_2 values (Group A = 80 patients), and those with normal SjO_2 values (Group B = 36 patients). Differences in IH and outcome between groups were analyzed. To assess patients' outcome the Glasgow Outcome Scale (GOS) was used and consigned at time of hospital discharge. Primary causes of low SjO_2 (desaturation) were also identified. For statistical assessment Chi-square test was used and statistical significance was considered with a p value less than 0.05.

Results

There were no differences between groups concerning age, gender, GCS after resuscitation, Injury Severity Score and Traumatic Coma Data Bank CT scan classification. IH developed in 66 of the 116 patients (56,9%) and it occurred between 12 and 48 hours from admission. As shown in Table 1, Incidence of IH observed was higher in group A (60 patients – 75%) than Group B (6 patients – 16,6%) ($p < 0,001$). Patients from Group A had a risk of IH development 4.5 fold higher than those in Group B. Also, patients in Group A showed a worse outcome (GOS 1 and 2) than those in Group B ($p < 0,005$) (Table 1). Considering the 66 patients who developed IH, those with a previous abnormal SjO_2 value had a 2.3-fold higher risk of death than those patients who developed IH without previous SjO_2 disturbances. Causes of jugular desaturation episodes are shown in Table 2.

Discussion

This series showed a high IH incidence and its relationship with poor outcomes. Also, the present data indicate that SjO_2 disturbances are common in patients with sTBI and that occurrence of these disturbances impaired the prognosis of the patients. All these

Table 2. *Primary Causes of Desaturation*

Causes of desaturation	Episodes (%)
Hyperventilation	40.7%
Hypovolemia	28.4%
Anemia	21%
Hypotension	8.6%
Hypoxemia	1.2%

features are coincident with those reported previously by several authors [3, 4, 6].

Also, in this series a higher incidence of IH was found in those patients who experienced SjO_2 disturbances prior to the IH development, than in those without such disturbances. SjO_2 reflects the interconnection between cerebral oxygen delivery (arterial oxygen content and CBF) and cerebral oxygen demands. When occurring in higher than normal values (> 75%) it reflects an uncoupled relationship with an elevated CBF as compared to cerebral metabolic requirements, the "luxury perfusion syndrome" described by Lassen [8]. This "hyperemia" might be "absolute" if CBF values are higher than normal, as demonstrated recently by Martin and colleagues and earlier by others [1, 9, 10], or it might be "relative", if CBF shows normal values with low cerebral oxygen requirements [9, 10]. The link between hyperemia and raised ICP was explained through an increase in cerebral blood volume with an increment in intracranial content [10], or by an exacerbation of edema when autoregulation is impaired (the "vasomotor paralysis" described by Langfitt and coworkers) and capillary hydrostatic pressure is increased [7]. The relationship between hyperemia and outcome hasn't been well defined yet. The present data showed a high incidence of bad outcome in those who experienced early hyperemia, even without simultaneous IH. These results didn't agree with other reports, such as that of Kelly's and colleagues [12] who reported a 75% favorable outcome in patients who experienced hyperemia without simultaneous IH. However, it is important to point out that we didn't measure CBF or $CMRO_2$, and those patients with high SjO_2 values might have had such values because of an extremely low $CMRO_2$ being related with an "ischemia-infarct" state, as described by Robertson and coworkers [12], and with the expected bad prognosis. Cormio and colleagues [3] reported recently, that among patients with high SjO_2 values those with lower $CMRO_2$ measurements attained a worse outcome. Jugular lactate determinations [11, 12] or Transcranial Doppler assessment [2] could help distinguish these two states (hyperemia or ischemia-infarct).

A low value of SjO_2 usually indicates a cerebral oligoemic state or ischemia due to an inadequate arterial oxygen content (hypoxia, anemia) and/or a CBF too low to supply oxygen cerebral demands. This cerebral oligoemia has been demonstrated by several authors and it has been related to poor outcome [4]. An insufficient cerebral oxygen delivery might amplify the ischemic damage in a brain with increased vulnerability. Gopinath and coworkers [4] reported that the occurrence of one episode of jugular desaturation was associated with a two-fold increase in the risk of poor outcome, and multiple episodes were associated with a fourteen-fold increase. These episodes of low cerebral oxygen delivery, even if transient, may cause infarction of cerebral tissue increasing brain swelling, leading to an increase in ICP and further deterioration.

The present data showed a high incidence of jugular venous desaturation, higher than reported in the literature [4, 13]. This may be due to SjO_2 measurements being taken from the first 24 hours after traumatic injury. Bouma and coworkers [1] reported low CBF values during the first 12 hours from trauma with coincident high values of arterio-jugular differences of oxygen. One third of patients analyzed before 6 hours of primary injury had CBF values below the ischemia threshold. Those patients experienced a poor outcome. Recently, Martin and colleagues [9] have also found low CBF values during the first day after injury in most patients. However, they found relatively normal arterio-jugular oxygen proportions (mean $5{,}4 \pm 0{,}5$ vol%).

In this series, the most frequent causes of jugular desaturation were related with disturbances decreasing CBF: hypocapnia and hypovolemia-related low CPP. Hypocapnia occurred because of unnoticed hyperventilation due to inadequate sedation or relaxation. Hypovolemia was recorded as the cause of desaturation when a low repleted intravascular space was recorded producing a low CPP, but out of the range was considered as "hypotension" (SBP < 90 mmHg). When hypovolemia was present, most cases were due to insufficient initial fluid resuscitation or, in some patients, because of negative fluid balance due to "blind" mannitol administration before ICU admission. Hypoxemia was the least cause of desaturation (1,2% of episodes). Probably, it was due to the fact that first jugular venous saturation measurements were obtained when all patients had already been mechanically ventilated. These results are coincident with previous reports, except hypotension which in most of these reports was significantly more frequent [13].

The present data indicate that SjO_2 disturbances are common in patients with sTBI. They also showed that their occurrence is related to high IH development and poor outcome. SjO_2 monitoring in a real-time fashion, allowed the detection of secondary insults which, if present, improve outcome. Early detection of disturbances in oxygen supply-demand relationship and prevention or resolution of secondary insults producing those disturbances, may lead to a reduction in the incidence of Intracranial Hypertension.

References

1. Bouma G, Muizelaar J, Choi S *et al* (1991) Cerebral circulation and metabolism after severe traumatic brain injury: the elusive role of ischemia J Neurosurg 75: 685–693
2. Chan K, Dearden N, Miller J *et al* (1993) Multimodality monitoring as a guide to treatment of intracranial hypertension after severe brain injury. Neurosurgery 32: 547–553
3. Cormio M, Valadka A, Robertson C (1999) Elevated jugular venous oxygen saturation after severe head injury. J Neurosurg 90: 9–15
4. Gopinath S, Robertson C, Contant C *et al* (1994) Jugular venous desaturation and outcome after head injury. J Neurol Neurosurg Psychiatry 57: 717–723
5. Kelly D, Kordestani R, Martin N *et al* (1996) Hyperemia following traumatic brain injury: relationship to intracranial hypertension and outcome. J Neurosurg 85: 762–771
6. Lang E, Chesnut R (1995) Intracranial pressure and cerebral perfusion pressure in severe head injury. New Horizons 3: 400–409
7. Langfitt T, Tannanbaum H, Kassel N (1966) The etiology of acute brain swelling following experimental head injury. J Neurosurg 24: 47–56
8. Lassen N (1966) The luxury-perfusion syndrome and its possible relation to acute metabolic acidosis localised within the brain. Lancet 2: 1113–1115
9. Martin N, Patwardhan R, Alexander M *et al* (1997) Characterization of cerebral hemodynamic phases following severe head trauma: hypoperfusion, hyperemia, and vasospasm. J Neurosurg 87: 9–19
10. Obrist W, Langfitt T, Jaggi J *et al* (1984) Cerebral blood flow and metabolism in comatose patients with acute head injury. Relationship to intracranial hypertension. J Neurosurg 61: 241–253
11. Robertson C, Grossman R, Goodman J *et al* (1987) The predictive value of cerebral anaerobic metabolism with cerebral infarction after head injury. J Neurosurg 67: 361–368
12. Robertson C, Narayan R, Gokaslan Z *et al* (1989) Cerebral arteriovenous oxygen difference as an estimate of cerebral blood flow in comatose patients. J Neurosurg 70: 222–230
13. Robertson C, Valadka A, Hannay J *et al* (1999) Prevention of secondary ischemic insults after severe head injury. Crit Care Med 27: 2086–2095

Correspondence: Pablo Schoon M.D., Intensive Care Unit, "Prof. Dr. Luis Güemes" General Hospital, Rivadavia 15.000 (1706) Haedo, Buenos Aires, Argentina.

Acta Neurochir (2002) [Suppl] 81: 289–293

Detection of Early Ischemia in Severe Head Injury by Means of Arteriovenous Lactate Differences and Jugular Bulb Oxygen Saturation. Relationship with CPP, Severity Indexes and Outcome. Preliminary Analysis

A. Chieregato[1], **M. Marchi**[2], **R. Zoppellari**[2], **E. Fabbri**[2], **G. Cianchi**[4], **E. Forini**[3], and **L. Targa**[1]

[1] Neurorianimazione, Ospedale Civile M. Bufalini, Cesena, Italy
[2] Servizio di Anestesia e Rianimazione, Ospedale S. Anna, Ferrara, Italy
[3] Servizio di Biostatistica, Ospedale S. Anna, Ferrara, Italy
[4] Servizio di Anestesia e Rianimazione, Ospedale Careggi, Firenze, Italy

Summary

Early ischemia may be highly relevant in patients with severe head injuries. The aims of the study were: 1) to define if abnormal arteriovenous lactate difference (AVDL) and jugular bulb oxygen saturation (SjO2) are found in the early 24 hrs post injury; 2) to compare if abnormalities of SjO2 and of AVDL were associated with a specific typology of severity indexes and outcome; 3) to detect any association between abnormal AVDL and SjO2 with levels of cerebral perfusion pressure (CPP). The study involved 29 patients, with CPP, AVDL and SjO2 measured within 24 hours post-injury. Results: 1) Abnormal AVDL was found in 21% while abnormal SjO2 was detected in 38% of the patients; 2) abnormal AVDL was associated with cases of most severe injury; 3) CPP level below 60 mmHg was associated with abnormal AVDL and SjO2. Low CPP appeared to be the most likely measurable cause of early ischemia. Abnormalities of AVDL appeared to be more sensitive, than SjO2, with regard to detection of the most severe cases.

Keywords: Arteriovenous lactate difference; early ischemia; jugular bulb oxygen saturation; cerebral perfusion pressure.

Introduction

In recent years evidence has suggested that, in the first 24 hours post-injury, global and regional cerebral blood flow (CBF) is reduced, frequently to levels considered critical for cerebral viability and with a potentially negative consequence on outcome [1, 2]. Ischemia is the result of an imbalance between cerebral oxygen delivery and the cerebral metabolic oxygen rate (CMRO2). Ischemia begins with a reduction of SjO2, followed by an increase of lactate production. The measurement of AVDL may potentially help to detect ischemia. Currently, early ischemia is detected by CBF or SjO2 measurement. However, the measured CBF values do not take into account the extent of coupling with CMRO2, if this is not simultaneously measured. SjO2 interpretation also has limits. Low SjO2 may be associated with compensated hypoperfusion [8], early ischemia [1, 7] or cerebral viability [4, 5]. High SjO2 values can be the expression, not only of a supernormal CBF [8], but also of a low post-traumatic or even ischemic CMRO2 [4]. AVDL measurement may be an easy way to detect global ischemia and correctly interpret the recorded values of CBF or SjO2 found. Nevertheless, AVDL measurements were rarely adopted in early phases [7, 9]. The relationships between levels of AVDL and cerebral perfusion pressure (CPP) or levels of severity indexes and type of outcome were not studied. The objectives of the present study are: 1) to define whether abnormal AVDL and low SjO2 measurements are found within 24 hrs post injury; 2) to compare SjO2 and AVDL data with severity indexes and outcome data; 3) to detect a possible threshold of CPP for SjO2 and AVDL abnormalities.

Materials and Methods

The study involved patients with severe head injury (GCS ≤ 8 post-stabilization) on arrival were excluded. Twenty nine consecutive patients, who underwent AVDL, SjO2 and CPP monitoring within 24 hours post-injury, were included in the study. The neurology of the patient was categorized for mGCS ≤ 3 or ≥ 4. Pupillary reactivity to light was defined as normal or abnormal. The worst CT were classified in two categories: a) low risk CT including DI I and II (according to Marshall classification) and b) high risk CT including DI III and IV (according to Marshall classification) and mass lesion.

Table 1. *Physiological Data*

	AVDL			SjO2		
	Abnormal	Normal		Abnormal	Normal	
N	6	23		11	18	
AVDL mmol/L	−0.67 (−0.76/−0.41)	−0.06 (−0.17/−0.045)	<0.05	−0.1 (−0.58/−0.06)	−0.09 (−0.19/0.03)	Ns
SjO2 %	57.7 (42.3/63.1)	59.5 (55.1/65.7)	Ns	54 (40.7/55.2)	64.5 (60/67.2)	<0.01
CPP mmHg	44 (30/50)	71 (65/77)	<0.05	59 (50/69)	73.5 (67/82)	<0.01
Hb gr/dl	10.11 (7.5/12)	11.5 (10.2/12.4)	Ns	9.2 (8.2/11.7)	11.6 (11/12.3)	0.059
PaCO2 kPa	3.51 (3.3/4.3)	4.33 (3.8/4.7)	0.07	3.62 (3.4/4.3)	4.33 (3.4/4.6)	0.09
SaO2 %	97.6 (97.5/97.9)	97 (95.1/97.6)	Ns	97.2 (96.7/97.6)	97.55 (96.5/97.8)	Ns
MAP mmHg	90.5 (80/108)	86 (81.3/92.7)	Ns	85 (80/93.5)	88 (83/93)	Ns
ICP mmHg	48.5 (38/53)	15 (9/22)	<0.01	26 (17.2/43.2)	12 (8/22)	<0.01

Two kinds of outcome measurements were obtained. The first was the occurrence of brain death within 48 hrs post injury [2]. The second was outcome at one year, measured with the GOS scale. It was dichotomized into two classes: poor outcome (including: dead, vegetative state and severe disability), and good outcome (including moderate disability and good recovery). AVDL measurement was not involved in the decision making protocol of treatment, but was considered as a physiological warning signal of actual ischemia. The main structure of the research should only be considered as observational. Patients were analyzed according to the abnormality of the SjO2 and AVDL values. On the basis of the limits of confidence obtained from the analysis of Gibbs data [3], the threshold for abnormal SjO2 was 56% and for abnormal AVDL −0.36 mmol/L. Physiological data was described by median, 25% and 75% percentile. The Mann-Whitney test was applied to compare median values. Categorical data was compared using the Fischer exact test. P values below 0.05 were considered significant.

Results

The median age of the patients was 32 years (21/45); there were 23 males out of a total of 29. Sixteen patients had associated multiple injuries. The median delay of measurements form injury was 16 hrs (13/19). Objective 1: No useful information was obtained from descriptive analysis of all AVDL (−0.09 mmol/L, −0.23/0.01) and SjO2 values (59.5%, 55/65.5). Abnormal AVDL was found in 21% of the patients, while abnormal SjO2 was detected in 38% (Table 1). Objective 2: AVDL abnormalities were more frequently associated with a high risk grade of first Ct, with mGCS ≤ 3 and abnormalities in pupillary reactivity (Table 2). Patients with abnormal AVDL values had a higher frequency of early death (Fig. 1). Differences (even if not statistically confirmed) were found when comparing the outcome at one year of the two AVDL categories (Fig. 1). Early and late outcome appeared to differ between abnormal and normal SjO2, even if these differences were not statistically confirmed (Fig. 1). Objective 3: AVDL and SjO2 abnormalities were associated with differences in CPP and ICP (Table 1). From the analysis of categorical data, both abnormal SjO2 ($p < 0.05$) and abnormal AVDL ($p < 0.01$) were more frequent when CPP was below 60 mmHg. A comparison of median values (for AVDL, Fig. 2) confirmed the differences. Lower CPP was also associated with lower haemoglobin (hb), but not to differences in mean arterial pressure (MAP). CPP abnormality appeared to be associated with abnormal ICP values and not to differences in MAP levels.

Discussion

The present study showed that AVDL and SjO2 are frequently abnormal in the first 24 hours post-injury. The early abnormalities of SjO2 were described in recent years [1, 5, 7, 9, 10]. The association of low SjO2 with worse outcomes is not definitively defined. Some data suggests that low SjO2 values may be associated to better CMRO2 and improved final outcome [4, 5]. Our results suggest an association of low SjO2 values with the most severe cases and with those with the worst outcome, but without reaching a statistically significant level. This may be due to the reduced level of the sample or to the fact that some cases with high SjO2 may be associated with the same severity of those with low SjO2. It is well known that established ischemia or extensive neurological damage may be associated with high SjO2 levels, as a consequence of hyperemia [8] or marked depression of CMRO2 [4]. The differences between the various studies concerning early SjO2 measurement may be partly explained by differences in the case mix adopted.

The most original data of the study is the detection of abnormalities of AVDL in about 1/5 of the patients. Contrarily to the subgroup of low SjO2, patients with

Table 2. *Severity Indexes and Outcome*

N		AVDL Abnormal 6	AVDL Normal 23		SjO2 Abnormal 11	SjO2 Normal 18	
First CT	high risk	5	6	<0.05	5	6	Ns
	low risk	1	17		6	12	
Worst CT	high risk	5	12	Ns	8	9	Ns
	low risk	1	11		3	9	
Motor GCS	≤3	5	7	<0.05	7	5	Ns
	≥4	1	16		4	13	
Pupils	normal	1	18	<0.05	6	4	Ns
	abnormal	5	5		5	14	
Hypotension	yes	0	3	Ns	1	2	Ns
	no	6	20		10	16	
Hypoxia	yes	2	8	Ns	3	7	Ns
	no	4	15		8	11	
Multiple injuries	yes	2	14	Ns	7	9	Ns
	no	4	9		4	9	
Age	years	29.5	32 (20/50)	Ns	23 (19/59)	33 (24/36)	Ns
Delay	hours	13	16 (8/19)	<0.01	16 (13/18.5)	16 (13/20)	Ns
Early death	yes	4	2	<0.01	3	3	Ns
	no	2	21		8	15	
Final outcome	poor	5	10	Ns	8	7	Ns
	good	1	13		3	11	

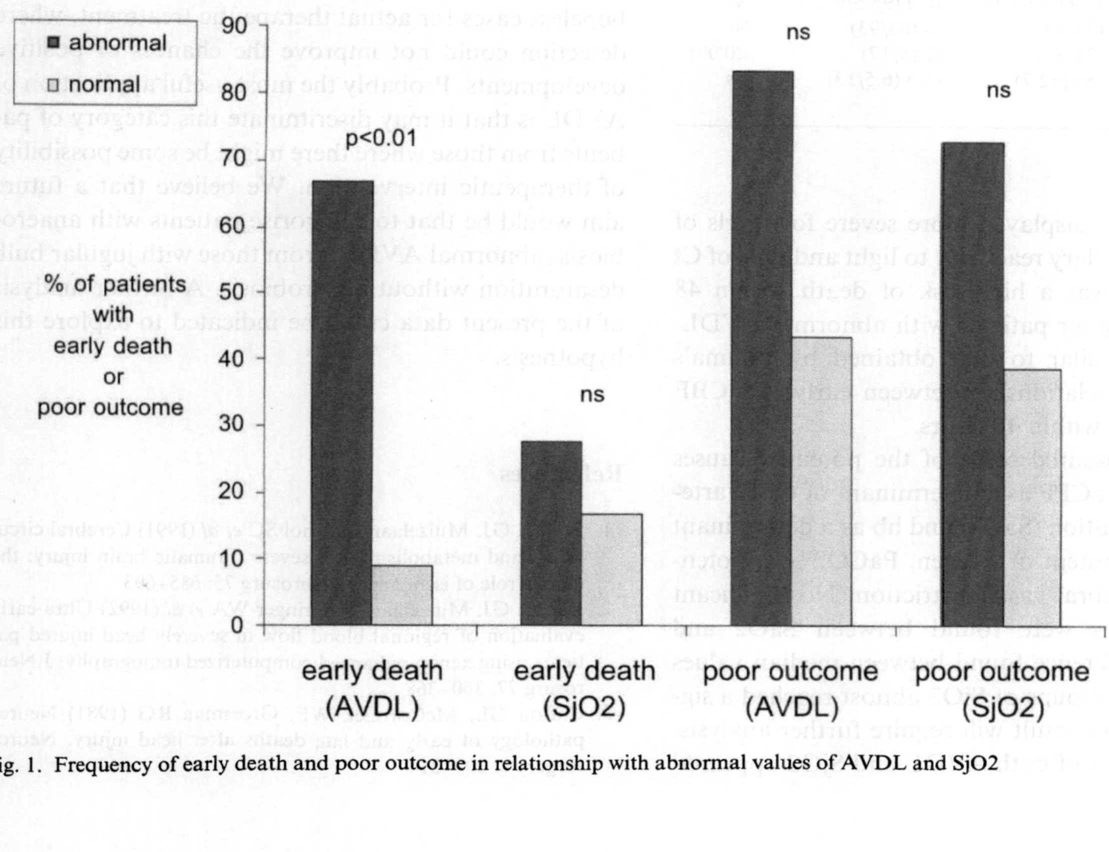

Fig. 1. Frequency of early death and poor outcome in relationship with abnormal values of AVDL and SjO2

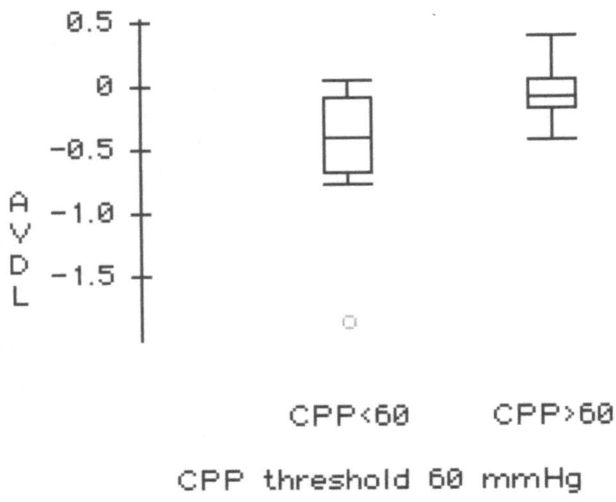

Fig. 2. Different levels of AVDL in relationship with a threshold of CPP equal to 60 mmHg

Table 3. *Classes of CPP: Main Physiological Data*

	CPP < 60 mmHg	CPP > 60 mmHg	
N	9	20	
AVDL mmol/L	−0.4 (−0.7/−0.08)	−0.08 (−0.18/0.04)	<0.01
SjO2 %	55.1 (40.1/60.4)	62.3 (56.1/66.3)	<0.05
CPP mmHg	48 (37/54)	75 (68/80)	<0.0001
Hb gr/dl	9.2 (7.9/11.5)	11.7 (10.6/12.6)	<0.05
PaCO2 kPa	3.79 (3.3/4.4)	4.3 (3.7/4.7)	Ns
SaO2 %	97.6 (97.1/97.7)	96.9 (95.6/97.7)	Ns
MAP mmHg	86 (79/94)	88 (83/93)	Ns
ICP mmHg	47 (31/51)	12 (8/17)	<0.001
Delay from injuries (hours)	16 (6.8/12.7)	16.5 (6.5/13)	Ns

abnormal AVDL displayed more severe for levels of motor GCS, pupillary reactivity to light and type of Ct findings. There was a high risk of death within 48 hours post injury for patients with abnormal AVDL. This result is similar to that obtained by Bouma's [2] study of the relationship between early low CBF values and death within 48 hours.

Our study measured some of the potential causes of early ischemia: CPP as a determinant of CBF, arterial oxygen saturation (SaO2) and hb as a determinant of the arterial content of oxygen, PaCO2 as a potential cause of cerebral vasoconstriction. No significant group differences were found between SaO2 and PaCO2. The difference found between median values of hb in the two groups of SjO2 almost reached a significant level. This result will require further analysis. The abnormalities of both AVDL and SjO2 appeared to be associated to abnormal levels of CPP. As CPP is the most probable measurable cause of early ischemia, data was analyzed whilst looking for a common threshold of CPP for abnormalities of AVDL and SjO2. A CPP value equal to 60 mmHg appeared to be significantly associated with both AVDL and SjO2 differences. These differences were more pronounced for AVDL. As CPP is an established determinant of CBF, the data suggests that both AVDL and SjO2 may detect the condition of low perfusion associated with abnormal low CPP levels. The threshold used for CPP analysis is not substantially different from that currently applied to the management of patients with severe head injury.

The results of the study suggest that AVDL was able to detect the condition of early ischemia to a greater extent than SjO2. AVDL appeared to be more informative regarding the consequence of low CPP condition, and corresponded better to the clinical and prognostic severity of the patient. Most patients with AVDL abnormalities resulted in early death. Patients who underwent an early poor outcome demonstrated substantial differences in primary damage from patients who survived [3]. In this case early ischemia should probably be considered as a epiphenomena of the first damage. The practical aspect of the problem is that most patients with abnormal AVDL are regarded as hopeless cases for actual therapeutic treatment, where detection could not improve the chances of positive developments. Probably the most useful application of AVDL is that it may discriminate this category of patients from those where there might be some possibility of therapeutic intervention. We believe that a future aim would be that to categorise patients with anaerobiosis (abnormal AVDL) from those with jugular bulb desaturation without anaerobiosis. A further analysis of the present data could be indicated to explore this hypothesis.

References

1. Bouma GJ, Muizelaar JP, Choi SC *et al* (1991) Cerebral circulation and metabolism after severe traumatic brain injury: the elusive role of ischemia. J Neurosurg 75: 685–693
2. Bouma GJ, Muizelaar JP, Stringer WA *et al* (1992) Ultra-early evaluation of regional blood flow in severely head-injured patients using xenon-enhanced computerized tomography. J Neurosurg 77: 360–368
3. Clifton GL, McCormick WF, Grossman RG (1981) Neuropathology of early and late deaths after head injury. Neurosurgery 8: 309–314

4. Cormio M, Valadka AB, Robertson CS (1999) Elevated jugular venous oxygen saturation after severe head injury. J Neurosurg 90: 9–15
5. Cruz J (1996) Relationship between early patterns of cerebral extraction of oxygen and outcome from severe acute traumatic brain swelling: cerebral ischemia or cerebral viability? Crit Care Med 24: 953–956
6. Gibbs EL, Lennox WG, Nims LF *et al* (1942) Arterial and cerebral venous blood. Arterial-venous differences in man. J Biol Chem 144: 325–332
7. Gopinath SP, Cormio M, Ziegler J *et al* (1996) Intraoperative jugular desaturation during surgery for traumatic intracranial hematomas. Anesth Analg 83: 1014–1021
8. Roberston CS, Narayan RK, Gokaslan ZL *et al* (1989) Cerebral arterovenous differences as an estimate of cerebral blood flow in comatose patients. J Neurosurg 170: 222–230
9. Sahuquillo J, Poca MA, Garnacho A *et al* (1993) Early ischemia after severe head injury. Preliminary results in patients with diffuse brain injuries. Acta Neurochir 122: 204–214
10. Vigué B, Ract C, Benayed M *et al* (1999) Early SjvO2 monitoring in patients with severe brain trauma. Intensive Care Med 25: 445–451

Correspondence: Dr. Arturo Chieregato, Via Boccacanale di S. Stefano n° 25, 44100 Ferrara, Italy.

Acta Neurochir (2002) [Suppl] 81: 295–297

Non Invasive Local Cerebral Oxygenation Monitoring Using a Combination of Light and Ultrasound

A. Lev[1], Z. Kotler[1], B. Sfez[1], J. Soustiel[2], and M. Feinsod[2]

[1] Optronic Materials and Technologies, Electro-Optics Division Soreq, Research Center Yavneh Israel
[2] Head Injury Applied Research Center Department of Neurosurgery, Rambam (Maimonides) Medical Center Faculty of Medicine, The Technion Israel Institute of Technology Haifa, Israel

Summary

Objectives. We present a new imaging technology that will allow to obtain three-dimensional maps of oxygen saturation in the brain tissues. This technology is not invasive and not ionizing, and can lead to small, portable device that can be brought to bedside.

Methods. The technology uses a combination of near-infrared laser light and ultrasound. Like for other near-infrared spectroscopy techniques, light gives the information on the hemoglobin species present in the tissues. However, since tissues are turbid media, light alone cannot give precise local information. In the technique that we demonstrate, localization is obtained using a focussed ultrasound that locally shifts the laser wavelength, similarly to laser doppler techniques. The frequency-shifted light can be precisely detected and attributed without ambiguities to a specific location. By scanning the ultrasound focus, we can obtain a mapping of the oxygen saturation.

Results. We present preliminary results on a phantom showing the detection of an absorbing object buried more than two centimeters within the phantom. Scanning the ultrasound on the phantom allows to determine precisely the object position and absorption. Scattering and absorption parameters of the phantom are similar to the brain's. The probe works in the reflection mode, meaning that no trans-illumination is needed. The ultrasound frequency is 1.25 MHz, ensuring relatively good ultrasound penetration within the skull.

Conclusions. The method is very promising for brain imaging of trauma or tumors. It is particularly suited for monitoring, since the use of the ultrasound removes the well-recognized problem of light propagation in the CSF.

Keywords: Laser doppler; near infrared; oxygen saturation.

Introduction

Much effort has been undertaken in recent years to use light for brain function imaging. Near-infrared spectroscopy (NIRS) that started in 1977 with the pioneering work of Jobsis [6] has tremendously developed since then. Based on the different absorption coefficients of the oxy- and deoxyhemoglobin forms in the blood, this technique gave information on abnormal functions in injured brain tissues. Two major steps have then pushed these optical techniques forward: one, in the time domain [1, 2, 5], allows determining also scattering coefficients through delays of short pulses in the tissue. The second, in the frequency domain [3, 4], gives the same kind of information through phase measurement of the properly modulated incident light.

These techniques have proven successful in the simultaneous determination of both scattering and the absorption coefficients of tissues. However the *local* detection of the oxygen saturation still proves to be a very difficult task. This is due to the highly complex propagation of light in tissues. Contrarily to X-rays that propagate in straight line in tissues, optical photons show a random-walk like behavior that makes standard reconstruction algorithms difficult to apply. Thus complex inverse back-scattering algorithms must be employed, which very often are model dependent, unstable, and lack resolution.

We present here a new imaging technology that will allow obtaining three-dimensional maps of oxygen saturation within the brain tissues. This technology is not invasive and not ionizing, and can lead to small, portable devices that can be brought to the bedside.

Materials and Methods

The technology uses a combination of near-infrared laser light and ultrasound. As for other near-infrared spectroscopy techniques, light gives the information on the hemoglobin species present in the tissues. However, contrarily to other near-infrared imaging techniques, light is not used for the localization. In the technique that we demonstrate, localization is obtained by using a focused ultrasound that

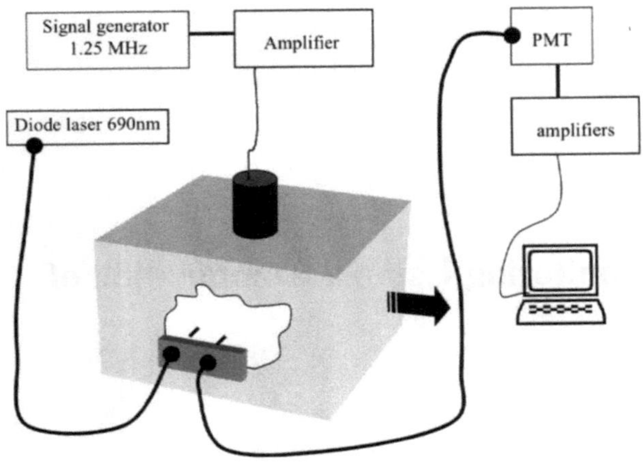

Fig. 1

locally shifts the laser wavelength, in a mode similar to laser Doppler techniques. The frequency-shifted light can be precisely detected and attributed without ambiguities to a specific location. By scanning the ultrasound focus, we can obtain a mapping of the oxygen saturation.

In order to ascertain the concept feasibility, we have devised the following experimental procedure on a phantom.

The phantom is an 8 cm edge cube of Agar gel with 98% water content and 20% Intralipid solution (dilution: 14.5 ml per liter). The diffusion coefficient of this gel is then similar to tissues' ($\mu_s' = 17.5\ \mathrm{cm}^{-1}$). A dye is also introduced in the gel in order to mimic average tissue absorption (Pelikan 4001). The resulting absorption factor is $\mu_a \sim 0.05 \pm 0.01\ \mathrm{cm}^{-1}$.

The experimental set-up is shown in Fig. 1. Light from a 690 nm diode laser (Melles Griot) is focused onto an optical fiber. This fiber is then coupled to the phantom using a (light) index-matching gel. This allows both good light coupling to the phantom and free transversal movement of the fiber with respect to the phantom. Another fiber, also plugged into the index-matching gel, collects light from the phantom and redirects it towards a photomultiplier. The distance between the fibers is about 19 mm.

A focused ultrasound transducer (Panametrics A392S, focal length 63 mm, waist size ~4 mm) is coupled to the phantom using ethylene glycol as an (ultrasound) index match gel between the transducer and the phantom. The ultrasound wave is purely continuous (cw mode). The ultrasound frequency (1.25 MHz) has been chosen in order to allow good penetration in the skull. It should be noted that in this imaging technique, contrarily to ultrasound imaging, the ultrasound crosses the skull only once, which reduces the distortions that make ultrasound imaging impossible in the brain.

Results

Two experiments have been performed: without and with absorbing object. The absorbing object was introduced by drilling a small hole (~9 mm diameter) in the phantom (see dimensions in Fig. 2) and partially filling it with a mixture of Agar and carbon black (10 mm height). The rest of the hole was filled with the same surrounding "white" Agar gel.

The optical signal detected at the ultrasound frequency contains the absorption information at the ultrasound focus. The phantom is then scanned in the direction perpendicular to the fibers. The fibers and the ultrasound transducers are staying fixed. In fact it is a way to scan the absorbing object, in a fashion similar to the one described in references [7] and [8].

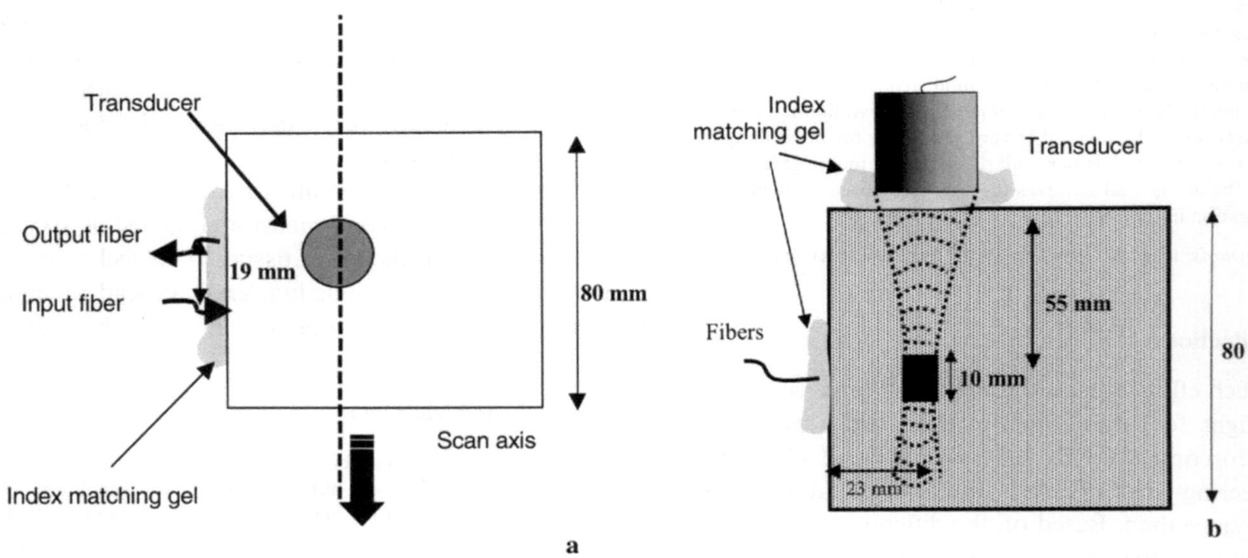

Fig. 2

The ultrasound crossing of the object and the attenuation of about 40%. This attenuation is compatible with the relative geometries of the ultrasound and the object and can be improved by using shorter focal zone transducers, ultrasound pulses or chirped cw ultrasound waves [9].

Conclusions

The method is very promising for brain imaging of trauma. It is particularly suited for monitoring, since the use of the ultrasound removes the well-recognized problem of light propagation in the CSF.

References

1. Andersson-Engels SR, Berg R, Svanberg S, Jarlman O (1990) Opt Lett 15: 21
2. Benaron DA, Stevenson DK (1993) Science 256: 1463–1466
3. Chance B, Yodh A (1995) Phys Tod 48: 34–40
4. Fishkin JB, Gratton E (1992) J Opt Soc Am A 10: 127
5. Hebden JC, Delpy DT (1994) Opt Lett 19: 311
6. Jobsis FF (1977) Science 198: 1264–1267
7. Kempe M, Larionov M, Zaslavski D, Genack AZ (1997) J Opt Soc Am A 14: 5–1151
8. Wang L, Jacques SL, Zhao X (1995) Opt Lett 20: 629
9. Wang LV, Ku G (1998) Opt Lett 23: 975

Correspondence: M. Feinsod, M.D., Department of Neurosurgery, Rambam (Maimonides), Medical Center, Haifa 31096 Israel.

Acta Neurochir (2002) [Suppl] 81: 299–301

Brain Tissue PO_2: Correlation with Cerebral Blood Flow

A. B. Valadka, R. Hlatky, Y. Furuya, and C. S. Robertson

Department of Neurosurgery, Baylor College of Medicine, Houston, Texas

Summary

This investigation analyzed 22 xenon CT cerebral blood flow (CBF) studies from 18 severely head-injured patients (Glasgow motor score < 6) who underwent xenon CT scanning while brain tissue oxygen tension ($PbtO_2$) was being monitored. CBF was determined both in a localized region of interest around the actual or estimated location of the tip of the $PbtO_2$ probe and in the entire corresponding CT slice. Linear regression analysis was used to examine the relationship between these CBF measurements and $PbtO_2$ values recorded immediately prior to the xenon CT CBF study. $PbtO_2$ varied linearly with both regional CBF (rCBF) and global CBF measurements, but the average global CBF value was significantly higher than the average rCBF value. Very low values were significantly less common for global CBF than for rCBF. Further investigation is necessary to determine how probe placement near contused areas vs. in normal tissue affects our understanding of the relationship between rCBF, global CBF, $PbtO_2$, and cerebral oxygen consumption.

Keywords: Brain tissue oxygen tension; cerebral blood flow; ischemia; xenon CT.

Introduction

The partial pressure of oxygen in the cerebral extracellular space ($PbtO_2$) reflects the balance between oxygen delivered to the brain and that consumed during cerebral metabolism. Because oxygen is transported to the brain via the blood stream, changes in cerebral blood flow (CBF) should directly affect cerebral oxygen delivery. The hypothesis tested by this investigation was that $PbtO_2$ serves as an indicator of regional CBF (rCBF).

Materials and Methods

Eighteen severely head-injured patients (Glasgow motor score < 6) who underwent a total of 22 xenon CT scans (Diversified Diagnostic Products, Houston, TX) while $PbtO_2$ was being monitored constitute the study population. Licox $PbtO_2$ probes (Kiel-Mielkendorf, Germany) were used in all patients. On the xenon CT scan slice that most closely approximated the location of the tip of the $PbtO_2$ probe, a region of interest was drawn around the actual or estimated location of the tip of the $PbtO_2$ probe. Custom software developed using IMAQ Vision for Labview 5.1 (National Instruments, Austin, TX) was used to calculate the mean CBF within each of these regions of interest. Linear regression analysis (SigmaStat for Windows 2.03, SPSS, San Rafael, CA) was used to examine the relationship between these rCBF measurements and the $PbtO_2$ values recorded immediately prior to the xenon CT CBF study.

Results

The mean age of the patients was 29.5 ± 11.0 years. Fifteen of the 18 were male (83.3%). Nine patients had cerebral contusions, either in isolation or in association with other lesions. Craniotomy was performed in 11 patients: seven had emergency evacuation of subdural and/or epidural hematomas, three had evacuation of enlarging contusions, and one underwent debridement of a gunshot wound to the head.

The xenon CT CBF studies were performed an average of 57.7 ± 42.7 hours after injury. The areas of the localized regions of interest averaged 1.75 ± 0.77 cm^2. $PbtO_2$ values ranged from 2.2 to 60.2 mm Hg. Regional CBF values ranged from 8.1 to 53.0 ml/100 g/min. CBF in the entire CT slice that contained the region of interest was also measured; these global CBF values ranged from 17.9 to 73.0 ml/100 g/min.

As shown in Figs. 1 and 2, linear regression analysis revealed that $PbtO_2$ varied directly with both rCBF and global CBF ($p \leq 0.001$ and r = approximately 0.65 both for rCBF vs. $PbtO_2$ and for global CBF vs. $PbtO_2$). The mean rCBF was significantly lower than the mean global CBF: 29.4 ± 11.7 vs. 36.4 ± 11.6 ml/100 g/min ($p = 0.05$, t-test). Seven of the 22 rCBF

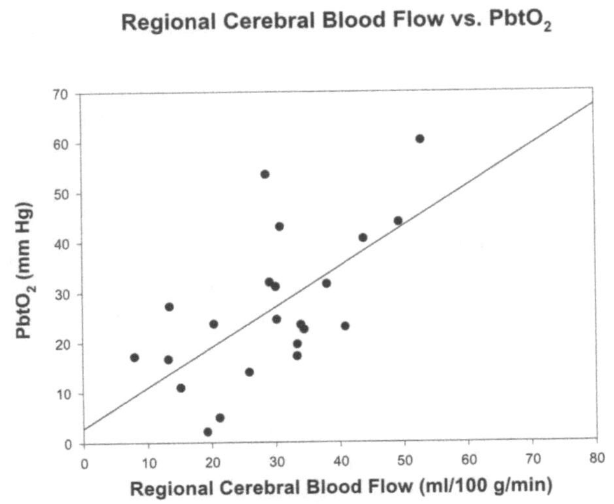

Fig. 1. Linear regression plot of brain tissue oxygen tension ($PbtO_2$) as a function of regional cerebral blood flow

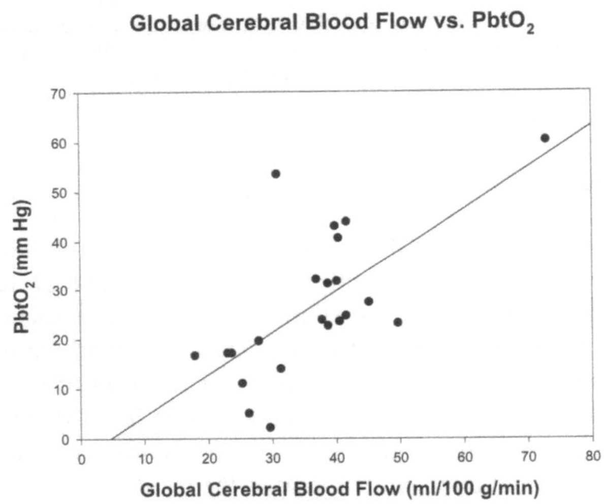

Fig. 2. Linear regression plot of brain tissue oxygen tension ($PbtO_2$) as a function of global cerebral blood flow

measurements (32%) were below 22 ml/100 g/min, as compared to one of the 22 global CBF measurements (4.5%). This difference was significant ($p < 0.05$, Fisher exact test).

Discussion

The injured brain may demonstrate considerable regional heterogeneity of cerebral metabolism [3]. Thus, global monitors of cerebral physiologic function may not accurately measure the status of a brain region with atypical metabolic activity.

In our small group of patients, $PbtO_2$ varied directly with both regional and global CBF. However, very low values were much less common for global CBF than for rCBF, and the average global CBF was significantly higher than the average rCBF. Because a global CBF value represents an average of all regions in a given CT slice, the influence of small areas of unusually high or low CBF becomes diluted. When the existence of areas of abnormal cerebral metabolism is suspected, such as by identification of cerebral contusions on a CT scan, monitoring should include the at-risk abnormal tissue as well as the entire brain. The tissue in such injured areas, although potentially viable, is the most vulnerable to secondary ischemic or hypoxic insults. Aggressive monitoring for prompt detection and treatment of secondary insults would seem to be most indicated in these regions [1]. $PbtO_2$ probes are well suited to such focal monitoring because they indicate the oxygen tension in only a very localized region of tissue [2].

Bullock and colleagues have also reported a correlation between $PbtO_2$ and rCBF [4]. However, they described a nonlinear relationship between rCBF and $PbtO_2$, with $PbtO_2$ remaining slightly higher than in a linear plot as rCBF decreases into the ischemic range. One possible reason for this discrepancy between their results and ours is that they used a different type of $PbtO_2$ probe than we did. Another difference between the present study and that of Bullock and colleagues is that they avoided CT-demonstrated primary traumatic lesions when they inserted their $PbtO_2$ sensors. $PbtO_2$ measurements obtained in this way most likely reflect global cerebral metabolism. In contrast, we tried, whenever possible, to place the $PbtO_2$ probes in brain adjacent to contusions or other abnormalities [1].

Several potential sources of error in this work must be acknowledged. Perhaps the most significant of these is the need to estimate the location of the tip of the $PbtO_2$ probe on xenon-enhanced CT slices. Because only four CT slices are produced with each xenon CT scan, the actual tip of the oxygen sensor is not always shown. In such cases, the most closely corresponding slice (based on a simultaneously obtained conventional CT scan) must be used. The relatively small number of patients is another drawback, but ongoing accrual will minimize this problem in future communications. Data from additional patients may help to elucidate the manner in which probe location near contusions vs. in grossly uninjured tissue affects our interpretation of the relationship between $PbtO_2$, rCBF, and global CBF.

Acknowledgments

Supported by Grant NS-38660 from the National Institutes of Health of the Public Health Service, United States Department of Health and Human Services.

References

1. Gopinath SP, Valadka AB, Uzura M, Robertson CS (1999) Comparison of jugular venous oxygen saturation and brain tissue PO_2 as monitors of cerebral ischemia after head injury. Crit Care Med 27: 2337–2345
2. Hoffman WE, Charbel FT, Portillo GG, Edelman G, Ausman JI (1998) Regional tissue pO_2, pCO_2, pH and temperature measurement. Neurol Res 20 [Suppl] 1: S81–S84
3. Marion DW, Darby J, Yonas H (1991) Acute regional cerebral blood flow changes caused by severe head injuries. J Neurosurg 74: 407–414
4. Menzel M, Doppenberg EM, Zauner A, Soukup J, Reinert MM, Clausen T, Brockenbrough PB, Bullock R (1999) Cerebral oxygenation in patients after severe head injury: monitoring and effects of arterial hyperoxia on cerebral blood flow, metabolism and intracranial pressure. J Neurosurg Anesthesiol 11: 240–251

Correspondence: Alex B. Valadka, M.D., 6560 Fannin Street, Suite 944, Houston, Texas, USA 77030.

Acta Neurochir (2002) [Suppl] 81: 303–305

Coexistence of Regional Cerebral Hypoxia with Normal or Hyperemic Brain Detected by Global Monitoring Methods. Analysis of Apparently Contradictory Findings Based on the Siggaard-Andersen Model of Tissue Hypoxia

J. Sahuquillo[1], S. Amorós[2], M. A. Poca[1], M. P. Mena[2], J. Ibañez[1], M. Báguena[3], and L. Domínguez[3]

[1] Department of Neurosurgery, Vall d'Hebron University Hospitals, Barcelona, Spain
[2] Neurotraumatology Intensive Care Unit, Vall d'Hebron University Hospitals, Barcelona, Spain
[3] Neurotraumatology Research Unit, Vall d'Hebron University Hospitals, Barcelona, Spain

Summary

The aim of our study was to perform and in-depth analysis of several episodes of regional brain hypoxia detected by monitoring brain partial pressure of oxygen ($PtiO_2$) in which simultaneous measurements of cerebral oxygen extraction fraction (O_2EF) suggested a normally perfused or even a hyperemic brain. To gain deeper insight into these episodes, we used the model of tissue hypoxia described by Siggaard-Andersen. In 244 simultaneous measurements, 31 episodes (12.7%) of brain hypoxia ($PtiO_2 \leq 15$ mmHg) were detected simultaneously with an O_2EF within the normal range or below the lowest normal percentile. Using Siggaard-Andersen methodology, we classified 6 episodes (19%) as *high-affinity hypoxia* and 25 (81%) as *shunt hypoxia* or *dysperfusion hypoxia*. Siggaard-Andersen's comprehensive classification of tissue hypoxia can be used as an integrative model to build coherent algorithms for diagnosing and managing neurocritical patients that are at risk of brain hypoxia due to either intracranial or extracranial conditions.

Keywords: Brain hypoxia; shunt hypoxia; dysperfusion hypoxia; head injury.

Introduction

Because ischemic and/or hypoxic brain damage is an almost constant finding in patients who die from head injury, the main goal of their management is to ensure that oxygen delivery to the brain is sufficient for or exceeds the oxygen demand of the brain cells.

Our capacity to monitor brain tissue oxygenation has improved in the last decade because of the introduction of reliable monitors that can measure both global hemometabolic parameters and regional tissue oxygenation through probes inserted directly into the brain parenchyma. However, the simultaneous monitoring of both regional and global oxygen-related variables has produced many conflicting data. In the absence of relevant focal lesions, regional measurements represent fairly well the oxygenation of the brain hemisphere in which the probe has been implanted. The relatively frequent finding of regional cerebral hypoxia coexisting with a normal or reduced global cerebral extraction of oxygen has not yet been adequately addressed. This paradox may reflect methodological artifacts (regional versus global monitoring measurements) or, as we believe, true physiopathological events. The aim of this study was to perform and in-depth analysis of several episodes of regional brain hypoxia detected by monitoring brain partial pressure of oxygen ($PtiO_2$). In these episodes, simultaneous measurements of cerebral oxygen extraction fraction (O_2EF) suggested a normally perfused or even a hyperemic brain. To gain deeper insight into these episodes, we used the model of tissue hypoxia described by Siggaard-Andersen in 1995 [5, 7].

Clinical Material and Methods

In 61 severely head-injured patients, Licox® probes (GMS, Mielkendorf, FRG) were implanted in the macroscopically normal frontal white matter. Retrograde catheters placed in the dominant jugular bulb were also inserted to monitor cerebral extraction rate of oxygen. We took 244 simultaneous measurements of $PtiO_2$, SjO_2, total hemoglobin content, half-saturation tension (P_{50}), arterial oxygen extraction tension (P_x), arterial and jugular partial pressure of oxygen (PaO_2, PjO_2), and arterial oxyhemoglobin saturation (SaO_2) at different time-points within the first 72 hours after injury. From the information obtained, comprehensive systemic and cerebral hemometabolic variables were calculated. Cerebral oxygen extraction fraction (O_2EF) was calculated as $O_2EF = (CaO_2 - CjO_2/CaO_2)*100$. The normal range for O_2EF was considered to be from 26–41% [2]. Siggaard-Andersen's software (Oxygen Status Algo-

Table 1.

Hypoxia type	Primary disturbance	$PTiO_2$ (mm Hg)	O_2EF (%)	P_x (mm Hg)	P_{50} (mm Hg)
High-affinity hypoxia	low P_{50}	≤15	N/⬇	⬇	≤24
Shunt hypoxia	increased arterio-venous shunting	≤15	N/⬇	N	>24
Dysperfusion hypoxia	increased diffusion distance, reduced diffusion area	≤15	N/⬇	N	>24

Summary of the main characteristics of the three types of brain tissue hypoxia studied. For abbreviations see text. Adapted from Siggaard-Andersen (5). *N* Within the normal range.

rithm version 3.0) was used to calculate all relevant variables [4]. To make a causal diagnosis of cerebral hypoxia, we applied an adapted version of Siggaard-Andersen's classification of tissue hypoxia to the brain (Table 1).

Results

In these 244 measurements, 31 episodes (12.7%) of brain hypoxia ($PtiO_2 \leq 15$ mmHg) were detected simultaneously with a normal or reduced O_2EF. These 31 episodes were detected in 12 patients. The mean age for these 12 patients was 32.5 ± 15.5 years. Using Siggaard-Andersen methodology, we classified 6 episodes (19%) as *high-affinity hypoxia* and 25 (81%) as *shunt hypoxia* or *dysperfusion hypoxia*. Of the 6 episodes of high-affinity hypoxia 4 were attributed to therapeutic hypothermia (temperature $< 33\,°C$), 1 was attributed to hypothermia and associated hypocapnia, and another episode was related to low temperature and anemia.

Discussion

In the injured brain, low $PtiO_2$ may coexist fairly frequently with global oxygen-derived variables that show normal or even increased oxygen delivery. Our main hypothesis is that in these cases abnormalities in hemoglobin-oxygen affinity or alterations in the diffusion of oxygen from hemoglobin to the brain tissue could be the cause of such apparent discrepancies. Siggaard-Andersen's conceptual framework of tissue hypoxia described in 1995 is, in our opinion, extremely useful for differentiating between different forms of brain hypoxia [5, 7].

The main advantage of using P_x when evaluating oxygen status is that it summarizes the integrated effect of changes in PaO_2, in oxygen capacity and in the affinity of hemoglobin to oxygen [6]. Furthermore, calculating P_{50} is helpful in detecting hypoxia secondary to the high-affinity of hemoglobin to oxygen. The possibility of dysperfusion hypoxia or shunt hypoxia has been very well established in studies of systemic tissue oxygenation [1] and should be considered in the injured brain. The swollen brain is characterized both by intracellular and extracellular edema, which increases the distance of diffusion from the capillaries to the cell. In addition, cell swelling or interstitial edema may compress the microcirculation, reducing the effective perfusion of capillaries. A second hypothesis that might explain shunt hypoxia in the brain is that because the white matter is much less perfused than the gray matter, the white matter may behave as a *microcirculatory weak unit* (MWU) [3]. According to the definition introduced by Ince, MWUs are areas in the microcirculation that are especially vulnerable to hypoxia due to anatomic or physiological characteristics.

Clinically, shunt hypoxia cannot be differentiated from dysperfusion hypoxia. Both types of hypoxia are characterized by low O_2EF and low $PtiO_2$. According to Ince and Sinaasappel, four different types of shunting may be defined: 1) convective arteriovenous shunting through anatomical anastomosis, 2) direct diffusion of oxygen from arterioles to venules lying in close proximity, 3) vascular steal where certain microcirculatory units steal flow from MWUs, 4) inability of oxygen to off-load oxygen fast enough to the tissues. This last type of shunting could be included in the category of high-affinity hypoxia described by Siggaaard-Andersen [3]. One hypothesis we propose is that white brain matter may behave as a MWU. Theoretically, blood can be shunted from the white matter by channels in the gray matter, or directly by channels in the white matter. Further studies are necessary to confirm or refute this hypothesis.

Siggaard-Andersen's comprehensive classification of tissue hypoxia can be used as an integrative model to build coherent algorithms for diagnosing and managing neurocritical patients at risk of brain hypoxia. We believe that the routine use of variables such as P_{50} and P_x allow the clinician to diagnose clinical situations of covert brain hypoxia in patients in whom the additive effects of multiple but mild alterations in different variables coexist (hypothermia, respiratory alkalosis, anemia etc.). The routine use of this paradigm could be very helpful in changing the future management of the neurocritical patient.

Acknowledgments

The authors wish to acknowledge Prof. O. Siggaard-Andersen for his generous and continuous help in adapting his classification of tissue hypoxia to the brain and for correcting our many errors and misunderstandings in this process. We also thank Gail Craigie for correcting the manuscript. This work was supported by *Fondo de Investigaciones Sanitarias de la Seguridad Social* (FIS) grants numbers 00/0827 and 1031/97 from the *Fundació La Marato de TV3* to Dr. J. Sahuquillo.

References

1. Dantzker DR (1993) Adequacy of tissue oxygenation. Crit Care Med 21: S40–S43
2. Gibbs EL, Lennox WG, Nims LF, Gibbs FA (1942) Arterial and cerebral venous blood. Arterial-venous differences in man. J Biol Chem 144: 325–332
3. Ince C, Sinaasappel M (1999) Microcirculatory oxygenation and shunting in sepsis and shock. Crit Care Med 27: 1369–1377
4. Siggaard-Andersen M, Siggaard-Andersen O (1995) Oxygen status algorithm, version 3, with some applications. Acta Anaesthesiol Scand 39: 13–20
5. Siggaard-Andersen O, Fogh-Andersen N, Gothgen IH, Larsen VH (1995) Oxygen status of arterial and mixed venous blood. Crit Care Med 23: 1284–1293
6. Siggaard-Andersen O, Gothgen IH, Wimberley PD, Fogh-Andersen N (1990) The oxygen status of the arterial blood revised: relevant oxygen parameters for monitoring the arterial oxygen availability. Scand J Clin Lab Invest [Suppl] 203: 17–28
7. Siggaard-Andersen O, Ulrich A, Gothgen IH (1995) Classes of tissue hypoxia. Acta Anaesthesiol Scand 39: 137–142

Correspondence: Dr. Juan Sahuquillo, Osona 6, 2-4, 08023 Barcelona, Spain.

Acta Neurochir (2002) [Suppl] 81: 307–309

Therapeutic Aspects of Brain Tissue pO_2 Monitoring after Subarachnoid Hemorrhage

A. Väth[1], E. Kunze[1], K. Roosen[1], and J. Meixensberger[2]

[1] Department of Neurosurgery, University of Würzburg, Germany
[2] Department of Neurosurgery, University of Leipzig, Leipzig, Germany

Summary

Prolonged phases of brain tissue hypoxia ($p_{ti}O_2 < 10$ mmHg) lead to cerebral infarction. Therefore, the present study investigates the role of $p_{ti}O_2$ – monitoring to guide hypervolemic hypertensive therapy in patients suffering from severe subarachnoid hemorrhage (SAH). Besides transcranial doppler, neuromonitoring of ICP/CPP was supplemented by $p_{ti}O_2$ monitoring. The $p_{ti}O_2$ catheter was inserted into viable tissue in the vascular territory with the highest risk for vasospasm. Patients were divided in an infarction ($n = 21$) and a non-infarction group ($n = 11$). Critical CPP (< 70 mmHg) as well as hypoxic ptiO2 (< 10 mmHg) was significantly more frequent in the infarction group (CPP: 25 vs 13%, $p < 0.001$; ptiO2: 16 vs 7%, $p < 0.001$). In both groups, over 25% of the critical ptiO2 values occurred at a CPP > 90 mmHg. In the infarction group, 13 patients showed transient phases of hypoxia which normalized under induced hypervolemic hypertension and 5 patients developed persistent hypoxia. In the non-infarction group 6 patients showed transient hypoxia and in 5 patients no hypoxic values could be found. In conclusion, monitoring of $p_{ti}O_2$ provides an additional independent parameter to detect hypoxic events and to guide therapy.

Keywords: Subarachnoid hemorrhage; tissue-pO_2; ischemia; hypervolemic hypertension.

Introduction

Inadequacy of cerebral perfusion leading to prolonged phases of hypoxia and cerebral infarction worsens the outcome of patients suffering from subarachnoid hemorrhage (SAH) [2]. Monitoring of brain tissue pO_2 ($p_{ti}O_2$) is an established technology in head injured patients which allows detection of critical, hypoxic cerebral oxygenation [3, 6]. Additionally, different studies could demonstrate guidance of therapy [4, 5]. This study is focused on the therapeutic aspects of $p_{ti}O_2$ in severe SAH patients. Monitoring of $p_{ti}O_2$ may be helpful to recognize critical oxygenation due to vasospasm. Our interest was especially focused on the question whether $p_{ti}O_2$ – supplemented monitoring of cerebral perfusion pressure (CPP) allows balance of hypervolemic, hypertensive hemodilutive (HHH) – therapy.

Patients and Methods

According to a protocol approved by the local ethics committee neuromonitoring of ICP, CPP and $P_{ti}O_2$ was performed on thirty two patients suffering from subarachnoid hemorrhage (SAH) who had either an initial Hunt and Hess grade of 4 or secondarily deterioration to grade 4. For each patient age, initial Hunt and Hess grade and incidence of initial pupillary disturbances were noted and the severity of SAH was classified from initial CT scans using the Fisher score. Angiography was used to detect the source and location of the hemorrhage. All patients were intubated and artificially ventilated to maintain a $p_aO_2 \approx 100$ mmHg and a $p_aCO_2 \approx 35–40$ mmHg. To reduce the risk of rebleeding, aneurysms were clipped as early as possible.

For neuromonitoring ICP (Camino Laboratories, San Diego, USA) and $P_{ti}O_2$ sensors (LICOX, Kiel-Mielkendorf, Germany) were used. The $P_{ti}O_2$ sensor was inserted into initially viable tissue in the area at risk for vasospasm or close to a developing cerebral infarction. The standard position of the $P_{ti}O_2$ catheter was 22–27 mm subdurally in white matter. Mean arterial blood pressure was measured in the radial artery referenced to the Foramen of Monroi, and CPP was calculated from MAP-ICP. All monitoring parameters were synchronously digitized at a rate of 4/minute (Neurox, Kiel-Mielkendorf, Germany) and stored on a computer. In addition to stabilization of arterial blood gases the major therapeutic targets were: (1) avoidance of raised ICP (> 20 mmHg) by liquor drainage/decompression and mannitol and (2) HHH therapy to avoid hypoxic $P_{ti}O_2$ (< 10 mmHg) due to vasospasm. Ca^{2+} antagonists were only administered, if blood pressure was not affected. For further analyses artifacts due to nursing and therapeutic interventions were manually removed from neuromonitoring time series using self made software (SCILAB, INRIA, France; Visual C++, Microsoft Corp.).

Results

For analysis the patients were divided into two groups: an infarction group ($n = 21$) and a non-

Table 1. *Final Response of Induced Hypervolemic Hypertension after Detection of Hypoxic $P_{ti}O_2$ Event ($p_{ti}O_2 < 10$ mmHg, Duration > 10 min) in Patients Suffering from SAH. Values Given as Median/Standard Deviation*

		Infarction group n = 21	Non-infarction group n = 11
Transient hypoxia			
CPP (mmHg)	N	13	6
		89.9/15	83.7/9.7
Persistent hypoxia			
CPP (mmHg)	N	5	0
		89.5/18	
No hypoxia			
CPP (mmHg)	n	3	5
		78/15	78.9/9.7

infarction group. Between both groups no significant difference could be found concerning age, Hunt & Hess grade, amount of subarachnoid blood according to the Fisher classification and aneurysm location, almost in the anterior part of the circle of Willis. Ten patients (48%) of the infarction group died, none of the non-infarction group. Therefore the duration of monitoring was significantly shorter in the infarction group in comparison to the patient group without cerebral ischemia (median value 3.8 days vs 7.8 days). Analysing the median values over the whole monitoring time, no significant difference between the infarction/non-infarction group could be detected (median CPP/mmHg: 87 vs 82; $p_{ti}O_2$/mmHg: 23 vs 25). However, critical CPP episodes (<70 mmHg, > 10 minutes) as well as hypoxic $p_{ti}O_2$ periods (<10 mmHg, >10 minutes) occurred significantly more frequently in the infarction group (CPP: 25% vs 13%, $p < 0.001$; $p_{ti}O_2$: 16% vs 7%, $p < 0.001$). In the infarction group thirteen patients revealed transient phases of hypoxia which could be normalised inducing HHH therapy (Table 1). Five patients developed persistent hypoxia despite the fact that cerebral perfusion pressure was increased in the individual case. Three patients showed no critical values of cerebral oxygenation. In these cases $p_{ti}O_2$-catheters were not positioned in the vascular territory where infarction could be seen on CT scan. In the non-infarction group, in six patients transient cerebral hypoxia could be treated by volume expansion and increase of arterial blood pressure. Figure 1 shows a typical example of a patient where transient episodes of hypoxic $p_{ti}O_2$ occur and who responds to hypertensive therapy, while the second case demonstrated development of persistent hypoxia leading to cerebral infarction. Finally, the fractions of hypoxic $p_{ti}O_2$ (<10 mmHg) were analysed above different CPP thresholds (Fig. 2). Critical values of cerebral oxygenation could be detected in about 78% at a CPP threshold above 70 mmHg. If CPP was above 80 mmHg, 55% of critical $p_{ti}O_2$ values occurred. At a CPP threshold over 90 mmHg, 27% of critical cerebral oxygenation could be found in both groups. Individual analysis revealed a change of CPP threshold to maintain sufficient oxygenation from day to day.

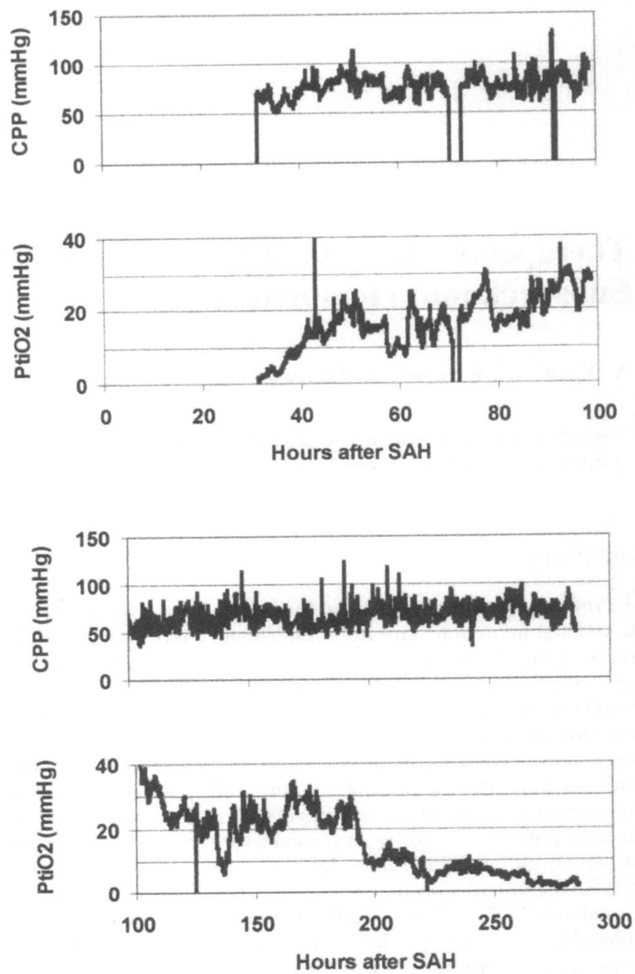

Fig. 1. Original data curves of a patient with $P_{ti}O_2$ returning to normal values after a hypoxic event following induced hypervolemic (responder, upper curves) hypertension and a patient developing infarction (non-responder, lower curves)

Discussion

Monitoring of brain tissue pO_2, reflecting local cerebral oxygenation, is a safe and reliable technology,

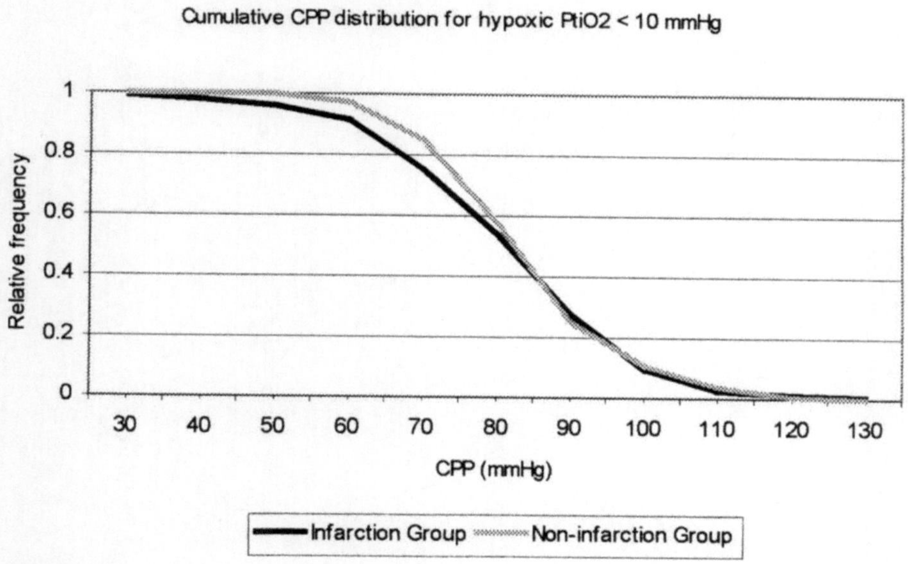

Fig. 2. Proportion of hypoxic $P_{ti}O_2 \leq 10$ mmHg above different CPP thresholds for infarction (n = 21) and non-infarction group (n = 11)

which has the potential to detect cerebral hypoxia in vascular territory at risk of cerebral infarction, if catheter could be inserted in the region of interest. In this series tissue catheters were in correct position in over 90% of the patients. Vascular territory at risk of ischemia/vasospasm was chosen based on operation site of aneurysm, morphological changes on repeated CT scans (development of hypodensity) and TCD findings (critical increase of blood flow velocity). However, in three cases cerebral infarction occurred although $p_{ti}O_2$ was in normal range indicating the limitations of a local monitoring technology. Nevertheless, monitoring of $p_{ti}O_2$ allows real-time detection of hypoxic cerebral oxygenation in critically ill SAH patients, who are at risk for ischemia and vasospasm. Additionally, the effect of therapy (induced hypertension in combination with volume expansion) to maintain sufficient oxygenation could be balanced in the individual patients. Our data confirm Xenon-CT studies which demonstrated increase of territorial local CBF above the ischemic range in more than 90% of uninfarcted territories using dopamin-induced hypertension [1]. However, $p_{ti}O_2$-monitoring enables continuous determination of the critical CPP threshold, which may vary from day to day.

Acknowledgments

This work was supported by the Vera und Volker Doppelfeld-Stiftung and DFG Me-1020/3-2.

References

1. Darby JM, Yonas H, Marks EC, Durham S, Snyder RW, Nemoto EM (1994) Acute cerebral blood flow response to dopamine-induced hypertension after subarachnoid hemorrhage. J Neurosurg 80: 857–864
2. Dorsch NWC (1994) A review of cerebral vasospasm in aneurysmal subarachnoid hemorrhage. Part 2: management. J Clin Neurosci 1: 78–92
3. Dings J, Meixensberger J, Jäger A, Roosen K (1998) Clinical experience with 118 brain oxygen partial pressure catheter probes. Neurosurgery 43: 1082–1094
4. Kiening KL, Hartl R, Unterberg AW, Schneider GH, Bardt T, Lanksch WR (1997) Brain tissue pO2-monitoring in comatose patients: implications for therapy. Neurol Res 19: 233–240
5. Meixensberger J, Jäger A, Dings J, Baunach S, Roosen K (1997) Quality and therapeutic advances in multimodality neuromonitoring following head injury. In: Bauer BL, Kuhn TJ (eds) Severe head injuries. Springer, Berlin Heidelberg New York Tokyo, pp 99–108
6. Zauner A, Doppenberg E, Woodward JJ, Allen C, Jebraili S, Young HF, Bullock R (1997) Multiparametric continuous monitoring of brain metabolism and substrate delivery in neurosurgical patients. Neurol Res 19: 265–273

Correspondence: Prof. Dr. Jürgen Meixensberger, Department of Neurosurgery, University of Leipzig, Johannisallee 34, D-04103 Leipzig, Germany.

Acta Neurochir (2002) [Suppl] 81: 311–313

Dynamic Correlation Between Tissue PO2 and near Infrared Spectroscopy

R. D. Rothoerl, R. Faltermeier, R. Burger, C. Woertgen, and A. Brawanski

Department of Neurosurgery, University of Regensburg, Germany

Summary

Multimodal O2 monitoring including tissue pO2 measurements and near infrared spectroscopy (NIRS) are techniques increasingly employed for monitoring patients on neurosurgical intensive care units. NIRS measures a mixed venous arterial oxygen saturation, whereas tissue pO2 evaluates the oxygen pressure in the white matter. In contrast to the tissue pO2 measurements, the NIRS at the moment has not been completely established in clinical practice. We wanted to evaluate whether both techniques are monitoring different dynamic changes. Thirteen patients were included (SAH n = 3, TBI n = 10), 12 patients were male and 1 was female. Mean age was 34 years with a range from 16–76 years. Tissue pO2 probes (Licox, GMS, Germany) were implanted in the frontal lobe showing most pathological changes on the initial CT scan. A near infrared spectroscopy sensor (Invos, Somanetics, USA) was placed simultaneously at the patient's forehead. Due to the drift of the tissue pO2 probe, only data sets were taken into further account in which a tissue pO2 value above 15 mmHg was measured. 66 data sets were analyzed by calculating the spectral coherence with multi taper methods. The coherence of two independent white noise signals were defined as an observation by chance. The significance level for correlated frequencies was 90%. In the spectral long time regime (frequency ≥ 0.02), more than 80% of the data sets showed a higher percentage of correlated frequencies as compared to the observation by chance. The assumption that tissue pO2 and near infrared spectroscopy probes are measuring different dynamic changes in neurosurgical intensive care patients could not be supported by our data.

Keywords: NIRS; Tissue PO2; frequency analysis.

Introduction

Episodes of insufficient cerebral oxygenation are considered to enhance secondary brain damage in severely head injured patients [6]. Thus several new continuous hemodynamic monitoring technologies like regional, invasive measurement of brain tissue pO2 as well as regional non invasive NIRS (rSO2; regional oxygen saturation) and global jugular bulb oximetry (SjO2; jugular venous saturation) have been introduced in the last few years into clinical practice in order to monitor the oxygen metabolism and enable to treat ischemic episodes.

In case of the tissue pO2 it could be demonstrated that measurements were reliable and hypoxic values were correlated to other monitoring modalities [1, 2, 5]. These results seem to be generally accepted. In case of the near infrared spectroscopy the reports in the literature appear to be contradictory. Kirckpatrick *et al.* correlated desaturation episodes detected with the jugular bulb oximetry to desaturation episodes detected with the NIRS. The authors found a good correlation of both methods [4]. In contrast to this study. Lewis *et al.* desribed a low correlation of both methods [5]. When comparing the near infrared spectroscopy to tissue pO2 measurements, Meixenberger described a restricted reliability and sensitivity of the near infrared spectroscopy when analyzing desaturation episodes. Thus the tissue pO2 measurements seem to be generally accepted. In the case of near infrared spectroscopy most authors seem to doubt reliability and data quality of this method.

We think that evaluation of dynamic changes of these signals allow a comparison of data quality and reliability of both methods. Aim of this study was not to compare values at defined episodes but to analyze dynamic changes in both signals in order to evaluate whether both techniques monitor different or similar dynamic changes in the cerebral oxygen metabolism.

Materials and Methods

Patients and Monitoring Devices

A multimodality recording system was used in 13 ventilated patients with closed head injury (n = 10) or SAH (n = 3); 12 patients were male and 1 was female. Mean age was 34 years with a range from 16–76 years. Tissue pO2 probes (Licox, GMS, Germany) were implanted in the frontal lobe showing most pathological changes on the initial CT scan. A near infrared spectroscopy sensor (Invos, Somanetics, USA) was placed simultaneously at the patient's forehead. Signals of intracranial pressure, cerebral perfusion pressure, brain tissue pO2, and NIRS-derived changes in the chromophores of oxy- and deoxyhemoglobin were digitized and stored simultaneously.

Mathematical Methods

In both time series tissue pO2 and NIRS data were split into segments of 1920 points at a sample rate of 15 seconds, i.e. every segment covers eight hours of monitoring. Three independent spectral estimates of each data segment were calculated at each inducible frequency (f). A confidence test similar to Thompsons F variance ratio test was used to determine the significance level of the coherence amplitude at each inducible. In order to quantify the common long term dynamics of both signals, the density of coherent frequencies was calculated for $f \leq 0.02$ at a significance level of 0.9. These results were compared to two completely uncorrelated white noise signals treated in the same manner.

Results

In the spectral long time regime (frequency ≤ 0.02) more than 80% of the data sets showed a higher percentage of correlated frequencies as compared to uncorrelated white noise.

Discussion

Several authors describe the tissue pO2 measurement as a save and reliable method in detecting ischemic episodes after traumatic brain injury. For example Kiening concludes in 1996 that monitoring brain tissue pO2 is a safe, reliable, and sensitive diagnostic method to follow cerebral oxygenation. In comparison to SjvO2, tissue pO2 is more suitable for longterm monitoring. It can be used to minimize episodes of secondary cerebral maloxygenation after severe head injury and may, hopefully, improve the outcome in severely head injured patients. These results seem to be generally accepted. In case of the near infrared spectroscopy the reports in the literature, however, are contradictory. Kirckpatrick *et al.* correlated desaturation episodes detected with the jugular bulb oximetry to desaturation episodes detected with the near infrared spectroscopy. They included 14 patients after severe head injury and found 38 desaturation episodes in the jugular bulb oximetry and 37 desaturation episodes in the near infrared spectroscopy [3]. In contast to this study, Lewis examined 10 patients suffering from severe head injury with NIRS and jugular bulb oximetry and concluded that tissue oxygen saturation determined by near-infrared spectroscopy does not reflect significant changes in cerebral oxygenation detected by the global measurement of jugular venous bulb oximetry and cannot be routinely recommended for assessment of cerebral oxygenation in patients with acute head injury [4].

Only a few reports in the literature compare the near infrared spectroscopy and tissue pO2 devices. For example Meixensberger *et al.* concluded that long-term-measurements of rSO2 using near infrared spectroscopy reached, if possible, a restricted reliability in comparison to tissue pO2. In comparison of both methods a restricted reliability and sensitivity of the near infrared spectroscopy when analyzing desaturation episodes is reported. Thus the authors concluded that only the tissue pO2 measurements supplements the standard neuromonitoring [5]. However our results suggest that dynamical changes in the tissue pO2 measurements are well reflected in the NIRS. This correlation of dynamic changes in both methods is higher than an observation by chance as demonstrated by the spectral coherence analysis. It seems that both methods are able to reflect dynamical changes in the cerebral oxygen metabolism with a dependent reliability. The assumption that tissue pO2 and near infrared spectroscopy probes reflect different dynamic changes in neurosurgical intensive care patients could not be supported by our data.

References

1. Dings J, Meixensberger J, Jager A, Roosen K (1998) Clinical experience with 118 brain tissue oxygen partial pressure catheter probes. Neurosurgery 43: 1082–1095
2. Kiening KL, Unterberg AW, Bardt TF, Schneider GH, Lanksch WR (1996) Monitoring of cerebral oxygenation in patients with severe head injuries: brain tissue PO2 versus jugular vein oxygen saturation. J Neurosurg 85: 751–757
3. Kirkpatrick PJ, Smielewski P, Czosnyka M, Menon DK, Pickard JD (1995) Near-infrared spectroscopy use in patients with head injury. J Neurosurg 83: 963–970
4. Lewis SB, Myburgh JA, Thornton EL, Reilly PL (1996) Cerebral oxygenation monitoring by near-infrared spectroscopy is not clinically useful in patients with severe closed-head injury: a comparison with jugular venous bulb oximetry. Crit Care Med 24: 1334–1338

5. Meixensberger J, Jager A, Dings J, Baunach S, Roosen K (1998) Multimodal hemodynamic neuromonitoring – quality and consequences for therapy of severely head injured patients. Acta Neurochir (Wien) [Suppl] 71: 260–262
6. Robertson CS, Contant CF, Gokaslan ZL, Narayan RK, Grossman RG (1992) Cerebral blood flow, arteriovenous oxygen difference, and outcome in head injured patients. J Neurol Neurosurg Psychiatry 55: 594–603

Correspondence: Ralf Dirk Rothoerl, M.D., Departments of Neurosurgery, University of Regensburg, Franz Josef Strauss Allee 11, 93053 Regensburg, Germany.

Acta Neurochir (2002) [Suppl] 81: 315–317

Effects of Hyperoxia on Brain Tissue Oxygen Tension in Cerebral Focal Lesions

L. Longhi, V. Valeriani, S. Rossi, M. De Marchi, M. Egidi, and **N. Stocchetti**

Department of Anesthesia and Intensive Care, Ospedale Maggiore Policlinico IRCCS, Milano, Italy

Summary

We evaluated the systemic and cerebral effects induced by an increase to 100% of the inspired oxygen fraction (FiO2) on 20 comatose patients with head injury (9 patients) and SAH (11 patients). Brain tissue oxygen tension (PtiO2) was measured through a Clark electrode inserted in penumbra-like areas. We performed 55 hyperoxia tests by increasing FiO2 from 35 ± 8% to 100% in one second and calculating the PtiO2 index as: PtiO2 variation from baseline at 1 minute/arterial oxygen tension (PaO2) variation from baseline at 1 minute × 100. One hundred percent FiO2 caused an increase of both arterial (from 139 ± 28 to 396 ± 77 mmHg) and cerebral (from 22.6 ± 14 to 65.4 ± 60 mmHg) oxygenation after 1 minute. The range of the PtiO2 response was not uniform and two groups were identified. The change was small, 0.8 mmHg/min/100 mmHg PaO2 (±0.7; range 0–2) when mean PtiO2 was 19.7 ± 13.1 mmHg, while a stronger response, 8 mmHg/min/100 mmHg PaO2 (±5; range 3–18) ($p < 0.01$) was found when mean PtiO2 was 31.7 ± 14.3 mmHg. Since O2 diffusion should follow the gas diffusion law, the increase in diffusion distance due to a reduction of capillary density in focal lesions may explain this relationship.

Keywords: Head injury; cerebral oxygenation; cerebral ischemia; hyperoxia.

Introduction

Cerebral ischemia is one of the major factors influencing the prognosis and outcome in acute head injured patients [5]. Continuous measurement of cerebral oxygen tension (PtiO2) has been suggested as a reliable method for assessing the adequacy of oxygen supply to the brain [1]. Low PtiO2 values are associated with poorer outcome and hyperoxia tests have been proposed in the clinical setting for determination of the oxygen diffusion from the microcirculation to the tissue. Some authors have suggested that the PtiO2 response to an increase in the inspired oxygen fraction (FiO2) can be used to assess cerebral autoregulation. A relation between this response and outcome has been described [6, 7]. Little is known about the changes induced systemically and to the brain by a rapid increase of the FiO2. Our aim is to characterize the systemic modifications induced by the increase of the inspired oxygen fraction, to define the PtiO2 behavior after hyperoxia and to clarify the mechanisms involved in this response for potential clinical applications.

Material and Methods

Twenty (11 female) comatose (median GCS = 7) patients admitted to our intensive care unit for head injuries (9 cases) or SAH (11 cases), age 40 ± 18 years (range 13–70) were studied. Mean Arterial Pressure (MAP), Intracranial Pressure (ICP), Cerebral Perfusion Pressure (CPP = MAP − ICP) were continuously monitored and samples of blood from the jugular bulb and from an arterial catheter were analyzed. Surgical mass lesions were removed and patients were treated according to a protocol including sedation, curarization, mannitol and moderate hyperventilation for ICP control. PtiO2 was measured using a Clark electrode (Licox, GMS, Germany) placed in penumbra-like areas, identified with a CT scan. A second CT scan was performed for assessment of the correct positioning of the probe. FiO2 was increased from baseline to 100% in one second under stable conditions; arterial and jugular blood samples were collected at baseline and 1, 3, 5, 10, 15 minutes thereafter. The PtiO2 response was calculated using the following formula:

PtiO2 response = (PtiO2 at 1 minute − PtiO2 baseline) × 1/(PaO2 at 1 minute − PaO2 at baseline)*100.

Data are referred as mean values and standard deviation. T-test was used for comparison between groups.

Results

In 55 tests FiO2 was increased from a mean value of 35 ± 8.6% (range 25–65) to 100%. In all cases a significant ($p < 0.01$) increase in PaO2 was detected (from 139.5 ± 28 to 396 ± 77 mmHg). The response reached a maximum in the first phase of the test and rapidly decreased within a few minutes. The curve has a loga-

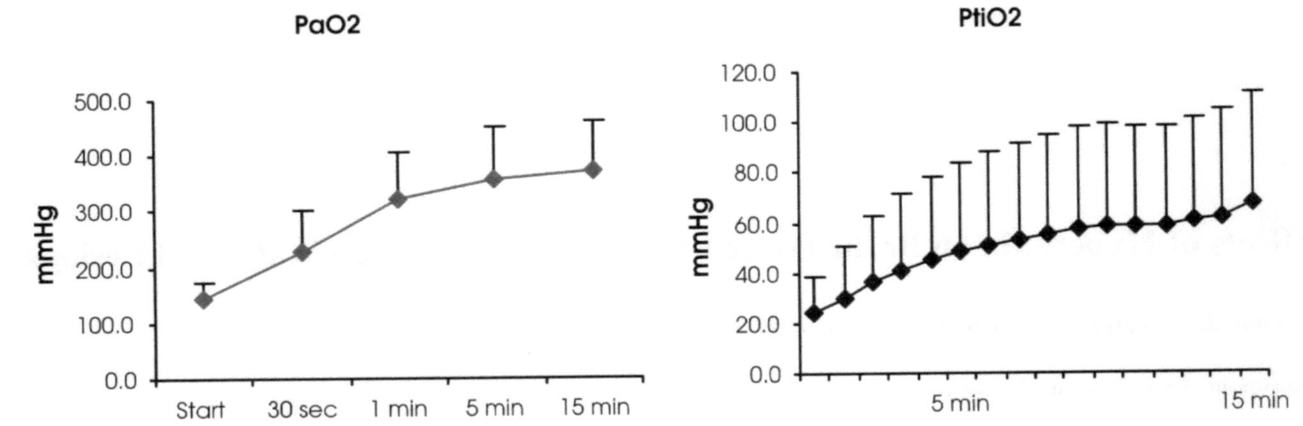

Fig. 1. Arterial (left) and cerebral (right) modifications of oxygen tension induced by increasing FiO2 to 100%

rithmic shape in accordance with a "wash in" function as described in Fig. 1.

The PtiO2 response to 100% FiO2 has a logarithmic morphology, and the maximum increase could be detected at 1 minute from baseline (mean increase at 1 minute $= 6.2 \pm 9.7$ mmHg). The PtiO2 response to hyperoxia showed a great variability and depended on the PtiO2 baseline value. The change was weak, 0.8 mmHg/min/100 mmHg PaO2 (± 0.7; range 0–2) when mean PtiO2 was 19.7 ± 13.1 mmHg (42 tests in 18 patients). A stronger response ($p < 0.01$) of 8 mmHg/min/100 mmHg PaO2 (± 5; range 3–18) was found when mean PtiO2 was 31.7 ± 14.3 mmHg (13 tests in 8 patients). No differences in PaO2, CPP, ICP and PaCO2 among cases with weak or strong response were detected.

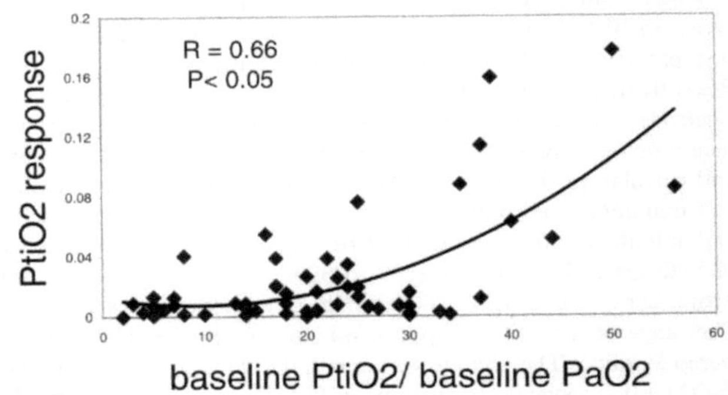

Fig. 2. Relation between baseline PtiO2 values corrected for baseline oxygen tension and PtiO2 response to hyperoxia

Discussion

Hyperoxia increases arterial oxygen tension and the oxygen gradient between capillaries and cerebral tissue without concurrent systemic alterations. The PtiO2 response is well described by a logarithmic curve with a maximum increase at 1 minute from baseline. The PtiO2 response to hyperoxia is variable and two different patterns could be identified: the index is elevated when associated with normal basal PtiO2 values and is smaller when associated with lower basal PtiO2 values. Since O2 diffusion should follow the gas diffusion law, the increase in diffusion distance due to a reduction of capillary density in focal lesions may explain this relationship.

However the polinomial curve describing the relation between the PtiO2 index and PtiO2 baseline values (Fig. 2) explains 66% of tests performed ($P < 0.05$) and a cluster of tests could be identified where even with a baseline PtiO2 in the normal range the response was weak. In this group we hypothesize that the PtiO2 response is the results of vasoconstriction secondary to an increase in cerebral oxygen tension. PtiO2 and its response to hyperoxia might be useful for assessing the microcirculation in penumbra-like areas, but further work is necessary to elucidate the mechanisms involved in its regulation [2, 3, 4].

References

1. Gopinath SP, Valadka AB, Uzura M, Robertson CS (1999) Comparison of jugular venous oxygen saturation and brain tissue Po2 as monitors of cerebral ischaemia after head injury. Crit Care Med 11: 2337–2345
2. Harris RJ, Richards PG, Symon L, Habib AHA, Rosenstein J (1987) pH, K and PO of the extracellular space during ischamia of primate cerebral cortex. J Cereb Blood Flow Metab 5: 599–604

3. Jacobson I, Harper AM, McDowall DG (1964) The effects of oxygen at 1 and 2 atmospheres on the blood flow and oxygen uptake of the cerebral cortex. Surgery Gynecology Obstetrics 4: 737–742
4. Nair P, Whalen WJ, Buerk D (1975) PO of cat cerebral cortex: response to breathing N2 and 100% O2. Microvascular Research 9: 158–165
5. Teasdale GM, Graham DI (1998) Craniocerebral trauma: protection and retrieval of the neuronal population after injury. Neurosurgery 43: 723–738
6. Valadka AB, Gopinath SP, Contant CF, Uzura M, Robertson CS (1998) Relationship of brain tissue pO2 to outcome after severe head injury. Crit Care Med 26: 1576–1581
7. Van Santbrink H, Maas AIR, Avezaat CJJ (1996) Continuous monitoring of partial pressure of brain tissue oxygen in patients with severe head injury. Neurosurgery 38: 21–31

Correspondence: Dr. Nino Stocchetti, Ospedale Policlinico di Milano IRCCS, Neurosurgical Intensive Care, Via F. Sforza 35, 20122 Milan, Italy.

Acta Neurochir (2002) [Suppl] 81: 319–321

Detection of Secondary Insults by Brain Tissue pO_2 and Bedside Microdialysis in Severe Head Injury*

A. S. Sarrafzadeh, O. W. Sakowitz, T.-A. Callsen, W. R. Lanksch, and A. W. Unterberg

Department of Neurosurgery, Charité Campus Virchow Medical Center, Humboldt University of Berlin, Germany

Summary

We evaluated bedside cerebral on-line microdialysis for early detection of cerebral hypoxia in patients with traumatic brain injury. 24 severely head injured patients (Glasgow Coma Score ≤ 8) were studied. Patients underwent continuous brain tissue PO_2 ($PtiO_2$) monitoring using the LICOX (GMS mbH, Germany) microcatheter device. The catheter was placed into the non-lesioned frontal white matter within 32.2 (7–48) hrs post injury. The microdialysis catheter (CMA 100, Sweden) was placed close to the $PtiO_2$ probe via a 2- or 3-way skull screw, connected to a pump and perfused with Ringer solution (0.3 µl/min). The microdialysis samples were collected hourly and analyzed at the bedside for glucose, lactate, lactate-pyruvate-ratio and glutamate (CMA 600, Sweden). We identified 252 episodes of impending hypoxia ($PtiO_2 < 15$ mm Hg; 11810 minutes) and 38 episodes of cerebral hypoxia ($PtiO_2 < 10$ mm Hg; 1996 minutes). Before cerebral hypoxia, glucose decreased significantly. Glutamate was unchanged when no hypoxia or impending hypoxia occurred but increased 3–4fold before a hypoxic episode appeared. We conclude that early metabolic detection of cerebral hypoxia before a critical decrease in brain tissue $PtiO_2$ is seen and possibly allows earlier changes in treatment (e.g. reduction of hyperventilation therapy).

Keywords: Cerebral metabolism; microdialysis; cerebral oxygenation; severe head injury.

Introduction

Ischemia and hypoxia are insults to the brain tissue that frequently occur in neurointensive care patients. Inherent physiological thresholds of brain tissue probably determine the extent of damage that results. Time, temperature, blood flow, metabolic substrates, and many other variables influence ultimately the severity of cerebral lesion and outcome. Continuous monitoring of local brain tissue PO_2 is an accepted method for the early detection of impending hypoxia/ischemia [1, 3, 7, 8]. The longer the presence of impending ($PtiO_2 < 15$ mm Hg) or present hypoxia ($PtiO_2 < 10$ mm Hg) the higher the likelihood of an adverse outcome [7]. Recently, bedside microdialysis, a method to evaluate on-line cerebral metabolism in a clinical setting, has become available [6]. Energy metabolites as glucose, pyruvate and lactate, the excitatory amino acid and indicator of ischemia glutamate as well as glycerol, a marker of cell membrane damage can be measured immediately in the patient room. The combination of the brain tissue PO_2 monitoring and microdialysis may help to index cerebral damage, reflecting prognosis, clinical course, critical thresholds and response to therapy. The purpose of this study was to determine the regional metabolic changes monitored by microdialysis before cerebral hypoxia in patients with severe head injury in order to evaluate microdialysis for early detection of cerebral hypoxia.

Patients and Methods

Patient Characteristics and Management

24 severely head injured patients (Glasgow Coma Score < 9) admitted to the Dept were included into the study. There were 6 females and 18 males with age ranging from 6 to 75 years (mean age 37 years). On admission, traumatic lesions were confirmed by computerized tomography (CT) scanning. Mass lesions were immediately evacuated. Thereafter a standardized protocol followed. The patients were not paralyzed, but sedated and ventilated to achieve normoventilation ($PaCO_2 > 35$ mm Hg). Intracranial hypertension (ICP > 20 mm Hg) was managed according to the AANS-guidelines for the management of severe head injury with cerebrospinal fluid drainage, boluses of mannitol (0,5 g^{-1} g/kg body weight over a period of 20 minutes) and moderate hyperventilation ($PaCO_2$ 30–35 mm Hg). Barbiturate coma was induced in otherwise uncontrollable intracranial hypertension and guided by a "burst-

* Supported by Deutsche Forschungsgemeinschaft Un-56/7.

suppression"-EEG pattern. Cerebral perfusion pressure was maintained above 60 mm Hg using colloidal and noncolloidal agents, blood products and catecholamines if necessary.

Monitoring Devices

Mean arterial pressure (MAP) was monitored continuously using an intraparenchymal fibre-optic transducer (Camino Laboratories, San Diego, CA; Codman, Johnson&Johnson). Patients underwent continuous brain tissue PO_2 ($PtiO_2$) monitoring using the LICOX (GMS mbH, Germany) microcatheter device. The catheter was placed into the non-lesioned frontal white matter within 32.2 (7–48) hrs post injury. Correct position of the $PtiO_2$ catheters tip was verified by CCT. The microdialysis catheter (CMA 100, Sweden) was located close to the $PtiO_2$ probe via a 2- or 3-way skull screw connected to a pump and perfused with Ringer solution (0.3 µl/min). The microdialysis samples were collected hourly and analyzed at the bedside for glucose, lactate, lactate-pyruvate-ratio and glutamate (CMA 600, Sweden). Total monitoring time including $PtiO_2$ and microdialysis was 5.2 (1–11) days. After monitoring, the $PtiO_2$ catheters were checked for sensitivity drifts.

Data Analysis

Analog signals of MAP, ICP, $etCO_2$ (Modul M1020A, Hewlett Packard, Waltham, MA) and $PtiO_2$ were continuously digitized, displayed and stored on a Windows-platform running a LabVIEW (National Instruments, Austin, TX) based software for multimodal data acquisition. Data were stepwise analyzed according to the following criteria: 1. Identification of episodes of impending ($PtiO_2$ 10–15 mm Hg, >5 min duration) and present hypoxia ($PtiO_2$ <10 mm Hg, >5 min duration). The end of an episode was defined as following 5 minutes of normal brain tissue PO_2 values. 2. Occurrence of hypoxic episodes in relation to the day after trauma. 3. Presence of intracranial hypertension (ICP > 20 mm Hg), arterial hypotension (MAP < 70 mm Hg), low cerebral perfusion pressure (CPP < 60 mm Hg), presence of hyperventilation (endtidal CO_2 <30 mm Hg, $etCO_2$) during impending/present hypoxia. Microdialysis (sampled hourly) values within 60 minutes before the onset of impending/present hypoxia were analyzed (SPSS 8.0). The first 12 hours after insertion of the microdialysis and $PtiO_2$-probe were excluded from analysis. Data are given as mean values with sem. A one-way ANOVA was used for normally distributed data. For non normally distributed data, non parametric tests were used. A $p < 0.05$ was statistically significant.

Results

Occurrence of Impending/Present Hypoxia

252 episodes of impending hypoxia ($PtiO_2$ < 15 mm Hg; 11810 minutes) and 38 episodes of present hypoxia ($PtiO_2$ < 10 mm Hg; 1996 minutes) were identified. Mean duration of impending hypoxia was 65 ± 33 minutes and of present hypoxia 85 ± 21 minutes. Intracranial hypertension was the parameter most frequently associated with impending hypoxia (77%), while in cerebral hypoxia ($PtiO_2$ < 10 mm Hg) in most cases was associated with hyperventilation (97%).

Microdialysis Changes Before Impending/Present Hypoxia

Microdialysis data collected before the occurrence of impending/present hypoxia (within 60 minutes after sampling) were divided into 3 groups: no hypoxia present after sampling ($PtiO_2$ > 15 mm Hg, n = 2083 hrs), impending hypoxia present after sampling ($PtiO_2$ 10–15 mm Hg, n = 310 hrs), hypoxia present after sampling ($PtiO_2$ < 10 mm Hg, n = 120 hrs).

In Figs 1 and 2 mean values of glucose and glutamate of these groups are shown. Baseline glucose levels were extremely low (<0.5 mmol/l) and further decreased before impending (p = 0.069) or present hy-

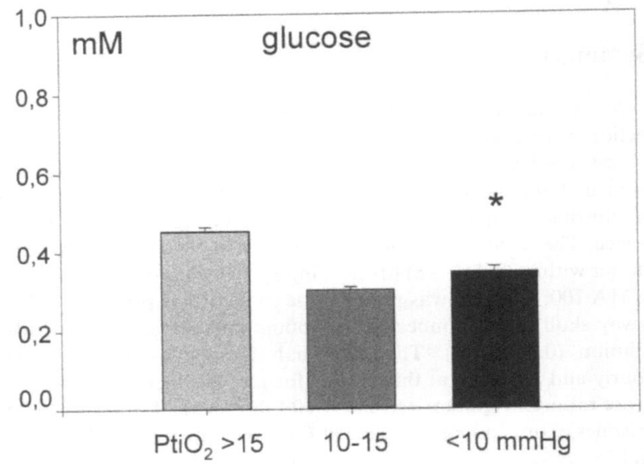

Fig. 1. Extracellular glucose concentrations (mean + sem) before different brain tissue PO_2 ranges are shown. Baseline glucose levels were extremely low (<0.5 mmol/l) and further decreased before impending (p = 0.069) or before present hypoxia (p = 0.015)

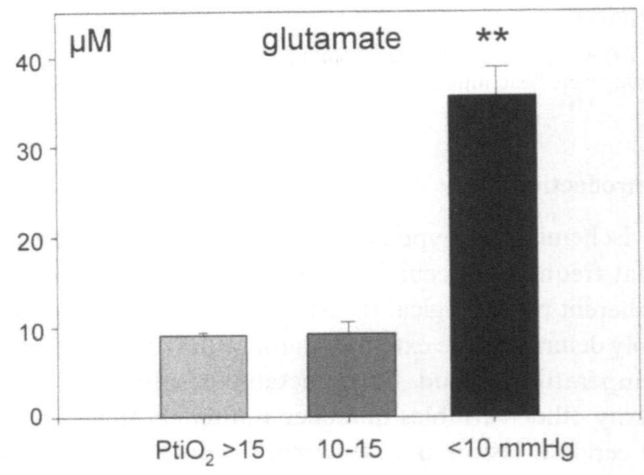

Fig. 2. Extracellular glutamate concentrations (mean + sem) before different brain tissue PO_2 ranges are shown. Glutamate was unchanged when no hypoxia or impending hypoxia followed but increased 3–4fold before a hypoxic episode occurred (p < 0.001)

poxia ($p = 0.015$). Glutamate was unchanged when no hypoxia or impending hypoxia occurred but increased 3–4fold ($p < 0.001$) before a hypoxic episode appeared. Lactate (mean range 2.3–4.1 mmol/l) and the lactate-pyruvate-ratio (mean range 23.2–34.5) did not increase before the presence impending or present hypoxia, suggesting no anaerob metabolism.

Discussion

Cerebral hypoxia/ischemia is a major contributor of poor outcome in severe head injury [4]. New monitoring devices have been developed for early detection of cerebral ischemia/hypoxia to minimize secondary bain damage. Measurement of brain tissue oxygen tension ($PtiO_2$) has been shown to reliably monitor regional cerebral oxygenation and to be closely correlated to cerebral perfusion [1, 3, 8]. When inserted into non lesioned white matter, a good correlation between global ischemia monitored by jugular venous oxygen saturation ($SjvO_2$) and regional brain tissue $PtiO_2$ is found [3]. When cerebral desaturation ($SjvO_2 < 50\%$), indicative for global ischemia occurrs, brain tissue-$PtiO_2$ is below 10 mm Hg (a so called "hypoxic episode"). In our study, the major contributors to impending and present hypoxia were the presence of intracranial hypertension and hyperventilation. Both conditions are known to correlate with metabolic changes [2, 5]. In severely head injured patients, secondary increases of glutamate have been observed to correlate with intracranial hypertension [2, 9]. Hyperventilation therapy has the risk of inducing ischemia, especially in already critically perfused areas. Bedside microdialysis allows to monitor cerebral metabolism "on-line" next to the patient. During transient regional or global ischemia, relevant metabolic changes with an increase in lactate and decrease in glucose were found [5]. The authors concluded that microdialysis adds a measure of how severely the reduction in oxygenation is affecting the brain's metabolism.

Our data clearly show that there are metabolic changes occurring already before the decrease in brain tissue $PtiO_2$ is observed. Before cerebral hypoxia, glucose decreased and glutamate increased 3–4fold compared to values when "normal oxgyenation" episodes (brain tissue $PtiO_2 > 15$ mm Hg) followed. We conclude that the early metabolic detection of cerebral hypoxia before a critical decrease in brain tissue $PtiO_2$ is seen possibly allows earlier changes in treatment (e.g. reduction of hyperventilation therapy).

Acknowledgments

We thank Miss Sabine Seidlitz and Adelina Stössel for their technical assistance and the nurses of the neurointensive care unit for their excellent help in collecting the microdialysis samples.

References

1. Dings J, Meixensberger J, Roosen K (1997) Brain tissue PO2-monitoring: catheter stability and complications. Neurol Res 19: 241–245
2. Hillered L, Persson L, Ponten U, Ungerstedt U (1990) Neurometabolic monitoring of the ischaemic human brain using microdialysis. Acta Neurochir (Wien) 102: 91–97
3. Kiening KL, Unterberg AW, Bardt TF, Schneider G-H, Lanksch RW (1996) Monitoring of cerebral oxygenation in severely head-injured patients: brain tissue PO_2 vs jugular venous oxygen saturation. J Neurosurg 85: 751–757
4. Miller JD, Becker DP (1982) Secondary insults to the injured brain. J R Coll Surg Edinburgh 27: 292–298
5. Robertson CS, Gopinath SP, Uzura M, Valadka AB, Goodman JC (1998) Metabolic changes in the brain during transient ischemia measured with microdialysis. Neurol Res 20 [Suppl] 1: 591–594
6. Ungerstedt U, Hallstrom A (1987) In vivo microdialysis – a new approach to the analysis of neurotransmitters in the brain. Life Sci 41: 861–864
7. Valadka AB, Gopinath SP, Contant CF, Uzura M, Robertson CS (1998) Relaionship of brain tissue PO_2 to outcome after severe head injury. Crit Care Med 26: 1576–1581
8. Van den Brink WA, Van Santbrink H, Steyerberg EW, Avezaat CJJ, Carmona Suazo JA, Hogesteeger C, Jansen WJ, Kloos LMH, Vermeulen J, Maas IR (2000) Brain oxygen tension in severe head injury. Neurosurgery 46: 868–876
9. Zauner A, Bullock R, Kuta AJ, Woodward J, Young HF (1996) Glutamate release and cerebral blood flow after severe human head injury. Acta Neurochir (Wien) [Suppl] 67: 40–44

Correspondence: Asita S. Sarrafzadeh, Department of Neurosurgery, Charité Campus Virchow Medical Center, Humboldt University of Berlin, Augustenburger Platz 1, 13353 Berlin, Germany.

Acta Neurochir (2002) [Suppl] 81: 323–325

Intraoperative Monitoring of Brain Tissue Oxygen and Carbon Dioxide Pressure in Peritumoural Oedema by Stereotactic Placement of Multiparameter Microsensors

F. A. Pennings[1], G. J. Bouma[1], M. Kedaria[2], and G. Jansen[2]

[1] Department of Neurosurgery, Academic Medical Center, University of Amsterdam, The Netherlands
[2] Department of Anaesthesiology, Academic Medical Center, University of Amsterdam, The Netherlands

Summary

Ischaemia may play an important role in peritumoural brain oedema and swelling, but little data exist so far on brain tissue oxygenation adjacent to a tumour mass. We have monitored brain tissue oxygen tension ($ptiO_2$) and brain tissue CO_2 tension ($ptiCO_2$) in 19 patients undergoing craniotomy for resection of a brain tumour using a multiparameter sensor placed in the brain parenchyma. Accurate placement of this probe in the peritumoural area was accomplished with the aid of a 3-D neuronavigation system. Due to various problems we obtained useful data in only 13/19 patients.

The presence of brain swelling was associated with a significant rise in $ptiO_2$ upon opening of the dura from 7.1 ± 7.8 to 23.6 ± 14.7 mm Hg. The average $ptiO_2$ before tumour resection was 18.1 ± 10.8 mm Hg. A significant improvement in $ptiO_2$ occurred after tumour resection to an average $ptiO_2$ of 29.7 ± 15.2 mm Hg.

From these preliminary data, we conclude that $ptiO_2$ is depressed in the peritumoural area, and improves following tumour resection. Stereotactic placement of sensors for intraoperative $ptiO_2$ monitoring is feasible and may enhance data quality. Nevertheless, the high incidence of failures with this type of sensor remains a matter of concern.

Keywords: Brain oedema; brain oxygen pressure; brain tumour; stereotactic techniques.

Introduction

Peritumoural brain oedema often aggravates neurological symptoms and makes surgery more difficult, which adversely affects outcome. Ischaemia is thought to be an important mechanism in the pathogenesis of oedema around brain tumours [3]. Hypoperfusion in the peritumoural area may result from abnormal angiogenesis or from increased local tissue pressure [1]. To date, little is known about the perfusion and oxygenation of the brain during surgery for brain tumours.

Monitoring of jugular venous oxygen saturation may considerably underestimate regional ischaemia [6]. Direct measurement of brain tissue oxygen pressure using conventional Clark type electrodes or a multiparameter sensors employing fiberoptic techniques to detect pO_2, pH and pCO_2 may overcome this limitation [5]. This technique has been applied during aneurysm surgery and in patients with severe head injury [4, 9]. Attempts have been made to define critical thresholds for ischaemia but consensus on this subject has not been reached yet [2, 9]. In this study, we have monitored brain tissue pO_2 ($ptiO_2$) and pCO_2 ($ptiCO_2$) in oedematous peritumoural brain tissue during surgery for tumour removal. Specifically, we have investigated the effects on tissue oxygenation of bulk resection of the tumour mass.

Patients and Methods

This study was approved by the Medical Ethics Committee of the Academic Medical Center, and written informed consent was obtained from each patient. Patients undergoing craniotomy for removal of a supratentorial intracranial tumour were recruited. A total of 19 patients were studied, thirteen males and six females, age ranging from 20 to 74 years. The histological diagnosis was malignant glioma in 10 patients, metastasis in 5 patients and meningioma in 4 patients. Patients were anaesthetised with Thiopental (5 mg/kg) or Propofol (2 mg/kg) and intubation was facilitated with 0.5 mg/kg Rocuronium. Anaesthesia was maintained with 1–2% Sevoflurane/O_2 air-mixture with an inspired oxygen fraction (FiO_2) of 0.4. A radial artery catheter was inserted for continuous mean arterial pressure measurement. Ventilation was adjusted to maintain an arterial pCO_2 at 4.0–4.5 kPa (30–35 mm Hg). A multiparameter sensor (Neurotrend®, Codman, USA) was used for continuous measurement of $ptiO_2$, $ptiCO_2$ and pH. Preoperatively a trajectory was planned on MRI images for stereotactic placement of the sensor into the peritumoural tissue using a 3-D neuronavigation system (Surgiscope®, Elekta, Stockholm, Sweden). Before placement in the patient, the sensor was calibrated using sterile precision gases, according to the manufacturer's specifications. Using the neuronavigation system, the exact entry site and angle of probe insertion were determined. A burr hole was made accordingly, and a stainless steel bolt with a Luerlock was placed into the skull. The dura was perforated with a needle and the brain tissue with a blunt-tipped stylet, thus creating a path for insertion of the sensor. A "peel-away" catheter of appropriate length was used to introduce the probe. In this way, accurate placement of the sensor in the peritumoural zone was accomplished in all patients. Following probe insertion, approximately 60 min. were allowed to obtain stable and reliable measurements. During this time, the surgery proceeded as planned.

The presence of swelling of the brain tissue upon opening of the dura as noted by the surgeon was recorded. The ptiO_2 and ptiCO_2 were monitored continuously throughout the surgical procedure. All recorded data were stored in a computer database every 10 seconds using a Labview program (National Instruments, Austin, TX).

Data are expressed as mean $\pm$ standard deviation (SD). Comparisons of means before and after dura opening and before and after tumour resection were made using the Wilcoxon Signed Rank Test. Statistical significance was defined as $P < 0.05$.

Results

Of the 19 patients recruited for this study, two were excluded from analysis due to a computer failure and a multiparameter sensor failure (no display of ptiO_2). Three other patients were only suitable for analysis of the effect of dura opening on ptiO_2, because the ptiO_2 reading fell to zero during the operation for no apparent reason, without a concomitant change in ptiCO_2. Brain swelling ($n = 8$) was associated with very low ptiO_2 values before opening of the dura (7.1 ± 7.8 mm Hg). After dura opening, a steep rise in ptiO_2 occurred to 23.6 ± 14.7 mm Hg ($p < 0.05$). This effect was not seen in patients without brain swelling ($n = 8$) (Fig. 1).

Thirteen patients were suitable for analysis of the effect of tumour resection. The average ptiO_2 and ptiCO_2 prior to tumour resection was 18.1 ± 10.8 mm Hg and 47.5 ± 7.2 mm Hg respectively. A marked improvement in ptiO_2 was seen to 29.7 ± 15.2 mm Hg ($p < 0.05$) without a significant change in ptiCO_2. In 9/13 patients an increase in ptiO_2 was observed following tumour removal. In three patients, ptiO2 remained virtually unchanged. In two of those patients, progressive swelling of the brain occurred during surgery after an initial improvement in ptiO_2. One patient showed a decline in ptiO_2 following tumour removal. The presence of brain swelling at the start of the operation had no relation with the level of ptiO_2 before, during and after tumour resection (Fig. 2).

Discussion

We studied ptiO_2 and ptiCO_2 levels intraoperatively in peritumoural oedema using microsensors inserted under guidance of image-guided neuronavigation. We feel that this technique enhances the safety and accuracy of intracranial placement of the multiparameter sensor. The high malfunction rate of the multiparameter sensor in 4/19 cases (21%) in this study, however, remains a matter of concern. This problem was also encountered by other investigators, who reported a malfunction rate of 16% [9]. In three cases, a sudden drop in ptiO_2 to values near zero was noted during surgery without any apparent reason. A possible explanation for this intraoperative ptiO_2 decline could be the presence of microhaemorrhages around the sensor tip, although one would expect a malfunctioning starting directly after insertion [10]. Other possible reasons for malfunction such as reduction in blood flow due to brain retraction, swelling or manipulation, were not

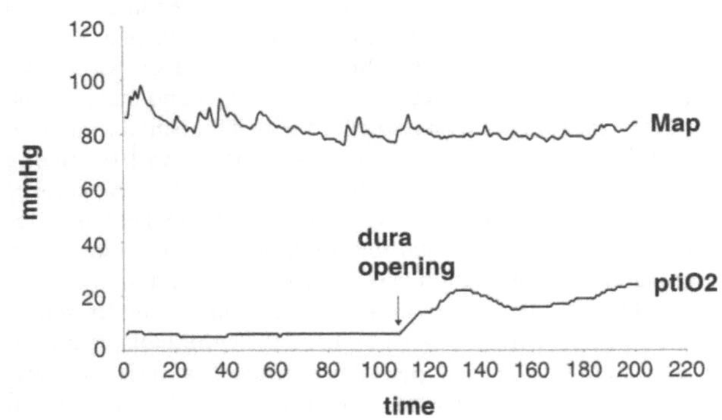

Fig. 1. Graph showing the course of mean arterial blood pressure (MAP, upper) and brain tissue pO_2 (ptiO_2, lower) during opening of the dura in a patient with severe brain swelling X-axis: time in minutes

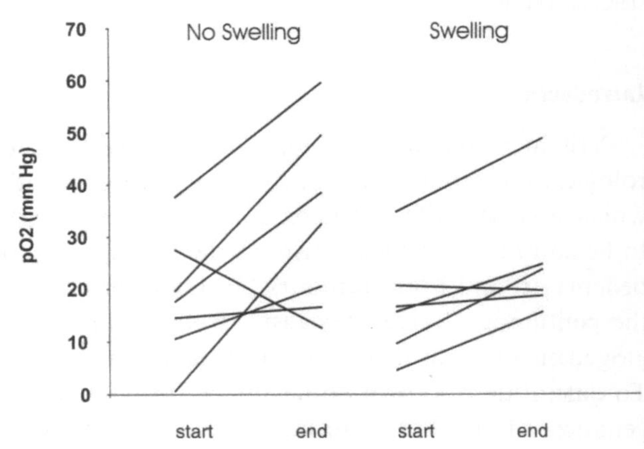

Fig. 2. Graph showing the change in peritumoural ptiO_2 during tumour resection in patients without brain swelling (left) and patients with brain swelling (right)

associated with this event. Moreover, the drop of $ptiO_2$ was not accompanied by an increase in $ptiCO_2$ suggesting no metabolic derangements at that time. Therefore, we conclude that the observed decrease to zero of $ptiO_2$ in our cases most likely was an artefact caused by some malfunction of the probe. The fragility of the instrument may have contributed to this problem, although in all cases care was taken that the catheters were not severely bent or twisted.

The present data indicate low $ptiO_2$ values in the peritumoural area. This finding is in agreement with the results of Meixensberger *et al.* [7] and with other studies of cerebral blood flow, showing decreased flow in hypodense areas around brain tumours on CT [8]. Furthermore, we found that both dura opening and tumour removal had a beneficial effect on tissue oxygenation. The effect of dura opening was particularly present in patients who had severe brain swelling as noticed by the surgeon upon opening of the dura. This observation may indicate that high intracranial pressure is in part responsible for the low tissue oxygenation, which is relieved after decompression. In cases where progressive swelling occurred during the course of surgery, a decline in $ptiO_2$ was seen, again demonstrating the influence of swelling on regional brain perfusion and the ability of the multiparameter sensor to detect tissue changes in a real-time fashion.

In conclusion, these preliminary data suggest that cerebral perfusion and brain tissue oxygenation are compromised in the peritumoural area. This finding emphasises the need for maintaining adequate cerebral perfusion pressure during neuroanesthesia, especially when brain swelling is present. Monitoring of $ptiO_2$ may enhance safety during neurosurgical anaesthesia and provide better understanding of the pathophysiology of peritumoural brain swelling, but its value is still limited by technical failures. Hopefully, further product improvements and refinements will help to solve these problems.

References

1. Arbit E, DiResta GR, Bedford RF, Shah NK, Galicich JH (1989) Intraoperative measurement of cerebral and tumour blood flow with laser-Doppler flowmetry. Neurosurgery 24: 166–17
2. Doppenberg EM, Zauner A, Watson JC *et al* (1998) Determination of the ischemic threshold for brain oxygen tension. Acta Neurochir (Wien) [Suppl] 71: 166–169
3. Fishman RA (1975) Brain oedema. New Engl J Med 293: 706–711
4. Hoffman WE, Charbel FT, Gonzalez-Portillo G, Ausman JI (1999) Measurement of ischemia by changes in tissue oxygen, carbon dioxide, and pH. Surg Neurol 51: 654–658
5. Lubbers DW (1996) Oxygen electrodes and optodes and their application in vivo. Adv Exp Med Biol 388: 13–34
6. Marion DW, Darby J, Yonas H (1991) Acute regional cerebral blood flow changes caused by severe head injuries. J Neurosurg 74: 407–414
7. Meixensberger J, Dings J, Kuhnigk H, Roosen K (1993) Studies of tissue PO_2 in normal and pathological human brain cortex. Acta Neurochir (Wien) [Suppl] 59: 58–63
8. Nakamura O, Segawa H, Tanaka H, Yoshimasu N, Nagai M, Takakura K (1987) rCBF in brain tumours as measured by xenon enhanced CT. Neurol Res 9: 24–29
9. Valadka AB, Gopinath SP, Contant CF, Uzura M, Robertson CS (1998) Relationship of brain tissue PO_2 to outcome after severe head injury. Crit Care Med 26: 1576–1581
10. van den Brink WA, Haitsma IK, Avezaat CJ (1998) Brain parenchyma/pO_2 catheter interface: a histopathological study in the rat. J Neurotrauma 15: 813–824

Correspondence: Gerrit. J. Bouma, M.D., Ph.D., Department of Neurosurgery, Academic Medical Center Amsterdam, P.O. Box 22600, 1100 DD Amsterdam, The Netherlands.

Acta Neurochir (2002) [Suppl] 81: 327–329

Effects of Variation in Cerebral Haemodynamics During Aneurysm Surgery on Brain Tissue Oxygen and Metabolism

R. Kett-White, P. J. Hutchinson, M. Czosnyka, P. Al-Rawi, A. Gupta, J. D. Pickard, and P. J. Kirkpatrick

Academic Department of Neurosurgery and the Wolfson Brain Imaging Centre, Addenbrooke's Hospital, Cambridge, UK

Summary

Objectives. This study explores the sensitivities of multiparameter tissue gas sensors and microdialysis to variations in blood pressure, CSF drainage and to well-defined periods of ischaemia accompanying aneurysm surgery, and their predictive value for infarction.

Methods. A Neurotrend sensor [brain tissue partial pressure of oxygen (P_BO_2), carbon dioxide (P_BCO_2), brain pH (pH_B) and temperature] and microdialysis catheter were inserted into the appropriate vascular territory prior to craniotomy.

Results. Baseline data showed a clear correlation between P_BO_2 and mean arterial pressure (MAP) below a threshold of 80 mmHg. P_BO_2 improved with CSF drainage in 20 out of 28 (Wilcoxon: $P < 0.05$) cases where data was available. In 26 patients the effects of temporary vascular clipping (TC) (mean duration 16 minutes) were assessed. 2 patients subsequently declared infarction in the region of the probes. P_BO_2 fell from a mean 3.2 (95% CI 2.4–4.1) kPa to a minimum of 1.5 (95% CI 1.0–2.0) kPa in the non-infarct group. There was a lower baseline P_BO_2 (mean 0.8 kPa) in the patients who infarcted. P_BCO_2 mirrored P_BO_2 changes, whereas pH_B did not change significantly in either group. Microdialysis changes associated with decreased P_BO_2 included a delayed increase in lactate, a raised lactate/pyruvate ratio and more rarely an increased glutamate. These changes were seen in 11 patients but were not predictive of infarction.

Conclusion. Hypotension during aneurysm surgery is associated with a low P_BO_2. Multiparameter sensors can be sensitive to acute ischaemia. Microdialysis shows potential in the detection of metabolic changes during tissue hypoxia.

Keywords: Cerebral ischaemia; temporary clipping; clinical microdialysis; glutamate.

Introduction

Traditional methods of monitoring patients at risk for ischaemia are either indirect or insensitive to focal ischaemia. Patients in a poor grade are often paralysed and sedated on the intensive care ward allowing neurological deterioration to occur undetected. Additionally, in the treatment of ischaemia, there are considerable risks associated with the use of hypervolaemia, inotropes and endovascular intervention. There is therefore a need for instruments that can continuously and directly detect focal ischaemia at a reversible stage and guide potentially hazardous therapeutic manoeuvres.

Temporary clipping (TC) of the parent artery during aneurysm surgery is an accepted method of facilitating dissection and clipping of aneurysms [7]. Without direct cerebral monitoring there is a paucity of information about how well the brain is tolerating these periods. Additionally, TC provides a fortuitous opportunity to study in humans the effects of clearly identifiable episodes of acute ischaemia on new monitors in a controlled environment. We have combined the use of a probe that measures P_BO_2, P_BCO_2, pH_B and temperature with a microdialysis system that determines changes in the extracellular concentrations of glucose, lactate, pyruvate and glutamate. Although changes in some of these parameters with TC have already been reported [3, 6, 2], we wished to examine not only the changes detected by each monitoring system during episodes of ischaemia, but also their interrelations and their reproducibility in a larger group of patients.

Materials and Methods

41 patients undergoing craniotomy to clip an aneurysm were studied. Patients who presented with large or complex unruptured aneurysms were particularly recruited because of the anticipated likelihood of TC. The mean age was 54 (range 29–78). 33 patients had suffered SAH. The WFNS [9] grade was poor (grade 3–5) in 14. The ICA was the parent artery in 18, MCA in 10, ACA in 11 and basilar artery in 2. 7 aneurysms were giant and 3 recurrent (2 previously coiled). Aneurysms were approached via a standard pterional craniotomy. Thorough drainage of CSF from the basal cisterns

and reduction of the gyrus rectus minimised the effects of retraction. TC was used on clinical grounds and was kept to a minimum. Postoperatively, patients were examined for any new neurological deficit and CT scans were examined for any evidence of infarction, with particular reference to the monitored region.

Monitoring Technique

A triple lumen bolt [5] was inserted over the vascular territory on interest prior to craniotomy. A Neurotrend (Codman, Bracknell, UK) sensor and a 10-mm CMA 70 (CMA, Solna, Sweden) microdialysis catheter (Ringer's solution at 1 μl/min^{-1}) were introduced in to the cortex (Neurotrend depth = 40 mm, CMA 70 depth = 20 mm). The vials were changed every 10–20 minutes and processed by a CMA 600 analyser. Data was downloaded on-line to a personal computer using our own acquisition software. A contemporaneous operation log was kept. Mean values from 5 minutes after dural opening, 20 minutes after the start of CSF drainage and mean, minimum/maximum values during the whole period of TC were compared against those over 5 minutes before each event (Student's t-test for paired samples). In order to acquire baseline data, periods when the above manoeuvres clearly affected parameters were excluded. The first 10 minutes of Neurotrend data after insertion was excluded.

Results

Technical Difficulties

There were no clinical complications. The Neurotrend was damaged during insertion in 2 patients and calibration failed in 4. A CMA 70 catheter had a faulty inlet tube, one was broken during craniotomy and one failed for an unknown reason. P_BO_2 usually became stable within 10 minutes of insertion. pH_B tended to start low and P_BCO_2 high before gradually settling, usually within one hour. Glutamate values were initially high in nearly all patients (mean 65 μmol/l), and decreased exponentially, mostly in the first hour. Glucose, lactate and pyruvate were steadier and concentrations tended to be stable by the time of aneurysmal dissection.

Baseline Data

5,500 minutes of data was amalgamated. Figure 1 shows a threshold relationship between P_BO_2 and MAP. P_BO_2 was independent of MAP above 80 mm Hg. P_BO_2 was significantly lower at MAP < 60 mm Hg (ANOVA $P < 0.025$).

Effects of Opening the Dura and of CSF Drainage

There was a statistically significant increase in P_BO_2 (paired 2-tail t-test: $P = 0.02$, Wilcoxon: $P < 0.02$) after opening the dura during craniotomy. During CSF drainage P_BO_2 improved (paired 2-tail t-test: $P = 0.01$, Wilcoxon: $P < 0.05$). There were no significant changes in MAP, SaO_2 or $ETCO_2$ over these times.

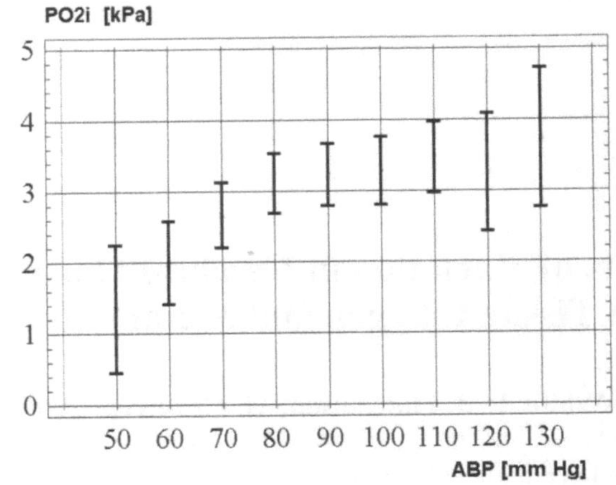

Fig. 1. Relationship between MAP (grouped in intervals of 10 mm Hg) and P_BO_2 for 30 patients. At MAP < 60 mm Hg, P_BO_2 was significantly decreased (ANOVA $P < 0.025$)

Temporary Arterial Occlusion: Thresholds for Infarction

30 patients required parent artery TC (17 to facilitate dissection, 10 for intraoperative rupture, 3 for thrombectomy). The mean total duration was 14 minutes (range 3 to 52 minutes). Perioperative neurological deterioration was observed in 11 patients (permanent in 7, transient in 4) and was not observed in any patient not requiring TC. Infarcts were seen subsequently in the monitored region in 2 cases.

Overall, TC caused significant reductions in mean P_BO_2 ($P < 0.05$) and mean pH_B ($P < 0.02$) and an increase in mean P_BCO_2 ($P < 0.01$) (t-tests for paired samples, $n = 28$). The minimum P_BO_2 recorded tended to be lower the longer temporary clips were applied. The minimum P_BO_2 during occlusion in those that did *not* infarct in the monitored region was 1.5 kPa (95% CI: 1.0–2.0 kPa). The lower 95% confidence interval was 1.0 kPa. In the 2 monitored-region infarcts P_BO_2 was lower than this before and during TC (mean 0.8 kPa) (Fig. 2). P_BCO_2 increased and pH_B decreased in both, but remained within the range of non-infarct cases. Typical microdialysis changes associated with decreased P_BO_2 included a delayed increase in lactate, a raised lactate/pyruvate ratio and an

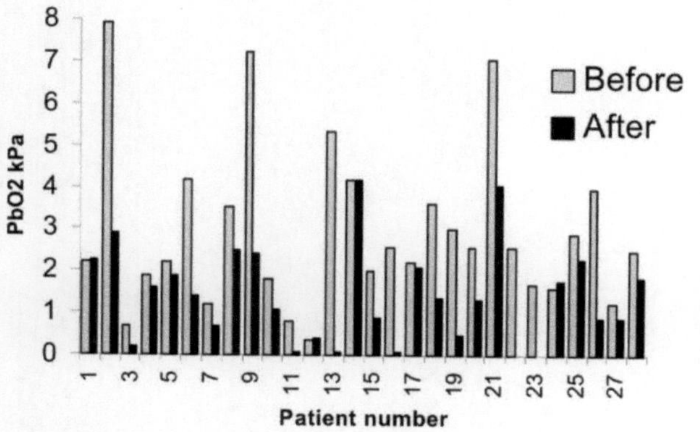

Fig. 2. Chart showing P_BO_2 just before and the minimum P_BO_2 during the whole period of temporary parent artery occlusions. Patients 3 & 11 infarcted in the monitored region

increased glutamate. These changes were seen in 11 patients but were not predictive of infarction.

Discussion

The principle findings are the relationship between P_BO_2 and perfusion pressure and the establishment of a threshold value for P_BO_2 during episodes of ischaemia.

P_BO_2 and Perfusion Pressure

Previously, in common with other authors [10], we have been unable to demonstrate good correlation between P_BO_2 and CPP or ICP in the majority of head-injured patients [1]. In the present study, the threshold relationship with hypotension is clearer, possibly because the operating theatre is a more controlled environment or because of different pathophysiology. This finding is clear evidence of the potential harm of hypotension during aneurysm surgery. If one accepts the threshold value for P_BO_2 of 1 kPa, then Fig. 1 shows that at MAP below 59 mm Hg, P_BO_2 overlaps the range of infarction.

Threshold Value for P_BO_2

Because few cases suffer neurological deterioration, small series have been unable to draw conclusions regarding thresholds [2, 4]. In studies on head-injuries, the difference in outcome between the patients with and without P_BO_2 values below 0.7 kPa was significant [10]. In another series, patients, with a mean P_BO_2 above 4.7 kPa experienced a good recovery, whereas those with a mean $P_BO_2 < 3.3$ kPa died or were vegetative [11]. It is encouraging that our threshold value of 1 kPa is identical to that calculated against a jugular venous oxygen saturation threshold of 50% during episodes of hypotension [8].

P_BCO_2 increased and pH_B decreased in both our patients who infarcted in the monitored region, but remained within the range of non-infarct cases and were therefore not predictive of infarction.

Acknowledgments

The Stroke Association generously sponsored this work. We also thank Mr S. Piechnik, the nursing staff, Mrs Maskell and Dr N. Higgins FRCR for their help. The bolts were made by Centrax Limited (Newton Abbott, Devon, UK).

References

1. Al Rawi P, Hutchinson PJ, Gupta AK *et al* (2000) Multiparameter brain tissue monitoring-correlation between parameters and identification of CPP thresholds. Zentralblatt Fur Neurochirurgie
2. Doppenberg E, Watson JC, Broaddus WC *et al* (1997) Intraoperative monitoring of substrate delivery during aneurysm and hematoma surgery: initial experience in 16 patients. J Neurosurg 87: 809–816
3. Hoffman WE, Charbel FT, Edelman G (1996) Brain tissue oxygen, carbon dioxide, and pH in neurosurgical patients at risk for ischemia. Anesth Analg 82: 582–586
4. Hoffman WE, Charbel FT, Gonzalez-Portillo G *et al* (1999) Measurement of ischemia by changes in tissue oxygen, carbon dioxide, and pH. Surg Neurol 51: 654–658
5. Hutchinson PJA, Hutchinson DBA, Barr RHH *et al* (2000) A new cranial access device for cerebral monitoring. Br J Neurosurg 14: 46–48
6. Hutchinson PJ, Al RP, O'Connell MT *et al* (1999) Monitoring of brain metabolism during aneurysm surgery using microdialysis and brain multiparameter sensors. Neurol Res 21: 352–358
7. Jabre A, Symon L (1987) Temporary vascular occlusion during aneurysm surgery. Surg Neurol 27: 47–63
8. Kiening KL, Unterberg AW, Bardt TF *et al* (1996) Monitoring of cerebral oxygenation in patients with severe head injuries: brain tissue pO2 versus jugular vein oxygen saturation. J Neurosurg 85: 751–757
9. Teasdale GM, Drake CG, Hunt W *et al* (1988) A universal subarachnoid haemorrhage scale: report of a committee of the World Federation of Neurosurgical Societies. J Neurol Neurosurg Psychiatry 51: 1457
10. van Santbrink H, Maas AI, Avezaat CJ (1996) Continuous monitoring of partial pressure of brain tissue oxygen in patients with severe head injury. Neurosurgery 38: 21–31
11. Zauner A, Doppenberg EM, Woodward JJ *et al* (1997) Continuous monitoring of cerebral substrate delivery and clearance: initial experience in 24 patients with severe acute brain injuries. Neurosurgery 41: 1082–1091

Correspondence: R. Kett-White, Academic Neurosurgery, Box 167, Addenbrooke's Hospital, Cambridge CB2 2QQ, UK.

Acta Neurochir (2002) [Suppl] 81: 331–333

Microdialysate Nitrate/Nitrite Levels Following Severe Head Injury

R. Hlatky[1,2], Y. Furuya[1,3], A. B. Valadka[1], J. C. Goodman[1], and C. S. Robertson[1]

[1] Department of Neurosurgery, Baylor College of Medicine, Houston, USA
[2] Department of Neurosurgery, University Hospital, Hradec Kralove, Czech Republic
[3] Department of Neurosurgery, St. Marianna University School of Medicine, Kawasaki, Japan

Summary

Nitric oxide (NO) has important regulatory functions within the central nervous system. The purpose of this study was to measure the concentration of nitric oxide in the brain after severe traumatic brain injury. NO is oxidized in vivo to nitrate and nitrite. Measurement of these products gives an index of NO production. Laboratory studies have shown a good correlation between NO measured directly with an electrode, and indirectly by microdialysis nitrate/nitrite. Using chemiluminescence method we measured nitrate/nitrite levels in 2024 microdialysate samples obtained from 24 patients during the first five days following severe head injury. We used CMA 70 probe (AB Microdialysis, Sweden) perfused by normal saline at a rate of 2 μl/min. The median values of nitrate/nitrite for the whole group were highest on day 1 and gradually decreased over the 5 day monitoring period (day 1 – 19.2 μmol/l, day 5 – 12.7 μmol/l). Average values were lowest in the patients that died of their injury (14.3 μmol/l), and highest in patients who recovered by 3 months after injury with a moderate or severe disability (25.8 μmol/l or 31.9 μmol/l). In addition, there was a strong interaction between the severity of neurological injury and the change in dialysate nitrate/nitrite over time. The results suggest that nitric oxide may have a role in secondary injury mechanisms, but that this role is complex and varies as the injury evolves over time.

Keywords: Nitric oxide; head injury; microdialysis.

Introduction

Nitric oxide (NO) is a mediator of cellular and vascular effects in the brain, and has been implicated in some of the pathophysiological processes induced by traumatic brain injury. The purpose of this study was to measure the concentration of nitric oxide in the brain after traumatic brain injury in severely head-injured patients. To accomplish this, we measured extracellular concentrations of nitrate and nitrite, which are end products of nitric oxide metabolism, in microdialysis samples.

Methods

We studied 24 patients with severe head injury (2 females, 22 males). The demographic characteristics of the patients studied were typical of a head injury population. The average admission GCS was 5.1 (range 3–8). Fifteen patients required surgery for evacuation of a mass lesion. By 3 months after injury 8 patients had a good recovery or moderate disability, 4 patients died of their injury.

All study patients were managed by a standard protocol. A microdialysis probe (CMA-70) was placed usually for 5 days in frontotemporal region of brain. The position of the probe was noted on follow-up CT scan. The probe was perfused at 2 μl/min with normal saline and samples were collected every 30 min. From the 24 patients a total of 2024 microdialysate samples (average 84/patient) were analyzed. Measurement was performed using chemiluminescence following vanadium stripping for reduction of nitrate and nitrite back to nitric oxide.

Results

Changes in Nitrate/Nitrite Levels Over the Time

The median concentration of nitrate/nitrite in the 2024 dialysate samples was 14.3 μmol/l. Sixty-five percent of the samples were between 5–20 μmol/l, but the values ranged from a low of 0.3 to a high of 461 μmol/l.

Table 1 shows the average nitrate/nitrite concentrations on days 1–5 after injury. When the whole group of 24 patients was examined together, the median values were highest on day 1 and gradually decreased over the 5 day monitoring period (time effect, $p = 0.018$). There was a wide distribution of values, especially on days 3–4 (day 3 – min. 8.2 μmol/l, max. 89.4 μmol/l; day 4 – min. 9.2 μmol/l, max. 291.5 μmol/l), suggesting that there may be more than one pattern of change in nitrate/nitrite concentrations over time.

Table 1. *Daily Median Concentration of Nitric Oxide per Whole Group of 24 Patients*

	Nitrate/nitrite values [μmol/l]		
	Median	25%	75%
Day 1	19.2	16.2	34.1
Day 2	16.5	11.6	25.8
Day 3	16.9	10.5	21.5
Day 4	15.1	12.6	17.8
Day 5	12.7	10.0	14.3

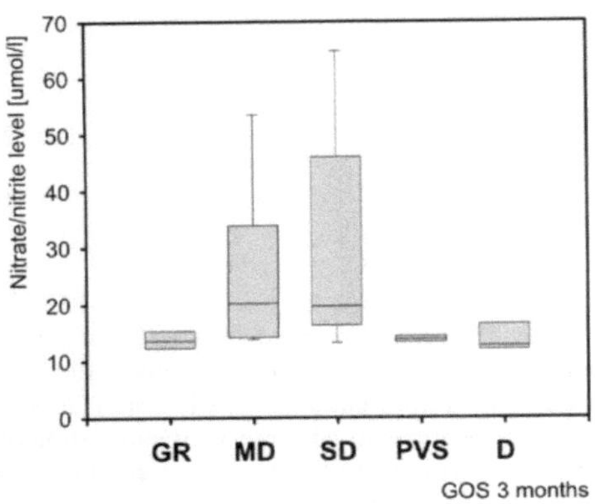

Fig. 1. Nitrate/nitrite levels by 3 month Glasgow Outcome Score

Outcome and Nitrate/Nitrite Levels

Neurological outcome was one of the factors that significantly interacted with the distribution of nitrate/nitrite concentrations over time. Figure 1 shows the values for nitrate/nitrite concentrations by 3 months Glasgow Outcome Score. The median values were lowest in the patients that died of their injury (14.3 μmol/l), and highest in patients who recovered with a moderate or severe disability (25.8 μmol/l or 31.9 μmol/l-group effect, $p = 0.075$).

Initial value for patients who died of their head injury was 17.2 μmol/l and initial level for patients who survived was 30.9 μmol/l. In the patients who died of their head injury, the nitrate/nitrite levels gradually decreased over days 1–3. In patients who survived, nitrate/nitrite levels increased over the first 3 days postinjury (time effect, $p = 0.144$, time by group interaction, $p = 0.185$).

Discussion

Because nitric oxide has important regulatory functions within the central nervous system, there is interest in examining any changes in nitric oxide metabolism that might occur after traumatic brain injury. Low levels of nitric oxide are associated with vasoconstriction of cerebral vessels, resulting in decreased cerebral blood flow or even ischemia. Increased production of nitric oxide is associated with free radical damage to the brain as nitric oxide is metabolized to peroxinitrite. Despite this interest, relatively few studies have been published regarding nitric oxide metabolism after human traumatic brain injury [2]. Part of the reason for this may be the difficulty in measuring nitric oxide. In experimental models, nitric oxide can be measured directly with a NO electrode or by using a method for trapping NO in a stable form [1]. In humans, direct measurement is not practical and some indirect method must be used. One method is to measure the end products of NO metabolism, nitrate and nitrite, as an index of nitric oxide production. In experimental studies, simultaneous measurement of NO after TBI by both NO electrode and by microdialysis nitrate/nitrite assays show similar changes [1].

We do not have any normal data for microdialysate nitrate/nitrite levels in humans, however, there are several studies in the literature where nitrate and nitrite concentrations have been measured in the CSF of normal subjects [5]. Levels of approximately 10–15 μmol/L appear to be normally present in CSF. Clark *et al.* have examined CSF levels of nitrate/nitrite following traumatic injury and observed the highest levels in the first few hours after injury. These levels averaged 26 μmol/L [2]. Our studies demonstrate intracerebral dialysate levels that are comparable to those that have been observed in CSF.

In experimental brain injury models, a characteristic pattern of change in NO has been observed. Immediately after the injury, there is a marked release in NO in the brain. Within a few minutes, NO levels fall to levels that are significantly lower than baseline, and remain that way for at least 3 hours after injury [1]. After a time, there is a second increase in NO levels, which is probably related to the inflammatory response to injury [3, 4]. In these human studies, we observed more complex patterns of change in NO in the brain, which were dependent on the severity of the neurological injury.

It is possible that the reason that the nitrate/nitrite concentrations in the patients with a good recovery are relatively low is that these patients tended to be monitored for a shorter period of time, and therefore the second increase in nitric oxide was not captured. Another possibility is that both high and low levels of nitric oxide reflect pathological changes. The patients with a good recovery then have near normal physiological concentrations of NO. The patients with a moderate or severe disability have secondary injury caused by increased nitric oxide concentrations. The patients who die from their injury have the most severe secondary injury caused by ischemia associated with low NO levels. This suggests that both high and low nitric oxide values may have pathological effects.

Our studies show that nitrate/nitrite concentrations can be measured in human head injury using the microdialysis technique. The results suggest that nitric oxide has a role in secondary injury mechanisms, but that this role may be complex and may vary as the injury evolves over time.

References

1. Cherian L, Goodman JC, Robertson CS (2000) Brain nitric oxide changes after controlled cortical impact injury in rats. J Neurophysiol 83: 2171–2178
2. Clark RS, Kochanek PM *et al* (1996) Cerebrospinal fluid and plasma nitrite and nitrate concentrations after head injury in humans. Crit Care Med 24: 1243–1251
3. Licinio J, Prolo P, McCann SM, Wong ML (1999) Brain iNOS: current understanding and clinical implications. Mol Med 5: 225–232
4. Wada K, Chatzipanteli K, Busto R *et al* (1998) Role of nitric oxide in traumatic brain injury in the rat. J Neurosurg 89: 807–818
5. Zecca L, Rosati M, Renella R *et al* (1998) Nitrate and nitrite levels in cerebrospinal fluid of normal subjects. J Neural Transm 105(6–7): 627–633

Correspondence: Prof. C. S. Robertson, Dept. of Neurosurgery, Baylor College of Medicine, 6560 Fannin Ste 944, Houston, TX 77030, USA.

Acta Neurochir (2002) [Suppl] 81: 335–338

Neurochemical Changes in Ventilated Head-Injured Patients with Cerebral Perfusion Pressure Treatment Failure

W. S. Poon[1], S. C. P. Ng[1], M. T. V. Chan[2], C. H. S. Leung[1], and J. M. K. Lam[1]

[1] Neurosurgical Unit, Department of Surgery, Prince of Wales Hospital, The Chinese University of Hong Kong, Shatin, New Territories, Hong Kong

[2] Department of Anaesthesia and Intensive Care, Prince of Wales Hospital, The Chinese University of Hong Kong, Shatin, New Territories, Hong Kong

Summary

The goal of intensive care management of patients with head injury is to provide them with a favourable physiological and metabolic environment for recovery of injury-compromised cells, and to prevent secondary brain insults. Clinical intracerebral mircodialysis has enabled documentation of the metabolic derangement after head injury. Treatment targeted at this derangement has emphasized maintenance of optimal cerebral perfusion pressure (CPP). To determine the relationships between CPP and five clinically relevant intracerebral extracellular metabolites (glucose, lactate, glycerol, glutamate and pyruvate) in relation to different therapy intensities, 23 moderate to severe head-injury patients with hourly microdialysis samples were studied. These five metabolites were correlated with CPP and showed a biphasic relation at CPP of 65 to 67 mmHg, which was believed to be the critical CPP indicating irreversible brain damage. Relationship between intracerebral metabolites and CPP in relation to different therapy intensities was studied and suggests the critical CPP threshold in head-injured patients with high ICP and maximum therapy is elevated and should be maintained above 70 mmHg to prevent irreversible brain damage.

Keywords: Head injury; microdialysis; cerebral perfusion pressure.

Introduction

After head injury, metabolic disturbances at the cellular level are common. This may potentiate further brain damage [1, 3]. The goal of treatment for head-injured patients is to provide a physiologically favourable environment for recovery of these compromised cells. Previous studies indicated that impaired cerebral blood flow (CBF) regulation, which is common after head injury, may lead to ionic and energy failure at the cellular level resulting in secondary brain insults. Targeted treatment has focussed on maintaining cerebral perfusion pressure (CPP) above a critical threshold. This would, in theory, maintain an adequate CBF, which in turn would normalise the metabolic disturbances.

The aim of this study is to determine the relationships between CPP and the five clinically relevant metabolites (glucose, lactate, glycerol, glutamate and pyruvate) in the intracerebral extracellular fluid in relation to different therapy intensities [2] in ventilated patients with moderate to severe head injury requiring intracranial pressure (ICP) monitoring.

Materials and Methods

23 patients (20 males and 3 females; mean age: 41.3 ± 18.4 years) with moderate to severe head injury, as defined by admission post-resuscitation Glasgow Coma Scale (GCS) scores of 12 or lower (median GCS 8), were prospectively studied. After surgical treatment of brain pathology, all patients were managed in the intensive care unit according to a standard protocol including artificial ventilation with muscle paralysis and sedation.

Patients were divided into 3 groups based on their therapy intensities. Group I (n = 5): required no specific therapy; Group II (n = 8): standard therapy of ventricular drainage within 4 times per hour and/or mannitol administration less than 1 gm/kg/hr; and Group III (n = 10): maximum therapy including ventricular drainage more than 4 times per hour, mannitol administration more than 1 gm/kg/hr mannitol and barbiturates at any dosage.

Via the same burr hole, ventricular catheter placement was followed by insertion of a microdialysis catheter (CMA 70: 60 mm shaft length, 10 mm-membrane length) into the frontal lobe anterior to the ventricular catheter. The right frontal lobe or the side of maximum injury was chosen for placement of the microdialysis probe. The probe was perfused at 0.3 µl/min using sterile lactate-free standard Ringer solution. Microdialysates were collected hourly and concentrations of the metabolites were measured by spectrophotometry (CMA 600 analyser).

Routine continuous monitoring included heart rate, arterial blood pressure by an arterial line inserted in the radial artery, ICP by an intraventricular catheter, arterial oxygen saturation by pulse oximeter, end-tidal carbon dioxide concentration by capnograph, jugular venous bulb oxygen saturation by Oximetrix 3 system and blood flow velocity in the middle cerebral artery by transcranial Doppler sonography.

Results

3536 microdialysis samples were collected in 23 patients. Correlation between glucose (1.70 ± 1.25 mmol/L), lactate (5.57 ± 3.74 mmol/L), glycerol (188.92 ± 405.30 μmol/L), glutamate (58.65 ± 146.21 μmol/L), pyruvate (141.71 ± 100.28 μmol/L) and CPP (66.9 ± 19.3 mmHg) were 0.27, −0.36, −0.61, −0.67 and 0.47 (all correlation coefficient (r)) respectively. Analysis of variance showed biphasic relationships at CPP of 65 to 67 mmHg. As CPP decreased below the breakpoint, there was a strong correlation between glucose ($r = 0.401$), lactate ($r = -0.468$), glycerol ($r = -0.682$), glutamate ($r = -0.757$), pyruvate ($r = 0.541$) and CPP. Above the CPP breakpoint, lactate correlation was weaker with CPP ($r = -0.042$), and the other four metabolites: glucose ($r = 0.042$), glycerol ($r = -0.040$), glutamate ($r = -0.005$) and pyruvate ($r = -0.004$) did not correlate with CPP.

Data were then subdivided into 3 groups according to their therapy intensities. The characteristics of the three patient groups are shown in Table 1. Group I patients required no specific therapy and were associated with normal ICP (11.6 ± 5.3 mmHg) and no mortality. No biphasic relationship was found between metabolites and CPP. Group II patients required standard therapy associated with moderate ICP (18.4 ± 11.8 mmHg) and 25% mortality where CPP breakpoints of 53 to 56 mmHg were found. Group III patients required maximum therapy and were associated with high ICP (30.1 ± 22.8 mmHg), an 80% mortality and CPP breakpoints of 64 to 67 mmHg.

Table 1. *Patient Characteristics of the three Therapy Intensity Groups: Group I (no Specific Therapy), Group II (Standard Therapy) and Group III (Maximum Therapy)*

Parameter		Group I (n = 5)	Group II (n = 8)	Group III (n = 10)
Microdialysis samples		347	1764	1425
Sex	male	5	6	9
	female	0	2	1
Age (years)		31.0 ± 20.3	45.0 ± 21.0	46.5 ± 16.7
Median GCS		8	8	6
ICP (mmHg)		11.6 ± 5.3	16.6 ± 9.5	30.9 ± 22.3
CPP (mmHg)		71.9 ± 9.9	72.5 ± 13.4	58.6 ± 23.8
Outcome	died	0	2	8
	survive	5	6	2

Discussion

In this group of moderate-to-severe ventilated head injury patients, we have demonstrated an optimal CPP threshold of 65–67 mmHg, below which intracerebral metabolic disturbances were exaggerated. However, in Groups I and II patients, where only minimum ICP manipulation was required, CPP breakpoints either did not exist or were 10 mm Hg below those of Group III patients, where maximum CPP therapy was required. Critical CPP in patients with high ICP and maximum therapy intensity (Group III) is elevated and should be maintained above 70 mmHg. The majority of those patients who died succumbed to overwhelming primary brain injury (8/10, 80%). The survivors were associated with successful targeted and aggressive CPP management. Clinical microdialysis in this group of patients has been shown to generate clinically relevant and useful information.

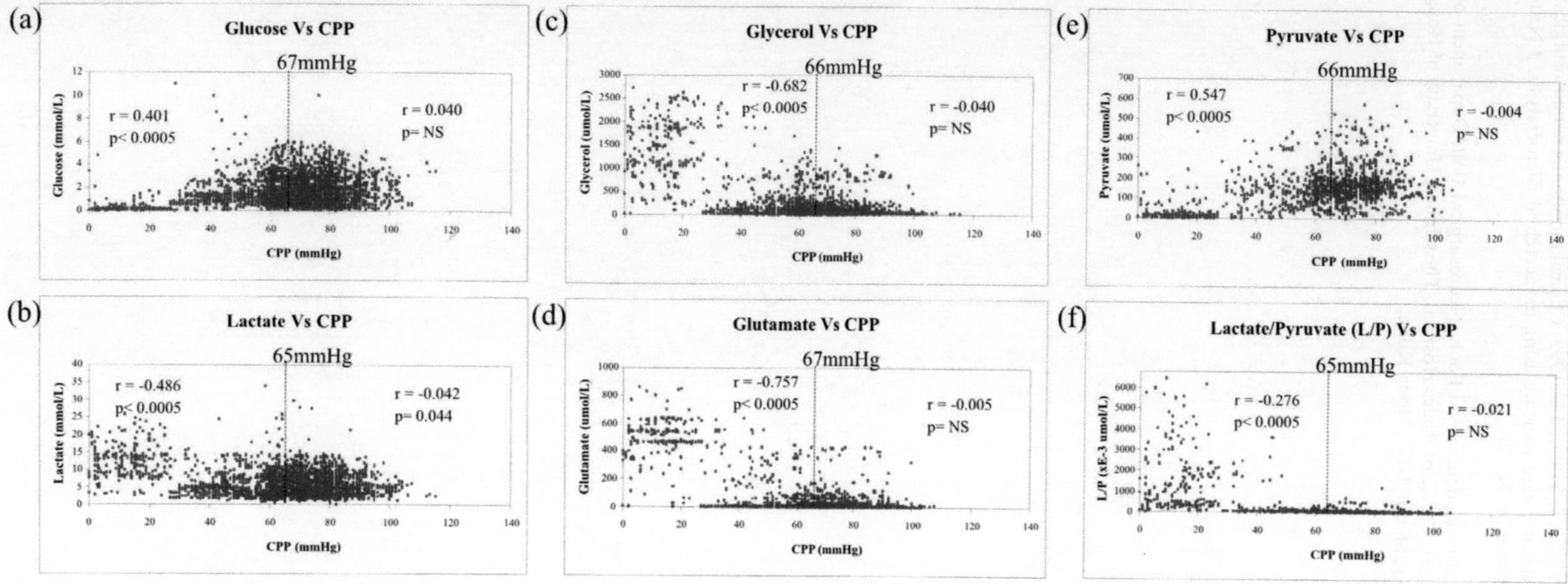

Fig. 1. (a–f) Groups plotting cerebral perfusion pressure (*CPP*) versus metabolites: glucose (a), lactate (b), glycerol (c), glutamate (d) and pyruvate (e), and lactate/pyruvate (L/P) ratio (f) in 23 patients with moderate to severe head injury. The vertical dotted lines represent the CPP breakpoints found

References

1. Katayama Y, Becker DP, Tamura T, Hovda DA (1990) Massive increases in extracelluear potassium and the indiscriminate release of glutamate following concussive brain injury. J Neurosurg 73: 889–900
2. Marmarou A, Anderson RL, Ward JD, Choi SC, Young HF (1991) NNDS Traumatic coma data bank: intracranial pressure monitoring methodology. J Neurosurg 75: S21–27
3. Persson L, Hillered L (1992) Clinical monitoring in neurosurgical intensive care patients using intracerebral microdialysis. J Neurosurg 76: 72–80

Correspondence: Wai Poon, Neurosurgical Unit, Department of Surgery, Prince of Wales Hospital, The Chinese University of Hong Kong, Shatin, N.T., Hong Kong.

Satellite-Neurochemical Monitoring

Acta Neurochir (2002) [Suppl] 81: 341–342

Third International Satellite Conference on Neuro-Chemical Monitoring

Proposed Guidelines for Neuro-Chemical Monitoring

P. Hutchinson

Department of Neurosurgery, University of Cambridge, UK

The satellite meeting concluded with a panel discussing the applications and limitations of neuro-chemical monitoring and addressing key points, in particular ethics and consent, standardisation, catheter location, interpretation for management, prognosis and statistical analysis.

Ethics and Consent

The consensus of the panel was that local ethics committee approval should be obtained for each institution. Currently, individual patient consent is obtained from the patient or next-of-kin in the UK, although this is not necessary in Sweden. Obtaining individual consent can delay implementation of monitoring techniques resulting in missing early and important derangements in metabolism. Now that extensive world-wide experience has shown that microdialysis is safe, it was felt that the best way forward is to request approval for deferred consent.

Standardisation

Implementation of microdialysis in different neurosurgical centres has resulted in variations in which the technique is applied i.e. membrane length, type of perfusion fluid, flow rate. For example, different fluids currently in use include normal saline, Ringer's solution and artificial CSF. It was the consensus of the panel that standardisation of these variables would facilitate comparison of results between centres.

Catheter Location

Controversy over ideal catheter location, both for microdialysis catheters and oxygen/multi-parameter sensors continues. In subarachnoid haemorrhage, the position is clearer than in head injury, with the catheters ideally monitoring brain supplied by the parent vessel of the aneurysm. In head injury, there are two scenarios. Firstly, in diffuse injury, catheter location in non-eloquent frontal cortex is appropriate. Secondly, in focal injury e.g. contusions, it was felt that monitoring the centre of the contusion (core) is not useful. Monitoring of the penumbra is probably the best location enabling the chemistry to be determined as a contusion evolves. However, this will not determine the metabolism of brain distant from the contusion which appears uninjured on imaging but is nevertheless at risk. The Swedish concept of two cerebral catheters ("better" and "worse" side) is the gold standard and overcomes this problem but may not be practical, particularly when using both microdialysis and oxygen/multiparameter sensors. The use of peripheral reference catheters e.g. monitoring the chemistry of the adipose tissue of the anterior abdominal wall is performed in several centres. However, the benefit from this is not clear at present. It was suggested that the use of an intravenous reference catheter may be more suitable.

Interpretation for Management

It was recognised that overall it is too early to apply microdialysis changes directly to patient management, although some centres, particularly in Sweden are beginning to make such management decisions based on the cerebral chemistry. Specific hypothesis-driven studies are still required to examine the effects of therapeutic manoeuvres on the chemistry.

Prognosis

Further work is required to establish which of the parameters are likely to be the most useful in terms of predicting prognosis. Currently, the lactate/pyruvate ratio appears to be a valuable index. Prognosis should be expressed both in terms of patient and "tissue" outcome.

Statistical Analysis

Monitoring of physiological and chemical parameters generates enormous numbers of data points. Better education and possibly some form of standardisation of the description of results was proposed, particularly with regard to the influence of individual variables on tissue and patient outcome.

**Panel*

R. Bullock
A. Gupta
P. J. Hutchinson (secretary)
P. J. Kirkpatrick
A. Marmarou
C. Hendrik-Nordstrom
L. Persson
J. D. Pickard (chairman)
C. Robertson
U. Ungerstedt

Correspondence: Dr. P. Hutchinson, Department of Neurosurgery, University of Cambridge, UK

Acta Neurochir (2002) [Suppl] 81: 343–345

Measurement of the Nitric Oxide Metabolites Nitrate and Nitrite in the Human Brain by Microdialysis

J. C. Goodman[1,2], Y.-Q. Feng[1], A. B. Valadka[1], R. J. Bryan[3], and C. S. Robertson[1]

[1] Department of Neurosurgery, Baylor College of Medicine, Houston, Texas
[2] Department of Pathology, Baylor College of Medicine, Houston, Texas
[3] Department of Anesthesiology, Baylor College of Medicine, Houston, Texas

Summary

To examine the feasibility of measuring the nitric oxide (NO) metabolites nitrate and nitrite in microdialysate samples from the human brain, microdialysis probes were placed in normal appearing cerebral cortex of severely head injured patients in the Neurosurgical Intensive Care Unit at Ben Taub General Hospital. Nitrate/nitrite analysis was performed using NO chemiluminescence. Low micromolar levels of NO metabolites were consistently and easily detected. These levels seen are comparable to levels reported in CSF but tissue tortuosity and probe recovery considerations suggest that the absolute concentrations at the probe site are probably ten fold higher. Microdialysis with measurement of nitric oxide metabolites is technically feasible and may provide valuable insights into both normal neurochemistry and neurochemical derangements in disease.

Keywords: Microdialysis; nitric oxide; head injury.

Introduction

The gaseous signaling molecule, nitric oxide (NO), is critical in vasomotor control, inflammation, and neuronal communication. Peroxidation products of NO may be produced in a variety of pathophysiological states including head trauma and lead to damage of nucleic acids, proteins and lipids [5, 6, 7]. NO is produced by tissue specific isoforms of nitric oxide synthetase (NOS) from arginine, and rapidly and radially diffuses to adjacent target cells where it interacts with iron centers stimulating cGMP synthesis. NO has a short half-life and is oxidized to nitrate and nitrite. NO can be measured directly in vivo using NO selective electrodes, but in physiological fluids and in microdialysis samples, its metabolites, nitrate and nitrite, are measured as surrogate markers. These metabolites can be measured using chemiluminescence, spectrophotometric detection following the Greiss reagent reaction, or fluorometric methods [8]. We measured nitrate/nitrite in microdialysis samples from the cerebral cortex of head injured patients using chemiluminescence.

Material and Methods

Microdialysis probes were placed in grossly normally appearing cerebral cortex of 24 severely head injured patients as part of a high intensity neuromonitoring protocol in the Neurosurgical Intensive Care Unit at Ben Taub General Hospital. Physiological saline was pumped through the probes at 2 microliters/minute, and 30-minute epochs were collected for lactate/glucose, amino acid and nitrate/nitrite analysis. Nitrate/nitrite analysis was performed using NO chemiluminescence (Antek Instruments, NO Analysis System, Houston, TX) following vanadium stripping (reduction of nitrate and nitrite back to NO in a heated vanadium chloride solution) of 10 microliter microdialysate samples.

The NO chemiluminescence assay is based on the fact that some of the NO_2 produced by the reaction of NO with ozone (O_3) is in an excited state (NO_2^*) and as the unstable electrons return to their ground state; they dissipate energy and emit electromagnetic radiation in the red light and infrared range (640–900 nm). The intensity of this chemiluminescent emission is proportional to the amount of NO in the original sample [3, 4].

A schematic of the NO analyzer is shown in Figure 1. The chemiluminscence detector system consists of NO ozone reaction chamber, a thermoelectrically cooled photomultiplier tube that collects the emitted light and transforms it to an electrical signal, and an integrator that measures the peak height and area of the signal. O_3 is produced by a high-voltage electrostatic discharge through O_2 supplied to the O_3 generator at a constant rate. The effluent from the reaction chamber is passed through a charcoal filter to eliminate O_3. The sample injection trap contains heated vanadium (III) reagent that reconstitutes NO by reducing the nitrate and nitrite in the microdialysate samples. This newly generated NO is carried through 1 N NaOH acid vapor trap to the chemiluminescence reaction chamber by nonreactive helium carrier gas. The vanadium (III) re-

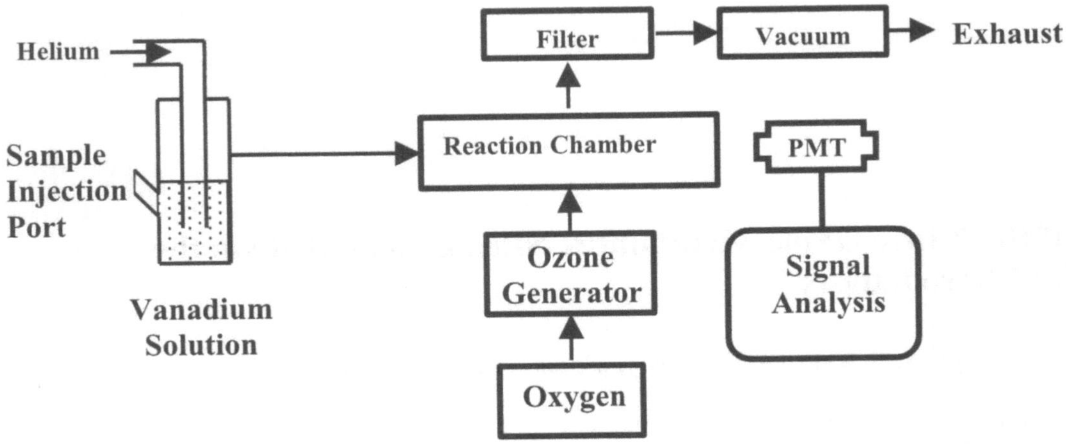

Fig. 1. A schematic diagram of the NO chemiluminescence analysis system. The sample is injected into the vanadium solution where nitrate and nitrite are reduced back to nitric oxide. The NO is carried by non-reactive helium to the reaction chamber where it mixes with ozone to produce an unstable intermediate that releases light when it decays. The light emission is proportional to the NO concentration and is detected by a cooled photomultiplier tube (*PMT*). Gas flow throughout the system is rapid and constant because it is "pulled" by a vacuum pump at the exhaust port of the apparatus

agent is prepared by converting vanadium (IV) to vanadium (II) using mossy zinc, and then converting vanadium (II) to vanadium (III) by bubbling O_2 through the solution.

Results

Low micromolar levels NO metabolites were easily and consistently detected in all 2269 microdialysate samples. The mean was 23.72 micromoles/L, standard error of the mean 1.70, and standard deviation 81.15. Low background levels were present in the microdialysate perfusate and were subtracted for analysis purposes. The background levels probably represent dissolved atmospheric NO and contaminated plastic materials. Calibration solutions were injected every 10th sample to verify instrument stability. Using linear regression analysis, the calibration curve was fitted ($y = 364.23x + 2.41$) and the correlation coefficient (r^2) of the regression line calculated ($r^2 = 0.999$).

Discussion

Nitrate and nitrite can be easily measured in human brain microdialysis samples by chemiluminescence. The levels seen are comparable to levels reported in CSF in humans but it must be recognized that tissue tortuosity and probe recovery considerations would indicate that the absolute concentrations at the probe site are probably at least ten fold higher [2, 9]. It must also be realized that these samples were obtained from damaged brains with variable ongoing pathophysiological processes. Nevertheless, while the levels of nitrate and nitrite we measured in humans are considerably higher than have been seen in rodents, the levels are almost identical to values reported in sheep – another large brained mammal [1]. Microdialysis with measurement of nitric oxide metabolites is technically feasible and may provide valuable insights into both normal neurochemistry and neurochemical derangements in disease.

Acknowledgments

Supported by NIH NINDS PO1 NS27616) The efforts of the research fellows, residents, technical staff and nurses of the Ben Taub General Hospital are gratefully acknowledged. The Baylor College of Medicine Institutional Review Board approved this work and informed consent was obtained in all cases.

References

1. Cherian L, Goodman JC, Robertson CS (2000) Brain nitric oxide changes after controlled cortical impact injury in rats. J Neurophysiol 83: 2171–2178
2. Clark RS, Kochanek PM *et al* (1996) Cerebrospinal fluid and plasma nitrite and nitrate concentrations after head injury in humans. Crit Care Med 24(7): 1243–1251
3. Hampl V, Walters CL, Archer SL (1996) Determination of nitric oxide by the chemiluminescence reaction with ozone. In: Feelisch

M, Stamler JS (eds) Methods in nitric oxide research. Wiley, New York, pp 309–318
4. Michelakis ED and Archer SL (1998) The measurement of NO in biological systems using chemiluminescence. In: Titheradge MA (ed) Nitric oxide protocols. Humana Press, Totowa, New Jersey, pp 111–127
5. Wada K, Dietrich WD, Chatzipanteli K *et al* (1997) L-arginine, but not SIN-1 reduces contusion volume after fluid percussion brain injury in rats. J Neurotrauma 14: 760–760
6. Wada K, Chatzipanteli K, Busto R *et al* (1999) Effects of L-NAME and 7-NI on NOS catalytic activity and behavioral outocme after traumatic brain injury in the rat. J Neurotrauma 16: 230–212
7. Wada K, Chatzipanteli K, Busto R *et al* (1998) Role of nitric oxide in traumatic brain injury in the rat. J Neurosurg 89: 807–818
8. Wishnok JS, Glogowski JA, Tannenbaum SR (1996) Quantitation of nitrate, nitrite, and nitrosating agents. Meth Enzymol 268: 130–41
9. Zecca L, Rosati M, Renella R *et al* (1998) Nitrate and nitrite levels in cerebrospinal fluid of normal subjects. J Neural Transm 105(6–7): 627–633

Correspondence: J. Clay Goodman, M.D., Department of Pathology, Baylor College of Medicine, One Baylor Plaza, Houston, TX 77030.

Acta Neurochir (2002) [Suppl] 81: 347–349

Comparison of Microdialysate Arginine and Glutamate Levels in Severely Head-Injured Patient

R. Hlatky[1,2], Y. Furuya[1,3], A. B. Valadka[1], J. C. Goodman[1], and C. S. Robertson[1]

[1] Department of Neurosurgery, Baylor College of Medicine, Houston, USA
[2] Department of Neurosurgery, University Hospital, Hradec Kralove, Czech Republic
[3] Department of Neurosurgery, St. Marianna University School of Medicine, Kawasaki, Japan

Summary

L-arginine concentrations in the brain are of interest following TBI because L-arginine is the immediate precursor of nitric oxide (NO). In addition, in vitro studies suggest that glutamate, which is a mediator of secondary injury after TBI, may stimulate release of arginine from glial cells. This study examines arginine concentrations in brain tissue using the microdialysis technique after human TBI. From 78 TBI patients, a total of 1739 microdialysate samples were collected using a CMA-70 probe perfused with normal saline at 2 μl/min and concentrations of amino acids in microdialysate were determined. Amino acid concentrations for each patient were averaged for 8-hour periods during the first 3 days after injury, and daily for postinjury days 4 and 5. Following an initial rapid decrease in arginine, the dialysate arginine concentrations were low on days 1–3 and then increased over the days 4–5 after injury. In contrast, the microdialysate glutamate levels decreased slowly over the first 48 hours after TBI and thereafter remained low. Thirty-five episodes of jugular venous desaturation ($SjvO_2 < 50\%$) occurred during monitoring. Arginine and glutamate levels simultaneously doubled during desaturation and decreased as the clinical episode resolved. The low concentrations of arginine during the first 3 days after TBI may indicate that substrate unavailability could contribute to the decreased NO concentrations that have been observed after TBI. The simultaneous increase in glutamate and arginine during ischemic events is consistent with experimental data which has observed that glutamate induces release of arginine.

Keywords: Brain injury; arginine; glutamate; microdialysis.

Introduction

Concentrations of NO are decreased in the brain after TBI. Possible mechanisms for this decreased NO after TBI could include decreased production of NO because of substrate depletion (arginine, which is the precursor of NO, or oxygen) or inhibition of nitric oxide synthase, or because of rapid inactivation of NO.

TBI induces many processes, which could alter arginine levels. Ischemia, which occurs as a secondary complication of TBI, can limit conversion of arginine to NO because this is an O_2-dependent reaction. In vitro studies suggest that glutamate, which is often released in high concentrations after TBI, may stimulate release of arginine from glial cells [3]. This study examines arginine and glutamate concentrations in microdialysate samples after TBI.

Methods

All study patients were managed by a standard protocol that emphasized prompt evacuation of intracranial mass lesions and prevention of secondary insults to the brain. The research protocol was approved by the Baylor Institutional Review Board and informed consent was obtained from each patient's nearest relative for participation in the study.

Microdialysis probes were placed in fronto-temporal region (injured but not clearly necrotic tissue), either by direct vision at surgery (n = 44) or by CT scan in the ICU (n = 34). The probes were perfused at 2 μl/min with normal saline and samples were collected every 30 min. Amino acids (AA) were measured in every fifth sample during time periods where the patients were stable and, in addition, in all samples surrounding clinical events. From the 78 patients a total of 1739 microdialysate samples (average 22/patient) were analyzed. Concentrations of AA were determined by pre-column phenylisothiocyanate derivatization, reverse phase gradient separation, and absorbance detection (Waters PICO-TAG).

Results

Changes in Glutamate and Arginine Concentrations over Time:

The individual glutamate and arginine concentrations were summarized for every 8 hour time period from admission through day 3 after injury and then for each 24 hour time period on days 4 and 5 postinjury. Because the data were not normally distributed in this

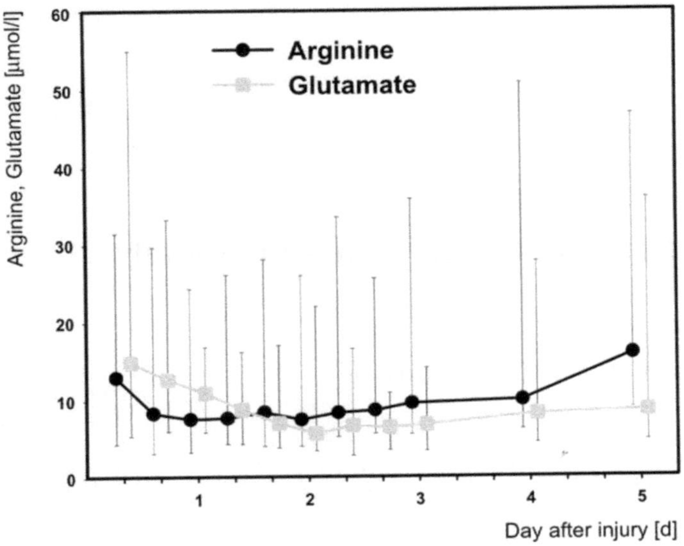

Fig. 1. Median microdialysate values of arginine and glutamate in 8 hour blocks during five days after injury

analysis, the summaries are represented by the median and interquartile ranges. After an initial rapid decrease in the microdialysate concentration of arginine, the values remained low from days 1–3, and then increased again on the fourth and fifth days postinjury. The concentrations of glutamate were highest on the first day after injury, and gradually decreased over the first 3 days postinjury. Median and interquartile range values for arginine and glutamate over time are presented in Fig. 1.

Changes in Glutamate and Arginine during jugular venous desaturation episodes:

Thirty-seven episodes of jugular venous desaturation ($SjvO_2 < 50\%$) occurred during the microdialysis monitoring in these 78 patients. Thirty of the episodes were transient and reversible and seven episodes were terminal and irreversible. The changes in glutamate and arginine levels that occurred during the 37 episodes of jugular desaturation are summarized in Table 1.

With the transient ischemic episodes, the microdialysis concentration of glutamate and arginine doubled during the time that $SjvO_2$ was low and then returned to the pre-desaturation baseline as the clinical episode resolved. Seven episodes of terminal desaturation occurred as the patient died of refractory intracranial hypertension and therefore represented irreversible global ischemia. As the ischemia developed, the concentration of arginine in the microdialysate samples increased ten times and concentration of glutamate increased 63 times.

Table 1. *Median Arginine (ARG) and Glutamate (GLU) Microdialysate Values [µmol/l] During Changes in Jugular Venous Saturation*

		Transient desaturation			Terminal desaturation	
		Pre	During	Post	Pre	During
	75th	15.1	29.6	16.8	12.3	139.5
ARG	med	*5.7*	*13.5*	*8.3*	*5.5*	*50.5*
	25th	3.2	7.7	4.9	4.3	27.0
	75th	9.6	48.4	9.3	9.5	529.8
GLU	med	*4.9*	*12.8*	*4.8*	*5.4*	*427.3*
	25th	3.1	6.1	2.9	3.4	224.3

Discussion

Nitric oxide (NO) is synthesized in the brain from L-arginine by the enzyme nitric oxide synthase (NOS). Following TBI, NO concentrations in the brain are decreased for several hours to days [2]. This reduction in NO is associated with a decrease in cerebral blood flow. The metabolism of NO is complex, and production of NO can be altered by a number of factors that are known to be abnormal after TBI.

It is not clear what causes the reduced concentrations of NO in the early phase of TBI, but reduced production because of limited availability of substrates or by inhibition of NOS, and increased utilization of NO are general categories of possible mechanisms. Administration of L-arginine after TBI restores cerebral blood flow to near-normal levels, suggesting that there may be some limitation in arginine availability [1]. In addition, NO production is an oxygen-dependent reaction and hypoxia can inhibit NOS activity [4]. Ischemia is a common secondary event after TBI.

The first goal of this study was to examine the concentrations of arginine in the brain, to determine if a decrease in availability of L-arginine was a likely contributing factor in the reduced NO that has been observed after TBI. Because the concentrations of L-arginine are relatively low during the first 3 days after injury, the time when NO concentrations are known to be low, reduced availability of L-arginine could play a role. However, extracellular concentrations of arginine may not always reflect local availability. Increased utilization of L-arginine could be another explanation of this finding.

The second goal of this study was to examine arginine levels during ischemic episodes. Jugular venous desaturation was used as the indicator of significant cerebral ischemia. During these periods of reduced oxygen availability, the concentrations of arginine in the brain increased significantly. The increased levels of arginine could reflect reduced utilization, i.e. decreased production of NO. However, another explanation is equally possible. Grima *et al.* demonstrated that arginine is released from cerebellar and cortical slices and from cortical astroglial cultures upon activation of ionotropic non-NMDA glutamate receptors [3]. During the ischemic episodes in the present study, the increase in arginine paralleled the increase in glutamate and is therefore, consistent with this experimental study.

The dynamics of arginine concentrations during the acute post-injury period are probably the result of complex interactions, and many factors are probably responsible for the alterations in NO metabolism, which occur after trauma. These studies suggest that reductions in arginine availability could play a role, particularly during the first 3 days after injury.

References

1. Cherian L, Chacko G, Goodman JC, Robertson CS (1999) Cerebral hemodynamic effects of phenylephrine and L-arginine after cortical impact injury. Crit Care Med 27: 2512–2517
2. Cherian L, Goodman JC, Robertson CS (2000) Brain nitric oxide changes after controlled cortical impact injury in rats. J Neurophysiol 83: 2171–2178
3. Grima G, Benz B, Do KQ (1997) Glutamate induced release of nitric oxide precursor arginine, from glial cells. Eur J Neurosci 9: 2248–2258
4. Kim N *et al* (1993) Oxygen tension regulates the nitric oxide pathway: physiological role in penile erection. J Clin Invest. 91: 437–442

Correspondence: Prof. C. S. Robertson, Dept. of Neurosurgery, Baylor College of Medicine, 6560 Fannin Ste 944, Houston, TX 77030, USA.

Acta Neurochir (2002) [Suppl] 81: 351–354

Temporal Profiles of Extracellular Nitric Oxide Metabolites Following Aneurysmal Subarachnoid Hemorrhage

O. W. Sakowitz[1], **S. Wolfrum**[2,3], **A. S. Sarrafzadeh**[1], **J. F. Stover**[1], **W. R. Lanksch**[1], and **A. W. Unterberg**[1]

[1] Department of Neurosurgery, Charité – Humboldt University Berlin, Berlin, Germany
[2] Institute of Pharmacology and Toxicology, Medical University Lübeck, Lübeck, Germany
[3] Medical Clinic II, Medical University Lübeck, Lübeck, Germany

Summary

The temporal profile of nitric oxide metabolite concentrations i.e. nitrite and nitrate (NO_x) was investigated in brain parenchyma of patients following aneurysmal subarachnoid hemorrhage (SAH).

In a subset of ten patients (7F/3M, age: 47 ± 14 yrs) included in a prospective clinical trial on neurochemical intensive-care monitoring, microdialysis (MD) probes (CMA70, Sweden) were implanted at time of aneurysm surgery. Samples from patients clipped electively (n = 3) were considered "normal" in regard to SAH patients (n = 7). MD was performed for 162 ± 63 hrs. NO_x was measured off-line using a highly sensitive, fluorometric assay (2–3-diaminonaphtalene, DAN). NO_x concentrations determined from electively operated patients averaged 36.7 ± 9.6 μM (n = 59, pooled data). Regardless of the development of delayed ischemic neurological deficits (DIND), SAH patients showed a specific temporal profile of NO_x consisting of an initial peak followed by an exponential decay. In detail, NO_x decreased from initial values of 46.2 ± 34.8 μM to 23.5 ± 9.0 μM on day 6–7 after SAH ($p < 0.05$).

Following SAH extracellular concentrations of NO metabolites decrease over time. This is in agreement with hypothetical NO scavenging by products of hemolysis. However, subsequent development of DIND cannot be explained by a lack of vasodilatory NO alone.

Keywords: Cerebral vasospasm; ischemia; microdialysis; nitric oxide.

Introduction

In the post-operative phase following aneurysm occlusion cerebral vasospasm (VSP) is the major complication of SAH, potentially leading to infarction and thus long-term morbidity and mortality. Despite of extensive research the pathomechanisms of SAH-induced VSP still remain unclear.

During the last decade there has been increasing awareness that NO may play an essential role in the development of VSP. However, both reduced and excessive NO-metabolism have been suggested as important factors in the pathophysiology of VSP [5, 10]. Pioneering studies of experimental VSP in primates have implied that a lack of NO due to scavenging by liberated hemoglobin might be the cause for VSP [3, 8]. Recently experimental studies of VSP reversed by NO replacement have triggered substantial interest [9, 12].

In SAH patients, NO-metabolites (mainly nitrite and nitrate, NO_x) have been measured in cerebrospinal fluid (CSF) [11]. However, it has been reported that VSP extends up to the distal parenchymal branches of cerebral arteries where CSF-NO_x might be an insufficient estimator of the local conditions [6]. Microdialysis (MD) provides an elegant way to study the microenvironment of the brain.

The present study aimed to define the temporal profile of cerebral NO_x concentrations in aneurysm patients with or without recent SAH.

Materials and Methods

Patients

In 10 aneurysm patients with (n = 7) or without (n = 3) recent SAH, cerebral metabolism was monitored post-operatively by bedside MD. On admission SAH was confirmed by computerized tomography (CT) scanning. SAH was graded by distribution and pattern of hemorrhage according to the Fisher-Scale and by clinical presentation according to the WFNS-Scale, respectively.

Blood flow velocities were obtained at least once daily by TCD (TC2-64, EME, Tubingen, Germany). Cerebral angiography was performed routinely in all patients upon admittance. According to the time course of VSP control angiography was performed on day 7–8 after bleeding or earlier in case of neurologic deterioration.

Only patients presenting with DIND were treated with "triple-H" (hypertension, hypervolemia and hemodilution) therapy. Insidious onset of confusion, appearance of a focal neurological deficit or both, were judged as symptomatic vasospasm. Cranial CT scans were obtained to rule out acute ischemic events or development of post-hemorrhagic hydrocephalus.

Ethics

Intensive-care monitoring of SAH patients using the microdialysis-technique was approved by the local medical ethics comittee. Written informed consent was obtained from the patient or the closest relative.

Microdialysis of NO_x

MD catheters (CMA70, CMA, Sweden; 10 mm membrane) were inserted immediately after clipping of the aneurysm. Catheters were placed 25–35 mm into the brain parenchyma of the vascular territory most likely to be affected by VSP, e.g. the temporal lobe in patients with a middle cerebral (MCA) or an internal carotid artery (ICA) aneurysm or into the frontal lobe in patients with anterior communicating artery (Acom) aneurysms. Catheters were perfused (CMA106 microdialysis pump, CMA, Sweden) with sterile Ringer's solution at a fixed flow rate of 0.3 $\mu l\ min^{-1}$.

Extracellular concentrations of NO_x were determined off-line with a sensitive method by using 2,3-diaminonaphtalene (DAN, Sigma, Deisenhofen, Germany) as described previously [4].

Data Analysis

All statistics were done using SPSS 8.0 (SPSS Inc., Chicago, IL, USA). Data averaged among groups are reported as means and standard deviation. For statistical testing of NO_x time-courses a repeated measurements ANOVA with post-hoc analysis by one-sided paired t-tests was employed. A p-value less than 0.05 was considered significant.

Results

Demography

MD monitoring was performed in 10 aneurysm patients who underwent microsurgical clip ligation (demographic data summarized in Table 1). In 7 of these, recent hemorrhage had been confirmed by CT. Probes were inserted in vascular territories at risk for delayed ischemia according to aneurysm location. Of three patients who were operated electively none had experienced clinical symptoms of SAH prior to operation.

Table 1. *Demographic Data of 10 Aneurysm Patients With or Without Aneurysmal SAH (n = 7 and n = 3, Respectively)*

Patient characteristics	
Age	47 ± 14 (25–65) yrs
Gender	7F/3M
WFNS Grade	[0] [1] [2] [3] [4] [5]
n =	3 2 1 3 1 0
Fisher Grade	[1] [2] [3] [4]
n =	3 3 2 2
Total time of MD	162 ± 63 (36–235) hrs

Of the SAH patients, 4 presented with DIND. This was confirmed by secondary deterioration of MD values (n = 4), significant angiographic vessel narrowing (n = 3) and elevated blood flow velocities (n = 3). In three SAH patients without DIND significant angiographic vessel narrowing and elevated blood flow velocities were observed once. None of the electively operated patients deteriorated secondarily.

All of the patients with DIND received "triple-H" therapy. Permanent resolution of DIND was achieved in all cases except one patient, who retained a mild left-sided hemiparesis.

Temporal Profile of NO_x

In 3 patients without SAH extracellular concentrations of NO_x stabilized within 4 hours after insertion of the probe. Following stabilization, amounts of total NO_x averaged 36.7 ± 9.6 μM (95% CI: 34.2–39.2, pooled samples, n = 59). These values were regarded as "normal" for comparison with SAH patients. In Fig. 1 they are plotted in comparison with results reported for samples of arterial and venous blood [13] and ventricular CSF [1].

Regardless of the development of DIND, SAH patients showed a specific temporal profile of NO_x consisting of an initial peak with an exponential decay following. Overall, values of NO_x averaged 46.2 ± 34.8 μM (n = 7) on days 1–3. Up to days 4–5 and 6–7 these significantly decreased to 28.8 ± 12.6 μM and 23.5 ± 9.0 μM respectively (n = 7, $p < 0.05$) (cf. Fig. 2). Initial values varied intra-individually with 3 of 7 patients presenting with

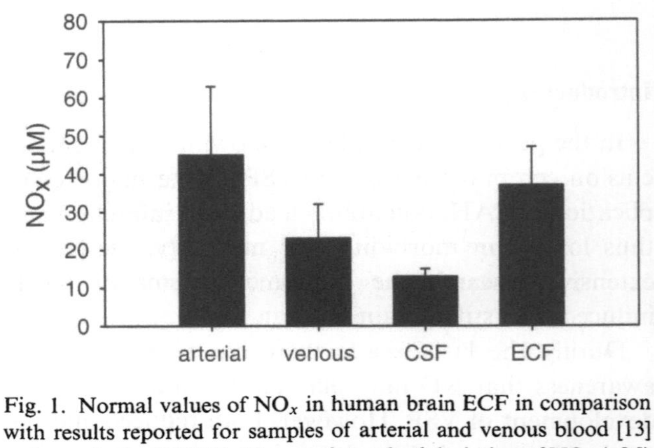

Fig. 1. Normal values of NO_x in human brain ECF in comparison with results reported for samples of arterial and venous blood [13] and ventricular CSF [1]. Mean and standard deviation of NO_x (μM)

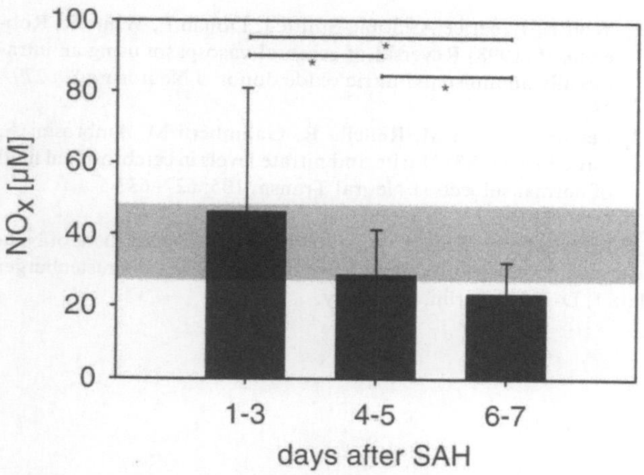

Fig. 2. Average temporal profile of brain ECF NO_x in SAH patients. Mean and standard deviation of NO_x (µM) on days 1–3, 4–5 and 6–7 following SAH. Shaded area depicts normal values. *: $p < 0.05$

supranormal NO_x-concentrations, wheras NO_x decreased to less than normal values in 6 of 7.

Discussion

In the present study cerebral microdialysates of aneurysm patients with and without recent SAH were analyzed for stable metabolites of NO.

Experimentally, measurements of NO_x have been proven effective using microdialysis [7]. The main benefit of this method is the ability to recover NO_x in-vivo in the cerebral extracellular space. A sensitive fluorometric assay fitted for aqueous samples was employed in this study. Compared with methods based on the Griess-reaction it is approximately 50–100 times more sensitive making it ideal for small-volume, ultrafiltrated samples with micromolar concentrations of NO_x [4].

Samples from patients without SAH were analyzed in order to estimate "normal" values. In patients following SAH NO_x appeared to decrease over time. This pattern is consistent with the assumption that lowered ECF-NO_x leads to an imbalance of vasoconstrictive and vasodilative factors and thus to vasoconstriction and subsequent decreases in local cerebral perfusion.

In cisternal CSF samples of SAH patients tended to higher than normal concentrations of NO_x [11]. In comparison with the current study concentrations in CSF might well be different from those in other compartments (perivascular, vascular, intravascular, brain parenchyma). For CSF samples it appears that the increase of NO-metabolites over time is a function of SAH-extent [11] or acute injury severity as it has been shown in severely head-injured patients [2].

In the perivascular or parenchymal environment following SAH the picture differs. In a primate model of cisternal hemorrhage, Pluta *et al.* [8] provided in vivo evidence that the concentrations of oxyhemoglobin and deoxyhemoglobin, both potent NO-scavengers, increase in the cerebral subarachnoid perivascular space during the development of delayed cerebral vasospasm. In the SAH group perivascular concentrations of oxyhemoglobin and deoxyhemoglobin peaked (about 100-fold higher than control) on day 7 the time where prevalence of VSP is highest. Hence, NO-scavenging by products of hemolysis might theoretically account for the temporal profile of NOx in the current study.

Following SAH extracellular concentrations of NO metabolites decrease over time. This is in agreement with hypothetical NO scavenging by products of hemolysis. However, subsequent development of DIND cannot be explained by a lack of vasodilatory NO alone.

References

[1] Cicinelli E, Ignarro L, Schonauer L, Matteo M, Galantino P, Falco N (1999) Different plasma levels of nitric oxide in arterial and venous blood. Clin Physiol 19: 440–442

[2] Clark R, Kochanek P, Obrist W, Wong H, Billiar T, Wisniewski S, Marion D (1996) Cerebrospinal fluid and plasma nitrite and nitrate concentrations after head injury in humans. Crit Care Med 24: 1243–1251

[3] Edwards D, Byrne J, Griffith T (1992) The effect of chronic subarachnoid hemorrhage on basal endothelium-derived relaxing factor activity in intrathecal cerebral arteries. J Neurosurg 76: 830–837

[4] Lei B, Adachi N, Nagaro T, Arai T (1999) Measurement of total nitric oxide metabolite (no(x)(-)) levels in vivo. Brain Res Brain Res Protoc 4: 415–419

[5] Medele R, Stummer W, Reulen H, Steiger H (1996) Evidence for peroxidative damage by nitric oxide in experimental chronic cerebral vasospasm. Neurol Res 18: 277–280

[6] Ohkuma H, Itoh K, Shibata S, Suzuki S (1997) Morphological changes of intraparenchymal arterioles after experimental subarachnoid hemorrhage in dogs. Neurosurgery 41: 230–235

[7] Ohta K, Araki N, Shibata M, Hamada J, Komatsumoto S, Shimazu K, Fukuuchi Y (1994) A novel in vivo assay system for consecutive measurement of brain nitric oxide production combined with the microdialysis technique. Neurosci Lett 176: 165–168

[8] Pluta R, Afshar J, Boock R, Oldfield E (1998) Temporal changes in perivascular concentrations of oxyhemoglobin, deoxyhemoglobin, and methemoglobin after subarachnoid hemorrhage. J Neurosurg 88: 557–561

[9] Pluta R, Oldfield E, Boock R (1997) Reversal and prevention of cerebral vasospasm by intracarotid infusions of nitric oxide donors in a primate model of subarachnoid hemorrhage. J Neurosurg 87: 746–751
[10] Pluta R, Thompson B, Dawson T, Snyder S, Boock R, Oldfield E (1996) Loss of nitric oxide synthase immunoreactivity in cerebral vasospasm. J Neurosurg 84: 648–654
[11] Suzuki Y, Osuka K, Noda A, Tanazawa T, Takayasu M, Shibuya M, Yoshida J (1997) Nitric oxide metabolites in the cisternal cerebral spinal fluid of patients with subarachnoid hemorrhage. Neurosurgery 41: 807–811
[12] Wolf E, Banerjee A, Soble-Smith J, Dohan F, White R, Robertson J (1998) Reversal of cerebral vasospasm using an intrathecally administered nitric oxide donor. J Neurosurg 89: 279–288
[13] Zecca L, Rosati M, Renella R, Galimberti M, Ambrosini A, Fariello R (1998) Nitrite and nitrate levels in cerebrospinal fluid of normal subjects. J Neural Transm 105: 627–633

Correspondence: Oliver W. Sakowitz, M.D., Department of Neurosurgery, Charité – Campus Virchow Med. Ctr., Augustenburger Platz 1, D-13353 Berlin, Germany.

Acta Neurochir (2002) [Suppl] 81: 355–357

Delayed Increase in Extracellular Glycerol with Post-Traumatic Electrographic Epileptic Activity: Support for the Theory that Seizures Induce Secondary Injury

P. Vespa, N. A. Martin, V. Nenov, T. Glenn, M. Bergsneider, D. Kelly, D. P. Becker, and **D. A. Hovda**

UCLA, Department of Neurosurgery, Los Angeles

Summary

Early post-traumatic seizures occur commonly and may have adverse clinical consequences. In order to determine the significance of post-traumatic seizures, we performed a prospective assessment of the consequences of epileptic activity by assessing the change in extracellular glycerol levels. Glycerol is a marker of cellular membrane breakdown. Thirteen patients underwent combined electroencephalography (EEG) and cerebral microdialysis monitoring. Two patients had seizures on EEG with associated delayed elevations of glycerol associated with the seizure activity. Higher mean levels of glycerol were present in those patients with seizures compared to those without seizures ($p < 0.001$). Preliminary evidence suggests that post-traumatic seizures lead to additional membrane injury as reflected by elevated extracellular glycerol levels.

Keywords: Head injured; seizures; EEG; microdialysis.

Introduction

Post traumatic seizures and epileptiform activity occurs commonly during a critical window of time after the primary traumatic insult [6, 9] and have been related to increased extracellular glutamate levels [8]. Acute changes in glucose metabolism and extracellular levels of glucose occur in response to brain trauma and membrane depolarization or irritability [2–5, 7]. The influence of post-traumatic epileptiform activity on these neurochemical changes is not well defined. Moreover considerable controversy exists as to whether epileptiform activity can independently induce additional brain injury in the setting of a primary insult or long-standing epilepsy. The aim of this study is to illustrate the influence of seizures on the extracellular levels of glucose and to determine if additional membrane injury occurs with seizures, as indicated by changes in extracellular glycerol.

Methods

Patients with traumatic brain injury were enrolled under the University of California, Los Angeles Institutional Review Board consent process. A microdialysis probe (CMA 70 – CMA Stockholm, Sweden) was inserted into the cortex in the peri-contusional site under direct observation or into the right frontal lobe adjacent to the ventriculostomy catheter. The microdialysis catheter was perfused with sterile 0.9% NaCl using an infusion pump at 2 μL/minute with hourly fractions collected and immediately analyzed. The hourly samples were analyzed using the CMA600 automated analyzed (CMA – Stockholm) for glycerol. Quality control repeat analysis of analyzed samples was implemented for those samples in which >30% change in the value occurred compared to a previous 4 hour baseline in order to eliminate artifactual measurements.

Continuous Electroencephalography (cEEG) was performed on all patients using the methods previously described [9]. Epileptiform activity was identified using standard criteria. The timing of the EEG abnormalities was correlated with the matched hourly sample of microdialysis adjusting for dead space considerations.

Results

Thirteen patients underwent cerebral microdialysis during the initial 10 days after injury. The median GCS was 7, with 6 females and 7 males, mean age of 41.5 ± 19.5 years. The traumatic lesion types were single or multiple contusions (8), subdural hematoma (3), diffuse shear and subarachnoid hemorrhage (1) and epidura hematoma (1). Two patients died, 4 were severely disabled, 3 were moderately disabled and 2 made a good outcome at 30 days.

Two patients with electrographic seizures had large contusions involving the frontal and temporal lobes. In each case, the seizures began within 24 hours of injury and were characterized as electrographic spike and wave discharges that had a focal onset with secondary

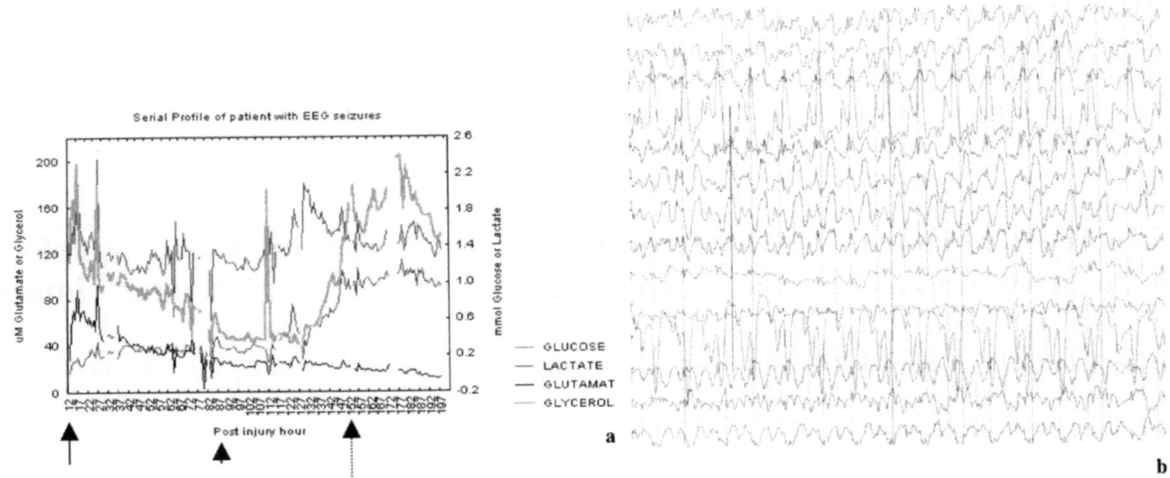

Fig. 1. (a) This is a time course of hourly microdialysis values in a patient with generalized electrographic seizures (b). At the onset of seizure (arrow) there is an elevation of glycerol (200 μM) and glutamate (80 μM) associated with reduced glucose (0.2 mmol) and elevated lactate (1.4 mmol). With propofol, the EEG went into burst suppression (arrowhead), with reduction in glycerol. With cessation of propofol, seizures recurred and glycerol increased again (dotted arrow)

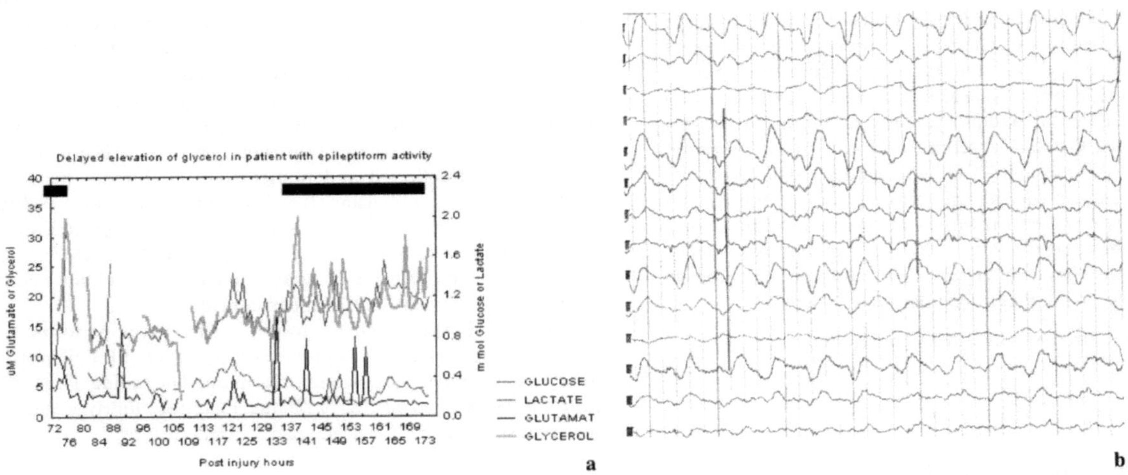

Fig. 2. (a) This hourly time plot shows elevated glycerol (25 μM) at time 72 hours after injury in conjunction with a seizure. Between hours 84 and 130, the glycerol level if <15 μM, but increases again to >20 μM in several transient peaks between hours 137 and 173, in association with transient epileptiform activity (b). Elevated glutamate levels ranging from 5–10 μM occur in conjunction during hours 137–157

generalization. Patient 1 (Fig. 1) had status epilepticus and required high dose continuous infusion of propofol and high levels of phenytoin and phenobarbital to stop the seizures. Figure 1a demonstrates the serial changes in glycerol and glutamate with the initial seizure activity and the reduction of glycerol and glutamate with propofol induced burst-suppression. Glycerol was initially elevated and slowly responded to treatment with a reduction from 200 μM to 40 μM (from hour 17 to hour 102, respectively). Glutamate similarly declined from 80 μM to 20 μM over the same time course. Intermittent interruption of propofol elicited recurrent seizures during this time frame. Later, at hour 152, propofol was stopped and the seizures recurred briefly but were controlled with high levels of phenytoin and phenobarbital.

Patient 2 had elevation of glycerol (30 μM) initially that came after a brief electrographic seizure. A delayed glycerol elevation (range 18–32 μM) occurred between 137 hours and 173 hours after injury, and were associated with delayed electrographic seizure activity at that time (Fig. 3a and b). No apparent

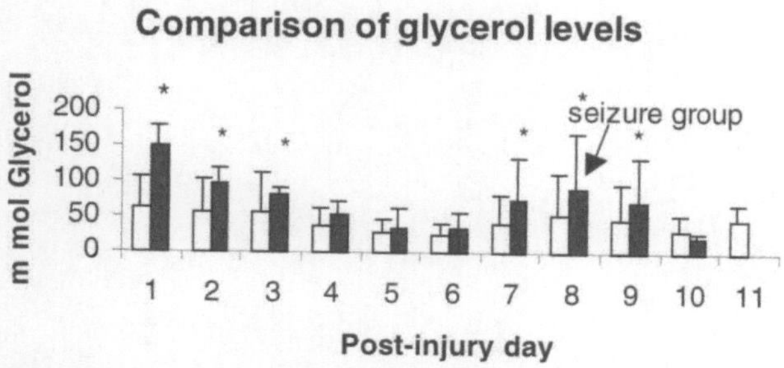

Fig. 3. A comparison of the mean daily glycerol levels between the 2 patients with seizures and the non-seizure group. Glycerol levels are higher during the initial 3 post-injury days ($p < 0.001$) and during days 7–9 ($p < 0.01$). These days correspond to the incidence of seizures

global hypoxic events were noted by jugular venous oximetry or intracranial pressure monitoring to explain these changes in glycerol.

When compared with the entire group, daily glycerol levels were statistically higher in the two patients with electrographic seizures during the initial 3 days after injury and on days 7–9. This global difference corresponds with the days on which electrographic seizures occurred.

Discussion

Post-traumatic electrographic seizures occur commonly in approximately 20% of patients [9]. Normal glycerol levels are 0–2 μM with elevation occurring with injury [1]. Elevation of glycerol occurs in conjunction with cellular membrane lipolysis [4]. We found secondary elevation of glycerol in the extracellular fluid during epochs of seizure activity. Patients with seizures had higher levels of glycerol during the initial 3 days after injury and during days 7–9 in comparison with those patients without post-traumatic seizures. Glutamate levels were elevated during seizures similar to previous reports [8].

Experimentally seizures can induce lipolysis [1] and injure cells, but seizures models have demonstrated no long term effect of prolonged seizures. The current data demonstrates elevation of glycerol levels above that expected with brain trauma alone and thereby indicates that seizures may potentiate lipolysis and membrane injury after trauma. Thus these preliminary data suggest that seizures may induce additional lipolysis in the setting of a primary brain trauma and may be injurious to cells that survived the initial insult.

References

1. Bazan NG (1971) Changes in free fatty acids of brain by drug-induced convulsions, electroshock and anesthesia. J Neurochem 18: 1379–1385
2. Bullock R, Zauner A, Myseros JS (1995) Evidence for prolonged release of excitatory amino acids in severe human head trauma: relationship to clinical events. Ann NY Acad Sci 59: 290–297
3. Goodman JC, Valadka A, Robertson C *et al* (1999) Simultaneous measurement of cortical potassium, calcium, and magnesium levels measured in head injured patients using microdialysis with ion chromatography. Acta Neurochir (Wien) [Suppl] 75: 35–37
4. Hillered L, Valtysson J, Enblad P, Persson L (1998) Interstitial glycerol as a marker for membrane phospholipid degradation in the acutely injured human brain. J Neurol Neurosurg Psychiatry 64: 486–491
5. Landolt H, Langemann H, Mendelowitsch A, Gratzl O (1994) Neurochemical monitoring and on-line pH measurements using brain microdialysis in patients in intensive care. Acta Neurochir (Wien) 60: 475–478
6. Nilsson P, Ronne-Engström E, Flink R, Ungerstedt U, Carlson H, Hillered L (1994) Epileptic seizure activity in the acute phase following cortical impact trauma in rat. Brain Res 637(1–2): 227–232
7. Robertson CS, Gopinath SP, Uzura M, Valadka AB, Goodman JC (1998) Metabolic changes in the brain during transient ischemia measured with microdialysis. Neurol Res 20 [Suppl] 1: S91–94
8. Vespa PM, Ronne-Engstrom E, Smith M, Hovda DA, Shalmon E, Martin NA, Becker DP (1998) Increase in extracellular glutamate caused by reduced cerebral perfusion pressure and seizures after human traumatic brain injury: a microdialysis study. J Neurosurg 89: 971–982
9. Vespa PM, Nuwer MR, Nenov V, Ronne-Engstrom E, Hovda DA, Martin NA, Becker DP (1999) Increased incidence and impact of nonconvulsive and convulsive seizures after traumatic brain injury as detected by continuous EEG in the intensive care unit. J Neurosurg 91: 750–760

Correspondence: Paul M. Vespa, Neurosurgical Department, UCLA, CHS 18-218, 10833 Le Conte Ave, Los Angeles, California 90095, USA.

Acta Neurochir (2002) [Suppl] 81: 359–362

Clinical Cerebral Microdialysis – Determining the True Extracellular Concentration

P. J. A. Hutchinson, M. T. O'Connell, P. G. Al-Rawi, R. Kett-White, A. K. Gupta, P. J. Kirkpatrick, and J. D. Pickard

Academic Department of Neurosurgery, Department of Neuro-Intensive Care and Wolfson Brain Imaging Centre, University of Cambridge, UK

Summary

Current monitoring of the cerebral extracellular chemistry of neurosurgical patients using microdialysis does not provide the true extracellular concentration because full equilibration across the membrane is not achieved. By varying the flow rate and extrapolating to zero flow, the relative recovery i.e. the concentration of the substance in the microdialysate as a proportion of the true concentration in the extracellular space may be calculated. The disadvantage of this method is that it depends on the underlying baseline chemistry being constant during measurements for the calculations, which is not the case in the changing environment of a neuro-intensive unit. We have therefore designed a modification of the extrapolation to zero flow method using an adjacent constant flow rate catheter to monitor the baseline. The results demonstrate that the relative recovery varies considerably with flow rate, and for the CMA70 10 mm membrane catheter, is approximately 70% at a rate of 0.3 μl/min and 30% at a rate of 1.0 μl/min for glucose, lactate, pyruvate and glutamate.

Keywords: Microdialysis; true extracellular concentration.

Introduction

Microdialysis is currently being applied to measure the concentration of chemicals in the cerebral extracellular space of neurosurgical patients. A fine tube lined with dialysis membrane and perfused with a physiological solution is placed within the cerebral parenchyma. Molecules diffuse from the extracellular space across the membrane into the solution which is then collected for analysis. It is important to appreciate that the concentration of substance measured in the microdialysis solution does not equate to the true extracellular concentration because full equilibration does not occur [1, 9]. The term relative recovery is applied to the concentration of the substance in the microdialysate as a proportion of the true concentration in the extracellular space and is defined by the equation:

$$\text{Relative recovery} = C_{md}/C_{ecf} = 1 - \exp - K_0\, A/F$$

where C_{md} is the microdialysis concentration, C_{ecf} is the extracellular concentration, K_0 is the average mass transfer coefficient, A is the membrane surface area and F is the flow rate [4, 5].

In practice, slow flow rates and long membrane lengths are used in order to increase the relative recovery. There have been several techniques applied in order to determine the true extracellular concentration [2, 6–8]. These include:

(i) Varying the flow, measuring the changes in concentration of substance coming out of the catheter and extrapolating to zero flow.
(ii) Perfusing the catheter with varying concentrations of the substance and calculating the concentration at which the substance concentration does not change.
(iii) Perfusing the catheter with a reference substance. Assuming that the recovery of the membrane is the same in both directions and that the diffusion properties of the reference substance in the perfusate and the substance to be recovered from the brain are the same, the percentage loss of the reference substance from the perfusate will be the same as the percentage recovery of the substance from the brain. This recovery value can then be

used to calculate the concentration in the extracellular fluid.

The extrapolation to zero flow method has the advantage in the clinical environment that during the course of the study the perfusion fluid does not need to be changed. However, it relies on the extracellular concentration being constant which is not true in patients on the neuro-intensive care unit. The objective of this study was to modify the extrapolation to zero flow method (by using an adjacent constant flow rate reference catheter) in order to determine the relative recovery at different flow rates varying from 0.1 to 1.5 μl/min for the 10 mm membrane CMA70 microdialysis catheter.

Methods

Ethical approval for the study was obtained from the Local Research Ethics Committee and consent obtained from the patients' relatives. This study was part of our on-going microdialysis monitoring program in neuro-intensive care and was performed in three patients. Microdialysis catheters were inserted into the frontal cortex using a cranial access device as described previously [3]. Two 10 mm membrane CMA70 catheters (CMA microdialysis, Stockholm, Sweden) were inserted through the same access device and perfused with Ringer's solution (4 mM K^+, 147 mM Na^+, 2 mM Ca^{++}, 155 mM Cl^-). The microdialysate was analysed for glucose, lactate, pyruvate and glutamate using the CMA600 microdialysis analyser.

Initially, both catheters were perfused at the same flow rate 0.3 μl/min to demonstrate concordance of the substance concentrations. For the flow rate study, the first catheter (control catheter) flow rate was kept constant at 0.3 μl/min. The second catheter (study catheter) flow rate was varied from 0.1 μl/min to 1.5 μl/min. The flow rate was changed every two hours with vial changes every 30 minutes. Four values were therefore collected for each flow rate step. The means of these four values were calculated to provide the concentration at each flow rate. Similarly, for the control catheter the vials were changed every 30 minutes and the means of each four values (equivalent to the flow rate steps for the study catheter) were calculated. The control catheter did demonstrate that there was variation in the underlying basal concentration. In order to correct for this, the mean concentration from the control catheter was determined for the duration of the study. A correction factor was calculated by dividing the mean concentration from the control catheter by the substance concentration for each flow rate from the study catheter.

$$CF = (\bar{x}_{cc}/\bar{x}_{sc}) @ F_{\infty}$$

where CF is the correction factor defined by $\bar{x}_{cc}$ the concentration determined by the control catheter and $\bar{x}_{sc}$ the concentration determined by the study catheter for each flow rate F_{∞}.

In order to determine the substance concentration corrected for variation in the baseline, the correction factor was multiplied by the study catheter concentration. Graphs were plotted of the corrected substance concentration against flow rate. This is an exponential relationship and therefore the natural log of the corrected substance concentration against flow rate was also plotted in order to determine a straight line. This line was then extrapolated to zero flow and the relative recovery determined for different flow rates.

Results

Comparison of Control and Study Catheters at 0.3 μl/min

The control and study catheters were perfused at the same flow rate (0.3 μl/min) in order to establish reproducibility. There was good correlation between the catheters with correlation r and % absolute differences (mean ± standard error of the mean) for glucose of $r = 0.89$, difference % 39 ± 5.7, glutamate of $r = 0.67$, difference % 26 ± 8.3, lactate of $r = 0.76$, difference % 14 ± 6.6 and pyruvate $r = 0.85$, difference % 19 ± 3.8.

Variation in Baseline Concentration Determined by Control Catheter

The control catheter was perfused at a constant rate of 0.3 μl/min. For each patient there was variation in the base-line concentrations. The mean and standard deviation for each of the three patients for glucose was (1.08 ± 0.12, 0.60 ± 0.13, 1.63 ± 0.22 mM), glutamate (6.19 ± 0.93, 2.10 ± 0.23, 5.32 ± 0.85 μM), lactate (3.07 ± 0.18, 6.38 ± 0.81, 3.29 ± 0.20 mM) and pyruvate (107 ± 6, 217 ± 23, 137 ± 13 μM).

Determination of the True Extracellular Concentration and Relative Recovery

Figure 1a shows an example of the glutamate concentrations for one patient. The study catheter (variable flow rate 0.1–1.5 μl/min) and control catheter (constant flow rate 0.3 μl/min) recordings are shown. The baseline value was increasing during the study and this is taken account of by the glutamate corrected for variation in baseline recordings. Figure 1b shows the plot of all four substances for the same patient on a natural logarithmic scale. The flow rate which varied during the study from 0.1 to 1.5 μl/min is extrapolated to zero flow enabling the relative recovery to be calculated.

The results demonstrated that the relative recovery values for flow rates of 0.3 μl/min were between 63–69% for glucose, between 68–71% for lactate, between 68–73% for pyruvate and between 66–74% for glutamate. At 1.0 μl/min the relative recovery values were between 18–23% for glucose, between 23%–32% for lactate, between 32–38% for pyruvate and between 27–37% for glutamate. Figure 2 shows the relationship between flow rate and relative recovery for all three

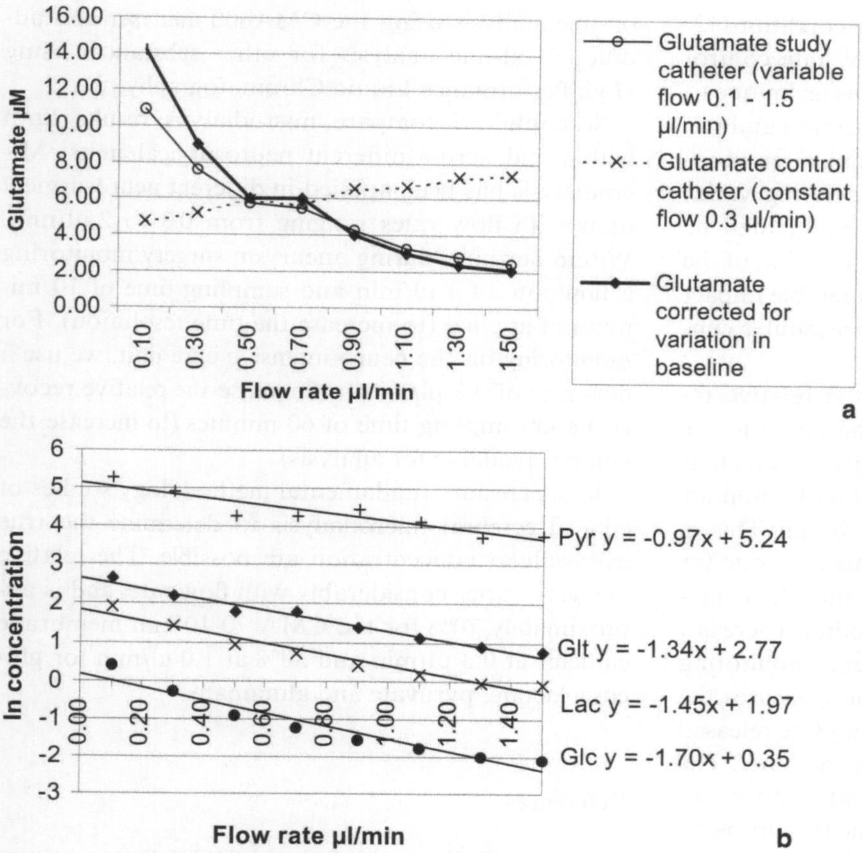

Fig. 1. (a) Effect of flow rate on extracellular glutamate concentrations. The study catheter is shown by the symbol o. As the flow rate increases from 0.1 to 1.5 μl/min, the glutamate concentration recovered in the microdialysate decreases. However, the underlying base-line concentration of glutamate detected by the constant flow rate 0.3 μl/min control catheter (symbol ×) is increasing. The study catheter glutamate concentration is therefore corrected for the increase in the base-line (shown by the symbol ◆). (b) Plot of pyruvate (pyr), glutamate (glt), lactate (lac) and glucose (glc) concentrations for the same patient on a natural logarithmic scale. The flow rate which varied during the study from 0.1 to 1.5 μl/min is extrapolated to zero flow enabling the relative recovery to be calculated. The equation for each line is shown on the right

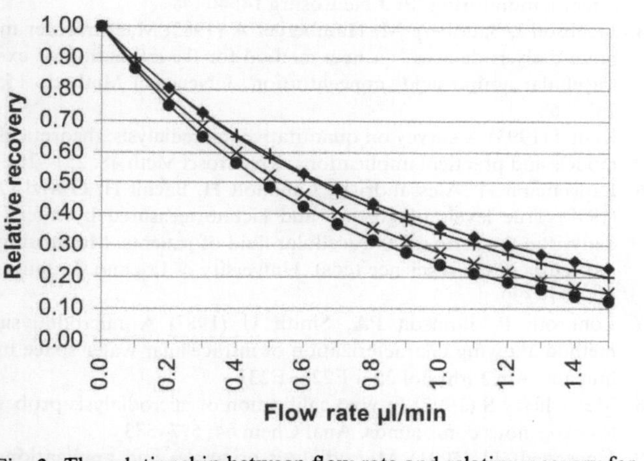

Fig. 2. The relationship between flow rate and relative recovery for all three patients (means – glutamate ◆, pyruvate +, lactate ×, glucose ●) using CMA70 microdialysis catheter 10 mm membrane. The findings demonstrate that variation in flow rate has a substantial effect on recovery. At 0.3 μl/min the relative recovery is approximately 70%, and at 1 μl/min approximately 30%. —◆— Glutamate, —+— Pyruvate, —×— Lactate, —●— Glucose

patients. The findings demonstrate that variation in flow rate has a substantial effect on recovery.

Solution for K_0

The equation relative recovery $= C_{md}/C_{ecf} = 1 - \exp - K_0\, A/F$ can now be solved. If the flow rate is 0.3 μl/min, relative recovery of 0.68 and membrane area 18.8 mm^2 (diameter 0.6 mm, length 10 mm), the value of K_0 is 1.81×10^{-5}. The 30 mm catheter has a membrane area of 56.5 mm^2 (diameter 0.6 mm, length 30 mm) and assuming the value of K_0 is the same, this would equate to a recovery of 0.97 at 0.3 μl/min.

Discussion

The extrapolation to zero flow method of determining the true extracellular concentration was pioneered in animal studies under relatively stable conditions [2, 8]. By adding an adjacent constant flow rate control catheter, we have been able to modify this technique to determine the true extracellular concentration and relative recovery in the more unstable clinical environment. The results did demonstrate underlying variation in the baseline chemistry which could then be corrected using the control catheter. Calculation of the relative recovery rates showed the considerable impact that flow rate does have on the true extracellular concentration.

This new method for determining the relative recovery does depend on assumptions additional to the classical extrapolation to zero flow model. Firstly, that the two catheters are close enough together to monitor the chemistry of the same region of brain. This is probably valid as the results for the same flow rate for both catheters were similar. Secondly, that the catheters are not so close that they are interacting. There is a potential risk that when two adjacent monitoring probes are placed in the brain that one measures the insertion artefact of the other and/or dialysate released from one catheter may be recovered for the other. The cranial access device was designed with divergent channel trajectories in order to overcome this problem. Thirdly, when the flow rates for the two catheters are different with simultaneous vial changes, the sampling time will not be exactly synchronised due to the different transit times along the outlet tubing. However, this difference is unlikely to be of clinical significance.

Determination of the relative recovery and true extracellular concentration is important for two reasons. Firstly, for the design of microdialysis catheters and methodology. Relative recovery rates in excess of 70% are desirable and this can be achieved using 10 mm membrane catheters and flow rates on 0.3 μl/min. Longer membranes are available and the solution for the relative recovery equation suggests that recovery rates approaching 100% may be achieved with a 30 mm catheter. However, longer catheters have the disadvantage that they are more difficult to implant and are likely to monitor more heterogeneous volumes of brain. The application of slower flow rates would also increase the recovery rates but at the expense of producing smaller volumes. Overcoming this by increasing the sampling time is undesirable as rapid fluctuations in chemistry may be missed. Vial changes every 60 minutes with a flow rate of 0.3 μl/min generates 18 μl of microdialysate which is sufficient for on-line analysis using the CMA600 analyser and additional off-line analysis for other substances using High Performance Liquid Chromatography.

Secondly, to compare microdialysis results both within and across different neurosurgical units. Microdialysis has been applied in different neurosurgical units with flow rates ranging from 0.3 to 2 μl/min. Within our unit, during aneurysm surgery monitoring a flow rate of 1 μl/min and sampling time of 10 minutes of applied (to increase the time resolution). For monitoring on the neuro-intensive care unit, we use a flow rate of 0.3 μl/min (to increase the relative recovery) and sampling time of 60 minutes (to increase the volume available for analysis).

In conclusion, fundamental methodology studies of clinical cerebral microdialysis to determine the true extracellular concentration are possible. The relative recovery varies considerably with flow rate, and is approximately 70% for the CMA 70 10 mm membrane catheter at 0.3 μl/min and 30% at 1.0 μl/min for glucose, lactate, pyruvate and glutamate.

References

1. Benveniste H, Hansen AJ, Ottoson NS (1989) Determination of brain interstitial concentrations by microdialysis. J Neurochem 52: 1741–1750
2. Fray AE, Boutelle M, Fillenz M (1997) Extracellular glucose turnover in the striatum of unanaesthetised rats measured by quantitative microdialysis. J Physiol 504: 721–726
3. Hutchinson PJ, Hutchinson DB, Barr RH, Burgess F, Kirkpatrick PJ, Pickard JD (2000) A new cranial access device for cerebral monitoring. Br J Neurosurg 14: 46–48
4. Jacobson I, Sandberg M, Hamberger A (1985) Mass transfer in brain dialysis devices – a new method for the estimation of extracellular amino acids concentration. J Neurosci Methods 15: 263–268
5. Kehr J (1993) A survey on quantitative microdialysis: theoretical models and practical implications. J Neurosci Meth 48: 251–261
6. Langemann H, Alessandri B, Landholt H, Bachli H, Gratzl O (1997) True levels of glucose and lactate measured by microdialysis in the cerebral extracellular fluid of patients. Monitoring molecules in neuroscience (eds). University of Loguno, Loguno, pp. 397–399
7. Lonnroth P, Jannson PA, Smith U (1987) A microdialysis method allowing characterization of intracellular water space in humans. Am J Physiol 253: E228–E231
8. Menacherry S (1992) In vivo calibration of microdialysis probes for exogenous compounds. Anal Chem 64: 577–583
9. Ungerstedt U (1991) Microdialysis-principles and applications for studies in animals and man. J Intern Med 230: 365–373

Correspondence: P. J. A. Hutchinson, F.R.C.S., Academic Department of Neurosurgery, University of Cambridge, Box 167, Addenbrooke's Hospital, Cambridge, UK, CB2 2QQ.

Acta Neurochir (2002) [Suppl] 81: 363–365

Extracellular Lactate/Pyruvate and Glutamate Changes in Patients During Per-operative Episodes of Cerebral Ischaemia

R. Kett-White, P. J. A. Hutchinson, P. G. Al-Rawi, A. K. Gupta, M. T. O'Connell, J. D. Pickard, and **P. J. Kirkpatrick**

Academic Department of Neurosurgery and the Wolfson Brain Imaging Centre, Addenbrooke's Hospital, Cambridge, UK

Summary

Objective. Temporary Internal Carotid Artery (ICA) clipping necessary during aneurysm surgery was used as a model to investigate metabolic changes in the human brain during defined episodes of ischaemia.

Design. An observational study using intracerebral monitors: P_BO_2 (Neurotrend) and microdialysis (CMA, Sweden).

Subjects. 16 patients monitored during complex aneurysm surgery.

Outcome Measures. Changes in extracellular concentrations of glucose, lactate, and glutamate and lactate/pyruvate ratio (L/P).

Results. Mean age was 55. 10 patients presented with subarachnoid haemorrhage and 6 with mass effect (4 giant). Temporary ICA occlusion was required for dissection (n = 9), intraoperative rupture (n = 5) or aneurysmal thrombectomy (n = 2). The mean total duration was 15 minutes (range 4–52 minutes). No infarcts developed in the monitored regions. Microdialysis was unsuccessful in 3 patients and Neurotrend in 1.

Patients were grouped according to the degree and duration of fall in P_BO_2: minimal brief falls were not associated with microdialysis changes (n = 5). More pronounced falls were associated with increases in L/P (n = 4). Only prolonged occlusions averaging 42 minutes (n = 3) with P_BO_2 sustained below 1 kPa were associated with rises in glutamate.

Conclusions. Brief temporary ICA occlusion caused an initial increased L/P. Glutamate increases were only seen after occlusion that was prolonged with P_BO_2 below 1.0 kPa.

Keywords: Temporary clipping; clinical microdialysis; brain tissue oxygen.

Introduction

Monitoring of the extracellular concentrations of substances has elucidated metabolic processes occurring in cerebral ischaemia in animal models [1, 2]. Subsequent studies in patients susceptible to ischaemia following SAH or head-injury have demonstrated microdialysis changes in isolated cases [8, 9, 10]. The first human model of ischaemia was in 4 patients undergoing frontal lobe tumour resection, producing progressive permanent ischaemia. Elevations in lactate and glutamate were seen amongst other changes [3]. However, it remains unclear what microdialysis changes occur during reversible episodes of human ischaemia and the reliability of such changes.

Temporary clipping (TC) of the parent artery during aneurysm surgery is an accepted method of facilitating dissection and clipping of aneurysms [6] and provides a fortuitous opportunity to study the effects of clearly identifiable episodes of acute ischaemia in humans. We have combined the use of a microdialysis system that determines changes in the extracellular concentrations of glucose, lactate, pyruvate and glutamate with a probe that measures P_BO_2. Analysis of P_BO_2 data over 41 patients, of which this group is a subset, has suggested a threshold for infarction of 1.0 kPa, in line with values obtained by different methods of estimation [7].

Materials and Methods

A subset of 16 patients requiring ICA TC was studied from a total of 41 patients monitored during craniotomy to clip an aneurysm. Patients who presented with large or complex unruptured aneurysms were particularly recruited because of the anticipated likelihood of TC. The mean age was 55 (range 32–74). 10 patients had suffered SAH. The WFNS(11) grade was poor (grade 3–5) in 4. 4 aneurysms were giant and 2 recurrent (1 previously coiled). Aneurysms were approached via a standard pterional craniotomy. TC was used on clinical grounds and was kept to a minimum. Post-operatively, patients were examined for any new neurological deficit and CT scans for any evidence of infarction, with particular reference to the monitored region.

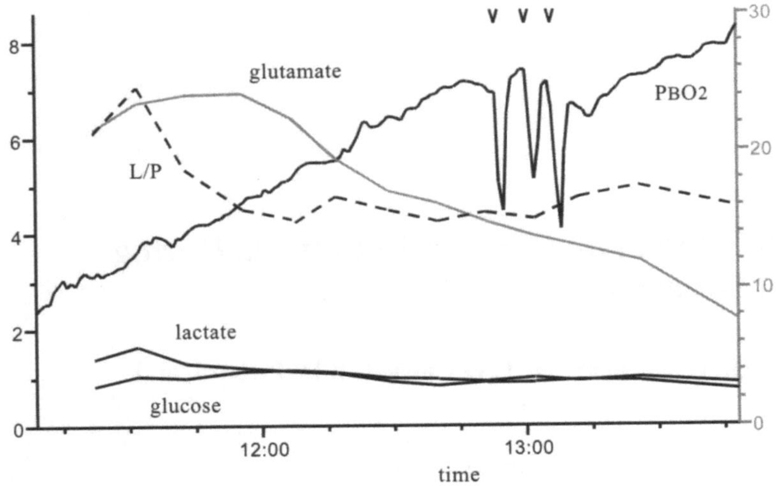

Fig. 1. Modest brain tissue oxygen (P_BO_2 kPa, left scale) decreases during 3 brief temporary ICA clips ('*V*') in a patient. There were no significant changes in microdialysis lactate/pyruvate ratio (*L/P*) or glutamate (μmol/l)(both right scale) or glucose and lactate (mmol/l, left scale)

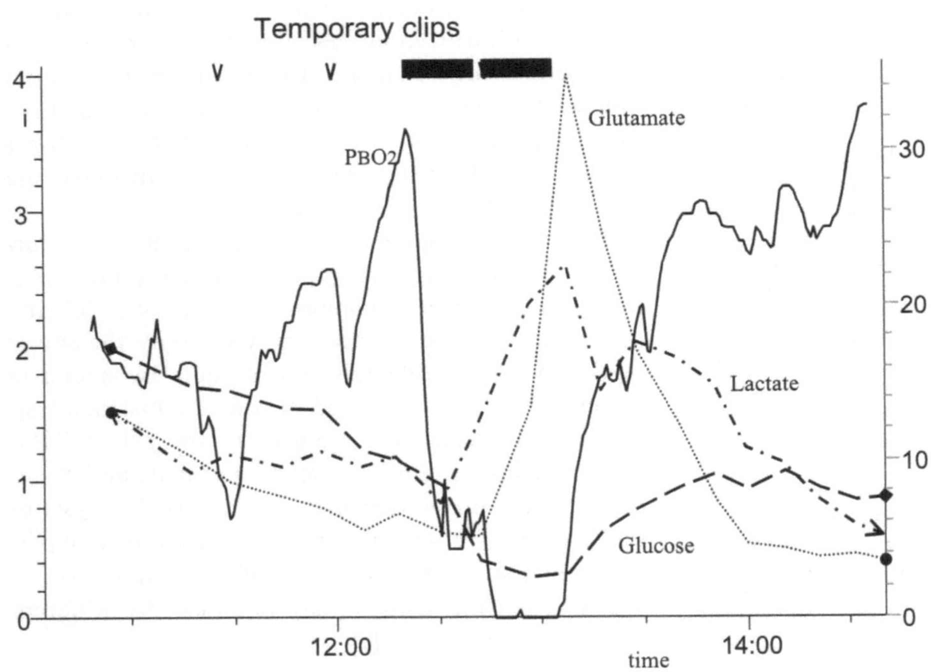

Fig. 2. Graph showing per-operative monitoring during surgery to clip a complex, giant ICA aneurysm. 2 short periods of temporary clipping ('*V*') caused brief falls in brain tissue oxygen (P_BO_2 kPa, left scale), without microdialysis changes. Subsequently, 2 more prolonged episodes of occlusion (black blocks) each just over 20 minutes caused a sustained fall in P_BO_2 and glucose (mmol/l, left scale) and rises in lactate (mmol/l, left scale) and glutamate (μmol/l, right scale)

Monitoring Technique

A triple lumen bolt(5) was inserted over the vascular territory on interest prior to craniotomy. A Neurotrend (Codman, UK) sensor and a 10-mm CMA 70 (CMA, Sweden) microdialysis catheter (Ringer's solution at 1 μl/min^{-1}) were introduced into the cortex (Neurotrend depth = 40 mm, CMA 70 depth = 20 mm). The vials were changed every 10–20 minutes and processed by a CMA 600 analyser. Microdialysis concentrations were examined graphically in each case.

Results

There were no clinical complications. One CMA 70 catheter had a faulty inlet tube; one was broken during craniotomy and one failed for an unknown reason. The Neurotrend calibration failed in 1 patient. Glutamate values were initially high in nearly all patients (mean 42 μmol/l), and decreased exponentially, mostly in the first hour. Glucose, lactate and pyruvate were steadier and concentrations tended to be reasonably stable by the time of aneurysm dissection.

The mean total duration of TC was 15 minutes (range 4–52 minutes). No infarcts developed in the monitored regions. Patients were grouped according to the degree and duration of fall in P_BO_2. In a group of 5 (Group A) in which TC was brief, averaging 7 minutes, and the P_BO_2 falls were small (by less than 50% and remaining above 1.0 kPa) there were no significant microdialysis changes. In groups B and C (mean TC 9 minutes) in which P_BO_2 falls were deeper [group B: over 50% from baseline (n = 2), or group C: briefly below 1 kPa (n = 2)] small transient rises in lactate and/or L/P ratio were seen, but without any change in glutamate or glucose. The 3 patients in group D [prolonged TC (mean of 42 minutes) with sustained decreases in P_BO_2 (below 1.0 kPa for over 30 minutes)] all showed transient increases in L/P ratio (in one case from 31 to 138) and glutamate (in the same case from 3 μmol/l to 25 μmol/l).

On regression analysis, there were linear correlations between % decreases in P_BO_2 and % increases in extracellular lactate (R^2 0.47, $P = 0.01$) and % decreases in glucose (R^2 0.35, $P = 0.05$). Increasing clip time was correlated with decreasing P_BO_2 (R^2 0.35, $P = 0.03$), decreasing glucose (R^2 0.6, $P = 0.003$) and increasing lactate (R^2 0.46, $P = 0.015$) and L/P ratio (R^2 0.38, $P = 0.02$).

Discussion

From this data it seems there is a predictable pattern of metabolic changes with ischaemia. Significant falls in P_BO_2 are followed within a few minutes by a rise in extracellular lactate and L/P concentrations, suggesting a shift towards anaerobic metabolism, with glucose levels falling as the delivery of substrate fails with arterial occlusion. Rises in glutamate were not seen at an early stage of TC, but only after prolonged periods of ischaemia. A loss of neuronal membrane integrity may partly explain this, but is unlikely to account for all of the increase, as monitored areas did not ultimately show infarction on post-operative CT, although in 2 out of 3 cases the probes were close to areas that did infarct.

A similar pattern of microdialysis changes has been reported in a patient monitored just with microdialysis following ACA TC resulting eventually in an infarction [9][(case 10)]. In this patient the L/P rise was almost immediate, but the total duration of TC and the delay in the glutamate rise was approximately 40 minutes. Raised extracellular glutamate has also been reported in a case following a period of low P_BO_2 [4]. It therefore seems that glutamate rises are uncommon, except after prolonged ischaemia. This information is of value before any clinical trial of the potential protective effects of glutamate antagonists during ischaemia.

Acknowledgments

The Stroke Association generously sponsored this work. We also thank Mr S. Piechnik, the nursing staff, Mrs Maskell and Dr N. Higgins FRCR for their help. The bolts were made by Centrax Limited (Newton Abbott, Devon, UK).

References

1. Benveniste H, Drejer J, Schousboe A *et al* (1984) Elevation of the extracellular concentrations of glutamate and aspartate in rat hippocampus during transient cerebral ischaemia monitored by intracerebral microdialysis. J Neurochem 43: 1369–1374
2. Hillered L, Hallstrom A, Segersvard S *et al* (1989) Dynamics of extracellular metabolites in the striatum after middle cerebral artery occlusion on the rat monitored by intracerebral microdialysis. J Cereb Blood Flow Metab 9: 607–616
3. Hillered L, Persson L, Ponten U *et al* (1990) Neurometabolic monitoring of the ischaemic human brain using microdialysis. Acta Neurochir (Wien) 102: 91–97
4. Hutchinson PJA, Al-Rawi PG, O'Connell MT *et al* (2000) Biochemical changes related to hypoxia during cerebral aneurysm surgery: combined microdialysis and tissue oxygen monitoring: case report. Neurosurgery 46: 201–206
5. Hutchinson PJA, Hutchinson DBA, Barr RHH *et al* (2000) A new cranial access device for cerebral monitoring. Br J Neurosurg 14: 46–48
6. Jabre A, Symon L (1987) Temporary vascular occlusion during aneurysm surgery. Surg Neurol 27: 47–63
7. Kiening KL, Unterberg AW, Bardt TF *et al* (1996) Monitoring of cerebral oxygenation in patients with severe head injuries: brain tissue pO2 versus jugular vein oxygen saturation. J Neurosurg 85: 751–757
8. Persson L, Hillered L (1992) Chemical monitoring of neurosurgical intensive care patients using intracerebral microdialysis. J Neurosurg 76: 72–80
9. Persson L, Valtysson J, Enblad P *et al* (1996) Neurochemical monitoring using intracerebral microdialysis in patients with subarachnoid haemorrhage. J Neurosurg 84: 606–616
10. Saveland H, Nilsson OG, Boris-Moller F *et al* (1996) Intracerebral microdialysis of glutamate and aspartate in two vascular territories after aneurysmal subarachnoid haemorrhage. Neurosurgery 38: 12–20
11. Teasdale GM, Drake CG, Hunt W *et al* (1988) A universal subarachnoid haemorrhage scale: report of a committee of the World Federation of Neurosurgical Societies. J Neurol Neurosurg Psychiatry 51: 1457

Correspondence: R. Kett-White, Academic Neurosurgery, Box 167, Addenbrooke's Hospital, Cambridge CB2 2QQ, UK.

Acta Neurochir (2002) [Suppl] 81: 367–371

The Evaluation of Brain CBF and Mitochondrial Function by a Fiber Optic Tissue Spectroscope in Neurosurgical Patients

A. Mayevsky[1], E. Ornstein[2], S. Meilin[1], N. Razon[3], and G. E. Ouaknine[3]

[1] Faculty of Life Sciences, Bar-Ilan University, Ramat Gan, Israel
[2] Department of Anesthesiology, College of Physicians and Surgeons, Columbia University, New York, NY, USA
[3] Department of Neurosurgery, Tel Aviv Medical Center, Tel Aviv, Israel

Summary

The brain of neurosurgical patients are exposed to various manipulations in the ICU or during surgery. Under such conditions brain O_2 balance may become negative and as a result brain vitality and function will deteriorate.

In order to evaluate brain vitality in real time it is important to measure more than one parameter. The multiparametric monitoring system used in our previous study to monitor comatose patients (Mayevsky *et al.*, Brain Res. 740: 268–274, 1996) was changed into a "simplified" tissue spectroscope for real time monitoring of brain O_2 balance.

Mitochondrial function was evaluated by monitoring the NADH redox state by surface fluorometry. Microcirculatory blood flow was assessed by laser Doppler flowmetry. The combined optical probe was located on the surface of the brain during various neurosurgical procedures and the responses were recorded and presented in real time to the surgeon. A total of 32 patients were monitored during various procedures.

The results could be summarized as follows: 1. Hypercapnia led to 3 different types of responses. In two patients the 'stealing' like event was recorded. In the other 7 patients the responses to high CO_2 was not detectable. In the last group of 6 patients a clear CBF elevation was recorded with variable response of mitochondrial NADH. 2. Our monitoring device was able to evaluate the efficacy of the STA-MCA anastomosis during aneurysm surgery. 3. A significant correlation was recorded between CBF and NADH redox state during changes in blood pressure, papaverine injection, spontaneous drop in blood supply to the brain or during releasing of high ICP levels.

We conclude that in order to evaluate the metabolic state of the brain during neurosurgical procedures it is necessary to monitor both CBF and mitochondrial NADH by using the tissue spectroscope.

Keywords: Brain O_2 balance; mitochondrial function; cerebral blood flow; tissue spectroscope; neurosurgical monitoring.

Introduction

In our previous publication [10], we showed that multiparametric monitoring of neurotrauma patients is feasible and has a significant contribution to the diagnosis of brain functional state. In neurosurgical patients, it is necessary to monitor brain function either in the operating room or in the neurosurgical ICU. The time available in the OR is much shorter and as a result, one should apply technology that will not disturb or significantly delay the surgical procedure. At the same time, a single parameter monitoring device such as laser Doppler flowmeter [4] will not be enough to provide valuable information in real time. Therefore, we have decided to apply the Tissue Spectroscope to be used in real time during various neurosurgical procedures.

Most of the neurochemical monitoring techniques applied to head injured patients (for details see [1] are not practical for the short time available in the OR.

As can be seen in Fig. 1, there are three components that may affect brain viability status, namely supply, demand and energy balance.

The intracellular organelle responsible for the major synthesis of ATP is the mitochondrion dependent upon O_2 availability [3].

Real-time evaluation of brain viability *in situ* could be done by monitoring different parameters, related to energy metabolism, which are complementary to each other. During the last 40 years the following 4 techniques were developed and applied to monitor, in real-time, the energy supply and balance in the brain *in situ*:

1. Cerebral Blood Flow (CBF) using laser Doppler flowmetry [5].
2. Hemoglobin oxygenation or saturation (HbO_2) by dual wavelength reflectometry [14] or spectral analysis.

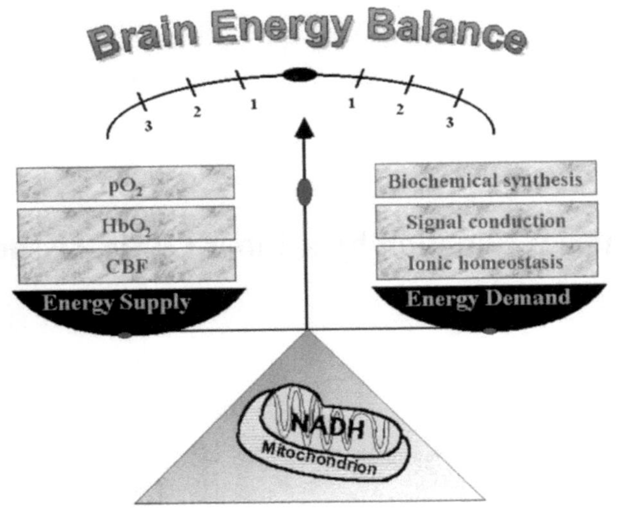

Fig. 1. Schematic presentation of the various components determine the energy or oxygen balance in the brain. pO_2 Partial pressure of oxygen; HbO_2 hemoglobin saturation; *CBF* cerebral blood flow; *NADH* mitochondrial NADH redox state

3. Tissue average oxygenation using oxygen electrodes [11].
4. Mitochondrial redox state by monitoring of NADH fluorescence using surface fluorometry [2].

All those techniques are based on the monitoring of a single parameter which make it very limited in terms of viability diagnosis in clinical situations. To monitor the second part of the equation, namely the energy demand of the brain, it is possible to evaluate the ionic homeostasis by monitoring the extracellular K^+ levels using ion specific electrodes in the brain [8].

In order to be able to evaluate the oxygen balance of the tissue *in situ* it is important to monitor more than 1 parameter simultaneously in real-time as shown in Fig. 1. Various combinations of the above mentioned parameters were made in the past and have been reported [9, 14]. We have developed and used a combination of two optical techniques, namely CBF and NADH redox state, in a single bundle of optical fibers thus enabling the correlation of the two optical parameters that could be monitored together.

The pioneering work published by Chance and Williams in 1955 and later on in 1962 by Chance *et al.* established the foundation for the close to 800 publications that have appeared since then on NADH fluorescence as an optical probe for mitochondrial function evaluation. In our previous work we combined the monitoring of the oxygenation of hemoglobin and NADH [14] or tissue pO_2 and NADH [11], but it seems to us that the best combination is to monitor CBF and NADH redox state simultaneously. This approach provides information about the two most important parameters that represent the regulated processes in brain's energy state, namely cerebral blood flow and mitochondrial function or redox state.

Since cerebral blood flow is a regulated process, it was hypothesized that simultaneous monitoring of cerebral blood flow and NADH redox state will provide significant knowledge as to the energy state of the brain. In order to evaluate in real time both mitochondrial NADH redox state and brain blood flow, we combined the optical fibers attached to the two instruments into one common bundle as shown also in Fig. 2 [9]. Using this approach we were able to correlate changes in CBF and mitochondrial redox state in the brain exposed to various pathological states in experimental animals [12] and in clinical research [9].

Methods

The multiparametric monitoring system used in the present study includes a minimal number of probes as compared to the one used in animal studies [12]. The tissue spectroscope is a combination of two optical based monitoring devices connected to the brain by a flexible light guide made of optical fibers. The common part connected to the brain includes the bundle of fibers transmitting light from the two instruments to the brain and the reflected light from the brain to the two instruments. All measurements were performed after approval by the ethical committees of the medical centers involved.

Results

Clinical Monitoring

The optical multiprobe was used in clinical situations, and a significant correlation was found between CBF and NADH redox state. In a group of patients that underwent various neurosurgical procedures (aneurysm correction or tumor removal) we monitored CBF and mitochondrial NADH redox state. In each patient we induced a short hypercapnic episode and the response to the change in CO_2 was recorded. We analyzed the responses and found that the patients could be divided into a non-responsive and a responsive group. In the non-responsive group, elevation of the end tidal CO_2 did not change the CBF or the NADH significantly. In the responsive group two types of responses to changes in the end tidal CO_2 were recorded. The averages of the responses measured in 6 patients revealed that the CBF increased significantly without any significant response in the NADH trace.

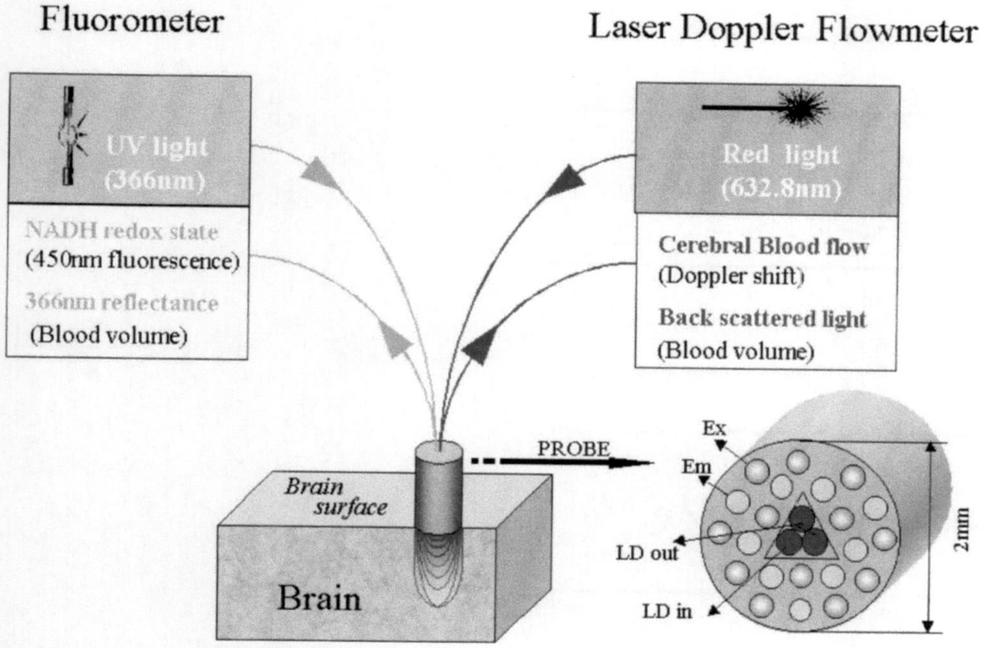

Fig. 2. The tissue spectroscope used in the present study enables to monitor simultaneously cerebral blood flow (laser Doppler Flowmeter) and mitochondrial NADH redox state (by surface fluorometry). E_x, E_m Excitation and emission transmitting fibers of the fluorometer; LD_{in}, LD_{out} Fibers connecting the brain to the laser Doppler flowmeter

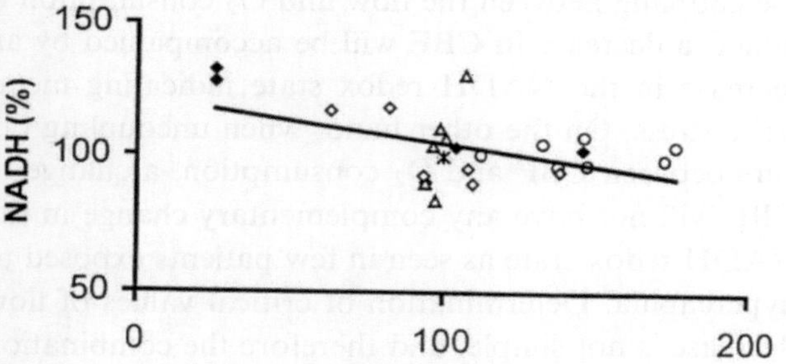

Fig. 3. The correlation between CBF and NADH redox state measured in neurosurgical patients exposed to hypercapnia during the operation

In two patients, the change in end-tidal CO_2 led to the phenomenon of blood steeling. When the data recorded in the responsive group of patients was analyzed (Fig. 3), the correlation between the two signals was found to be statistically significant ($R = -0.5$, $p < 0.05$, $n = 15$).

In order to demonstrate the potential use of our technology in clinical neurosurgery the results obtained are presented. The patient underwent carotid artery aneurysm correction procedure (Fig. 4). As

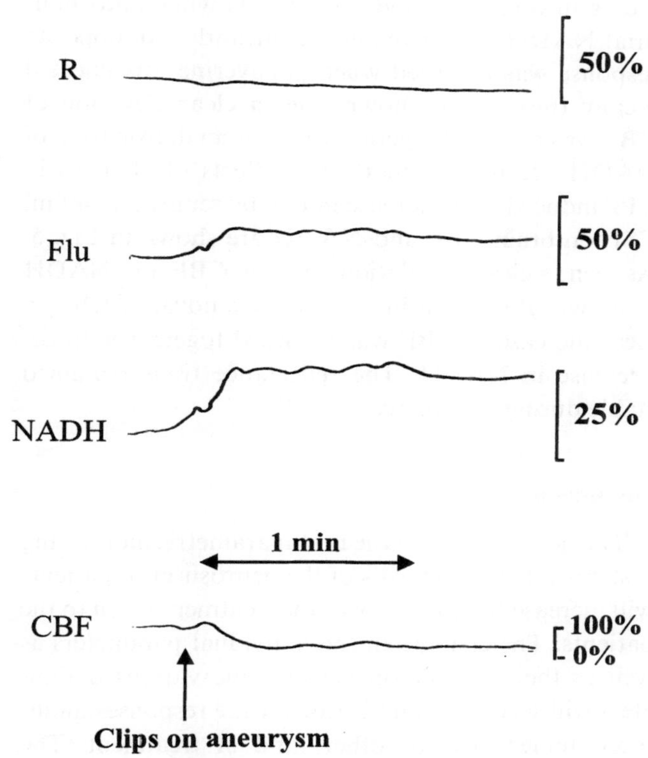

Fig. 4. Metabolic and hemodynamic responses to occlusion of an aneurysm located in one of the brain arteries

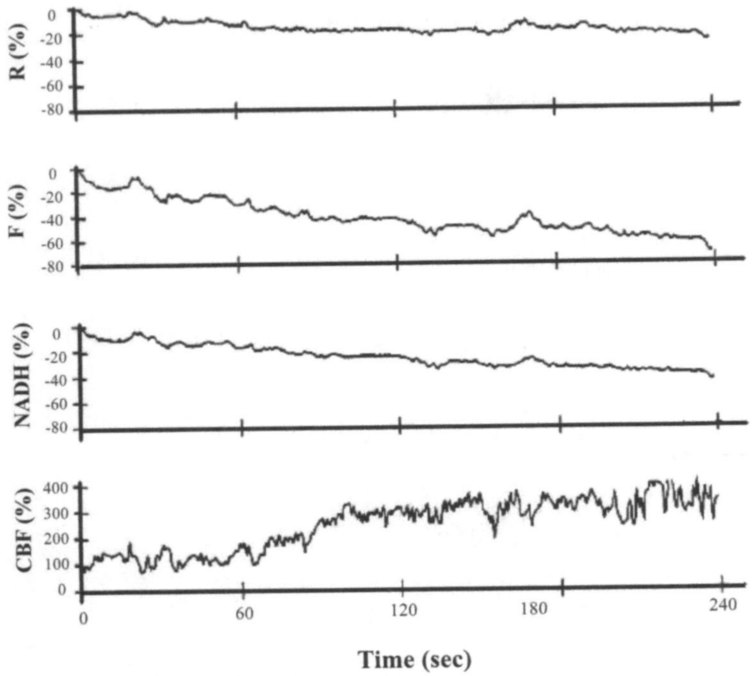

Fig. 5. Effects of a change in CPP induced by withdrawal of CSF on brain CBF and NADH

seen, occlusion of aneurysm area led to a clear decrease in cerebral blood flow (CBF) while mitochondrial NADH was increased significantly. An opposite response was recorded when papaverine was injected locally (results not shown) and a clear elevation of CBF was recorded together with the small oxidation of NADH (decrease signal). The effects of changes in CPP induced by a decrease in ICP by removal of 40 ml CSF on brain CBF and NADH are shown in Fig. 5. As seen, a clear correlation between CBF and NADH is shown. By decreasing the ICP (removal of CSF) a clear increase in CBF was recorded together with the decrease in NADH. The reflectance trace remained stable during the changes in CPP.

Discussion

The development of the multiparametric monitoring systems for the diagnosis of the neurosurgical patients will increase the efficiency of the treatment given to the patients. The changes in the individual parameters as well as the interrelation between the various parameters will serve as an indicator for the responses monitored under drug or other kind of treatment. The changes in CBF may identify a vascular event alone, namely an increase or a decrease without direct connection to the utilization of this blood by the tissue. If the coupling between the flow and O_2 consumption is intact, a decrease in CBF will be accompanied by an increase in the NADH redox state indicating metabolic stress. On the other hand, when uncoupling occurs between CBF and O_2 consumption, a change in CBF will not have any complementary change in the NADH redox state as seen in few patients exposed to hypercapnia. Determination of critical values of flow decrease is not simple, and therefore the combination with the NADH redox state data will enable the identification of critical transition points in the development of a pathological state.

The correlation between NADH redox state and CBF varies between various pathological states. The comparison point is the resting level of NADH and CBF measured in the normoxic brain after the stabilization period following the operation on the animal or location of the probe on the human brain. Under deep anesthesia, ischemia or death, the NADH increased toward state 4 and 5 simultaneously with the decrease in CBF. It is assumed that the primary effect was on CBF (a decrease) and the NADH response (an increase) is due to a decrease in O_2 delivery to the brain. When the brain is activated by seizures or by a spreading depression wave (SD) the demand for more energy may [6, 13] lead to oxidation of NADH (decrease) simultaneously with an increase in CBF to compensate for the extra O_2 needed. Under two other pathological conditions the NADH and CBF are inversely correlated. Exposing the brain to hypoxia may lead to an increase in NADH while CBF will increase. Under hyperoxia the NADH became more oxidized (decrease) while the CBF decreased [7] due to the vasoconstriction response.

In conclusion, these results demonstrate the importance of monitoring CBF and NADH, in order to provide enough data for evaluating energy or oxygen supply and balance for real time evaluation of brain vitality.

Acknowledgments

This study was supported by the Health Sciences Research Fund, the Charles Krown Research Fund in the Faculty of Life Sciences, and the Research Authority, Bar-Ilan University, Israel.

References

1. Bullock R, Marmarou A, Alessandri B, Watson J (1999) Neuromonitoring in Brain Injury. Acta Neurochir (Wien) [Suppl] 75
2. Chance B, Cohen P, Jobsis F, Schoener B (1962) Intracellular oxidation-reduction states in vivo. Science 137: 499–508
3. Chance B, Williams GR (1955) Respiratory enzymes in oxidative phosphorylation. I. Kinetics of oxygen utilization. J Biol Chem 217: 383–393
4. Dirnagl U, Kaplan B, Jacewicz M, Pulsinelli W (1989) Continuous measurement of cerebral cortical blood flow by Laser Doppler Flowmetry with a rat stroke model. J Cereb Blood Flow Metab 9: 589–596
5. Haberl RL, Heizer ML, Marmarou A, Ellis EF (1989) Laser Doppler assessment of brain microcirculation: Effect of systemic alterations. Am J Physiol 256: H1247–H1254
6. Mayevsky A (1983) Metabolic, ionic and electrical responses to experimental epilepsy in the awake rat. In: Baldy M *et al* (eds) Proceedings First International Congress of Cerebral Blood Flow, Metabolism & Epilepsy. John Libbey, pp 263–270
7. Mayevsky A (1984) Brain oxygen toxicity. Invited review. In: Bachrach AJ, Matzen MM (eds) Underwater physiology. 8th Symposium Undersea Medical Society, Bethesda, Maryland, pp 69–89
8. Mayevsky A (1993) Biochemical and physiological activities of the brain as in vivo markers of brain pathology. In: Bernstein EF *et al* (eds) Cerebral, revascularization. Med-Orion Pub, pp 51–69.
9. Mayevsky A, Doron A, Manor T, Meilin S, Zarchin N, Ouaknine GE (1996) Cortical spreading depression recorded from the human brain using a multiparametric monitoring system. Brain Res 740: 268–274
10. Mayevsky A, Doron A, Meilin S, Manor T, Ornstein E, Ouaknine GE (1999) Brain viability and function analyzer: Multiparametric real-time monitoring in neurosurgical patients. Acta Neurochir (Wien) [Suppl] 75: 63–66
11. Mayevsky A, Lebourdais S, Chance B (1980) The interrelation between brain PO_2 and NADH oxidation-reduction state in the gerbil. J Neurosci Res 5: 173–182
12. Mayevsky A, Meilin A, Rogatsky GG, Zarchin N, Thom SR (1995) Multiparametric monitoring of the awake brain exposed to carbon monoxide. J Appl Physiol 78: 1188–1196
13. Mayevsky A, Weiss HR (1991) Cerebral blood flow and oxygen consumption in cortical spreading depression. J CBF Metab 11: 829–836
14. Rampil IJ, Litt L, Mayevsky A (1992) Correlated, simultaneous, multiple-wavelength optical monitoring in vivo of localized cerebrocortical NADH and brain microvessel hemoglobin oxygen saturation. J Clin Monit 8: 216–225

Correspondence: E. Ornstein, Department of Anesthesiology, College of Physicians and Surgeons, Columbia University, New York, USA.

Acta Neurochir (2002) [Suppl] 81: 373–375

Application of Chemical Shift Imaging for Measurement of NAA in Head Injured Patients

S. Signoretti[1], A. Marmarou[1], P. Fatouros[2], R. Hoyle[2], A. Beaumont[1], S. Sawauchi[1], R. Bullock[1], and H. Young[1]

[1] Division of Neurosurgery, Virginia Commonwealth University, Richmond, Virginia, USA
[2] Division of Radiation Physics, Medical College of Virginia, USA

Summary

Neurochemical damage following brain injury can be assessed non-invasively by measurement of N-Acetyl-Aspartate (NAA) using Proton Magnetic Resonance Spectroscopy (^{1}HMRS). This report documents results of applying Chemical Shift Imaging (CSI) post-processing for measuring NAA in traumatically injured brain.

Following stabilization, severely head-injured patients (GCS 8 or less) were transported to the MRI suite. Semi-quantitative measurement of NAA, creatine (Cr/PCr) and choline (Cho) were obtained from single voxels (8 cm^3) and CSI for acquisition of smaller voxels (2 cm^3) throughout areas of the brain. Studies were completed with no complication.

In focal injury, SVS positioned at the site of lesion demonstrated reduced NAA, compared to contralateral hemisphere. In diffuse injury, CSI demonstrated uniform reduction of NAA throughout the brain. NAA/Cho showed normal levels within 24 hours of injury averaging 2.4 and decreased over the next 10 days reaching a plateau of 0.75. At 30 days, NAA showed no recovery in poor outcome patients. In patients with good outcome, NAA initially low recovered near baseline levels.

CSI provides a comprehensive neurochemical assessment of neuronal damage. NAA decreases and remains low in patients with poor outcome. NAA recovers in patients with favorable outcome, suggesting marginal metabolic impairment and possible re-synthesis of the NAA pool.

Keywords: Traumatic brain injury; N-acetylaspartate; mitochondrial dysfunction; magnetic resonance spectroscopy.

Introduction

Predicting outcome after traumatic brain injury remains yet an unresolved issue and a primary matter of debate in Neurotraumatology. Glasgow Coma Scale for the assessment of injury severity, and "neuroimaging" technology strongly improved the initial management of critically injured patient [7]. However, none of these methods is currently able to distinguish among the wide range of post-traumatic conditions: from mild neuropsychological disturbances to persistent vegetative state [5].

Recently, Proton Magnetic Resonance spectroscopy (^{1}HMRS) techniques have became a powerful clinical tool providing insights of the neurochemistry of the brain. These non-invasive methods probe specific cerebral areas and are useful in detection of tissue at risk. N-acetylaspartate (NAA), present in very high concentration within the brain is considered a neuron-specific metabolite and its reduction observed with many neurological diseases that cause neuronal and axonal degeneration [6]. Although the physiologic role of NAA is still debated, there is strong evidence that its decrease reflects neuronal damage, in particular mitochondrial dysfunction [1]. The objective of this study was to measure NAA in the traumatically injured brain to relate the severity of neurochemical damage with outcome and to provide information for potential recovery, by applying the recently developed Chemical-Shift Imaging (CSI) post-processing technique.

Material and Methods

Following stabilization, fifteen severely brain injured patients (GCS 8 or less) were transported from the Neuroscience ICU to the MR suite. During transportation and the time of MRI-MRS, appropriate ventilation, sedation and continuous monitoring of blood pressure (arterial line), pulse oximetry, end-tidal CO2 and ICP was performed through MR compatible devices. Semi-quantitative analysis of NAA, creatine containing compounds (Cr/PCr), and choline (Cho), were extracted from proton spectra using ^{1}HMRS in a 1.5 T (Vision/Siemens) system. In patients with focal lesions the location of an eight cm^3 single voxel was determined from T1-weighted images. For diffusely injured patients the voxel was placed bilaterally, in a standard region of the frontal lobes. Following localized shimming and water suppression a spectrum was obtained using the PRESS pulse sequence with 1500/135 TR/TE and 256 acquisitions. After measurement of the single voxel, a specific standard slice of the brain adjacent to the roof of the corpus callosum was selected for CSI analysis, carefully avoiding the lateral ventricles and consequent CSF artifacts. CSI technique, measuring smaller voxels (2 cm^3) throughout this standard area, allowed studying also the spatial distribution of NAA within the hemispheres. In six comatose patients, the exam was repeated to analyze the time course of the metabolic changes and to investigate the degree of potential recovery of NAA. These results were compared with proton ^{1}HMRS studies performed in five normal, age-matched, control volunteers previously screened to exclude prior head injuries.

Results

Twenty-one studies were completed with no complication. All trauma patients exhibited normal NAA/Cho and NAA/Cr ratios of 2.4 ± 0.4 within the first 72 hours. Patients with poor outcome revealed a consistent decrease of this value over the next 10 days reaching a minimal level of 0.75 ± 0.2 with no recovery during the next 30 days. Single voxel positioned at the site of lesion demonstrated markedly reduced NAA spectra compared to contralateral hemisphere and volunteer controls. In patients with good outcome, NAA showed an initial reduction followed by a gradual restoration within 30 days to near baseline levels. Comatose patients with relatively "normal" radiological aspect at the MRI and poor outcome showed a markedly depressed NAA/Cho throughout the brain equaling a 50% reduction compared to the normal distribution. In this subgroup, no recovery was observed up to 60 days. Patients with good outcome showed early NAA/Cho reduction followed by total recovery at 60 days post-injury. CSI analysis in focal injury demonstrated a reduction in the lesion hemisphere and either near normal or depressed NAA levels at distant sites.

Discussion

Our data showed that NAA/Cho and NAA/Cr ratios assessed by single voxel ^{1}HMRS gradually decline following TBI and do not recover in patients with poor outcome. This data is consistent with previous studies in which single voxel data were correlated to prognosis after TBI [3].

Application of CSI post-processing technique allowed us to study the spatial distribution of NAA in the normal brain and the consequent variations following TBI. In diffuse brain injury, NAA/Cho reduction occurred uniformly throughout the brain and did not recover in poor outcome patients. In contrast, the NAA/Cho ratio in focal injury was less uniform with maximal NAA/Cho reduction occurring in the ipsilateral hemisphere adjacent to the lesion site. In patients that experienced good outcome, ratio values were never below unity, thus identifying a threshold effect of 50% reduction beyond which restoration of NAA is less likely to occur. To our knowledge, these data are the first multi-voxel measures of NAA/Cho following TBI.

There is overwhelming experimental and clinical evidence confirming the utility of NAA as a surrogate marker of neuronal loss. However, several studies have furnished strong evidence to support the view that NAA reduction is not only related to neuronal death, but also reflects mitochondrial dysfunction [1]. Recent data from our laboratories (Signoretti *et al. submitted for publication*) provided supportive evidence that following TBI post-traumatic energetic unbalance is the leading cause of NAA reduction. These data suggested a metabolic threshold effect beyond which NAA loss is irreversible. Most importantly, when the mitochondrial impairment was overcome [8], as signified by return of ATP, NAA spontaneously recovered.

In several neurological diseases reduced NAA levels have been restored following therapeutic intervention and NAA recovery found to coincide with resolution of neurological deficits [2, 4]. This evidence suggests that NAA reduction can be a transient, reversible phenomenon, and is not solely due to neuronal cell death. Our data supports this hypothesis demonstrating that NAA recovers in patients with favorable outcome suggesting marginal impairment of mitochondria and possible re-synthesis of the NAA pool.

In conclusion, NAA/Cho ratio is reduced following TBI and is related to outcome. Application of Chemical Shift Imaging provides greater resolution and sensitivity in identifying tissue less likely to recover. The opportunity to monitor NAA in brain injured patients, yields important insights to clarify the optimal window for therapeutic intervention.

References

1. Clark JB (1998) N-acetyl aspartate: a marker for neuronal loss or mitochondrial dysfunction. Dev Neurosci 20: 271–276
2. De Stefano N, Matthews PM, Arnold DL (1995) Reversible decreases in N-acetylaspartate after acute brain injury. Magn Reson Med 34: 721–727

3. Friedman SD, Brooks WM, Jung RE *et al* (1999) Quantitative proton MRS predicts outcome after traumatic brain injury. Neurology 52: 1384–1391
4. Kalra S, Cashman NR, Genge A, Arnold DL (1998) Recovery of N-acetylaspartate in corticomotor neurons of patients with ALS after riluzole therapy. Neuroreport 9: 1757–1761
5. Lannoo E, Van Rietvelde F, Colardyn F, Lemmerling M, Vandekerckhove T, Jannes C, De Soete G (2000) Early predictors of mortality and morbidity after severe closed head injury. J Neurotrauma 17: 403–414
6. Sager TN, Laursen H, Fink-Jensen A *et al* (1999) N-Acetylaspartate distribution in rat brain striatum during acute brain ischemia. J Cereb Blood Flow Metab 19: 164–172
7. Servadei F, Murray GD, Penny K *et al* (2000) The value of the "worst" computed tomographic scan in clinical studies of moderate and severe head injury. European Brain Injury Consortium. Neurosurgery 46: 70–77
8. Vagnozzi R, Marmarou A, Tavazzi B *et al* (1999) Changes of cerebral energy metabolism and lipid peroxidation in rats leading to mitochondrial dysfunction after diffuse brain injury. J Neurotrauma 16: 903–913

Correspondence: Anthony Marmarou, Ph.D., Division of Neurosurgery, Medical College of Virginia, Virginia Commonwealth University, P.O. Box 950508, Richmond, Virginia 23298-0508, U.S.A.

Acta Neurochir (2002) [Suppl] 81: 377–379

Investigation of Extracellular Amino Acid Release in Children with Severe Head Injury Using Microdialysis. A Pilot Study

C. Tolias[1], **D. Richards**[2], **N. Bowery**[2], and **S. Sgouros**[1]

[1] Department of Neurosurgery and Institute of Child Health, Birmingham Children's Hospital, UK
[2] Department of Neuropharmacology, University of Birmingham, UK

Summary

Microdialysis has been used to investigate the pathophysiology of severe head injury in adults. No similar data exist, however, for children. As part of routine neuromonitoring, five children with severe, closed head injury (GCS < 8) were fitted with a microdialysis probe (CMA 70) at the time of intracranial pressure bolt insertion. Samples were collected at hourly intervals prior to analysis of amino acids by High Performance Liquid Chromatography. In contrast to adult patients, glutamate and aspartate did not correlate with structural amino acid levels and were inversely related to glutamine levels, suggesting that excitatory aminoacid release in children with severe head injury is likely to be an active process rather than an effect of indiscriminate cell destruction and that glutamate levels extracellularly may also depend on glutamate uptake and metabolism. The nitric oxide metabolite citrulline remained at similar levels in different patients throughout the monitoring period, indicating that nitric oxide metabolism may not follow the pattern of glutamate release. Our study is suggesting that amino acid release in severe head injury in children may not correspond to the recognised patterns from cell culture and animal studies and may also differ from that in adults.

Keywords: Children; severe head injury; microdialysis; glutamate.

Introduction

Severe head injury is an important cause of death in children. It is responsible for more deaths than all cancers and is the major cause of disability under the age of 30 [5]. Progressive brain cell death, also known as secondary brain injury, continues to occur following the acute impact. The mechanisms of brain cell death, however, remain poorly understood. Excitotoxic aminoacids have been implicated in the pathophysiology of severe head injury in both animals and humans [2, 4]. Microdialysis is a technique that allows direct sampling of the extracellular space of various tissues through a fine probe. Since the early '90s it has been used in neurochemical monitoring of adult patients with severe head injuries, especially in the intensive care environment, as well as stroke and subarachnoid haemorrhage [1, 3]. Until now no similar work on children has been published. Here we report the results of the first pilot study of microdialysis in children with severe head injury.

Methods

All children included in the study were admitted to the Birmingham Children's Hospital intensive care unit over a period of six months with severe head injury. As part of routine neuromonitoring they were fitted with an intracranial pressure (ICP) bolt (Camino, San Diego, Ca, USA) on admission. Following ethics committee approval and parental consent a microdialysis probe (CMA70, CMA/Microdialysis, Stockholm, Sweden) was also inserted at the time of ICP bolt insertion, through the same scalp incision and a separate twist-drill hole. The probe was tunnelled a few centimetres from the incision and was secured to the skin with sutures. The tip of the probe was inserted intraparenchymally at an approximate depth of 1 cm. Using a standard CMA microdialysis pump the probe was perfused with artificial CSF (CMA Perfusion Fluid, composition: Na^+ 147 mmol/L, K^+ 4 mmol/L, Ca^{2+} 2.3 mmol/L, Cl^- 156 mmol/L, pH 6, osmolality 290 mosm/kg) at a constant rate of 0.3 μL/min. Dialysate samples were collected hourly and immediately frozen to −20 °C. Analysis of the samples was performed using High Performance Liquid Chromatography (HPLC). The substances analysed were glutamate, aspartate, GABA, citrulline, glutamine, glycine, threonine, serine, tyrosine, histidine and beta-alanine. The microdialysis probes were left in situ for varying periods of time depending on the clinical need for ICP monitoring. Time of sampling ranged from 5 to 180 hours post-injury. No individual probe was left in situ for more than 60 h. Validation of recovery rate was performed on probes removed from patients and recovery rates of 90% were typically seen. Seven children with severe head injury were included in this study, 3 females and 4 males. Age ranged between 2 and 14 years. All patients had GCS < 8 before ventilation and the original CT scans confirmed diffuse brain injury with petechial haemorrhages, oedema and signs of raised ICP. A total of nine probes were used. One patient had the probe accidentally removed one hour after insertion and one probe was damaged on insertion. The remaining five patients are presented here. One patient had three different probes inserted in different brain regions with no significant changes

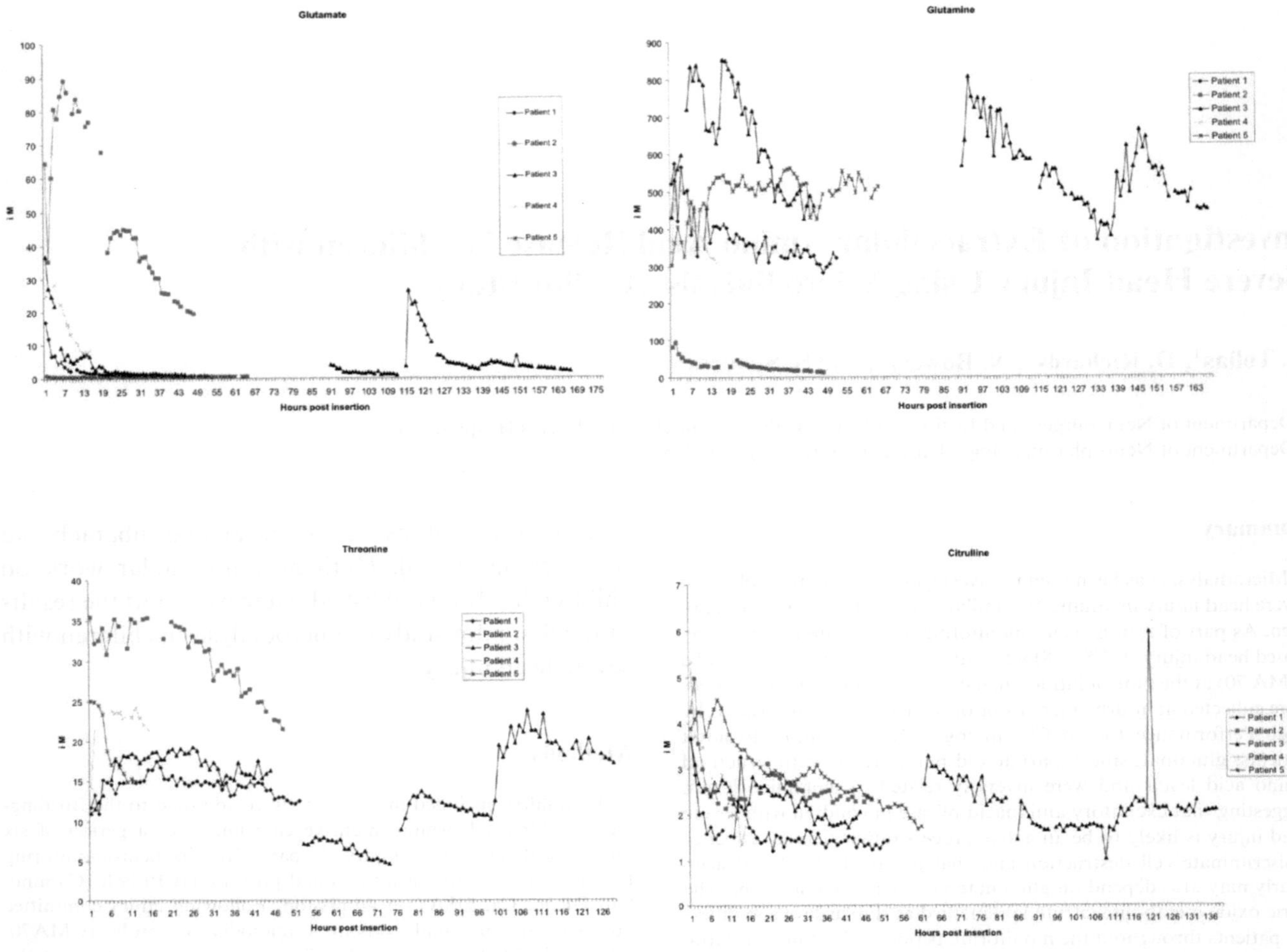

Fig. 1. Cumulative graphs of glutamate, glutamine, threonine and citrulline concentrations in all five patients during the whole monitoring period

in the levels of amino acids recorded. Clinical data were collected from the neuromonitoring charts of the intensive care unit. Hourly entries of ICP, cerebral perfusion pressure (CPP), mean arterial blood pressure (BP), central venous pressure (CVP), partial oxygen pressure (PO_2), partial carbon dioxide pressure (PCO_2), temperature and medications were plotted and correlated with dialysate concentrations. All patients survived their injuries and at 6 months have made full neurological recovery.

Results

Two distinct patterns of amino acid release were identified (Fig. 1). In four of the five children (patients 1,3,4,5) a gradual decline in glutamate and aspartate in the dialysate samples was evident in the first few hours after insertion. Levels reached a steady low value and remained at that level throughout the monitoring period. Concentrations of glutamate ranged between 0.55 μM–16.2 μM. No correlation with hour-to-hour ICP or any other clinical parameter was seen. In contrast, in one patient (Patient 2) very high concentrations of glutamate and aspartate were recorded. Hour to hour variations in ICP were also not associated with amino acid fluctuations, but glutamate and aspartate levels were reduced following evacuation of an intracranial clot. Although no hour-to-hour correlation of glutamate or aspartate concentrations were seen with the ICP in all patients, plotting mean ICP values with mean glutamate concentrations revealed a significant correlation, although this was based on data from five patients only (Fig. 2). More data is required before this relationship is consolidated. GABA concentrations followed a similar pattern to glutamate and aspartate in these patients, while if anything glutamine was inversely related to glutamate concentrations (Fig. 1). Citrulline remained at a constant level

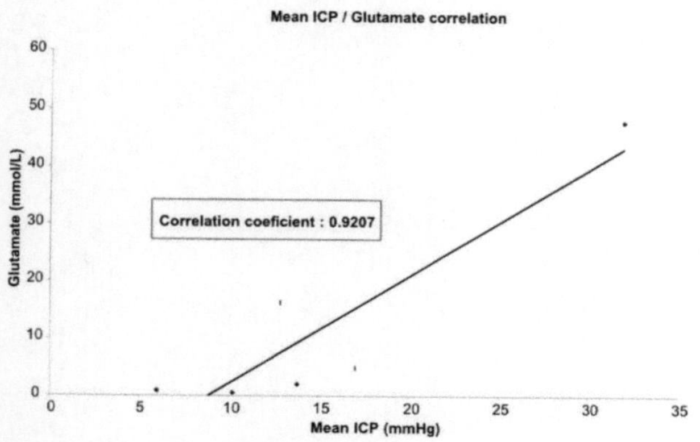

Fig. 2. Graph demonstrating the significant correlation of ICP with overall glutamate concentrations in all five patients

throughout the monitoring period in all patients (Fig. 1). Significantly, structural amino acids followed a different pattern in our patients. In all patients they remained at a steady level and did not mirror the fluctuations of the excitotoxic amino acids assayed (Fig. 1).

Discussion

We have performed a pilot study of microdialysis in children with severe head injury. Data from adult series have identified three subgroups of patients [1]. A minority with very high levels of amino acids (>20 μM), who are usually very severely injured patients. A larger group with intermediate levels (between 5–20 μM), who tend to exhibit fluctuations of glutamate concentrations correlating with ICP and the majority of patients with persistently low levels of extracellular amino acids (<5 μM). A similar pattern in structural amino acid concentrations had been observed in these patients indicating a cell destructive process, which resulted in release of substances in the extracellular space. Our findings suggested that in children a similar pattern of excitotoxic amino acid release was not mirrored by the structural amino acid concentrations. This can indicate that excitotoxic amino acids are released through an active rather than a destructive process in these patients. Furthermore, glutamine levels were inversely related with glutamate concentrations. As glutamine is a metabolite of glutamate, a process mainly involving astrocytes, we can hypothesise that alterations in glutamate metabolism and uptake might be responsible for the levels of glutamate extracellularly in severe head injury in children. The overall glutamate levels, however, correlated significantly with overall ICP values. The prognostic value of this observation is not clear from this study, as all patients survived their injuries. Finally citrulline levels remained constant throughout the monitoring period in similar levels in all patients. Although, citrulline is not the only metabolite of nitric oxide (NO), this finding indicates that NO may not be a main player in the pathophysiology of severe head injury in children. All these children had quite extensive brain injuries. They experienced neurological deterioration and had operative interventions. Although our study involved a small number of patients, the pattern of extracellular amino acid release is suggesting that the mechanisms underlying severe head injury in children may not follow the same pattern as in adults. More research is needed in order to explore this view further.

References

1. Bullock R, Zauner A, Woodward JJ, Myseros J, Choi SC, Ward JD, Marmarou A, Young HF (1998) Factors affecting excitatory amino acid release following severe human head injury. J Neurosurg 89: 507–518
2. Choi DW (1994) Glutamate receptors and the induction of excitotoxic neuronal death. Progr Brain Res 100: 47–51
3. Hillered L, Persson L (1999) Neurochemical monitoring of the acutely injured human brain. Scan J Clin Lab Invest [Suppl] 229: 9–18
4. Pettman B, Henderson CE (1998) Neuronal cell death. Neuron 20: 633–647
5. Working Party (1999) Report of the working party on the management of patients with head injuries. Royal College of Surgeons of England, London

Correspondence: S. Sgouros, M.D., F.R.C.S.(S.N.), Birmingham Children's Hospital, Steelhouse Lane, Birmingham B4 6NH, United Kingdom.

Author Index

Index of Keywords

Springer-Verlag
and the Environment

WE AT SPRINGER-VERLAG FIRMLY BELIEVE THAT AN international science publisher has a special obligation to the environment, and our corporate policies consistently reflect this conviction.

WE ALSO EXPECT OUR BUSINESS PARTNERS – PRINTERS, paper mills, packaging manufacturers, etc. – to commit themselves to using environmentally friendly materials and production processes.

THE PAPER IN THIS BOOK IS MADE FROM NO-CHLORINE pulp and is acid free, in conformance with international standards for paper permanency.

MIX
Papier aus verantwortungsvollen Quellen
Paper from responsible sources
FSC® C105338

If you have any concerns about our products,
you can contact us on
ProductSafety@springernature.com

In case Publisher is established outside the EU,
the EU authorized representative is:
Springer Nature Customer Service Center GmbH
Europaplatz 3, 69115 Heidelberg, Germany

Printed by Libri Plureos GmbH
in Hamburg, Germany